The Gravity of Weight

A CLINICAL GUIDE TO
Weight Loss and Maintenance

The Gravity of Weight

A CLINICAL GUIDE TO
Weight Loss and Maintenance

Sylvia R. Karasu, M.D.

*Clinical Associate Professor, Department of Psychiatry,
Weill Cornell Medical College; Associate Attending Psychiatrist,
New York–Presbyterian/Weill Cornell Medical Center, New York, New York*

T. Byram Karasu, M.D.

*Silverman Professor of Psychiatry and University Chairman, Department of
Psychiatry and Behavioral Sciences, Albert Einstein College of Medicine,
and Psychiatrist-in-Chief, Montefiore Medical Center, Bronx, New York*

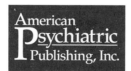

American Psychiatric Publishing, Inc.

Washington, DC
London, England

Disclosure of interests: The authors have no competing interests or conflicts to declare.

To purchase 25–99 copies of this or any other APPI title at a 20% discount, please contact APPI Customer Service at appi@psych.org or 800-368-5777. To purchase 100 or more copies of the same title, please e-mail bulksales@psych.org for a price quote.

Manufactured in the United States of America on acid-free paper
14   13   12   11   10   5   4   3   2   1
First Edition

Typeset in Adobe's Warnock Pro and Berthold's Akzidenz Grotesk.
American Psychiatric Publishing, Inc.
1000 Wilson Boulevard
Arlington, VA 22209-3901
www.appi.org

Acknowledgment: Excerpts from *The Art of the Commonplace: The Agrarian Essays of Wendell Berry*, ©2003, and "The Gift of Gravity," in *The Collected Poems of Wendell Berry*, ©1987, are reprinted by permission of Counterpoint.

Library of Congress Cataloging-in-Publication Data
Karasu, Sylvia R.
 The gravity of weight : a clinical guide to weight loss and maintenance / Sylvia R. Karasu, T. Byram Karasu. — 1st ed.
    p. ; cm.
Includes bibliographical references and index.
ISBN 978-1-58562-360-0 (alk. paper)
 1. Weight loss. 2. Weight loss—Psychological aspects. I. Karasu, Toksoz B. II. Title. III. Title: Clinical guide to weight loss and maintenance.
 [DNLM: 1. Obesity—psychology. 2. Obesity—therapy. 3. Body Weight—physiology. 4. Weight Loss—physiology. WD 210 K18g 2010]

RM222.2.K37 2010
613.2'5—dc22

2009045790

FSC
Mixed Sources
Product group from well-managed
forests and other controlled sources
Cert no. SW-COC-002283
www.fsc.org
© 1996 Forest Stewardship Council

British Library Cataloguing in Publication Data
A CIP record is available from the British Library.

All scientific work is incomplete—whether it be observational or experimental. All scientific work is liable to be upset or modified by advancing knowledge. That does not confer upon us a freedom to ignore the knowledge we already have, or to postpone the action that it appears to demand at a given time.

Sir Austin Bradford Hill (1965)

What has been one scientist's "noise" is another scientist's "signal."

Martin Moore-Ede (1986)

In memory of Cemil Karasu and Moses Rabson, M.D.

CONTENTS

FOREWORD

This book is a labor of love. As the authors state, it is "a tale of two fathers." The father of Sylvia Karasu suffered from morbid obesity all of his life, together with other risk factors for coronary heart disease, and lived to the age of 91. The father of Byram Karasu, also morbidly obese, died at the age of 56. This tale of two fathers is in the background of the volume as the authors seek to assess the many factors that contribute to obesity and its control.

The Gravity of Weight is a model of scholarly inquiry that describes and analyzes, in a critical manner, an enormous amount of information. With the possible exception of a few references that may have been cited twice, I estimate that the bibliography contains no fewer than 900 publications on every aspect of obesity, covering the field to an extraordinary extent. The book is well written and thoroughly up to date, with few references earlier than the year 2000.

The authors' goal in this volume is to integrate "the complex psychological and physiological aspects of the mind, brain, and body" and to explain why the control of body weight and its maintenance are "so daunting for so many people." The problems that they raise and the analyses that they conduct go far to realize this goal.

Early in the book, I was struck by the discussion of two problems in the understanding of obesity. The first problem is the alteration of the largely linear correlation between increasing body fat and mortality. It is the curious increase in mortality that occurs in underweight persons. The authors carefully analyze the data to show that the increase in mortality at the lower extent of fatness is not a function of this decreased fatness. Instead, it is due to independent risk factors.

The second question deals with the issue of "weight cycling," the widely held belief that cycles of weight loss and regain are a cause of morbidity and mortality. The authors deal with this belief by means of a thorough study of arguments for and against it. Their final answer, one with which I agree, is that the question requires such precision of measurement that it cannot be decided by currently available data in humans.

The section on physical activity benefits from the care with which accurate, quantitative measurements can be made. One such measure is the MET, or "metabolic equivalent." It is defined as the ratio of the activity performed compared to sitting quietly (which receives a standard MET of 1). Values in METs are available for essentially all activities and range from sleeping, at 0.9 MET, to running, at 18.0 METs.

Two articles in the *New England Journal of Medicine* point to the accuracy with which measurements of physical activity can be made (Florman 2000; Levine et al. 1999). The articles report that chewing gum for 12 minutes increased caloric expenditure by 11 ± 3 kcal/hour, a value similar to that of standing, as opposed to sitting. The experimenters make a playful estimate: if a person chewed gum during waking hours and changed no other component of energy balance, a yearly weight loss of 5 kilograms (11 pounds) should be expected.

The Gravity of Weight notes the three major components of energy expenditure: the basal metabolic rate, which accounts for about 60% of average daily caloric expenditure; the thermic effect of food (including its digestion, absorption, and storage), which accounts for about 10%–15% of daily expenditure; and physical activity. Physical activity is the most variable component, accounting for 15% (among sedentary people) to 50% (among active ones). Physical activity is thus the major factor on the energy output side of the energy balance equation, and it is important to consider. Less than 50% of the American population exercises on a regular basis, clearly a factor in the development of obesity but also an opportunity for favorable change. Even relatively small amounts of exercise have an effect, but it is exceptionally difficult to lose weight by exercise alone. To lose weight, exercise must be combined with caloric restriction and dieting, as discussed below.

Although exercise alone is of indifferent value in weight loss, it helps in the maintenance of weight loss. A great many treatment studies have made clear the strong tendency for weight loss programs to be followed by regain of the lost weight. The amount of exercise to prevent regain in the average person is, however, formidable: 45 to 60 minutes a day of walking.

In *The Gravity of Weight*, the section on circadian rhythms deals with a fundamental biological characteristic that is critical in weight control. We know about these rhythms primarily when they are disrupted, as in jet lag and shift work. The major biological clock, in the hypothalamus, is entrained to the 24-hour light/dark cycle. It is supplemented by additional clocks in the body and by a number of "clock genes." These additional mechanisms permit a finer degree of specialization among the activities of the various organs.

Prominent among disruptions of circadian rhythms is the night eating syndrome, characterized by a delay of 1½ hours in the circadian pattern of food intake. Night eaters consume at least 25% of their daily caloric intake after the evening meal and awaken during the night, with food intake, at least two to three times a week. Control subjects, on the other hand, awaken less frequently during the night and do not eat upon awakening. Night eating syndrome occurs in combination with binge eating disorder in some people, and when this occurs, it is associated with greater degrees of obesity. Night eating syndrome is present among nonobese persons, and its prevalence rises with increasing levels of obesity, leading to the observation that it is a pathway to obesity. The syndrome is readily diagnosed and effectively treated. Patients benefit from relief of their distressing behaviors and better control of their body weight. Unfortunately, the disorder usually goes unrecognized and untreated.

The authors devote a section to intensive forms of psychotherapy and present excellent short accounts of nine programs: Freud's original drive theory, ego psychology, object relations theory, self psychology, interpersonal relationship theory, neurolinguistic programming, gestalt therapy, cognitive-behavioral therapy, and dialectical behavioral therapy. Although the authors relate each of the therapies to its potential use in the treatment of obesity, outcome research is confined to one psychoanalytic study that included obese persons. Therapy was administered by practitioners of various schools of psychoanalysis, and the goals of treatment varied widely. The goals did not include weight reduction, but nevertheless significant weight losses were achieved. Clearly, the cost of weight reduction by these methods was high.

A thorough description of diets and weight provides a wealth of information. Diets are currently being followed by 54 million Americans. The review of diets begins with the famous self-selection diet experiment of Clara Davis in the 1920s and 1930s. Children, from weaning until 6 years of age, were permitted to select their meals from a wide variety of options. Davis reported that subjects chose to eat, over time, pretty much exactly what they needed for growth and development. The authors of *The Gravity of Weight* review this remarkable result, which had been accepted widely, including by me. They show that Davis's conclusion was not justified by the details of the study; the actual freedom of choice of the children was greatly constrained toward a healthy diet.

The section on diets opens a Pandora's Box. The authors mention "thousands" of publications on dieting, and it would seem that every possibility has been essayed: high-fat diets, low-fat diets; high-carbohydrate diets, low-carbohydrate diets; high-protein diets, low-protein diets; and so on. There are diets associated with good living: the South Beach diet, the Scarsdale diet, and the Beverly Hills diet. Diets are also associated with their authors, as with Pritikin (low fat), Atkins (low carbohydrate), and Stillman (high water).

The benefits of this extravagant panoply have been limited. It is not clear that any diet is any more effective than any other. The authors suggest two variables involved in weight loss. They are boredom with the diet, which leads to less consumption, and boredom with calorie counting, which leads to weight gain.

The section on pharmacotherapy for obesity describes the many medications that are currently available. *The Gravity of Weight* concisely describes their characteristics and problems. Only two, sibutramine and orlistat, have been well studied, and they have been shown to be modestly effective and safe. The description of a large number of less frequently prescribed medications is thorough and should be useful for the practitioner.

A promising new agent, not yet approved by the U.S. Food and Drug Administration, is rimonabant, a selective cannabinoid-1 receptor antagonist. It has been used widely in Europe for many years, but concern about depression as a possible side effect has interfered with its acceptance in this country.

The volume ends with a discussion of two very different surgical procedures. One is liposuction, a cosmetic measure designed for "body sculpting" or "body contouring." Liposuction usually removes about 3 kilograms (6.6 pounds) of fat, not enough to affect metabolic processes. Accordingly, the authors caution that "liposuction definitely should not be considered a clinical treatment for obesity." Liposuction is immensely popular; the number of procedures has risen from 100,000 in the 1980s to 400,000 in recent years. Its popularity is suggested by the report that 90% of liposuction patients would recommend it to other people.

Bariatric surgery is the second surgical procedure for obese persons. It is designed for individuals with "morbid" obesity, a body mass index value of at least 40 kg/m^2. The authors describe a number of reports on bariatric surgery, including many that involve untoward events. Perhaps as a result, the authors are able to contain their enthusiasm for this modality.

Several years ago, I studied a now outmoded surgical treatment of obesity and found a number of favorable behavioral changes (Stunkard et al. 1986). Accordingly, I was pleased to see reports of two large, well-controlled studies of bariatric surgery. Sjöström et al. (2007) and Adams et al. (2007) described studies of 2,000 and 7,900 obese persons, over periods of 10 and 7 years, respectively. Large weight losses were achieved as well as significant decreases in morbidity and mortality compared with their control groups. My conclusion from these results is that bariatric surgery is a highly specialized form of treatment and aftercare and that it requires teams with extensive experience with the method.

Who is the audience for *The Gravity of Weight*? I was a natural member of this audience, since the book deals so authoritatively with my long interest in obesity. But what other people may be drawn to this book?

As psychiatrists, the authors naturally had in mind fellow psychiatrists when they wrote the book. It should appeal to psychiatrists, not only because of its thorough discussion of clinical issues but also because of the basic behavioral science that is explicated in clear and well-written prose. Psychiatrists also often encounter the obesity that is caused by psychotropic medications, the atypical antipsychotics in particular. They are in the best position to modify medication to minimize side effects and maximize weight loss.

Other groups that should benefit from *The Gravity of Weight* are general practitioners, internists, and psychologists who specialize in obesity. These individuals today provide most of the professional care for obese persons, and they should find this volume particularly helpful. They too will benefit from the excellent description of the basic science of obesity as well as the description of how to treat obese people.

The Gravity of Weight is an authoritative account of obesity and its treatment. It deserves a place in the library of those who work on this disorder.

Albert J. Stunkard, M.D.

Professor of Psychiatry and Founder and Director Emeritus, Center for Weight and Eating Disorders, University of Pennsylvania School of Medicine

REFERENCES

Adams TD, Gress RE, Smith SC, et al: Long-term mortality after gastric bypass surgery. N Engl J Med 2007 357:753–761, 2007

Florman DA: More on chewing gum (comment on Levine et al. 1999). N Engl J Med 342:1531–1532, 2000

Levine J, Baukol P, Pavlidis I: The energy expended in chewing gum. N Engl J Med 341:2100, 1999

Sjöström L, Narbro K, Sjöström CD, et al: Effects of bariatric surgery on mortality in Swedish obese subjects. N Engl J Med 357:741–752, 2007

Stunkard AJ, Stinnett JL, Smoller JW: Psychological and social aspects of the surgical treatment of obesity. Am J Psychiatry 143:417–429, 1986

A TALE OF TWO FATHERS

…almost everyone knows some very obese person who died very early, possibly as the result of his or her obesity. At the same time, almost everyone knows some very obese individual who lived a very long and healthy life.

Kevin R. Fontaine and David B. Allison,
Handbook of Obesity: Etiology and Pathophysiology (2004, p. 776)

During the writing of this book, my father, a retired orthopedic surgeon, died of heart failure at the age of 91. Significantly, though, he had what we would consider class 3 obesity, or morbid obesity, his entire adult life, except for the years when he served in World War II and had to subsist on the army's K rations. My mother used to say my father had fought his own "Battle of the Bulge" his entire life. Because of his obesity and his perpetual struggles with his weight, I had always expected him to die fairly young. I would never have predicted that he would live into his 90s. In fact, he outlived most of his nonobese friends, many of whom had actually died years before.

My father had several of the risk factors that often lead to an earlier death, including chronic heart disease, abdominal obesity, a poor cholesterol profile (i.e., dyslipidemia), hypertension, adult-onset diabetes, and even gout, all symptoms of metabolic abnormalities. His own father had died at the age of 62 from a sudden myocardial infarction, so my father had a strong genetic risk factor as well. What was in my father's favor, though, was that he had always believed in the importance of exercise, particularly walking and weight lifting, well before it was fashionable. He also never drank very much, and he never smoked. In fact, he instilled in my brother and me the dangers of smoking well over 50 years ago, long before the Surgeon General's report.

Byram's father, a writer and diplomat, conversely, had a more predictable demise. He also had class 3 obesity, with fat predominantly accumulated in his abdominal area as well. But Byram's father was 56 years old when, after a dinner of a large omelet and lots of red wine, he died peacefully in his sleep after suffering a massive myocardial infarction. He had loved his cigarettes and cigars and his imported red wines, and he had never exercised. This was years before the availability of cardio-thoracic bypass surgery, stents, or even medications for abnormal lipid levels or hypertension.

Our fathers were worlds and cultures apart. My father lived most of his life in the Philadelphia area. Byram's father, born in Turkey, lived in France until he and his family fled back to Turkey during the Nazi occupation of France during World War II. Their lives, though, enable us to appreciate just how unpredictable—and even seemingly capricious—the consequences of obesity can be and how much we still do not know about the complex subject of weight. Statistics can never account for everyone.

Nevertheless, our book, *The Gravity of Weight: A Clinical Guide to Weight Loss and Maintenance*, is our attempt to explain some of these discrepancies and explore particularly why, for most people, it is so difficult to lose weight and maintain that loss. No one has all the answers, but an understanding of the science, of both mind and body, behind these complexities is a beginning. It is to our fathers that our book is dedicated.

Sylvia R. Karasu, M.D.

REFERENCES

Fontaine KR, Allison DB: Obesity and mortality rates, in Handbook of Obesity: Etiology and Pathophysiology. Edited by Bray GA, Bouchard C. New York, Marcel Dekker, 2004, pp 767–786

Hill AB: The environment and disease: association or causation? Proc R Soc Med 58:295–300, 1965

Moore-Ede MC: Physiology of the circadian timing system: predictive versus reactive homeostasis. Am J Physiol Regulatory Integrative Comp Physiol 250: R737–752, 1986

ACKNOWLEDGMENTS

The Gravity of Weight could not have been possible without the unwavering support and encouragement of Robert E. Hales, M.D., Editor-in-Chief at American Psychiatric Publishing, Inc. He and John McDuffie, Editorial Director, gave our book the structure it required amidst this overwhelming field of weight control. We also thank Roxanne Rhodes, our project editor, for her impressive, steadfast dedication, determination, and assistance; Tammy J. Cordova, Graphic Design Manager, for designing such an elegant cover; Greg Kuny, our Managing Editor; Bessie Jones, Acquisitions Coordinator; Susan Westrate, Prepress Coordinator, who created the book's typography and design; Bob Pursell, Director of Sales and Marketing; Ellie Abedi, Marketing Associate; and the indexers, whose work provides an essential component of a book such as ours. Most particularly, we owe considerable gratitude to the copyeditor, Carol Cadmus, who read our manuscript with an extraordinary and meticulous attention to detail. It is clear she had our best interests and the integrity of our project at heart throughout.

We also owe enormous appreciation to our wonderful secretaries, Mrs. Hilda Cuesta, who diligently typed all our references and tables, and Mrs. Josephine Costa, who wrote for permissions to use material; they both honored all our requests so pleasantly and identified with our project as if it were their own. And we owe particular thanks to Ms. Tina Bonanno and Ms. Angela Grosso, both of whom assisted us in the preparation of our manuscript.

We are grateful to those who read our manuscript despite their many other commitments. We are especially indebted to Albert J. Stunkard, M.D., Professor of Psychiatry, and founder and Director Emeritus of the Center for Weight and Eating Disorders at the University of Pennsylvania School of Medicine—who has been writing for over 55 years (in over 500 papers) on the subject of obesity, and without whose groundbreaking research this book could not have been written—for graciously and most generously accepting our invitation to write our Foreword. The pages of this book are suffused with Dr. Stunkard's contributions.

We also especially thank Brian Wansink, Ph.D., Director of the Food and Brand Lab at Cornell University, who creatively explores the relationship of human nature to portion control; Aaron T. Beck, M.D., Professor Emeritus at the University of Pennsylvania and the founder of the Beck Institute for Cognitive Therapy and Research; Antonio M. Gotto, Jr., M.D., D.Phil., the Stephen and Suzanne Weiss Dean of Weill Cornell Medical College; Frank B. Hu, M.D., Ph.D., Professor of Medicine, Nutrition and Epidemiology at Harvard; and David L. Katz, M.D., M.P.H., Associate Professor of Public Health at Yale and Director of the Prevention Research Center, all of whom not only kindly and charitably read but also provided valuable insights on prepublication copies of our manuscript.

Over the past years of preparation, we have discussed our text with many people whose input was important to us, particularly Allen M. Spiegel, M.D., the Marilyn and Stanley M. Katz Dean of Albert Einstein College of Medicine, whose earlier work as an endocrinologist at the National Institutes of Health led us to appreciate the important relationship of obesity to the brain; Robert Michels, M.D., former Dean and Chairman of Psychiatry at Weill Cornell Medical College, a longtime mentor and friend; Jack D. Barchas, M.D., Chairman of the Department of Psychiatry at Weill Cornell, who has been encouraging and enthusiastic about our work; Harvey Klein, M.D., an internist who is a physician's physician and as much a psychiatrist himself; Lawrence Friedman, M.D., who thoughtfully and supportively asked each week about our progress; Theodore Shapiro, M.D., David Shapiro, M.D., Kelly C. Allison, Ph.D., Namni Goel, Ph.D., Sanjay R. Patel, M.D., M.S., James Lomax, M.D., Mallay Occhiogrosso, M.D., and Ralph LaForge, M.Sc.; and Deena J. Nelson, M.D., internist and friend.

This book was also made so much more efficacious because of the Virtual Private Network (WebVPN) system at the medical library at Weill Cornell's Samuel J. Wood Library, where we could stream into our home or office literally hundreds of journal articles at all hours of the day or night. We single out Kevin Pain, Information Specialist, who always immediately and competently responded to our many requests and found any article we could not ourselves retrieve; Bruce Silberman, senior library assistant; and Edsel Watkins, Supervisor, both of the Interlibrary Loan Department.

Finally, there are personal appreciations to Joseph Rabson, M.D., who helped us understand the intricacies of plastic surgery and was the first to call our attention to "dieting dysphoria"; Mrs. Barbara Rabson, who has been (and continues to be) our diet partner for over 30 years; and Mrs. Frances Rabson, for her enthusiastic support for this project and for instilling in us the importance of a healthy lifestyle long before it was fashionable.

INTRODUCTION

To be able to write well on the regimen, one must study human nature, in all its complexity, its composition, its origin, its counterparts, and all there is to know about food and beverages, natural or artificial. But since man cannot live healthily on food without a certain proportionate amount of exercise, we must study all the factors concerning the virtues and influence of exercise on growth, and its relation to food, age, idiosyncrasy, seasons, and climate.

Hippocrates, *Regimen*, Book I
(Precope 1952, pp. 31–32)

THE UNBEARABLE HEAVINESS OF BEING

We tend to use the words *weight* and *fat* interchangeably; our weight, though, is really made up of our muscles, bones, organs, water, and other tissues as well as fat (Jain et al. 2007). Likewise, weight control and maintenance involve more than a study of adipose tissue: they involve every aspect of our psychology and physiology. In fact, obesity, the extreme condition of weight control and maintenance gone awry, has been called a brain disease, a metabolic disease, a genetic disease, and even a disease of inflammation. Bray (2004) considers obesity a "neurochemical" disease. There is even a debate about whether obesity should be considered a disease at all (Sturm 2002). For example, Albert J. Stunkard (personal communication, October 9, 2009), who has done research in the field of obesity for over 55 years, considers it a "disorder." Aronne et al. (2008) acknowledge that the question of whether obesity is a disease is "controversial," though not a new question. These authors support the idea that obesity "meets all the criteria of a medical disease, including a known etiology, recognized signs and symptoms, and a range of structural and functional changes that culminate in pathological consequences." On the other hand, rather than considering obesity a pathological condition, Power and Schulkin (2009, p. 11) think of it in terms of evolution, as "inappropriate adaptation." Of course, labeling obesity as a disease has many advantages and benefits, including garnering more public attention and potential sources of funding for its prevention and treatment, as well as decreasing the stigma attached to obesity (Allison et al. 2008).

Whether we call it a "disorder," a "disease," or "inappropriate adaptation," obesity essentially has multiple etiologies and has the primary sign of excess adipose tissue (i.e., fat). And obesity is a condition that is instantly obvious to everyone. We may not know the specific etiology of a person's obesity, but we can spot his or her adiposity immediately. Interestingly, though, besides the excess adipose tissue, there are no physical signs or symptoms that are characteristically seen in *everyone* who is obese (Allison et al. 2008).

Simplistically, obesity is a chronic (but sometimes relapsing) condition in which the amount of food eaten does not match the number of calories expended. In other words, it is an energy *imbalance* that is based on the first law of thermodynamics: when we take in more calories than we use, those excess calories are converted to fat (Bray 2004). But the study of obesity, as we will demonstrate, is far more complicated. For some, obesity is an unsightly crime. For example, in an editorial entitled "The Tyranny of Health," published years ago in the *New England Journal of Medicine*, Fitzgerald (1994) warned that we are inclined to assume those who are unhealthy have misbehaved, and we blame them for their illnesses. We see, she said, certain "failures of self-care" (e.g., obesity, substance abuse, heart disease) as "crimes against society" because society shoulders so much of the burden for the consequences of illness. In effect, she said, "we use illness as evidence of misbehavior" (Fitzgerald 1994).

Nowhere is this more evident than in the study of obesity. Two-thirds of a geographically diverse sample of hundreds of physicians still believe, from an etiological perspective, that obesity is primarily a "behavior problem" (Foster et al. 2003). For example, even the one of the most famous researchers in the field, Ancel Keys (see Chapter 10 for more on Keys's research) said, "And we can emphasize the fact that in both sexes and at all ages obesity is disgusting as well as a hazard to health" (Keys 1965). The obese suffer from this stigmatizing. Even many physicians and health care providers who treat the obese have overt prejudice against them (Foster et al. 2003). This is hardly surprising: after all, the *behaviors* of gluttony and sloth were among the "seven deadly sins" in early Christian theology. First delineated by Pope Gregory the Great in the sixth century and later depicted in literature in Dante's *Divine Comedy*, these sins could lead to eternal damnation ("Seven Deadly Sins" 2009).

In her editorial, Fitzgerald (1994) raises a provocative question: "How far will society go to regulate 'healthy behavior'?" But is it desirable or even possible for a society to regulate healthy behavior? Ironically, even what we consider "healthy behavior" can evolve and be modified over time, as Fitzgerald (1994) says:

> Clearly, our understanding of the scientific basis of health and disease changes
> over time. Many older people will remember when sunshine, milk, bread,

butter, and meat were good for you and recommended by physicians..... We must beware of developing a zealotry about health.

And what about labeling certain behaviors, as Fitzgerald says, "crimes against society"? Is it even a practically useful concept? Such oversimplified formulations hardly work, even in the criminal justice system.

Of course, those questions are even more relevant today, as the statistics on overweight and obesity have worsened dramatically, even since the mid 1990s. For example, statistics current as of 2007 revealed that one-third, or about 72 million, of the people in the United States were obese (C. L. Ogden et al. 2007). And the problem of obesity, of course, is not exclusive to the United States. For the first time worldwide, there are apparently more overweight people than there are those who go hungry (Brownell 2008; Newbold et al. 2007). Furthermore, King et al. (2009) reported that during the 18 years of their study (1988–2006), adherence to a healthy lifestyle, as manifested by keeping all five healthy habits (i.e., moderate alcohol use; no smoking; routine exercise; eating five or more fruits and vegetables a day; and a body mass index below 30 kg/m^2), actually decreased from being practiced by only 15% of their population to an even lower 8%!

Obesity has been called, perhaps more metaphorically, an "epidemic." Flegal (2006) questions the use of the word, even though obesity has a high prevalence rate as well as a rapid increase in frequency, both characteristic of typical epidemics. A classic epidemic, though, has a certain structure to it (Flegal 2006). Initially there is reluctance to accept what is happening "until admission of its presence is unavoidable." The second phase consists of attempting to provide "an explanatory framework," which may include making moral and social judgments and even blaming the victim. (And we may still be in this second phase.) In the third phase, there is pressure and urgency for some kind of response from the community. Eventually epidemics tend to end with a "whimper" rather than a "bang." The "whimper" ending for obesity does not seem all that likely. Flegal (2006) suggests that perhaps a better word would be *endemic* rather than *epidemic*, and she notes that although there has been a rise in the prevalence of obesity over the past twenty or so years, a survey done in the early 1960s actually found that 45% of the U.S. population was overweight at that time. In fact, back in the 1950s Breslow (1952) was already warning of the dangers of overweight and its relationship to increased mortality. He said, "The American people have learned that good hygiene does not permit spitting on the floor...but they have hardly begun to appreciate the importance of optimum weight in good hygiene. Here is clearly a task for public health."

And it is now more than fifty years ago that psychiatrist Albert Stunkard (1958), one of the earliest and most significant researchers in the field, noted the rarity of successful outcomes and warned, somewhat prophetically, of the extraordinary difficulties involved in treating obesity.

This "task for public health" is clearly upon us. According to a research report for the Strategies to Overcome and Prevent (STOP) Obesity Alliance, from the Department of Health Policy at the George Washington University School of Public Health and Health Services (Jain et al. 2007), medical expenditures related to obesity and overweight in the United States amount to $75 billion annually. Even more recently, Finkelstein et al. (2009) reported figures almost twice as high, noting that the "annual medical burden" for obesity could total $147 billion in 2008. This represents 10% of all medical spending in the United States and imposes a considerable economic burden on everyone. Significantly, this spending is mostly concerned with treating diseases associated with obesity, not with treating obesity itself. Some have gotten so concerned that there has even been the proposal of a "fat tax" health insurance premium for those with obesity (Leonhardt 2009, pp. 9–10). According to a study done by the Rand Corporation, obesity has approximately the same association with chronic health conditions as does twenty years of aging—and effects far worse than all the health problems related to smoking or drinking (Sturm 2002). Olshansky et al. (2005) have even predicted that obesity and its consequences may actually put an end to the steady rise we have seen in life expectancy over the past two centuries.

Louis Aronne (2002, p. 387), another leader in the field of obesity research, makes the point that the amount of weight loss most people can actually achieve and maintain is probably within a fairly limited range, but even a 5% to 10% loss of weight can have substantial health benefits. Nevertheless, many people cannot lose even the 10% that can be an achievable and reasonable goal and keep it off indefinitely. And many people have every wish to remain a certain weight yet find themselves overeating, often with considerable guilt before and regret afterwards.

So why is it that the U.S. population continues to grow fatter and fatter when each week new diet books appear on bookshelves and best-seller lists and American consumers spend about $60 billion a year on products designed for weight loss (Jain et al. 2007)?

There are several factors responsible. In part, variations on the typical prescription of diet and exercise for weight loss, weight control, and weight maintenance seem to apply better to animals that do not have the advanced cortical brains we have. We can limit an animal's food intake, for example, and give it regular exercise, and the animal will lose weight and maintain that loss, assuming its food and exercise regimens continue to be regulated. Human beings, however, are different. We are not only beneficiaries of our remarkable evolution but victims of it as well: our minds can override our knowledge, and we sabotage our own efforts, despite our best intentions, even when our food and exercise are regulated. For example, we can be quite conscious of the health benefits of exercise, but we can also be quite oppositional and just choose not to exercise. Or we can know a food is unhealthy and yet eat it or even eat too much of it, regardless of our knowledge. We have "shoulds" and "shouldn'ts" about eating. We actually make moral judgments about foods. We label foods as "good" and "bad," and even then disregard these judgments.

Even in nature, animals innately regulate their exercise and food intake, without the "should" or "shouldn't" internal dialogue that we humans often engage in. Imagine a lion's ruminating over whether he should or shouldn't eat more of that buffalo he just killed. Animals are on metabolic automatic pilot; we are often not. In fact, Berthoud (2007) suggests that our cognitive brain mechanisms are one of the major factors responsible for the obesity crisis we are now experiencing, and he believes that "neurophysiology is no less physiology than adipocyte or liver physiology."

Another factor is the genetic connection. Twin studies indicate that a major part of weight control, perhaps 70% or more, is genetically determined. Most researchers, though, such as Wardle et al. (2008), emphasize that much of the obesity epidemic is not due to changes in our genetic makeup, but rather is due to changes in our environment. In fact, our "obesogenic" (Wang et al. 2008) environment, with an emphasis on enormous portions and fast food choices, is still another major contributing factor to the obesity situation.

For example, even our cookbooks have changed over the years: Wansink and Payne (2009) surveyed recipes from the classic cookbook *The Joy of Cooking*, first published 70 years ago and reissued several times over the years. They found that in their sampling, the recipes, and particularly those published since 1996, had increased substantially in both portion size and use of higher-calorie ingredients. Overall, they found that the average calorie density had increased more than 35% per serving over the past 70 years.

People fail at weight maintenance because they do not sufficiently take into account both biological *and* psychological variables, simultaneously, when they initiate a sensible long-term eating plan. Essentially, notes Friedman (2003), "our drive to eat is to a large extent hardwired," and our body must have an "extraordinary level of precision," beyond merely conscious control, to be able to process the 10 million or so calories that we consume during the course of a decade. Nevertheless, our internal psychological state may "weigh in" just as heavily as our metabolic set point.

Some internal states are reflective of overt psychiatric pathology, such as undiagnosed anxiety or depression or even serious personality disorders; other states are reflective of maladaptive defenses. We are subject to temptations; we prefer short-term gratification to gratification that comes over the long term when we maintain our weight loss and preserve our physical health. We are prone to stress, which can work paradoxically: sometimes it makes us eat more, with subsequent weight gain, and sometimes less, with subsequent weight loss. Even transient feelings of anxiety and depression can complicate our eating behaviors.

THE "MINDED BRAIN"

The mind is the software program of the brain. In 1923, in his structural theory, Freud (1923/1961, pp. 1–66) conceptualized a mind divided into three parts, the *ego* (the rational, cognitive part), the *id* (the irrational, emotional part), and the *superego* (moral overseer, mediator between the two), all of which play a role in everyone's life. A component of Freud's ego is self-reflection—that is, our ability to anticipate, imagine, or argue. It is also our *self-consciousness*. As such, it is one of the major distinctions between humans and animals, as Leon Kass (1999, p. 93) says in his book *The Hungry Soul*.

Of course, not everyone believes in Freud's structural theory, but symbolically it is useful to divide the mind into its rational and irrational components. It is the rational mind, for example, that enables us to *contemplate* or *plan* what we want to eat or deliberately choose what not to eat and allows us to have *insight* into our behavior, both before and after we do something. The rational part of our mind is also involved with self-regulation, both conscious and nonconscious. Self-regulation is an executive function that involves not only memory, attention, choice, and decision making, but also control of emotion (Banfield et al. 2004, p. 62). Vohs and Baumeister (2004, p. 2) make the point that self-regulation is analogous to the body's homeostatic mechanisms. Failures of self-regulation may be seen in alcoholism, cigarette smoking, drug addiction, and other addictions, as well as overeating (Vohs and Baumeister 2004, p. 3). Self-regulation, of course, is a major factor not only in initiating weight control and a healthy lifestyle, but also in maintaining them over time.

It is the irrational part of the mind that makes us susceptible to temptations, that enables us to hear that piece of cake or box of cookies, as it were, calling out to us. And it is our moral compass that enables us to differentiate right from wrong, good from bad, and appreciate the pull of temptations.

Our personality, including our character, is also an aspect of our mind, as are the psychological defenses that we automatically employ to protect ourselves from feelings of unpleasure, such as anxiety and depression. Stunkard (1958), incidentally, found there is no one specific personality type or even specific psychopathology typical of all people with weight problems. More recently, obesity researcher Jules Hirsch (2003), of Rockefeller University, came to the same conclusion.

If the mind is our "software," the brain is our "hardware," or hardwiring. The mind, though, is part of the brain, of course, and not a separate anatomical structure. We have ideas about what parts of the brain contribute to our notion of mind, but we have yet to identify exactly what we mean by "mind," and sometimes it is more of a philosophical concept. In fact, it is very difficult to think of the mind without thinking of the brain. Neuroscientist Antonio Damasio (1997), for example, calls the brain the "minded brain." His view is that the mind, that is, all the mental phenomena we think of as the mind, is actually a composite of the physical and chemical states within neurons, the cells of the brain. And to make matters more complicated, we know the brain is part of the body. It is this intricate system of mind and brain and body, that is, this system of neural and biochemical connections, within the context of the environment, that makes the whole notion of weight control and maintenance so difficult and yet so intriguing.

THE DIETER AS WELL AS THE DIET

Jane Ogden (2003, p. 174), in discussing the psychological aspects of weight control, goes so far as to say that sometimes what a dieter believes is as important as what he or she does. In other words, those who want to preserve their weight loss not only must be motivated to change their behavior, they must also believe they can bring about change, and they must believe that the consequences of their own behavior are important and valuable.

It is our impression that no one book, so far, has integrated the complex psychological and physiological aspects of the mind, brain, and body sufficiently to explain why weight control and maintenance seem so daunting for so many people. As physicians who are psychiatrists, we offer that synthetic perspective.

Sometimes, though, a calorie is just a calorie. We therefore provide basic information about food (e.g., carbohydrates, protein, and fat) as well as the most recent medical research about the consequences of obesity and about the metabolic complexities of weight, including the concepts of set point and satiety; adipose tissue; and the many hormones involved in weight control. We also discuss the role of our "toxic" environment (e.g., portion size, the food industry) in sabotaging our best efforts at weight control, and the importance of exercise and sleep, as well as the complex circadian rhythms involved. Furthermore, we explain the principles behind various diets and explore the complications involved in starvation, and we also present some of the psychological approaches utilized for weight loss and maintenance.

Weight, a measure of the earth's gravitational pull, is one of the signals that alert us to the functioning not only of our body, but also of our mind. The poet Wendell Berry, who has written an essay on "The Pleasures of Eating," speaks about eating "as an agricultural act." He urges us to "eat responsibly," and he suggests that we must restore our "consciousness of what is involved in eating" (Berry 2003, pp. 321, 324). Weight loss and maintenance are, among other things, about eating responsibly. In his poem "The Gift of Gravity" (1987, pp. 257–258), Berry writes:

> In work of love, the body
> forgets its weight. And once
> again with love and singing
> in my mind, I come to what
> must come to me, carried
> as a dancer by a song.
> This grace is gravity.

REFERENCES

Allison DB, Downey M, Atkinson RL, et al: Obesity as a disease: a white paper on evidence and arguments commissioned by the Council of the Obesity Society. Obesity (Silver Spring) 16:1161–1177, 2008

Aronne LJ: Treatment of obesity in the primary care setting, in Handbook of Obesity Treatment. Edited by Wadden TA, Stunkard AJ. New York, Guilford, 2002, pp 383–394

Aronne LJ, Nelinson DS, Lillo JL: Obesity as a disease state: a new paradigm for diagnosis and treatment. Clinical Cornerstone: Obesity as a Disease State 9(4):9–29, 2009

Banfield JF, Wyland CL, Macrae CN, et al: The cognitive neuroscience of self-regulation, in Handbook of Self-Regulation: Research, Theory, and Applications. Edited by Baumeister RF, Vohs KD. New York, Guilford, 2004, pp 62–83

Aronne LJ, Nelinson DS, Lillo JL: Obesity as a disease state: a new paradigm for diagnosis and Berry W: The pleasures of eating, in The Art of the Common-Place: Agrarian Essays of Wendell Berry. Edited by Wirzba N. Berkeley, CA, Counterpoint, 2003

Berry W: The Collected Poems of Wendell Berry, 1957–1982. San Francisco, CA, North Point Press, 1987

Berthoud HR: Interactions between the "cognitive" and "metabolic" brain in the control of food intake. Physiol Behav 91:486–498, 2007

Bray GA: Obesity is a chronic, relapsing neurochemical disease. Int J Obes Relat Metab Disord 28:34–38, 2004

Breslow L: Public health aspects of weight control. Am J Public Health Nations Health 42:1116–1120, 1952

Brownell K: The Obesity Crisis: Psychiatry Weighs In. Speech delivered at Yale University, Anlyan Center for Medical Research and Education, October 3, 2008

Damasio AR: Exploring the minded brain. Speech delivered at the University of Michigan, November 14, 1997, in The Tanner Lectures on Human Values, Vol. 20. Salt Lake City, University of Utah Press, 1999, pp 169–187

Finkelstein EA, Trogdon JG, Cohen JW, et al: Annual medical spending attributable to obesity: payer and service specific estimates. Health Aff (Millwood) 28:w822–831, 2009

Fitzgerald F: The tyranny of health. N Engl J Med 331:196–198, 1994

Flegal KM: Commentary: the epidemic of obesity: what's in a name? Int J Epidemiol 35:72–74, 2006

Foster GD, Wadden TA, Makris AP, et al: Primary care physicians' attitudes about obesity and its treatment. Obes Res 11:1168–1177, 2003

Freud S: The ego and the id (1923), in The Standard Edition of the Complete Psychological Works of Sigmund Freud, Vol 19. Translated and edited by Strachey J. London, Hogarth Press, 1961, pp 1–66

Friedman JM: A war on obesity, not the obese. Science 299:856–858, 2003

Hirsch J: Obesity: matter over mind? The Dana Foundation. January 1, 2003. Available at: http://www.dana.org/news/cerebrum/detail.aspx?id=2908. Accessed July 6, 2009.

Jain A, Ferguson C, Mauery DR, et al: Re-visioning success: how stigma, perceptions of treatment, and definitions of success impact obesity and weight management in America. A research report for the Strategies to Overcome and Prevent (STOP) Obesity Alliance.

Washington, DC, George Washington University School of Public Health and Health Services, Department of Health Policy, November 2, 2007

Kass L: The Hungry Soul: Eating and the Perfecting of Our Nature. Chicago, IL, University of Chicago Press, 1999

Keys A: The Management of Obesity. Minnesota Medicine 48:1329–1331, 1965

King DE, Mainous AG III, Carnemolla M, et al: Adherence to healthy lifestyle habits in US adults, 1988–2006. Am J Med 122:528–534, 2009

Leonhardt D: Fat tax: should overweight people pay more for health insurance? New York Times Magazine, August 16, 2009, p 9

Newbold RR, Padilla-Banks E, Snyder RJ, et al: Developmental exposure to endocrine disruptors and the obesity epidemic. Reprod Toxicol 23:290–296, 2007

Ogden CL, Carroll MD, McDowell MA, et al: Obesity among adults in the United States—no statistically significant change since 2003–2004. NCHS Data Brief No 1. Hyattsville, MD, National Center for Health Statistics, U.S. Department of Health and Human Services, November 2007

Ogden J: The Psychology of Eating: From Healthy to Disordered Behavior. Malden, MA, Blackwell Publishing, 2003

Olshansky SJ, Passaro DJ, Hershow RC, et al: A potential decline in life expectancy in the United States in the 21st century. N Engl J Med 352:1138–1145, 2005

Power ML, Schulkin J: The Evolution of Obesity. Baltimore, MD, Johns Hopkins University Press, 2009

Precope J: Hippocrates on Diet and Hygiene. London, Zeno, 1952

Seven deadly sins, in Encyclopedia Britannica Online. 2009. Available at: http://www.britannica.com/EBchecked/topic/536446/seven-deadly-sins. Accessed September 1, 2009.

Stunkard AJ: The management of obesity. N Y State J Med 58:79–87, 1958

Sturm R: The effects of obesity, smoking, and drinking on medical problems and costs: obesity outranks both smoking and drinking in its deleterious effects on health and health costs. Health Aff (Millwood) 21:245–253, 2002

Vohs KD, Baumeister RF: Understanding self-regulation: an introduction, in Handbook of Self-Regulation: Research, Theory, and Applications. Edited by Baumeister RF, Vohs KD. New York, Guilford, 2004, pp 1–9

Wang Y, Beydoun MA, Liang L, et al: Will all Americans become overweight or obese? Estimating the progression and cost of the US obesity epidemic. Obesity (Silver Spring) 16:2323–2330, 2008

Wansink B, Payne CR: The joy of cooking too much: 70 years of calorie increases in classic recipes. Ann Intern Med 150:291–292, 2009

Wardle J, Carnell S, Haworth CH, et al: Evidence for a strong genetic influence on childhood adiposity despite the force of the obesogenic environment. Am J Clin Nutr 87:398–404, 2008

2

OBESITY IN
THE UNITED STATES

The Gravity of the Situation

There are several reasons why it is impossible to prescribe a rigorously perfect regimen, that is, one in which the amount of food will exactly counterbalance the amount of exercise.... Firstly, constitutions are not all alike. Secondly, individual requirements vary according to age, climate, season, etc.

Hippocrates, *Regimen,* Book III
(Precope 1952, p. 68)

DEFINITIONS OF OBESITY:
BODY MASS INDEX

There have been depictions in art of what we would consider obese people since mankind's earliest drawings and figurines. Over 23,000 years ago, in the Upper Paleolithic period, was created the famous Venus of Willendorf, a small statue with enormous, pendulous breasts and massive abdominal obesity. Many other examples of obese figures have been found through the Neolithic period, over 5,500 years ago, a period noted for the beginnings of agriculture and human settlements. And even though we think of Egyptians as angular and slender from hieroglyphic drawings made around 2,500 years ago, there is evidence from mummies that obesity was not uncommon in that culture as well (Bray 2003, pp. 2–5).

By the time of the fifth century B.C. in Athens, Hippocrates, in his treatise *Regimen* (Precope 1952, p. 32), was warning, uncannily and quite presciently, of the importance of watching one's food intake and getting proper exercise for maintaining health when he recommended "neither excess nor deficiency, between the two concomitants of health: food and exercise" and said that "however small the disproportion on either side [it] will ultimately, of necessity, lead to disease." And he even cautioned that those who are "constitutionally very fat are more apt to die quickly than those who are thin" (Hippocrates 1967, p. 199).

The word *obesity*, meaning fatness or stoutness, comes from Latin through the French and was first used in the middle of the 1600s (Oxford English Dictionary 1989). Through the years, some writers have waxed poetic in the use of the word, such as when Alexander Pope, in a note to his 1729 version of the *Dunciad*, spoke of one of his colleagues as a "martyr to obesity" ("who had fallen victim to the rotundity of his parts") or William Taylor (1812) spoke of writers having perished "of literary obesity." Even W. Somerset Maugham spoke of the vicar in *Of Human Bondage* as having a "slow, obese smile" (Oxford English Dictionary 1989).

Today, though, as populations around the world grow increasingly more obese, we are more interested in studying obesity and its consequences than waxing poetic about it. As measurements have become more scientific over the years, there have been more accurate ways of quantifying body composition and measuring obesity, that is, excessive fatness, specifically.

Years ago, people were more likely to use the word *corpulent* to describe someone obese by our standards today. Researchers Wadden and Didie (2003) described a study in which men and women who were obese (with a body mass index or BMI value of >35 kg/m^2) and an additional sample of women who were extremely obese (i.e., the morbidly obese, with BMI values of about 52.5 kg/m^2), who were being evaluated for bariatric surgery, rated the word *fatness* significantly the most undesirable description for their weight among eleven terms given them with a five-point rating scale. They also rated negatively the words *obesity, excess fat,* and *large size*. More neutral words included *weight problem, BMI, excess weight,* and *unhealthy body weight*. In this study, the ratings of men and women were fairly similar, though women rated the words *fatness, excess fat,* and *large size* even more significantly undesirable than the men in the study did. The researchers cautioned physicians that use of these terms, because of their pejorative connotations in our culture, could be "hurtful or offensive" and even "derogatory" and advised avoiding them when discussing a patient's weight condition. Their recommendation was that the "calling it what it is" confrontational approach just does

FAT BY ANY OTHER NAME

- Researchers have found that obese men and women rate the word *fatness* significantly the most undesirable description for their weight; they also don't like the words *obesity, excess fat,* and *large size*

- More neutral (and desirable) words: *weight problem, BMI, excess weight,* and *unhealthy body weight*

Source: Wadden and Didie 2003

not work, being "more likely to result in hurt feelings than in weight loss" (Wadden and Didie 2003).

It was around the turn of the twentieth century that scales became available for home use and life insurance companies began to gather data on weight and its relationship to mortality. One company in 1912, without standardization, gathered measurements of height with shoes on and weight with clothing on (Pai and Paloucek 2000). The Metropolitan Life Insurance Company charts were particularly popular throughout the middle of the century, even though they were not compiled very scientifically and also allowed for shoes and clothing. For example, the division of people into categories of frames (small, medium, or large build) was done arbitrarily without any corroborating data and was left to the subjective judgment of the examiner (Pai and Paloucek 2000). It was not until 1959 that body frame was later defined and "desirable weight" became synonymous with "ideal weight." From these charts, researchers agreed on a "simple rule" for estimating ideal weight: "for women, allow 100 pounds for the first five feet and five pounds for each additional inch; for men, allow 110 pounds for the first five feet and five pounds for each additional inch," with a 10% variation above or below allowed (Pai and Paloucek 2000). Further, the 1979 version of the Metropolitan tables included 10% who self-reported their weights and heights rather than having had them accurately measured, and of the 90% who were measured, again according to Harrison (1985), all were measured without standardizing clothing or shoes. Harrison also makes the point that our culture seems quite preoccupied with measurements of height and particularly weight. She notes that one of the first questions, after the question of sex, asked on the birth of a baby is its weight, and police always describe criminals by an estimate of their height and weight, as well as their sex and race.

One measurement that has been popular in recent years, though, actually dates back to the middle of the nineteenth century. This is the *Quételet index*, named after Adolphe Quételet, the father of modern statistics. Quételet, a Belgian mathematician and astronomer, was a so-called Renaissance man who studied normal weight populations in his effort to draw conclusions about statistical averages (Rössner 2007). He devised a formula, also now referred to as the *body mass index*, or BMI, in which one's weight in kilograms is proportional to one's height in meters squared. When using pounds and inches for measurements, as we do in the United States, we can use the same equation but need to multiply the quotient by 703. Essentially, the BMI is a measure of body fatness. How the BMI became so popular and the standard measure for obesity clinically as well as in most research studies is not clear. Keys et al. (1972), though, seem to have named it, in a paper in which they spoke of "the need for an index of relative body weight." In this same paper, Keys and his colleagues say, "What we here call the body mass index, weight/height^2," has a long history" and credits Quételet for first calculating that particular ratio.

The BMI table (Figure 2–1) is now commonly found in most texts on obesity and even in some physicians' offices next to their scales. This chart indicates the rela-

Figure 2–1. Body mass index table.[a]

Height (inches)	Normal						Overweight					Obese										Extreme obesity														
BMI	19	20	21	22	23	24	25	26	27	28	29	30	31	32	33	34	35	36	37	38	39	40	41	42	43	44	45	46	47	48	49	50	51	52	53	54
																	Body weight (pounds)																			
58	91	96	100	105	110	115	119	124	129	134	138	143	148	153	158	162	167	172	177	181	186	191	196	201	205	210	215	220	224	229	234	239	244	248	253	258
59	94	99	104	109	114	119	124	128	133	138	143	148	153	158	163	168	173	178	183	188	193	198	203	208	212	217	222	227	232	237	242	247	252	257	262	267
60	97	102	107	112	118	123	128	133	138	143	148	153	158	163	168	174	179	184	189	194	199	204	209	215	220	225	230	235	240	245	250	255	261	266	271	276
61	100	106	111	116	122	127	132	137	143	148	153	158	164	169	175	180	185	190	195	201	206	211	217	222	227	232	238	243	248	254	259	264	269	275	280	285
62	104	109	115	120	126	131	136	142	147	153	158	164	169	175	180	186	191	196	202	207	213	218	224	229	235	240	246	251	256	262	267	273	278	284	289	295
63	107	113	118	124	130	135	141	146	152	158	163	169	175	180	186	191	197	203	208	214	220	225	231	237	242	248	254	259	265	270	278	282	287	293	299	304
64	110	116	122	128	134	140	145	151	157	163	169	174	180	186	192	197	204	209	215	221	227	232	238	244	250	256	262	267	273	279	285	291	296	302	308	314
65	114	120	126	132	138	144	150	156	162	168	174	180	186	192	198	204	210	216	222	228	234	240	246	252	258	264	270	276	282	288	294	300	306	312	318	324
66	118	124	130	136	142	148	155	161	167	173	179	186	192	198	204	210	216	223	229	235	241	247	253	260	266	272	278	284	291	297	303	309	315	322	328	334
67	121	127	134	140	146	153	159	166	172	178	185	191	198	204	211	217	223	230	236	242	249	255	261	268	274	280	287	293	299	306	312	319	325	331	338	344
68	125	131	138	144	151	158	164	171	177	184	190	197	203	210	216	223	230	236	243	249	256	262	269	276	282	289	295	302	308	315	322	328	335	341	348	354
69	128	135	142	149	155	162	169	176	182	189	196	203	209	216	223	230	236	243	250	257	263	270	277	284	291	297	304	311	318	324	331	338	345	351	358	365
70	132	139	146	153	160	167	174	181	188	195	202	209	216	222	229	236	243	250	257	264	271	278	285	292	299	306	313	320	327	334	341	348	355	362	369	376
71	136	143	150	157	165	172	179	186	193	200	208	215	222	229	236	243	250	257	265	272	279	286	293	301	308	315	322	329	338	343	351	358	365	372	379	386
72	140	147	154	162	169	177	184	191	199	206	213	221	228	235	242	250	258	265	272	279	287	294	302	309	316	324	331	338	346	353	361	368	375	383	390	397
73	144	151	159	166	174	182	189	197	204	212	219	227	235	242	250	257	265	272	280	288	295	302	310	318	325	333	340	348	355	363	371	378	386	393	401	408
74	148	155	163	171	179	186	194	202	210	218	225	233	241	249	256	264	272	280	287	295	303	311	319	326	334	342	350	358	365	373	381	389	396	404	412	420
75	152	160	168	176	184	192	200	208	216	224	232	240	248	256	264	272	279	287	295	303	311	319	327	335	343	351	359	367	375	383	391	399	407	415	423	431
76	156	164	172	180	189	197	205	213	221	230	238	246	254	263	271	279	287	295	304	312	320	328	336	344	353	361	369	377	385	394	402	410	418	426	435	443

[a]Body weight fluctuates by 2%–3% during a normal day (Price 2002, p. 78).

Source. Adapted from National Heart, Lung, and Blood Institute: *Clinical Guidelines on the Identification, Evaluation, and Treatment of Overweight and Obesity in Adults: The Evidence Report* (NIH Publ No 98-4083). Bethesda, MD, National Institutes of Health, 1998.

tionship of weight and height and divides the results into categories of "normal" (BMI value, 18.5–24.9 kg/m^2), "overweight" (BMI 25.0–29.9 kg/m^2), and "obese" (BMI ≥30 kg/m^2). The category of obese is subdivided into Class 1 (BMI 30–34.9 kg/m^2), Class 2 (BMI 35–39.9 kg/m^2), and Class 3, also called morbid or extreme obesity (BMI ≥40 kg/m^2). More recently, with some patients seeking bariatric surgery, there is even a Class 4, called super-morbid obesity, with BMI levels greater than 50 kg/m^2 (Kalarchian et al. 2007). If someone's BMI value is less than 18.5 kg/m^2, that person is considered underweight, such as very thin models or those suffering from the eating disorder anorexia nervosa. An article in the *New York Times* (Ellin and Schwartz 2006) put these numbers in human form: model Kate Moss was reported as having a BMI value of 16.4 kg/m^2; actress

BODY MASS INDEX (BMI) RANGES	
Underweight	BMI <18.5 kg/m^2
Normal	BMI 18.5–24.9 kg/m^2
Overweight	BMI 25.0–29.9 kg/m^2
Obese	BMI ≥30 kg/m^2
Class 1	BMI 30–34.9 kg/m^2
Class 2	BMI 35–39.9 kg/m^2
Class 3 (extreme or morbid obesity)	BMI ≥40 kg/m^2
Class 4 (supermorbid obesity)	BMI ≥50 kg/m^2
Source: Devlin et al. 2000; Kalarchian et al. 2007	

Nicole Richie, just over 16 kg/m^2; George W. Bush, 26.6 kg/m^2; and actress Rosie O'Donnell, more than 31 kg/m^2. More recently, on a program on National Public Radio, host Scott Simon (2009) interviewed Keith Devlin, a professor from Stanford University who is critical of the use of BMI to measure obesity. Devlin noted that many professional actors and athletes, such as Johnny Depp, Brad Pitt, George Clooney, Will Smith, and Denzel Washington, would all be "officially classified as overweight" by BMI standards, and he believes that BMI measurements are "misleading."

These criteria have been set by the World Health Organization and the National Institutes of Health. Ogden and her colleagues (2006) studied a 6-year period from 1999 to 2004 in the United States and found that just over 17% of children and adolescents were overweight (above 95th percentile) and just over 32% of adults were obese, with a BMI value of 30 kg/m^2 or greater. By 2004, almost 3% of men and almost 7% of women had extreme obesity, with a BMI value of 40 kg/m^2 or greater. Ogden et al. also noted differences in prevalence rates among different races and ethnicities. Though over the 6-year period, rates of obesity in women seemed to be leveling off, rates for men and children and adolescents increased significantly.

Hu, in his book *Obesity Epidemiology* (2008, p. 16), noted that the prevalence of obesity in the adult U.S. population for 2005–2006 was 33.3% for men and 35.3% for women. The problem is such an acute one in the United States that the Centers for Disease Control and Prevention has actually drawn "obesity maps" that show that the Midwest and South have the highest prevalence of obesity in the United States. For example, Mississippi has the highest rate, with 37% of its population considered obese, and Virginia, Alabama, and Louisiana all have obesity rates hovering around 30% (Vinter et al. 2008). Of course, it is not just in the United States that obesity rates have skyrocketed. According to Hu (2008, p. 22), obesity has reached epidemic proportions in many parts of the world and is a problem particularly in developing countries. There is also a greater tendency toward and a dramatic rise in morbid obesity (BMI > 40 kg/m^2). Hu (2008, p. 23) notes that if the current trends continue, by 2025 the prevalence of obesity will exceed 40% in the United States and 30% in Great Britain. Wang and Beydoun (2007) give even more dire statistical predictions: they note that by 2015, 75% of adults will be either overweight or obese and 41% will actually be obese. In a more recent paper, Wang et al. (2008) even predicted that if the obesity trends continue, by 2030, over 86% adults will be either overweight or obese and 51% will actually be obese. These researchers are predicting that by 2048, *all* American adults will be overweight or obese!

Though BMI values have been correlated with cardiovascular disease, hypertension, and diabetes (Hu 2008, p. 67), there are several problems with using the BMI as a measurement. For one, O'Rahilly and Farooqi (2006) note that the division of obese from nonobese at a BMI of 30 kg/m^2 "has a certain degree of arbitrariness" to it and is not based on any specific biological (i.e., genetic) marker. Bouchard et al. (2004, p. 163) point out that BMI is a general measure of body build. As such, it includes fat mass, muscle mass, and skeletal mass. As a result, BMI may sometimes overestimate actual body fat in those with a more muscular build and may underestimate body fat in people who have lost muscle, a condition called *sarcopenia*, as may occur in older people. BMI also sometimes gives an inaccurate measure of body fat in people who are particularly short or tall, because height is part of the equation. Furthermore, it has been noted that when people are asked to self-report, men are more likely to exaggerate their height and women are more likely to underreport their weight. In fact, in one study by Nawaz et al. (2001), researchers found a tendency in about 100 overweight or obese women to underreport weight and overreport height. And for the same BMI value, women have a higher percentage of body fat than men. Deurenberg and colleagues (1991) note that the relationship of body fat and BMI is sex- and age-dependent as a result of the differences in body compo-

LIMITATIONS OF THE BODY MASS INDEX (BMI)

- As a measure of body build, includes muscle and bone as well as fat

- May overestimate body fat in muscular persons and underestimate body fat in older persons with muscle wasting (*sarcopenia*)

- Can be inaccurate in both very tall and very short people

- May be based on inaccurate self-reports of height and weight

sition between men and women as well as the increase in body fat as most people age. BMI values as a measure of body fat are also more problematic in children less than 16 years old because body fat generally remains constant (except in girls during puberty, when it increases slightly), but during this period BMI values increase. Further, these authors note that even when BMI (and body weight, specifically) remains the same as we age, our amount of body fat increases as we lose muscle mass.

An editorial in *The Lancet* even suggested that relatively recent research from the INTERHEART study indicates that "current practice with body mass index as the measure of obesity is *obsolete*, and results in considerable *underestimation* of the grave consequences of the obesity epidemic" (Kragelund and Omland 2005). More recently, Poirier (2007) suggested that use of the BMI as an obesity measurement has its limitations even though there is a correlation of greater risk factors for cardiovascular disease (i.e., comorbidities) with a higher BMI value. Poirier suggests use of waist circumference or even the waist-to-hip ratio as more predictive of increased mortality.

Several other measures have been used to assess obesity, including, as mentioned above, measurement of waist circumference and waist-to-hip ratio.

> Women with a waist circumference over 35 inches and men with a waist circumference over 40 inches (measured at the umbilicus) are considered obese and are more prone to obesity-related diseases.
>
> **Aronne 2002, p. 385**

However, anyone who has attempted to gather such data (even on oneself) realizes that it is sometimes easier said than done. In fact, this measurement procedure has not been standardized. The waist is usually measured at the level of the umbilicus because the so-called *natural waist*—the smallest circumference—is difficult to find in obese people. The hip is measured at the widest circumference over the rear.

Along these lines, it is not only whether someone has excess fat but where the fat is located that may be crucial to the health consequences of obesity. Jean Vague (1956), a French professor of medicine, noted that there are primarily two types of fat distribution, which are most likely genetically determined: the *gynoid* (as we delineate it more informally, the pear-shaped or bottom-heavy body)—named thus because it is more typical of women—and the *android* (the so-called apple-shaped or rounded body), with a much larger circumference at the waist than hips (think beer belly)—named thus because it is more typical of men. Vague did acknowledge that each type can be found in both sexes and that there are intermediate forms, but when there is fat accumulation around the waist there are clearly much more likely metabolic consequences, such as diabetes, gout, gallstones, and atherosclerosis. People with fat accumulation around the hips, on the other hand, are more likely to have what he called "mechanical complications," such as respiratory difficulty or circulatory problems (Vague 1956).

An indirect measure of fat accumulation is the measuring of skinfold thickness with special calipers to pinch skin in specifically designated areas, such as under the shoulder (subscapular area) or in the abdomen, thigh, triceps, or biceps. Snijder et al. (2006) suggest that the most accurate skinfold measurement is done in the sub-scapular region and "should be considered as an indicator of central fat distribution separately" from measurement of waist circumference. As we can imagine, these measurements may vary considerably from examiner to examiner and even from one examination to another. Often one examiner will take measurements several times in one area to get an average. The measurements are also difficult to obtain ac-curately in very obese people. Measurement of skinfold thickness is the least reliable of measurements, and it is not helpful in assessing fat within the abdominal cavity.

There are more precise measures of fat (adipose) tissue. The gold standard of measuring body composition is the procedure of underwater weighing, or *densi-tometry*. The principle here is that fat is less dense than water; the subject's weight is measured in air and then underwater. The technique is cumbersome and clearly not readily available, and it is not suitable for children or older people.

More recently, both computed tomography (CT) and magnetic resonance imag-ing (MRI) have been used to measure with considerable accuracy and high resolu-tion a person's percentage of body fat. CT, though, is less advantageous because it exposes the patient to radiation, whereas MRI does not. Though these techniques are expensive and not always available, both can provide a means of assessing fat distribution around bodily organs. In other words, they can distinguish so-called visceral fat from subcutaneous fat.

Another method for assessing body composition is dual-energy X-ray absorp-tiometry (DXA). It was originally used for assessing bone density and evaluating osteoporosis. Actually, women (and men) who have regular bone density examina-tions also have a record of their percentage of fat tissue. According to Hu (2008, p. 59), DXA is a highly accurate and reproducible measure of body composition and is based on the notion that X-ray beams pass differently through fat, bone, and muscle. However, it cannot be used on pregnant women (nor can a CT scan), and most machines cannot accommodate the extremely obese.

SOME METHODOLOGICAL PROBLEMS IN STUDYING OBESITY

When attempting to study, quantify, and research issues regarding obesity and weight in general, one has to consider several other limitations, some more par-ticular to obesity and others more general. In particular, measuring food intake, including calorie counts, can give extremely variable results, as can measuring daily physical activity and even exercise specifically. More generally, studies involv-ing lifestyle changes in diet and exercise often have very high dropout (attrition) rates—not uncommonly as much as 50% even within a year, let alone in long-term studies involving many years (see Hu 2008, p. 38, for a review). Along those lines, not only is the attrition rate high, this is further compounded by a high rate of noncompliance or sometimes incomplete compliance with the program. Further, many of these studies are not done under controlled conditions such as in a hospital setting, but rather in the community, so there are many variables not accounted for and only so much supervision is provided. Researchers are at the mercy of self-reports of diet and exercise that can, even with the best of intentions, be considerably inaccurate.

De Castro (2000) believes that laboratory research on obesity may miss "essential variables" that are seen only in real-life situations. For example, one variable that many people must consider is the cost of food, something that does not become part of most experimental protocols where

> **WHAT IS THE EYE-MOUTH GAP?**
>
> - Gap between how much people think they are eating per day and how much they are really eating, even when watching their food intake carefully
>
> - Even thin people may report only 80% of what they eat
>
> - Obese people report only one-half to two-thirds of what they actually eat
>
> **Source:** Lichtman et al. 1992; Tataranni and Ravussin 2002

food is provided. Further, obesity research is often conducted over a day or even over a meal, rather than over the two or three days that may be required for a "compensatory reaction" in eating variability to occur.

And people sometimes eat differently depending on external circumstances, such as the number of people present, their relationship (e.g., we tend to eat more with friends and relatives than with strangers), and even the gender of our eating companions, as well as the meal size and even the time of day. For example, de Castro (2000) notes that experiments in the lab are done at the convenience of the lab, that is, usually during the day, and thus important diurnal rhythms may be overlooked (see Chapter 9 in this volume, on circadian rhythms). Further, people tend to eat differently (and usually more) on weekends, differences that may be missed in a lab setting.

Brian Wansink (2006, p. 31), in his book *Mindless Eating: Why We Eat More Than We Think*, noted how easy it is to gain weight, particularly when people do not pay attention to everything they eat: "Just ten extra calories a day for a year—three small jelly beans—will make you a pound more portly a year from now!" The other problem is that most people, including thin people, underestimate how much they really eat. Studies are contradictory in terms of whether self-reporting of food intake is actually accurate enough. The *eye-mouth gap* is a term coined by researchers (Tataranni and Ravussin 2004, pp. 48–49) for the gap between what someone thinks he or she is eating and what is really eaten. Even under careful conditions of food intake assessment, Lichtman et al. (1992) found that obese people reported only one-half to two-thirds of their total calorie intake; even some lean subjects reported only 80% of their calorie intake (see also Chapter 3 in this volume, on food and calo-

GENETICS AND OBESITY

- Possibly more than 250 genes may influence weight
- Identical twins raised apart resemble each other in weight more than siblings raised together
- Genes account for as much as two-thirds of individual differences in adult obesity
- Obesity in one parent more than doubles the risk a child will be obese as an adult
- Risk is even greater if both parents are obese
- Childhood obesity doubles risk of obesity in adulthood
- Strongest predictor of adult obesity is a combination of child or adolescent obesity with family history of obesity (70%–75% of people with these two risk factors will be obese adults)
- Maternal obesity is a stronger risk factor than paternal obesity

Source: Price 2002; Wadden and Phelan 2002

ries). De Castro (2000) even suggests that people be given cameras to photograph their meals before eating, to get more accurate records of food intake!

There are also confounding or distorting variables to consider that may affect outcome. For example, Hu (2008, pp. 39–40) makes the point that smoking is one such variable that may distort an association between obesity and mortality, inasmuch as smokers tend to be thinner and have a higher mortality rate. Controlling for smoking, though, is more complicated than it sounds. One can control not only for smoking status, such as never, past, or current, but also for the number of cigarettes smoked per day and even the brands smoked and degree of inhaling of the smoke. Rarely are such details reported in a study.

Other confounding variables can include the notion of *clustering*, namely that many lifestyle behaviors, sometimes healthy, sometimes not, tend to cluster together. It makes it difficult, then, to sort out which variables are producing what effect. For example, in one study by Schulze et al. (2004), those who tend to be smokers may also tend to eat more red meat, be less physically active, and drink more sugared soft drinks.

GENETICS AND OBESITY

Genetic Loading for Obesity

Sandra, age 50 years, was exposed to a toxic food environment as a child, in the context of strong genetic loading for obesity, because both parents had serious weight issues. It was not until her parents' old age, when they developed sarcopenia (lost muscle mass), that they appeared as though they had lost weight. Sandra reported:

"I have always struggled with my weight. I was never really fat but always a little heavy as a child. As I got older, my weight increased slowly over the years.

"Both my parents, now in their late 80s, until recently have always been more than a little heavy. My mother would serve us all huge portions. Her Southern fried chicken was our favorite. And there were always huge bags of candy and boxes of chocolate-covered pretzels, my favorite, around. I guess you would call my father obese and my mother overweight by today's standards. My father was always embarrassingly overweight to me. He was an enormous eater who would eat anything and everything together since 'everything mixes up inside anyway,' and because he ate so quickly he would always be eyeing any leftover food on anyone else's plate. He always liked to save money, so he used to buy pretzels and potato chips in bulk. He would come home with enormous barrels, literally—the quantity, I later learned, that was sold to restaurants and bars—one filled with pretzels and the other filled with chips—and, of course, they became stale very quickly. For years, I did not realize you could buy small, individual bags that would remain fresh. In that environment, I guess I was primed to have a weight disorder."

It is through studies of thousands of monozygotic twins, who share all genes, and dizygotic (nonidentical) twins, who share about half of their genes, that researchers have noted the highest correlation of BMI values in monozygotic (identical) twins, whether raised together or apart. This correlation can run as high as 0.74 for monozygotic twins; for dizygotic twins, it is 0.32; and for siblings, it is 0.25 (Maes 1997). Adoption studies, with twins or siblings raised apart, have also verified the genetic component to obesity, with genetic factors accounting for 20%–60% of variation in BMI values (Hu 2008, p. 442). Albert Stunkard, one of the deans of psychiatric research in the field of obesity, did one of the early adoption studies in the 1980s (Stunkard et al. 1986). Stunkard and his colleagues found, from a sample of 540 Danish adoptees (out of a population of over 3,500 people) that there was a "strong relationship" between the weight (thin, medium weight, overweight, or obese) of the adoptees and the body mass index (BMI) of their biological parents. These researchers concluded that genetic influences "have an important role in determining human fatness in adults, whereas the family environment alone has no apparent effect." In general, Price (2002, p. 75) makes the point that genes probably account for as much as two-thirds of individual differences in adult obesity.

The exact nature of the genetics involved is not yet known, and it is very likely that many different genes (i.e., polygenic inheritance) are involved in the overwhelming majority of cases. Snyder and colleagues (2004), in the *human obesity gene map* update of 2003, noted that at least 430 genetic loci had been reported to be involved in obesity in mouse experiments. Pérusse et al (2005), in the 2004 human obesity gene update, noted "overall greater than 600 genes, markers, and chromosomal regions have been associated with or linked with human obesity phenotypes." In the 2005 human obesity gene map (Rankinen et al. 2006), the number of so-called *quantitative trait loci* for animals reached 408, and 253 separate trait loci had been reported for humans. The authors noted that there are possible loci on all human chromosomes except the Y chromosome. Bouchard et al. (2004, p. 162) make the point that it is also likely that the genetic factors leading to massive obesity are not the same as those leading to only moderate obesity. It is also likely that different genetics are responsible for fat distribution, namely the pear-shaped versus the apple-shaped distribution. And Price (2002, p. 75) makes the point that women, across different countries, cultures, and dietary habits, have a higher percentage of body fat than men. Further, though, many cultures are more prone to obesity than others. The Pima Indians of Arizona (as opposed to Pima Indians in Mexico) and some groups in the Pacific Islands, for example, are more prone to obesity. Mark (2008) points out that strong genetic factors underlie the development of obesity, by promoting either a sensitivity or a resistance to obesity in a "toxic environment" (due to overnutrition by the availability of low-cost/high-calorie food and an increasingly—by previous standards—sedentary lifestyle made possible by our increasing technology: e.g., computers, remote controls, and automobiles). Mark notes that there is a stronger genetic component for BMI values and the regulation of fat accumulation in humans than there is for height or arterial blood pressure, "where a large genetic contribution is widely recognized" (Mark 2008). And O'Rahilly and Farooqi (2006) suggest that from a genetics viewpoint obesity may be less of a metabolic disorder and more of a neurobehavioral disorder, with genes that are related to states of hunger and satiety as well as food intake.

It was in studying the Arizona Pima Indians, two-thirds of whose population has type 2 diabetes and obesity, that anthropologist James Neel (1962) came up in the 1960s with his *thrifty gene* hypothesis, namely that some groups have evolved to be able to resist times of famine by being more able to store energy as fat. The thrifty gene hypothesis remains just that: to date, no specific inheritance has been identified. Studies of obesity and genetics assume there is what is called a *shared environment*, namely that people living in a particular home live under similar circumstances, so that any differences between monozygotic and dizygotic twins would be of genetic, rather than environmental, origin (Hu 2008, p. 440).

Most likely, it is more advantageous to think of obesity as a condition that involves a complex interaction of genes and environment—what Mark (2008) called the "contribution of susceptibility genes/alleles to obesity." In other words, some people can be predisposed genetically to obesity but become obese only under certain environmental conditions. And others, no matter what the environment, are resistant and will not become obese. Hu (2008, pp. 469–470) reported on animal experiments involving gene–diet interactions, whereby genetically altered mice gained significantly less weight when fed a high-fat diet than those not lacking a specific gene. There have also been studies involving a carbohydrate diet–gene interaction, as well as suggestions that genes may be involved in energy expenditure, appetite regulation, glucose metabolism, and fat cell functioning, among other things (Moreno-Aliaga et al. 2005). Several studies, in fact, including the Quebec Overfeeding Study by Bouchard and colleagues in 1990, have demonstrated that genetic factors may be very much involved in how easily one individual gains weight as opposed to another, as well as how easily one is able to maintain weight loss. Nicklas and colleagues (1999) found that a group of subjects with carriers of a particular genetic allele regained significantly more weight over a 12-month follow-up period than those without that genetic makeup. And it is very likely that where we gain weight (android or gynoid distribution) is under genetic control. In fact, Lindgren et al. (2009) reported on their meta-analysis of genome studies that included over 70,000 Europeans to identify genetic loci that might affect fat distribution, particularly abdominal (i.e., central obesity), as well as waist circumference and waist-to-hip ratio. The researchers found three genetic loci that are "strongly implicated" in the regulation of fat distribution, among which one (waist-to-hip ratio) is gender specific to females. Even responses to weight loss medications may be genetically determined. For example, there is considerable variability in people's responses to sibutramine, a medication that induces satiety in some dieters; those who are homozygous for a particular gene are more likely to succeed in losing weight early in treatment (Hsia et al. 2009).

Such studies would suggest that genetic testing might eventually predict which dieting strategies and interventions will be successful in a particular individual. Moreno-Aliaga and colleagues (2005), though, raise two important caveats, namely whether a focus on genetics will divert attention away from environmental or lifestyle changes that may also be contributing to obesity and also whether knowledge of one's genetic susceptibility will change how a person approaches weight control (i.e., "weight loss self-efficacy"). In any case, the authors note that it is premature at this point to use genetic susceptibility to target weight loss strategies. O'Rahilly and Farooqi (2008) make the point that while genetics factor into processes like energy expenditure, it is the "heritable differences in neurobehavioral traits," such as those involved in hunger, satiety, and even the pleasurable (hedonic) aspects of eating, that are "likely to be more important." For O'Rahilly and Farooqi, even in the "midst of the obesity epidemic," the evidence that hereditary factors are important remains "unassailable" and heredity remains the "single most powerful determinant" of differences in weight among people.

THE NATIONAL WEIGHT CONTROL REGISTRY: WEIGHT LOSS VERSUS MAINTENANCE

In the late 1950s, Stunkard and McLaren-Hume (1959) studied 100 obese people and found that 2 years after treatment, almost no one (2%) was able to maintain a weight

loss of 20 pounds or more. Stunkard (1958), in a lecture to the departments of internal medicine and pharmacology at Cornell Medical College, noted that "preoccupations with problems of overweight have long since passed beyond any reasonable
concern with health benefits to assume the proportions of a national neurosis." He
spoke of how inadequate treatment was for obesity and summarized as follows:
"Most obese persons will not stay in treatment for obesity. Of those who stay in
treatment, most will not lose weight, and of those who do lose weight, most will
regain it." Though Stunkard's conclusions were unusually pessimistic, most people appreciate that it is far easier to lose weight than to maintain any weight loss over time.

DIFFERENCES BETWEEN WEIGHT LOSS AND WEIGHT MAINTENANCE

- Weight maintenance is less reinforcing (less encouragement and reinforcement from others).

- The process of weight maintenance is indefinite rather than time limited.

- Weight maintenance may involve accepting shape and weight previously regarded as still unacceptable.

Source: Cooper and Fairburn 2002, p. 475

In a more recent prospec-
tive, population-based study of
nearly 1,000 individuals (332
women and 579 men) from Finland with an initial BMI value of
greater than 27 kg/m^2 (Sarlio-
Lähteenkorva et al. 2000), the
authors concluded that "long-term weight loss maintenance is rare." Only 5% of the
overweight women and 7% of the overweight men were able to maintain a 5% weight
loss during 9 years of follow-up. Their conclusions were that predictors of successful
weight loss maintenance were gender specific, namely that medical problems for
men and psychosocial problems for women were involved. Many people have the
prejudice that it is actually impossible to maintain successful weight loss, regardless
of the motivating factors. As one patient who had initially been very successful at
her weight loss said, "It was as if the original switch turned off" when she began to
gain her weight back (Sarlio-Lähteenkorva et al. 2000).

In the early 1990s a group of researchers from Pittsburgh and Colorado (Klem et
al. 1997), who acknowledged that "surprisingly little is known about such successful
losers," began to study a group of people who had lost a significant amount of weight
and kept it off for a period of 5 years. Rather than investigate why dieters fail, these
researchers wanted to investigate and determine what it takes for a person to succeed at weight loss without significant weight regain. The initial group, in what has
come to be called the National Weight Control Registry (2009; http://www.nwcr
.ws), consisted of 629 women and 155 men, who were all more than 18 years old,
had lost at least 30 pounds, and had maintained the weight loss for at least 1 year
for eligibility. All participants were volunteers and none was compensated for participation in the study. The group, though, was not random, but was self-selected
and had been recruited through local and national media advertising, mailings to
some commercial weight loss programs, and articles in newsletters that dealt with

health. Eligibility was based on self-reports of height, weight, and weight change, but the subjects in this study were requested to provide some sort of documentation to verify their claims of weight loss. Some people sent in before-and-after photos and also provided names of doctors or others who could substantiate their claims. Of those in this original study, 19% did not provide any documentation, but because they "did not differ significantly from others with respect to primary variables under investigation," they were still included (Klem et al. 1997).

In general, the subjects in this study were not typical of the U.S. population: 80% were women and 97% were white; more than half had a college or even graduate degree; 67% were married at the time of the study. The average age at the time of the study was around 45 years. Almost half described themselves as being overweight as children, that is, before the age of 11, and another 25% reported becoming overweight between the ages of 12 and 18. The average lifetime BMI was 35 kg/m^2 for women and 37 kg/m^2 for men. Forty-six percent of study participants described one biological parent as overweight and almost 27% reported that both biological parents were overweight.

Significantly, 77% of those in the study reported that some event triggered their successful weight loss: 32% had either a medical trigger, such as back pain or sleep apnea, or an emotional trigger (more common in women; e.g., the husband left); others described a lifestyle trigger, such as a special anniversary approaching. Over 11% of women and almost 5% of men described seeing themselves in a photograph or a mirror as having triggered this weight loss.

About 55% of the subjects reported using a formal program to lose the weight. Organizations such as Weight Watchers and Overeaters Anonymous, and even individual counseling sessions with a professional, such as a physician or nutritionist, were mentioned (see Chapter 11, "Psychological Treatment Strategies").

NATIONAL WEIGHT CONTROL REGISTRY

- Now over 6,000 in study; majority women; begun in 1993 by Hill and Wing

- Nonrandom group of successful dieters who lost about 30 pounds and kept weight off for at least a year (most, for 6 years)

- Many diverse ways to lose weight (using diet and exercise) but many commonalities in keeping weight off

- The longer one has maintained weight loss, the easier it is to keep weight off

- Vast majority in the study had tried unsuccessfully to lose weight previously

- Medical trigger for weight loss is associated with long-term success

Source: Butryn et al. 2007; Daeninck and Miller 2006; Hill et al. 2005; Klem et al. 1997; McGuire et al. 1999

Significantly, 89% used modifications in both physical activity and diet to achieve their weight loss. Diet modifications included limiting certain types of food and limiting quantities. About a third of the sample restricted their daily fat intake to 20% or less. Over 43% actually counted calories. The researchers reported that 20% used liquid formulas as part of their diet. In this original group, from the early 1990s, only 4.3% used medication and only 1.3% used surgery to achieve their weight loss (Klem et al. 1997).

The authors note that physical activity was an important strategy used for the initial weight loss. The overwhelming majority (92%) reported they exercised at home during their weight loss phase; women preferred walking or aerobic dancing whereas men engaged in competitive sports or weightlifting. Often exercise occurred with a friend or in groups.

Of these successful losers, 91% had tried to lose weight before, often repeatedly. In other words, they were what are called *weight cyclers* or *yo-yo dieters*. Why were they more successful this time? The subjects noted they were "more committed to making behavioral changes" this time, sometimes for both social and health reasons, and they overwhelmingly noted that they took a stricter approach to diet and exercised more this time to maintain their weight loss over time. In other words, motivation—or psychological determination—was an important component of their weight loss program.

There were many commonalities, even though there were several different approaches to losing the weight. Most subjects ate the majority of their meals at home, and they ate at least three times a day (the average was actually five times a day). They tended to avoid fast food restaurants, and they continued to be quite physically active. On average, they walked the equivalent of 28 miles a week, and expended at least 1,000 calories in exercise a week (e.g., walking, cycling, running, hiking), and often many more calories. They also recognized the importance of self-monitoring in that they continued to weigh themselves regularly. About 75% of the sample weighed themselves at least once a week and almost one-third weighed themselves daily. There was no difference between men and women in regard to weighing themselves (Gorin et al. 2004; Klem et al. 1997; Wyatt et al. 2002).

Notably, a more recent study (Butryn et al. 2007) reported that daily weighing is an important part of weight loss maintenance and has not been associated with any adverse psychological effects. Another study, by Tanaka et al. (2004), described the importance of charting daily weight fluctuations in predicting weight regain. Subjects were asked to weigh themselves four critical times a day (on awakening, after breakfast, after dinner, and before bedtime). Researchers felt the repeated weighing enabled the obese to be more aware of "harmful food and fluid intake habits" and was an effective tool in preventing weight regain. In this study, the best predictor of weight regain was weight fluctuation measured immediately before bedtime, often resulting from the habit of some obese individuals to eat after dinner. Levitsky and colleagues (2006) found that monitoring weight by daily weighing on a scale enabled

---

COMMONALITIES AMONG SUCCESSFUL DIETERS IN THE NATIONAL WEIGHT CONTROL REGISTRY

- Consume low-calorie, low-fat food

- Do physical exercise daily (about 1 hour a day), mostly walking: 1,000–2,000 cal/week

- Eat breakfast daily

- Maintain diet consistently on weekdays, weekends, and holidays

- Weigh self daily or at least weekly and continue to do so, even during maintenance

Source: Gorin et al. 2004; Klem et al. 1997; Wyatt et al. 2002

---

a group of female freshman from Cornell University to avoid the "freshman fifteen" pounds of weight gain typically seen. The untreated control group, by the end of just one semester, had gained almost seven pounds (3.1 kg), whereas the group that weighed itself daily gained a negligible amount of weight that first semester of college.

In general, over 85% of the successful dieters in the National Weight Control Registry described their quality of life, including physical health, well-being, and self-confidence, as improved by their weight loss, though the study did note that 20% of the subjects reported spending more time thinking about weight and 15% spent more time thinking about food than they did before the weight loss. Maintaining one's weight loss for 2–5 years decreased the risk of subsequent weight gain by more than 50%.

Researchers have followed subjects in the National Weight Control Registry since the early 1990s, and the number of participants has grown considerably over time. One of the concerns of the researchers was to identify predictors of weight gain versus continued weight maintenance in those who were successful at initial weight loss. McGuire et al. (1999) noted that the average member of their group had lost over 65 pounds, with the average BMI decreasing from 35 to 25 kg/m^2, and had maintained the loss for more than 5 years. They were interested in investigating whether characteristics at study entry would predict weight gain over the subsequent year and "whether changes in behavior or psychological characteristics" would be seen in those who regained weight.

In McGuire et al. (1999), more than 700 individuals were assessed at 1-year follow-up and about one-third had gained more than 5 pounds since the initial assessment. The average weight gain among all gainers was over 15 pounds, with about 44% of them reporting a series of gains and losses over the year and slightly fewer than half reporting a steady gain over the year. Individuals who gained weight over the year were more likely to have had more episodes of weight cycling prior to entering the study, were more likely to have sought assistance (rather than losing weight on their own) for their initial weight loss, and were more likely to have used a liquid formula initially. Gainers were more likely to have been heavier at the beginning, more likely to have lost more weight initially (particularly if they had lost $\geq$ 30% of their initial weight), and more likely to have lost the weight for a shorter period of time. They were also more likely to have reported wishing to continue to lose weight than maintain their weight. There were no differences in behavioral characteristics initially in those who maintained their weight versus those who gained: all reported eating less than 1,500 calories per day (though the maintainers reported eating less protein) and all reported expending more than 2,500 calories per week in physical exercise.

RISK FACTORS FOR REGAINING WEIGHT

- More recent weight loss (<2 years)

- Larger weight loss (>30% of maximum weight)

- Higher levels of depression reported initially

- Binge eating initially and higher levels of dietary disinhibition initially

- Eating more fat

- Decline in self-monitoring over first year

- Expressing a wish to continue to lose weight (rather than maintain) initially

- Marked decrease in physical exercise over time

Source: McGuire et al. 1999

In terms of psychological characteristics initially, those who had gained weight at 1 year were more likely to have been binge eaters with higher levels of dietary disinhibition—"suggesting that subsequent gainers were already experiencing difficulty controlling dietary intake" even on entry—and were more likely to have depressive symptoms. In other words, higher depression and disinhibition scores "may be a consequence, not a cause, of their weight regain" (McGuire et al. 1999).

One of the major changes over the year, though, was that gainers were much less likely to continue their self-monitoring and were more likely to increase their intake of fat. They were also less likely to continue to exercise as much as before. They were more likely, too, to have higher levels of depression than maintainers. The study did suggest that those who had maintained their weight loss for 2–5 years decreased their risk of subsequent weight regain by more than 50%. The researchers concluded that though there may be physiological and metabolic factors involved in weight control, their data suggest that "a large part of regain may be due to inability to maintain healthy eating and exercise habits long term" (McGuire et al. 1999).

Jeffery et al. (2000) make the point that weight loss attempts are often "behavior changes of short duration." They note that weight regain occurs when there is a "deterioration in adherence" to behavioral changes. There seems to be a "natural history" to weight loss, with the maximum loss occurring around 6 months after beginning treatment. They note that weight regain begins and continues gradually until weight stabilizes at somewhat below baseline levels, and this particular temporal pattern is independent of the initial weight loss. The only difference is that large weight losers have a faster rate of initial weight loss rather than a difference in the duration of their weight loss efforts. They say biologically oriented scientists interpret the difficulty in weight maintenance as evidence of biological determinants of body weight, whereas behaviorally oriented scientists "view the same phenomena as evidence underscoring the difficulty of achieving lasting change in environmental factors that influence behaviors" (Jeffrey et al. 2000).

Over the years, the National Weight Control Registry has increased to over 6,000 self-selected participants (Daeninck and Miller 2006; Hill 2006; Phelan et al. 2006). As the study population has increased, it has become the largest ongoing study of those successful at weight loss maintenance. The focus has continued to be on examining behaviors common

SOME FACTS ABOUT WEIGHT LOSS

- Initial weight loss of 1–2 pounds a week over 6 months is the recommendation of most obesity specialists.

- The faster the weight loss, the more likely it will lead to fast weight regain.

- Losses of 5%–10% can lead to significant health benefits.

Source: Aronne 2002, p. 387

to those who are successful. Another important behavior, besides self-monitoring of weight and food intake and high levels of exercise, is eating breakfast regularly. In a study by Wyatt et al. (2002) of 2,959 Registry participants who maintained their weight loss over time, almost 90% reported eating breakfast (usually cereal and fruit) on most days of the week. Fewer than 5% reported never eating breakfast. The researchers speculated that eating breakfast may reduce hunger and overeating later in the day and may enable those who do so to have more energy for physical activity, though it may also just be a "marker for a low-calorie, low-fat eating style." Other studies (Masheb and Grilo 2006; Sitzman 2006) have also confirmed the importance of eating breakfast for weight maintenance in most people.

Another factor that seems to work in long-term control of weight is diet consistency. Gorin et al. (2004) reported that dieters who followed a similar behavioral strategy on weekends as on weekdays were more likely to maintain their weight than those who were less strict on certain days than others. Phelan et al. (2006) note that it is particularly difficult for those with a weight problem to maintain their weight strategies during the holiday season. They studied a group in the National Weight Control Registry and compared them to a group of individuals without any weight problem and found the Registry participants more vulnerable to weight gain during holidays than those without a weight problem, even though they worked harder to maintain their weight.

Yanovski et al. (2000), in a study using a population of National Institutes of Health employees, sought to estimate how much the average American actually does gain around the holiday season. Yanovski's group sampled 195 adults (51% women), with a median BMI value of 24.8 kg/m² (similar to the average U.S. BMI of 25.5 kg/m²), at four different times before and after the holiday season (September through January). They found that the average weight gain is not 5 pounds, as is commonly asserted. Instead, the subjects on average gained a little over 1 pound. What makes that weight gain more significant than it sounds, though, is that the subjects did not lose this weight after the holiday season, that is, during the spring and summer months. Potentially, then, year after year, this holiday weight accumulates. Further, the researchers found that those with a weight problem (i.e., already overweight or obese) were more likely to gain the 5 pounds typically attributed to the holiday. Wing and Phelan (2005) describe the importance of what they call *cognitive restraint*, namely "the degree of conscious control exerted over eating behaviors."

People who continue to maintain their weight loss do not change their behavior once they have lost the weight. Wing and Phelan (2005) have noted that the single best predictor of the risk of regaining weight was how long those in the study had maintained their weight loss. If they could maintain their weight loss for 2 years, they markedly increased their odds (by almost 50%) of keeping off the weight in the future. Those who regained the most weight at 1 year were least likely to recover from their relapse. These researchers caution that preventing small regains is crucial to maintaining weight loss over time. Though weight maintenance does become easier for most individuals over time, all researchers stress that weight difficulties are a chronic disorder and at present are not curable.

Finally, another study from the researchers in the National Weight Control Registry looked at changes in their participants' diet over time (Phelan et al. 2006). They found that diets did shift somewhat, but even with fads in diets, only a small minority consumed a low-carbohydrate diet. Mostly, their subjects continued to monitor their fat intake (although fat intake over time, from 1997 to 2003, increased from <25% to almost 30% of the diet) and limit fast food consumption. Although calorie intake remained stable over time, subjects reported decreasing their carbohydrate intake and increasing their fat intake. The researchers concluded that weight control "may be possible within a range of macronutrient composition," though all ate far less fat than recommended fat levels (Phelan et al. 2006).

THE MEDICAL CONSEQUENCES OF OBESITY

Having excess fat on one's body, particularly viscerally (i.e., abdominally or centrally), whether just being overweight or actually being obese, is associated with considerably higher risk for many diseases (i.e., for increased morbidity). Excess weight can affect every organ of the body. Diabetes, heart disease, gallbladder disease, gout, chronic kidney disease, osteoarthritis, many cancers, polycystic ovary disease, and sleep apnea, among others, have all been associated with obesity. In an editorial in the *New England Journal of Medicine*, Preston (2005) provocatively used the title "Deadweight? The Influence of Obesity on Longevity." Does obesity lead to a shortened life? Many studies over time have found a consistent relationship between increasing BMI values and mortality rates. Back in 1999, Allison and colleagues estimated that approximately 325,000 deaths in the United States per year were due to obesity. A study by Calle and colleagues (2005) with 20 years of follow-up found a persistent relationship between increased weight and mortality at all of the various points of measurement. After reviewing and summarizing many studies, Hu (2008, p. 224) made the strong statement that cumulative evidence supports the notion that obesity and mortality are linked and the strength of the association has not decreased over time, as some researchers have claimed.

More recently, Zhang and colleagues (2008) followed more than 44,000 women in the Nurses' Health Study for 16 years and found that abdominal obesity, as measured by waist circumference (measured at the umbilicus) and waist-to-hip ratio, is particularly detrimental. It is strongly and positively associated with mortality from any cause, including cancer and cardiovascular disease, and this is independent of the women's BMI values. What is important about this study is that it took into account a history of smoking, which many studies fail to do. In epidemiology research on weight, smoking is considered a strong negative confounder, that is, it tends to distort the connection between an exposure and obesity: in this case, primarily because smokers tend to be thinner in general, there may be an underestimation of the connection between obesity and mortality (Hu 2008, pp. 39–40).

Zhang et al. (2008) also found that even among normal-weight women, an elevated waist circumference and an elevated waist-to-hip ratio were associated with significantly increased cardiovascular disease mortality, as well as abnormal metabolic values such as higher total cholesterol levels, low-density lipoprotein cholesterol levels, triglyceride levels, and fasting blood glucose levels, and even higher systolic and diastolic blood pressure values. They also found that given a certain waist circumference, a greater hip circumference may even be associated with lower cardiovascular mortality, possibly because fat accumulation in the femoral and gluteal regions of the body may act as a "sink" for circulating free fatty acids and may prevent them from accumulating in tissue or around organs such as the liver or pancreas, or in skeletal muscle.

Can physical activity mitigate the effects of obesity? According to a study of women by Hu and his colleagues (2004), physically active women have lower mortality rates than those who are not active, but physical activity did not completely mitigate the mortality risk of having excess fat. Women who were lean and active had the lowest mortality rates. The authors' conclusion is that even among those who are physically active, gaining weight as an adult has its consequences. Hu (2008, p. 231) speaks of the particularly important *adiposity triad*, that is, BMI value, waist circumference, and weight gain during adulthood.

There has been controversy (Sui et al. 2007) about whether overweight is always associated with increased mortality, though. Some studies have suggested that either low *or* high BMI values are associated with increased mortality (the U-shaped curve). Romero-Corral et al. (2006) note how contradictory studies are in regard to the relation of obesity to mortality. In their meta-analysis review of over 250,000 patients from 40 studies, they concluded that BMI values might not be discriminating enough as a measure of body fat versus lean mass. They noted, as well, that when studies showed that a low BMI was associated with increased mortality, subjects tended to be older and chronic smokers. (A study by Grabowski and Ellis [2001], for example, concluded that a high BMI did not predict mortality, but they did not control for smoking.) Romero-Corral et al. (2006) did note that severely obese patients had a significant 88% increased risk for cardiovascular mortality. They concluded that the inability of BMI to discriminate between "excess of body fat and increments in lean mass" might explain the conflicting better outcomes in regard to mortality in some overweight and mildly obese patients.

Hu (2008, p. 216 et seq) summarizes all the methodological difficulties in evaluating studies regarding obesity and mortality. For example, reverse causation—that is, when a low BMI value is the result of an underlying illness rather than the cause of disease, such as diseases that cause wasting (e.g., chronic pulmonary disease, heart disease, smoking, or even psychological depression)—may complicate results. Hu makes the point that some of these chronic conditions may remain undiagnosed and hence unknown to the subjects and researchers at the time of the study (and for years after). He also notes, as have others, that precise measurements are often lacking, that studies that rely on self-reports can be notoriously inaccurate in that men exaggerate their height and women underreport their weight, and some studies do not even differentiate intentional weight loss from unintentional (i.e., disease-related) loss. Hu is confident that a review of studies supports the hypothesis that obesity can lead to increased mortality and there is "no evidence that the relative impact of obesity on mortality has decreased over time" (Hu 2008, p. 224) as some studies have maintained. He does acknowledge, though, that the evidence is less clear-cut with overweight than with obesity.

The most recent analysis of the relationship of obesity to BMI values to date (Prospective Studies Collaboration 2009) examined data from 57 studies (involving almost 900,000 people, 61% male). The researchers actually excluded the first 5 years of data results in order to attempt to limit reverse causation and still had 8 more years of follow-up data. They found, as Hu (2008) has suggested, that BMI is a strong predictor of overall mortality. For people with BMI values greater than 25 kg/m^2, death was usually due to vascular disease. When mortality was linked to lower BMI values, it was due to diseases related to smoking. They found that a person's survival is shortened by 2–4 years when the BMI is between 30 and 35 kg/m^2, and if it is between 40 and 45 kg/m^2, life can be shortened by 8–10 years!

Some researchers believe "cardiovascular fitness at any size" or the so-called *fitness-versus-fatness hypothesis* (Fontaine and Allison 2004, p. 770) may be more important than BMI values. Sui and colleagues (2007) studied more than 2,600 adults who were age 60 and older (though fewer than 20% were women) over a 12-year follow-up period. They assessed fitness by treadmill tests and measured BMI, waist circumference, and body fat percentage. Their conclusion was that cardiopulmonary fitness "predicted mortality risk, independent of overall or even abdominal obesity" (Sui et al. 2007). Those with higher levels of fitness, though, were less likely to have diabetes, hypertension, and high cholesterol levels. Those in their study (primarily white, well educated, and middle to upper middle class) who were obese—with BMI values of 30–34.9 kg/m^2, abdominal obesity, or excessive body fat percentage—but were fit, had a lower risk of all-cause mortality than normal-weight subjects who were unfit. How generalizable their findings are to the general population, however, remains to be seen. A study in women by Hu et al. (2004), for example, noted that women who were physically active and lean had the lowest mortality risk, but that "being physically active did not mitigate the mortality risk associated with body fatness." In general, though, it does seem to hold for obesity that the greater the BMI value (particularly values > 35 kg/m^2), the greater the risk is not only for certain diseases but also for a much higher mortality rate.

Other complications include that the BMI-mortality relationship is affected by age, race, and other variables. Fontaine and Allison (2004, p. 779) cautioned that it seems inadvisable to generalize from one study population, such as middle-aged white females, to other populations, and that "one should refrain from making broad statements." And Flegal et al. (2007), in revisiting data from an earlier study that found excess overall mortality associated with those underweight and obese but not just overweight, clarified that the association of BMI with mortality "varies considerably by cause of death."

Cardiovascular disease, including coronary artery disease, stroke, congestive heart failure, and hypertension, accounts for almost half (45.2%) of all deaths in the United States (Field et al. 2002, p. 7). As such, it is our leading cause of death. According to Hu (2008, p. 174), the relationship between excess fat and cardiovascular disease may be mediated through processes involving inflammation and platelet functioning, as well as those involving the endothelium, the cellular semipermeable barrier between human tissues and blood.

It is not just in the United States, though, that researchers have noted the connection between excess fat (adiposity) and disease. Hu (2008, pp. 174–177) reports there have been three meta-analyses, involving 92 prospective studies including over a million people worldwide, that have demonstrated a linear association between coronary artery disease and BMI, with increased mortality. Hu (2008, p. 177) makes the point that often the association of overweight and obesity with an increased risk of coronary artery disease is even stronger when the studies restrict themselves to those who have never smoked and when the studies have considerably longer follow-up. Because older people tend to lose muscle mass and accumulate fat abdominally, as we have noted above, some researchers believe that waist circumference or even the waist-to-hip ratio is more important than BMI for assessing coronary heart disease risk in older individuals. In other words, fat distribution, says Hu (2008, p. 179), is more important than overall fatness. Apparently Jean Vague's (1956) observations went unnoticed until the 1980s, when large Scandinavian studies confirmed that central body obesity (a high waist-to-hip ratio) is, in fact, correlated with cardiovascular disease and an increased risk of early mortality (Landsberg 2008).

Weight gain over time during adulthood seems also to be associated with coronary artery disease, and this is independent of BMI values. The adiposity triad (Hu 2008, p. 191) of increasing weight since early adulthood (since the age of 18), body fat distribution abdominally (i.e., waist circumference), and increased BMI should alert physicians to the possibility of a higher increase in coronary heart disease risk. Sometimes, though, because of decreasing muscle mass, weight may remain stable but a person may be still accumulating more fat and carry a greater risk of cardiovascular disease.

There is also convincing evidence, according to Hu (2008, p. 190), that increasing BMI values are associated with ischemic strokes, though not necessarily with hemorrhagic strokes, in both Asian and Western populations. For congestive heart failure, Hu (2008, p. 188) notes that waist circumference, that is, a measure of abdominal obesity, is the single most important predictor. Even cardiac arrhythmias, such as atrial fibrillation, are associated with obesity.

Obesity is also clearly associated with hypertension, and those with a higher BMI are at higher risk for developing it. The famous Framingham heart studies, with 38 years of follow-up (Moore et al. 2005), have shown that even modest weight loss

WHAT IS THE METABOLIC SYNDROME?

- Also called *syndrome X*

- It is a cluster of metabolic risk factors: obesity (especially abdominal), abnormal glucose regulation, abnormal lipid profile, high blood pressure
  - Abdominal obesity defined as a waist circumference > 40 inches in men and > 35 inches in women
  - High fasting blood glucose defined as ≥ 110 mg/dL
  - Increased triglycerides defined as > 150 mg/dL
  - High blood pressure defined as > 130/85 mm Hg

- It is estimated that 25% of U.S. adults have the metabolic syndrome

- It is associated with type 2 (but not type 1) diabetes, obstructive sleep apnea, chronic kidney disease, and polycystic ovary syndrome

- Patients with the metabolic syndrome are at markedly increased risk for coronary artery disease and diabetes

Source: Darsow et al. 2006; Ford et al. 2002; Sarafidis and Nilsson 2006

sustained over time lowers a person's risk for developing hypertension by almost 25%. One mechanism that may be involved in the connection between obesity and hypertension, we now know, is that fat cells (adipocytes) far from being inert, actually secrete, among many other cytokines, a precursor of angiotensin II, which is involved in the regulation of blood pressure.

Neter and her colleagues (2003) performed a meta-analysis of 25 randomized, controlled studies (from 1966 to 2002) involving almost 5,000 patients and concluded that there was "unequivocal evidence" that weight loss is an important component for the prevention and treatment of hypertension; significantly larger blood pressure reductions occurred in those subjects who had lost more than 10 pounds (>5 kilograms) than in patients who had lost less weight. Although a study by Aucott et al. (2005) did not find as significant an effect of weight loss on blood pressure, the investigators noted that factors such as a patient's initial blood pressure, the length of follow-up, and medication changes may have complicated the results. They also noted, incidentally, that bariatric surgery for the treatment of obesity, resulting in considerable weight loss, produced "undramatic blood pressure changes," even though a patient's metabolic profile may be considerably improved. They concluded that the "weight/hypertension relationship is complex."

The Metabolic Syndrome

Obesity has been associated with many metabolic disturbances. Though metabolic abnormalities associated with obesity were first noted many years earlier, it was in the late 1980s that a syndrome, called *syndrome X*, was described by Reaven (1988). It consisted of obesity, increased insulin secretion, glucose intolerance, and an abnormal blood lipid profile. Sarafidis and Nilsson (2006) note that Reaven apparently called it syndrome X in "an attempt to stress its unknown aspects." Since then, others have noted a cluster of abnormalities: specifically, abdominal (upper body) obesity, glucose intolerance, and even hypertension.

It was in 1998 that the World Health Organization began to use the term *metabolic syndrome*, which it defined as insulin resistance and/or impaired glucose regulation (i.e., type 2 diabetes) with at least two other symptoms, including hypertension, abnormal lipid levels (e.g., high triglyceride levels or low high-density lipoprotein [HDL] levels, the "heart healthy" kind), obesity, and protein in the urine (microalbuminuria). (In type 1 diabetes, which is not associated with the metabolic syndrome, the pancreas does not produce any insulin, whereas in type 2 diabetes, insulin is produced in excess, but the body is resistant to it.) Over the years, several other groups, including the International Diabetes Federation, have described certain metabolic disturbances seen in obese individuals that do not seem to occur randomly but rather seem to indicate some underlying pathological process, though researchers do not all agree on what constitutes the metabolic syndrome.

It is estimated that about one-quarter of adults in the United States have this syndrome (Ford et al. 2002). Criteria in Ford and colleagues' study included three or more of the following: abdominal obesity, with a waist circumference greater than 102 centimeters or 40 inches for men and greater than 88 centimeters or 35 inches for women (note that abdominal obesity is also defined as a waist-to-hip ratio of ≥ 0.95 for men and ≥ 0.85 for women [Kaplan 2008]); high trigylceride levels (> 150 mg/dL); low HDL levels (< 40 mg/dL in men and < 50 mg/dL in women); hypertension ($\geq 130/88$ mm Hg); and high fasting blood glucose levels (≥ 110 mg/dL). Worldwide, Grundy (2008) notes that between 20% and 30% of the adult population have the syndrome.

Janssen et al. (2008) found in their study that almost 14% of 949 women in the transition to menopause, as testosterone levels become higher relative to estrogen levels, developed the metabolic syndrome. This syndrome has also been called the *inflammatory syndrome* by Wisse (2004) because chronic inflammation, caused by cytokines secreted by excessive fat tissue, may be involved. Incidentally, microalbuminuria is a marker of enthothelial dysfunction (Hu 2008, p. 154). Hu (2008, p. 153) makes the point that insulin resistance, that is, reduced glucose uptake in the presence of insulin in tissues such as muscle or the liver that are sensitive to insulin, is the "defining pathophysiological defect" for the metabolic syndrome. With insulin resistance, blood glucose levels rise, which then triggers a release of insulin from the beta cells of the pancreas. Initially this mechanism works and blood glucose levels return to normal, but hyperinsulinemia (higher insulin levels) occurs. Eventually, though, this compensatory mechanism fails as the beta cell reserves are depleted, and overt type 2 diabetes develops. Ironically, though, insulin resistance preserves muscle function in times of starvation and thus provides a "survival advantage," according to Landsberg (2008): during starvation, glucose (the only fuel the brain can use) comes entirely from the breakdown of muscle protein (gluconeogenesis), whereas skeletal muscle can use the breakdown products from fat. Roth (2009) has even proposed that the metabolic and inflammatory disorders associated with obesity may have evolved advantageously over the centuries to offer certain protection against the ravages of tuberculosis, a disease historically responsible for more than 1 billion fatalities. Classically, tuberculosis, which still occurs at a rate of about 9 million new cases a year worldwide, has been associated with malnutrition, and Roth notes there is some suggestion that obesity may offer a decreased risk.

Björntorp (2004, p. 804) believes that the metabolic syndrome should be renamed because it is much more than a cluster of metabolic abnormalities (e.g., visceral obesity and hypertension). As a result, he feels it should be called the *central arousal syndrome* and that "disruptions of homeostasis in several neuroendocrine and autonomic pathways" may be involved (p. 805). He does acknowledge that given that many of the symptoms characteristic of the metabolic syndrome may disappear with weight loss, "obesity is probably the primary factor and the neuroendocrine and autonomic phenomena secondary" (p. 805).

Though the diagnostic criteria for the metabolic syndrome do vary, most researchers are in agreement that this cluster of symptoms strongly signifies the possibility of future cardiac disease. Darsow et al. (2006) do note other areas of disagreement among researchers and clinicians that include ambiguous diagnostic criteria, such as whether elevated diastolic and systolic blood pressure are both significant; whether to include risk factors like C-reactive protein (a nonspecific marker for disease) or microalbuminuria; and even how heavily to weigh the significance of certain criteria such as glucose intolerance.

A new study (Stefan et al. 2008), though, notes there is a subset of obese people who have what the researchers call "metabolically benign obesity;" that is, this subset did not have insulin resistance or early evidence of atherosclerosis. The researchers measured total body, visceral, and subcutaneous fat, as well as the thickness of the common carotid artery, and found that ectopic fat in the liver may be more problematic than visceral fat in some obese people. Along those lines, Wildman et al. (2008) reviewed data on over 5,000 participants in the National Health and Nutrition Examination Surveys from 1999 through 2004 and found that among U.S. adults, 24% of normal-weight adults over age 20 had metabolically abnormal profiles whereas 51% of overweight and 32% of obese adults had metabolically healthy profiles.

Clearly we are dealing with puzzling data—such as higher total cholesterol, low-density cholesterol, and triglyceride levels, higher blood pressures (both systolic and diastolic), and higher fasting blood glucose levels—that just confirm how complicated, even in normal-weight adults, metabolic abnormalities are. Seidell et al. (2001) also confirmed, in their study of over 700 men and women, that a narrow waist and large hips may actually protect against cardiovascular disease. The researchers concluded that variations in waist circumference reflect subcutaneous and visceral fat accumulation, whereas hip circumference may also reflect pelvic bone structure and gluteal muscle as well as subcutaneous gluteal fat.

Cancer

Obesity has also been associated with many cancers, such as endometrial, postmenopausal breast, kidney, esophagus, gallbladder, and colon cancers. It is not known why certain cancers are seen more frequently in those with excessive weight, but theories include increased production of, or stimulation by, hormones (e.g., estrogen, insulin, cortisol, leptin) by fat or other cells. Calle et al. (2003) noted that between 15% and 20% of all cancer deaths in the United States can be attributed to overweight and obesity. Their study included U.S. men and women from the more than one million participants (from all states) in the prospective mortality study begun in the 1980s by the American Cancer Society. From that group, this study had more than 400,000 men and almost 500,000 women (average age at time of the study, 57 years), participating with 16 years of follow-up. This study also separated out those who were smokers (there were about 375,000 nonsmokers) because smoking can obviously confound the results of obesity by decreasing body mass and increasing the risk of death. By the end of the follow-up period, there were 57,000 deaths from cancer in those who had not been diagnosed with cancer at the beginning. What Calle and her group found was that individuals with a BMI value of 40 or more had death rates from all cancers that were 52% higher in men and 62% higher in women than in those with normal weights, and these data were consistent with data from previous studies, but the magnitude of the effect was larger. They concluded that the proportion of all deaths from cancer that is attributable to overweight and obesity in U.S. adults 50 years of age or older may be "as high as 14% for men and 20% for women" (Calle et al. 2003). This translates into more than 90,000 avoidable deaths each year "if everyone in the adult population could maintain a BMI under 25 kg/m^2 throughout life" (Calle et al 2003).

Calle (2008, p. 203) emphasizes that obesity, particularly in heavier women, may also delay a cancer diagnosis. She notes there are "substantial data to suggest" that those women who are heavier may be more likely to have a more aggressive tumor, a larger tumor, and lymph node involvement by the time of diagnosis. They are also less likely to receive mammogram screenings. She further notes (p. 206) that adult weight gain, even more than BMI, is a strong predictor of postmenopausal breast cancer: "the women at greatest lifetime risk of breast cancer are those who are lean in the premenopausal period and become heavier in the postmenopausal period."

Other Medical Consequences of Obesity

Obesity has been associated with changes in the liver (fatty infiltration, inflammation, and fibrosis). Fan et al. (2005) reported that in their sample of over 3,100 people (about 22% of whom had the metabolic syndrome), those with the syndrome had a 40-fold greater chance of developing a fatty liver than those without the syndrome. Gallstone development in the gallbladder is also more common in heavier individuals. Manson et al. (2004), p. 819) noted that those with a BMI value of greater than 40 have a four- to fivefold higher prevalence of developing gallstones. Gallstone development is also particularly common among those with the metabolic syndrome. Hu (2008, p. 161) makes the point, as well, that rapid weight loss by liquid, very-low-calorie diets can also predispose some to the development of gallstones, as can weight cycling or the intentional loss of weight with regain (yo-yo dieting; see next section).

Osteoarthritis develops more commonly in those with excessive body weight. It makes sense that the heavier one is, the more wear and tear there is on the joints, particularly the weight-bearing ones. Manson et al. (2004, p. 819) report on results from the Framingham Heart Study that indicated obese women were twice as likely and obese men 1.5 times as likely to develop osteoarthritis as leaner people. And there is evidence that sometimes weight loss alone may alleviate some of the symptoms of the disease (Manson et al. 2004, p. 819).

Sleep apnea, the lack of air flow for 10 or more seconds during sleep, is also seen much more commonly in heavier individuals. And again, evidence indicates that weight loss alone is sometimes enough to alleviate or at least lessen these episodes. Even changes in brain structure may be seen in those who are overweight or obese. Gustafson et al. (2004) conducted a follow-up study in Sweden over 24 years (at various points), beginning in 1968 to assess the longitudinal relationship of body mass index to changes in brain tissue, as measured on CT scan. In their study of 275 elderly women born between 1908 and 1922, they found that a higher body mass index throughout life was associated with greater atrophy in the temporal lobes (but not other lobes) of the brain. The researchers acknowledge that they could not make causal inferences about the relationship between BMI and the atrophy found, but they note from their other studies that being overweight has been associated with Alzheimer's disease.

Reproductive health can also be compromised by excessive weight. Manson et al. (2004, p. 820) note that excessive weight may interfere with a woman's ability to conceive and, if she does become pregnant, may be responsible for a tenfold increase in hypertension during pregnancy as well as a threefold increase in gestational diabetes. Obesity also makes delivery more difficult: there can be more preterm deliveries, more cesarean section deliveries (babies are often heavier), and a greater possibility of anesthesia-related complications (see Chapter 7, "Medical Conditions and Weight").

Weight Cycling (Yo-Yo Dieting)

We do know that even a weight loss of only 5%–10% of body weight has been associated not only with considerable improvement in cardiovascular disease, diabetes, hypertension, and hyperlipidemia, but also with preventing the development of type 2 diabetes and hypertension in predisposed overweight individuals (Vidal 2002). Unfortunately, though, statistics on maintaining that weight loss over time can be dismal. Vidal (2002), for example, reports on one study of over 1,100 patients with hypertension in which only 13% maintained a weight loss goal of around 10 pounds 3 years later.

Weight cycling (yo-yo dieting) has its own medical consequences. Most people who have tried to lose weight, including even those who have been successful, such as those in the National Weight Control Registry, have tried previously (often repeatedly) and found themselves gaining weight (i.e., relapsing) again over time. As noted earlier, this pattern of weight loss and weight regain has been called weight cycling or yo-yo dieting. It is not known who first used the term *yo-yo dieting*, but it has been in the literature for years and aptly describes a particular, often disturbing, sequence. Weight cycling can occur in either sex and can occur both in those who are overweight and in those who are not. Weight cycling can also be part of one's profession, and as such can be an intentional pattern, as with professional wrestlers, boxers, or ballet dancers. It can also be considered a normal pattern in pregnancy, where weight is gained during the pregnancy and then lost in the postpregnancy phase. For purposes here, we are talking of intentional weight loss with subsequent regain, rather than an unintentional (e.g., related to a wasting disease or famine) cycle. Most commonly, though, it occurs—discouragingly, and seemingly out of control—in overweight people who struggle with their weight. For years, researchers have been trying to assess both the medical and psychological ramifications of a pattern of repeated weight loss and unintentional regain. Brownell and Rodin (1994) reviewed the early literature and found inconsistent results, sometimes because studies used different definitions for weight cycling. Weight cycling is particularly difficult to study because of the lack of a consistent definition for what constitutes weight cycling, namely how much weight is involved, over what time period it occurs, and how often it occurs in a person's life.

Both animal and human studies have sometimes (i.e., data are not consistent) found that subjects lose less weight (or lose weight more slowly) on a second or later trial. The data, of course, have serious consequences in that clinicians are constantly suggesting that their overweight and obese patients lose weight but wonder whether the failed attempts do more harm over time than good. Brownell and Rodin (1994) noted, for example, such as in the Framingham study where weight is measured every 2 years, that "weight variability is not identical to a measure of repeated cycles of weight loss and regain," so that total fluctuations within the 2-year period are not recorded. Brownell and Rodin (1994) also suggest that weight cycling may affect particular individuals, under particular circumstances, more than others, and there may be "periods of vulnerability" for a person. They caution that sometimes studies have not collected data specifically to study weight cycling. They recommend that future studies clarify why weight has changed, and they note that there is no uniformity in the data collection, such that different methods may be sensitive to different measurements (e.g., number of times for weight cycling vs. magnitude of a particular weight cycle).

Many of these studies are particularly prone to the methodological problems we have mentioned. For example, some large and even long-term studies (e.g., Søgaard et al. 2008) do not even differentiate between intentional and unintentional weight loss (i.e., do not ask participants about the nature of the weight cycling) or do not exclude smokers. Many others rely not only on self-reports, but on self-reports years after the fact, so data collection is subject to the inevitable memory distortions of older participants. Gorber et al. from Canada (2007), for example, reviewed 64 full-text articles of studies in both men and women and concluded that "the trend in studies where data were available was for height to be overestimated and weight and BMI to be underestimated."

Gorber et al. (2007) also note that studies often do not report the amount of time that elapsed between self-reports and direct measures, nor do most describe aspects such as who was conducting the measuring, what clothing was worn, whether the weight was a fasting one or after a meal, or at what time of day measurements were taken.

With these caveats in mind, clinicians must take the studies as provisional, without definite recommendations. All in all, it does seem prudent to recommend weight loss, even though weight may be regained. A study by Prentice et al. (1992) also refutes the notion that weight cycling is detrimental, at least in terms of body mass composition (though it may not be "an entirely benign phenomenon"). These authors argue that weight cycling would have been common in primitive humans in times of famine and plenty and our bodies have evolved to cope with these "periods of fluctuating energy balance and hence weight cycling." Their view is that adipose tissue, although important in thermal insulation and fertility, is most significantly an "energy buffer" closely related to survival during severe food shortages.

The National Task Force on the Prevention and Treatment of Obesity (1994) concluded that the currently available evidence is not compelling enough to dissuade people from losing weight and it should not "allow concerns about the hazards of weight cycling to deter the obese from losing weight." The study stressed the importance of lifelong changes in behavioral patterns, diet, and exercise, in order to attempt to prevent regaining weight. Now, some 15 years later, the data are still confusing and inconsistent.

Both Wing (1992) and Roybal (2005), in reviewing the literature, concluded that weight cycling has not had consistent effects on metabolic variables, such as metabolic rate, changes in body fat distribution, or even differences in weight loss patterns over time (i.e., ease or difficulty of weight loss in the second or third cycle). Nor has weight cycling seemed to affect blood pressure, cardiac function, lipid profiles, or even mortality consistently (especially when taking into account intentional vs. unintentional weight loss and cigarette smoking). For example, a study by Holme et al. (2007) in Norway, with 28 years of follow-up, did report that the risk of the metabolic syndrome and diabetes increased with increasing numbers of weight loss episodes after age 50 in a group of over 6,300 elderly men. This study, though, had several possible and typical methodological biases: the researchers did not specifically ask the men whether their weight loss was intentional or unintentional, and they were dealing with men ages 68–78 who were asked retrospectively to remember episodes of weight loss many years earlier. Their conclusion was that it may be the number of weight cycling episodes rather than the amount of weight lost that is most harmful.

Another study, by Li et al. (2007), studied 480 patients who repeatedly (some more than four times) entered a weight reduction program that offered severe calorie restriction (700–800 calories a day) for a period of several weeks. These researchers did not find that cardiovascular risk factors, such as blood pressure or lipid profiles (cholesterol or triglyceride levels), were adversely affected by repeat cycles. They also noted that the rate of weight loss in response to calorie restriction did not lessen over the repeated weight loss episodes. They concluded that weight cycling did not result in any long-term metabolic adaptations that would make successive attempts at weight loss more difficult. Nor did it change metabolic rate or lean body mass. And they noted that most of their patients maintained some of the weight they had initially lost in between their dieting periods. In their study, a maintenance of only 8.5 kilograms of weight loss resulted in improved cardiovascular risk factors like blood pressure and lipid profiles. Their conclusion was that all those who have tried to lose weight and regained their weight should be encouraged to try again.

In a large study in Germany, Kroke et al. (2002) followed over 18,000 men and women (almost twice as many women as men), nonsmokers, for 2 years. The researchers noted that weight cycling, which they defined as an unintentional weight gain and intentional weight loss of more than 5 kilograms during the 2-year period prior to the beginning of the study, was the best predictor of weight gain over time for men; for women, a prior weight loss was the strongest predictor of a subsequent large weight gain. The researchers stressed the importance of a thorough weight assessment history to identify those most likely to gain weight over time.

A cross-sectional study of almost 500 women (Olson et al. 2000) enrolled in the Women's Ischemia Syndrome Evaluation—a multicenter study to evaluate women suspected of having myocardial ischemia, sponsored by the National Heart, Lung, and Blood Institute—noted that 27% of the women reported some degree of weight cycling, from 10 pounds to as much as 50 pounds in 2% of them. In these cyclers (defined as having had a voluntary weight loss of ≥ 10 pounds at least three times, not including weight loss following pregnancy), the researchers found a "dose-response" effect: the larger the magnitude of weight cycling, the more significantly the woman's HDL (heart-healthy) cholesterol was lowered. Noteworthy, though, was the fact that the researchers did not find higher levels of coronary artery disease in those with lower HDL levels, so they were not able to make any causal inferences. They also acknowledged limitations of the study in that measurements were all self-reports and information was not gathered regarding how long ago the last weight cycling occurred, nor regarding the use of stimulant medications in the subjects' attempts to lose weight.

A prospective Swedish study (Luo et al. 2007), with over 7 years of follow-up on the incidence of renal cell carcinoma in almost 300 postmenopausal women, noted that those women who had central (i.e., abdominal) obesity and who had also experienced weight cycling of more than 10 pounds more than 10 times during their lives were 2.6 times more likely to develop renal cell carcinoma than women whose weight had been stable. Abdominal obesity, as noted earlier, is a risk factor for renal cell carcinoma in general, but obese women with a weight cycling history appear to be particularly vulnerable.

There is also conflicting literature that suggests weight cycling may have a deleterious effect on bone density. For example, Meyer et al. 1998, in a large prospective study of a population of 39,000 people in Norway, found a higher incidence of hip fracture in both men and women who showed "high weight variability" over the

11½ years of follow-up. Gallagher et al. (2002) did not find evidence of lower total body bone mineral content or bone density in almost 200 healthy sedentary women (ages 21–45) with BMI values ranging from 27 to 40 kg/m^2. The investigators cautioned that their results may not be generalizable to other populations, such as postmenopausal women or those with medical diseases.

Shapses and Riedt (2006) reviewed the literature on bone density and weight. They note that a 10% weight loss, recommended by clinicians for cardiac and metabolic health, can actually result in a 1%–2% bone loss at various sites. They further note that those who are losing weight often do not get enough calcium or vitamin D supplements and this can affect bone density. They caution that ghrelin, the hormone produced predominantly in the stomach that increases appetite and increases with weight loss, also stimulates bone cell proliferation and differentiation. Interestingly, ghrelin levels fall with gastric bypass surgery, and this may have a detrimental effect on bone. The authors recommend the possible inclusion of medications for osteoporosis, as well as calcium and vitamin D supplementation, for patients undertaking severe weight loss attempts or procedures (see Nguyen et al. 2007 regarding bone loss).

Though research results on the physical effects of weight cycling are conflicting, there is evidence that repeated bouts may have psychological consequences in some dieters (Brownell and Rodin 1994). As we have said, one of the problems with weight maintenance is that it is often considerably less reinforcing than weight loss, because significant others around the dieter may no longer give active encouragement as the process goes on indefinitely (Cooper and Fairburn 2002). Further, most dieters are fairly unrealistic in terms of the amount of weight they want to lose: weight maintenance may involve accepting a shape and weight previously regarded as unacceptable or "not good enough."

Some researchers who have studied weight cyclers, such as Foreyt et al. (1995), have described emotional and cognitive distress with dieting failure. This includes increased perceived stress, lowered sense of general well-being, and patterns of dysfunctional eating habits. Others, though, such as Kuehnel and Wadden (1994), have not found a significant association between dieting cycling and cognitive or emotional disturbances, including depression, or even control over eating. These researchers did not find a relationship between binge eating disorder and weight cycling specifically, and they noted that "the pernicious experiences of frustration, chronic ineffectiveness, and depression" that are assumed to be part of the weight cycling pattern should be more attributed to those who have a binge eating disorder. They did caution that perhaps their "measures…were not sensitive to the adverse emotional consequences of weight cycling." They noted that weight cyclers and those with binge eating disorder did share "dietary disinhibition" but it presented differently in each group: those with binge eating disorder were obviously binge eaters, with the ensuing shame, guilt, despair, and feelings of loss of control, whereas the weight cyclers were overeaters but they did not have a sense of loss of control.

Venditti and her colleagues (1996) studied the connection between weight cycling (a shift in weight of > 20 pounds) and psychological parameters in 120 obese women. The researchers divided their sample into four groups. The mean number of pounds lost ranged from just over 20 to over 450 pounds. In their sample, 24% said they had never had a cycle of losing and then regaining 20 pounds, whereas 19% said they had lost and regained at least 20 pounds four or more times, with an average of eight cycles. These investigators found a significant association between a self-reported history of weight cycling (with intentional weight loss) and the severity of binge eating. They cautioned, though, that they could not assess whether a history of weight cycling causes binge eating, whether binge eating causes weight cycling, or whether some third factor, such as psychological distress, is involved. They did not find any association between weight cycling specifically and depression ("either depressed mood or lifetime history of a diagnosable depressive disorder") (Venditti et al. 1996), but they did note that binge eating itself is strongly associated with greater psychological vulnerability. They concluded that weight cycling is not associated with negative psychological consequences, other than binge eating, and they recommended that further studies of weight cycling control for binge eating.

DISCRIMINATION AGAINST THE OBESE

In this age of political correctness, there are very few accepted bastions of prejudice and discrimination left. Discrimination against the overweight and obese, unfortunately, is one of them. And it is as strong today as it was 50 years ago, if not more so.

In the early 1960s Stephen Richardson, from the Association for the Aid of Crippled Children, and his colleagues devised a study to evaluate how children perceive others in regard to their physical characteristics and appearance. The boys and girls (ages 10 and 11) in this original study (Goodman et al. 1963; Richardson et al. 1961) were shown drawings of a child with no physical handicaps; one with crutches; another in a wheelchair but with legs covered; another with his left hand missing; one with facial disfigurement; and an obese child. The children were then asked to rank these drawings in order of preference and why. The study was repeated in public schools, in summer camps in New York, Montana, and California, and even with children who were themselves handicapped. Across the groups of children, including the handicapped children, the drawing of the child without any handicap was ranked first. The drawing of the obese child was ranked last.

This study was replicated 40 years later by Latner and Stunkard (2003) with over 450 children to assess any possible differences in acceptance, and in fact the results indicate that the obese child is still ranked last, and the ranking is even more polarized than in 1961 despite the fact that childhood obesity has increased exponentially. In general, boys tended to have a greater bias against disabilities that impair physical performance (or does this reflect castration anxiety as well?): they ranked the child with a missing hand and the child in a wheelchair lower. Girls tended to rank appearance-related disabilities lower: the facially disfigured child and the obese child. In reviewing the literature, the authors note that children as young as age 3 can have an anti-fat bias, and some of those ages 6 and 7 already place a value on thinness and dieting.

Latner and her colleagues (2005) also studied attitudes toward obesity in university students and found again that obesity was more stigmatized than physical disabilities, even among overweight and obese students. The authors note that African American women in the study had a greater acceptance of obesity, perhaps because of its higher prevalence among them, but they still rated obese peers lower than the nonobese, peers with crutches, and those with facial disfigurations. In this study, men in general liked their obese peers even less than the women did.

More recently, Andreyeva et al. (2008) found that discrimination and prejudice for height and weight has become significantly more prevalent over time, from over 7% in the mid 1990s to over 12% when they studied a large, nationally representative sample (>1,000 people) again from 2004 to 2006. During those years, incidentally, racial discrimination had not gotten worse. One speculation for the worsening statistics regarding the obese is that there has been a fivefold increase in media attention to the problems of obesity over the years. The focus in the media, though, has often been on obesity as a problem of personal responsibility or a disorder of individual choice, for which weight loss products from the diet industry are the solution, rather than a complex disorder involving individuals' genetics, the brain, the metabolic system, and the environment, among many other variables.

ANTI-FAT BIAS IN CHILDREN: THE STIGMA OF OBESITY

In the 1960s, researchers asked children to rate drawings: "Which child do you like best?"

- Besides a healthy child, there was a child with crutches, a child in a wheelchair, a child with a left hand missing, a child with a facial disfigurement, and an obese child. The obese child was liked least, not only by children from different socioeconomic and ethnic backgrounds, but even by children who themselves had physical disabilities (Goodman et al. 1963; Richardson et al. 1961).

- This study was replicated 40 years later (in 2001) with more than 400 children in the fifth and sixth grades, using the same drawings. Stigmatization of obesity had become even worse than in the original study: the healthy child was ranked even higher and the obese child was ranked even lower than in the earlier studies (Latner and Stunkard 2003).

- In both studies, boys and girls gave somewhat different rankings to drawings of functional impairment versus appearance-related impairment: boys rated lower the drawings of functional impairment (child in wheelchair and child with left hand missing), whereas girls rated lower the drawings of appearance-related impairment (child with facial disfigurement and obese child).

ANTI-FAT BIAS AMONG HEALTH PROFESSIONALS

- One study of more than 300 family physicians found that two-thirds reported their obese patients lack self-control and 39% considered them lazy.

- In another study, 100 physicians and students in a medical clinic viewed obese patients as *unintelligent, unsuccessful, inactive,* and *weak-willed,* and even indicated they preferred not to treat the obese.

- A study of more than 100 nurses found that 24% reported that caring for an obese person repulsed them, and 12% reported they preferred not to touch an obese patient.

- One study from Yale conducted with almost 400 clinicians and researchers attending an international conference on obesity found that even those who specialize in treating obesity have a "significant pro-thin, anti-fat bias" and implicitly endorsed typical stereotypes of the obese as *lazy, stupid, and worthless.*

Source: Maroney and Golub 1992; Puhl and Brownell 2001; Schwartz et al. 2003; Teachman and Brownell 2001

Puhl and Brownwell (2001) summarized the ways in which the overweight and obese experience discrimination, particularly in regard to employment, compensation, education, health care, and even jury selection. Those with a weight problem, because it is believed by others to be self-inflicted, receive less pay and fewer promotions. Puhl and Brownwell (2001) also note that the obese are less likely to receive acceptance to college. Most surprising, though, is that physicians and other health care professionals, even those in the obesity field, tend to have an anti-fat bias, the first step toward actual discrimination. Teachman and Brownell (2001) report on a study they did with 84 health care professionals who treat obesity and found their subjects, as well, shared a belief that the obese are lazy. A study of nurses by Maroney and Golub (1992) found that nurses felt obesity could be prevented by self-control and they felt uncomfortable caring for the obese. Similar results were seen in a study by Hoppé and Ogden (1997). Schwartz et al. (2003) surveyed clinicians and researchers attending an international conference on obesity and found that even they had a clear anti-fat bias, in which they "endorsed the implicit stereotypes of lazy, stupid, and worthless."

Foster et al. (2003) examined the attitudes of 600 physicians from different geographical areas and found significant prejudice against the obese. For example, two-thirds of the sample rated physical inactivity, overeating, and a high-fat diet as "very or extremely important" as etiologies for obesity. In other words, these physicians saw obesity as a behavior problem, and more than half of this sample described the obese as "awkward, unattractive, ugly, and noncompliant." And almost half of them believed that psychological problems were "very or extremely important" in the etiology of obesity. Significantly, these physicians were fairly pessimistic about treating their obese patients, with only 14% claiming success. They rated weight management treatment to be only as successful as treatment of drug addiction.

Most recently, studies by Puhl et al. (2008) confirm that prejudice and overt discrimination still exist for those who are overweight or obese. The investigators found that adults with a BMI value of 35 kg/m^2 or greater had a 40% chance of being the victim of discrimination, and women were three times more likely than their male peers to experience discrimination. And a study by Latner et al. (2008) suggests that pervasive discrimination against obese individuals seems more socially accepted than discrimination against other groups.

Maximova et al. (2008), in a study of over 3,500 children and adolescents, noted that overweight and obese youth are more apt to underestimate (i.e., misperceive the extent of) their own weight problems when they are surrounded by adults or peers (even more so with peers) who are themselves overweight or obese. These children and adolescents may then "develop false perceptions of what constitutes an appropriate weight status," the authors caution (Maximova et al. 2008). Obviously, one of the first steps in obesity prevention is having an accurate view of one's physicality. Over the years, there has been a growing movement to counteract discrimination against those who are "weight challenged." The National Association to Advance Fat Acceptance (NAAFA) was founded in the late 1960s to improve the quality of life for those who are overweight or obese (Neumark-Sztainer 1999). Fat acceptance will be discussed in Chapter 6, in the section on body image.

REFERENCES

Allison DB, Fontaine KR, Manson JE, et al: Annual deaths attributable to obesity in the United States. JAMA 282:1530–1538, 1999

Andreyeva T, Puhl RM, Brownell KD: Changes in perceived weight discrimination among Americans, 1995–1996 through 2004–2006. Obesity (Silver Spring) 16:1129–1134, 2008

Aronne LJ: Treatment of obesity in the primary care setting, in Handbook of Obesity Treatment. Edited by Wadden TA, Stunkard AJ. New York, Guilford, 2002, pp 383–394

Aucott L, Poobalan A, Smith WC, et al: Effects of weight loss in overweight obese individuals and long-term hypertension outcomes: a systematic review. Hypertension 45:1035–1041, 2005

Björntorp P: Etiology of the metabolic syndrome, in Handbook of Obesity: Etiology and Pathophysiology, 2nd Edition. Edited by Bray GA, Bouchard C. New York, Marcel Dekker, 2004, pp 787–811

Bouchard C, Tremblay A, Després JP, et al: The response to long-term overfeeding in identical twins. N Engl J Med 322:1477–1482, 1990

Bouchard C, Pérusse L, Rice T, et al: Genetics of human obesity, in Handbook of Obesity: Etiology and Pathophysiology, 2nd Edition. Edited by Bray GA, Bouchard C. New York, Marcel Dekker, 2004, pp 157–200

Bray GA: An Atlas of Obesity and Weight Control (The Encyclopedia of Visual Medicine Series). Baton Rouge, LA, Parthenon Publishing Group, 2003

Brownell KD, Rodin J: Medical, metabolic, and psychological effects of weight cycling. Arch Intern Med 154:1325–1330, 1994

Butryn ML, Phelan S, Hill JO, et al: Consistent self-monitoring of weight: a key component of successful weight loss maintenance. Obesity (Silver Spring) 15:3091–3096, 2007

Calle EE: Obesity and cancer, in Obesity Epidemiology. Edited by Hu FB. New York, Oxford University Press, 2008, pp 196–215

Calle EE, Rodriguez C, Walker-Thurmond K, et al: Overweight, obesity, and mortality from cancer in a prospectively studied cohort of U.S. adults. N Engl J Med 348:1625–1638, 2003

Calle EE, Teras LR, Thun MJ: Obesity and mortality (letter). N Engl J Med 353:2197–2199, 2005

Cooper Z, Fairburn CG: Cognitive-behavioral treatment of obesity, in Handbook of Obesity Treatment. Edited by Wadden TA, Stunkard AJ. New York, Guilford, 2002, pp 465–479

Daeninck E, Miller M: What can the National Weight Control Registry teach us? Curr Diab Rep 6:401–404, 2006

Darsow T, Kendall D, Maggs D: Is the metabolic syndrome a real clinical entity and should it receive drug treatment? Curr Diab Rep 6:357–364, 2006

De Castro JM: Eating behavior: lessons from the real world of humans. Nutrition 16:800–813, 2000

Deurenberg P, Weststrate JA, Seidell JC: Body mass index as a measure of body fatness: age- and sex-specific prediction formulas. Br J Nutr 65:105–114, 1991

Devlin MJ, Yanovski SZ, Wilson GT: Obesity: what mental health professionals need to know. Am J Psychiatry 157:854–866, 2000

Ellin A, Schwartz P: Fitness: quick, do you know your B.M.I.? The New York Times, December 28, 2006

Fan JG, Zhu J, Li XJ, et al: Fatty liver and the metabolic syndrome among Shanghai adults. J Gastroenterol Hepatol 20:1825–1832, 2005

Field AE, Barnoya J, Colditz GA: Epidemiology and health and economic consequences of obesity, in Handbook of Obesity Treatment. Edited by Wadden TA, Stunkard AJ. New York, Guilford, 2002, pp 3–18

Flegal KM, Graubard BI, Williamson DF, et al: Cause-specific excess deaths associated with underweight, overweight, and obesity. JAMA 298:2028–2037, 2007

Fontaine KR, Allison DB: Obesity and mortality rates, in Handbook of Obesity: Etiology and Pathophysiology, 2nd Edition. Edited by Bray GA, Bouchard C. New York, Marcel Dekker, 2004, pp 767–784

Ford ES, Giles WH, Dietz WH: Prevalence of the metabolic syndrome among US adults: findings from the third National Health and Nutrition Examination Survey. JAMA 287:356–359, 2002

Foreyt JP, Brunner RL, Goodrick GK, et al: Psychological correlates of weight fluctuation. Int J Eat Disord 17:263–275, 1995

Foster GD, Wadden TA, Makris AP, et al: Primary care physicians' attitudes about obesity and its treatment. Obes Res 11:1168–1177, 2003

Gallagher KI, Jakicic JM, Kiel DP, et al: Impact of weight-cycling history on bone density in obese women. Obes Res 10:896–902, 2002

Goodman N, Dornbusch SM, Richardson SA, et al: Variant reactions to physical disabilities. Am Sociol Rev 28:429–435, 1963

Gorber S, Connor MT, Moher D, et al: A comparison of direct vs. self-report measures for assessing height, weight and body mass index: a systematic review. Obes Rev 8:307–326, 2007

Gorin AA, Phelan S, Wing RR, et al: Promoting long-term weight control: does dieting consistency matter? Int J Obes Relat Metab Disord 28:278–281, 2004

Grabowski DC, Ellis JE: High body mass index does not predict mortality in older people: analysis of the longitudinal study of aging. J Am Geriatr Soc 49:968–979, 2001

Grundy SM: Metabolic syndrome pandemic. Arterioscler Thromb Vasc Biol 28:629–636, 2008

Gustafson D, Lissner L, Bengtsson C, et al: A 24-year follow-up of body mass index and cerebral atrophy. Neurology 63:1876–1881, 2004

Harrison GG: Height-weight tables. Ann Intern Med 103:989–994, 1985

Hill JO: Understanding and addressing the epidemic of obesity: an energy balance perspective. Endocr Rev 27:750–761, 2006

Hill JO, Wyatt H, Phelan S, et al: The National Weight Control Registry: is it useful in helping deal with our obesity epidemic? J Nutr Educ Behav 37:206–210, 2005

Hippocrates: Aphorisms, V, xlvi, in Works, Vol IV. Translated by Jones WHS. Loeb Classical Library. Cambridge, MA, Harvard University Press, 1967

Hsiao DJ, Wu LS, Huang SY, et al: Weight loss and body fat reduction under sibutramine therapy in obesity with the C825T polymorphism in the GNB3 gene. Pharmacogenet Genomics 19:730–733, 2009

Holme I, Sogaard AJ, Haheim LL, et al: Repeated weight loss is associated with the metabolic syndrome and diabetes: results of a 28 year re-screening of men in the Oslo Study. Metab Syndr Relat Disord 5:127–135, 2007

Hoppé R, Ogden J: Practice nurses' beliefs about obesity and weight related interventions in primary care. Int J Obes Relat Metab Disord 21:141–146, 1997

Hu FB: Obesity Epidemiology. New York, Oxford University Press, 2008

Hu FB, Willett WC, Li T, et al: Adiposity as compared with physical activity in predicting mortality among women. N Engl J Med 351:2694–2703, 2004

Janssen I, Powell LH, Crawford S, et al: Menopause and the metabolic syndrome: the study of women's health across the nation. Arch Intern Med 168:1568–1575, 2008

Jeffery RW, Drewnowski A, Epstein LH, et al: Long-term maintenance of weight loss: current status. Health Psychol 19 (1 suppl):5–16, 2000

Kalarchian MA, Marcus MD, Levine MD, et al: Psychiatric disorders among bariatric surgery candidates: relationship to obesity and functional health status. Am J Psychiatry 164:328–334, 2007

Kaplan NM: Obesity and weight reduction in hypertension. UpToDate, Edition 16.3, Reprint. 2008. Available (by subscription) at: http://www.uptodate.com/patients/content/topic .do?topicKey=~0cw6KBtHUt24j1. Accessed September 3, 2009.

Keys A, Fidanza F, Karvonen MJ, et al: Indices of relative weight and obesity. J Chronic Dis 25:329–343, 1972

Klem ML, Wing RR, McGuire MT, et al: A descriptive study of individuals successful at long-term maintenance of substantial weight loss. Am J Clin Nutr 66:239–246, 1997

Kragelund C, Omland T: A farewell to body-mass index? Lancet 366:1589–1591, 2005

Kroke A, Liese AD, Schulz M, et al: Recent weight changes and weight cycling as predictors of subsequent two year weight change in a middle-aged cohort. Int J Obes Relat Metab Disord 26:403–409, 2002

Kuehnel RH, Wadden TA: Binge eating disorder, weight cycling, and psychopathology. Int J Eat Disord 15:321–329, 1994

Landsberg L: Body fat distribution and cardiovascular risk: a tale of 2 sites. Arch Intern Med 168:1607–1608, 2008

Latner JD, Stunkard AJ: Getting worse: the stigmatization of obese children. Obes Res 11:452–456, 2003

Latner JD, Stunkard AJ, Wilson GT: Stigmatized students: age, sex, and ethnicity effects in the stigmatization of obesity. Obes Res 13:1226–1231, 2005

Latner JD, O'Brien KS, Durso LE, et al: Weighing obesity stigma: the relative strength of different forms of bias. Int J Obes (Lond) 32:1145–1152, 2008

Levitsky DA, Garay J, Nausbaum M, et al: Monitoring weight daily blocks the freshman weight gain: a model for combating the epidemic of obesity. Int J Obes 30:1003–1010, 2006

Li Z, Hong K, Wong E, et al: Weight cycling in a very low-calorie diet programme has no effect on weight loss velocity, blood pressure and serum lipid profile. Diabetes Obes Metab 9:379–385, 2007

Lichtman SW, Pisarska K, Berman ER, et al: Discrepancy between self-reported and actual caloric intake and exercise in obese subjects. N Engl J Med 327:1893–1898, 1992

Lindgren CM, Heid IM, Randall JC, et al: Genome-wide association scan meta-analysis identifies three loci influencing adiposity and fat distribution. PLoS Genet 5(6):e1000508, 2009

Luo J, Margolis KL, Adami HO, et al; Women's Health Initiative Investigators: Body size, weight cycling, and risk of renal cell carcinoma among postmenopausal women: the Women's Health Initiative (United States). Am J Epidemiol 166:752–759, 2007

Maes HH, Neale MC, Eaves LJ: Genetic and environmental factors in relative body weight and human adiposity. Behav Genet 27:325–351, 1997

Manson JE, Skerrett PJ, Willett WC: Obesity as a risk factor for major health outcomes, in Handbook of Obesity: Etiology and Pathophysiology, 2nd Edition. Edited by Bray GA, Bouchard C. New York, Marcel Dekker, 2004, pp 813–824

Mark AL: Dietary therapy for obesity: an emperor with no clothes. Hypertension 51:1426–1434, 2008

Maroney D, Golub S: Nurses' attitudes toward obese persons and certain ethnic groups. Percept Mot Skills 75:387–391, 1992

Masheb RM, Grilo CM: Eating patterns and breakfast consumption in obese patients with binge eating disorder. Behav Res Ther 44:1545–1553, 2006

Maximova K, McGrath JJ, Barnett T, et al: Do you see what I see? Weight status misperception and exposure to obesity among children and adolescents. Int J Obes (Lond) 32:1008–1015, 2008

McGuire MT, Wing RR, Klem ML, et al: What predicts weight regain in a group of successful weight losers? J Consult Clin Psychol 67:177–185, 1999

Meyer HE, Tverdal A, Selmer R: Weight variability, weight change, and the incidence of hip fracture: a prospective study of 39,000 middle-aged Norwegians. Osteoporos Int 8:373–378, 1998

Moore LL, Visioni AJ, Qureshi MM, et al: Weight loss in overweight adults and the long-term risk of hypertension: the Framingham study. Arch Intern Med 165:1298–1303, 2005

Moreno-Aliaga MJ, Santos JL, Marti A, et al: Does weight loss prognosis depend on genetic make-up? Obes Rev 6:155–168, 2005

National Task Force on the Prevention and Treatment of Obesity: Weight cycling. JAMA 272:1196–1202, 1994

National Weight Control Registry. Available at: http://www.nwcr.ws. Accessed March 11, 2009.

Nawaz H, Chan W, Abdulrahman M, et al: Self-reported weight and height: implications for obesity research. Am J Prev Med 20:294–298, 2001

Neel JV: Diabetes mellitus: a "thrifty" genotype rendered detrimental by "progress"? Am J Hum Genet 14:353–362, 1962

Neter JE, Stam BE, Kok FJ, et al: Influence of weight reduction on blood pressure: a meta-analysis of randomized controlled trials. Hypertension 42:878–884, 2003

Neumark-Sztainer D: The weight dilemma: a range of philosophical perspectives. Int J Obesity 23 (suppl 2):S31–S37, 1999

Nguyen ND, Center JR, Eisman JA, et al: Bone loss, weight loss, and weight fluctuation predict mortality risk in elderly men and women. J Bone Miner Res 22:1147–1154, 2007

Nicklas BJ, Tomoyasu N, Muir J, et al: Effects of cigarette smoking and its cessation on body weight and plasma leptin levels. Metabolism 48:804–808, 1999

Ogden CL, Carroll MD, Curtin LR, et al: Prevalence of overweight and obesity in the United States, 1999–2004. JAMA 295:1549–1555, 2006

Olson MB, Kelsey SF, Bittner V, et al: Weight cycling and high-density lipoprotein cholesterol in women: evidence of an adverse effect: a report from the NHLBI-sponsored WISE study. J Am Coll Cardiol 36:1565–1571, 2000

O'Rahilly S: Human obesity: a heritable neurobehavioral disorder that is highly sensitive to environmental conditions. Diabetes 57:2905–2910, 2008

O'Rahilly S, Farooqi IS: Genetics of obesity. Philos Trans R Soc Lond B Biol Sci 361:1095–1105, 2006

Oxford English Dictionary, 2nd Edition, s.v. "obesity," "W. Somerset Maugham; slow, obese smile." Oxford, UK, Oxford University Press, 1989

Pai MP, Paloucek FP: The origin of the "ideal" body weight equations. Ann Pharmacother 34:1066–1069, 2000

Pérusse L, Rankinen T, Zuberi A, et al: The human obesity gene map: the 2004 update. Obes Res 13:381–490, 2005

Phelan S, Wyatt HR, Hill JO, et al: Are the eating and exercise habits of successful weight losers changing? Obesity (Silver Spring) 14:710–716, 2006

Poirier P: Adiposity and cardiovascular disease: are we using the right definition of obesity? Eur Heart J 28:2047–2048, 2007

Precope J: Hippocrates on Diet and Hygiene. London, Zeno, 1952

Prentice AM, Jebb SA, Goldberg GR, et al: Effects of weight cycling on body composition. Am J Clin Nutr 56:209S–216S, 1992

Preston SH: Deadweight?—the influence of obesity on longevity. N Engl J Med 352:1135–1137, 2005

Price RA: Genetics and common obesities: background, current status, strategies, and future prospects, in Handbook of Obesity Treatment. Edited by Wadden TA, Stunkard AJ. New York, Guilford, 2002, pp 73–94

Prospective Studies Collaboration; Whitlock G, Lewington S, Sherliker P, et al: Body-mass index and cause-specific mortality in 900,000 adults: collaborative analyses of 57 prospective studies. Lancet 373:1083–1096, 2009

Puhl RM, Brownell KD: Bias, discrimination, and obesity. Obes Res 9:788–805, 2001

Puhl RM, Andreyeva T, Brownell KD: Perceptions of weight discrimination: prevalence and comparison to race and gender discrimination in America. Int J Obes (Lond) 32:992–1000, 2008

Rankinen T, Zuberi A, Chagnon YC, et al: The human obesity gene map: the 2005 update. Obesity (Silver Spring) 14:529–644, 2006

Reaven GM: Banting Lecture 1988: role of insulin resistance in human disease. Diabetes 37:1595–1607, 1988

Richardson SA, Goodman N, Hastorf AH, et al: Cultural uniformity in reaction to physical disabilities. Am Sociol Rev 26:241–247, 1961

Romero-Corral A, Montori VM, Somers VK, et al: Association of bodyweight with total mortality and with cardiovascular events in coronary artery disease: a systematic review of cohort studies. Lancet 368:666–678, 2006

Rössner S: Adolphe Quetelet (1796–1874). Obes Rev 8:183, 2007

Roth J: Evolutionary speculation about tuberculosis and the metabolic and inflammatory processes of obesity. JAMA 301:2586–2588, 2009

Roybal D: Is "yo-yo" dieting or weight cycling harmful to one's health? Nutrition Noteworthy 7(1):article 9, 2005. Available at: http://repositories.cdlib.org/uclabiolchem/nutrition-noteworthy/vol7/iss1/art9. Accessed September 3, 2009.

Sarafidis PA, Nilsson PM: The metabolic syndrome: a glance at its history. J Hypertens 24:621–626, 2006

Sarlio-Lähteenkorva S, Rissanen A, Kaprio J: A descriptive study of weight loss maintenance: 6 and 15 year follow-up of initially overweight adults. Int J Obes Relat Metab Disord 24:116–125, 2000

Schulze MB, Manson JE, Ludwig DS, et al: Sugar-sweetened beverages, weight gain, and incidence of type 2 diabetes in young and middle-aged women. JAMA 292:927–934, 2004

Schutz Y, Jéquier E: Resting energy expenditure, thermic effect of food, and total energy expenditure, in Handbook of Obesity: Etiology and Pathophysiology, 2nd Edition. Edited by Bray GA, Bouchard C. New York, Marcel Dekker, 2004, pp 615–653

Schwartz MB, Chambliss HO, Brownell KD, et al: Weight bias among health professionals specializing in obesity. Obes Res 11:1033–1039, 2003

Seidell JC, Pérusse L, Després JP, et al: Waist and hip circumferences have independent and opposite effects on cardiovascular disease risk factors: the Quebec Family Study. Am J Clin Nutr 74:315–321, 2001

Shapses SA, Riedt CS: Bone, body weight, and weight reduction: what are the concerns? J Nutr 136:1453–1456, 2006

Simon S: Interview with Keith Devlin. Weekend Edition Saturday, National Public Radio, July 4, 2009

Sitzman K: Eating breakfast helps sustain weight loss. AAOHN J 54:136, 2006

Snijder MB, van Dam RM, Visser M, et al: What aspects of body fat are particularly hazardous and how do we measure them? Int J Epidemiol 35:83–92, 2006

Snyder EE, Walts B, Pérusse L, et al: The human obesity gene map: the 2003 update. Obes Res 12:369–439, 2004

Søgaard AJ, Meyer HE, Tonstad S, et al: Weight cycling and risk of forearm fractures: a 28-year follow-up of men in the Oslo Study. Am J Epidemiol 167:1005–1013, 2008

Stefan N, Kantartzis K, Machann J, et al: Identification and characterization of metabolically benign obesity in humans. Arch Intern Med 168:1607–1608, 2008

Stunkard AJ: The management of obesity. N Y State J Med 58:79–87, 1958

Stunkard A, McLaren-Hume M: The results of treatment for obesity: a review of the literature and report of a series. Arch Intern Med 103:79–85, 1959

Stunkard AJ, Sorensen TI, Hanis C, et al: An adoption study of human obesity. N Engl J Med 314:193–198, 1986

Sui X, LaMonte MJ, Laditka JN, et al: Cardiorespiratory fitness and adiposity as mortality predictors in older adults. JAMA 298:2507–2516, 2007

Tanaka M, Itoh K, Abe S, et al: Irregular patterns in the daily weight chart at night predict body weight regain. Exp Biol Med (Maywood) 229:940–945, 2004

Tataranni PA, Ravussin E: Energy metabolism and obesity, in Handbook of Obesity. Edited by Wadden TA, Stunkard AJ. New York, Guilford, 2004, pp 42–72

Teachman BA, Brownell KD: Implicit anti-fat bias among health professionals: is anyone immune? Int J Obes Relat Metab Disord 25:1525–1531, 2001

Vague J: The degree of masculine differentiation of obesities: a factor determining predisposition to diabetes, atherosclerosis, gout, and uric calculous disease. Am J Clin Nutr 4:20–34, 1956

Venditti EM, Wing RR, Jakicic JM, et al: Weight cycling, psychological health, and binge eating in obese women. J Consult Clin Psychol 64:400–405, 1996

Vidal J: Updated review on the benefits of weight loss. Int J Obes Relat Metab Disord 26 (suppl 4):S25–S28, 2002

Vinter S, Levi J, St Laurent R, et al: F as in fat: how obesity policies are failing in America 2008. Robert Wood Johnson Foundation. August 19, 2008. Available at: http://www.rwjf.org/pr/product.jsp?id=33711. Accessed February 11, 2009.

Wadden TA, Didie E: What's in a name? Patients' preferred terms for describing obesity. Obes Res 11:1140–1146, 2003

Wadden TA, Phelan S: Behavioral assessment of the obese patient, in Handbook of Obesity Treatment. Edited by Wadden TA, Stunkard AJ. New York, Guilford, 2002, pp 186–226

Wang Y, Beydoun MA: The obesity epidemic in the United States—gender, age, socioeconomic, racial/ethnic, and geographic characteristics: a systematic review and meta-regression analysis. Epidemiol Rev 29:6–28, 2007

Wang Y, Beydoun MA, Liang L, et al: Will all Americans become overweight or obese? Estimating the progression and cost of the US obesity epidemic. Epidemiology 16: 2323–2330, 2008

Wansink B: Mindless Eating: Why We Eat More Than We Think. New York, Bantam, 2006

Wildman RP, Muntner P, Reynolds K, et al: The obese without cardiometabolic risk factor clustering and the normal weight with cardiometabolic risk factor clustering. Arch Intern Med 168:1617–1624, 2008

Wing RR: Weight cycling in humans: a review of the literature. Ann Behav Med 14:113–119, 1992

Wing RR, Phelan S: Long-term weight loss maintenance. Am J Clin Nutr 82:222S–225S, 2005

Wisse BE: The inflammatory syndrome: the role of adipose tissue cytokines in metabolic disorders linked to obesity. J Am Soc Nephrol 15:2792–2800, 2004

Wyatt HR, Grunwald GK, Mosca CL, et al: Long-term weight loss and breakfast in subjects in the National Weight Control Registry. Obes Res 10:78–82, 2002

Yanovski JA, Yanovski SZ, Sovik KN, et al: A prospective study of holiday weight gain. N Engl J Med 342:861–867, 2000

Zhang C, Rexrode KM, van Dam RM, et al: Abdominal obesity and the risk of all-cause, cardiovascular, and cancer mortality. Circulation 117:1658–1667, 2008

3

FOOD

The Basic Principles of Calories

Rather than double over with laughter at the sight of a candy bar that professes to boost the immune system, reduce stress, and burn fat, many Americans, some with college degrees, take out their wallets and spend $20 billion a year on foods with vitamins and herbs to ward off diseases.

Barry Glassner, *The Gospel of Food* (2007, p. 42)

FACTORS INVOLVED IN DAILY ENERGY REQUIREMENTS

During our lifetime, our bodies process about 70 million calories, or approximately 14 tons of food (Hirsch 2003). And according to the U.S. Department of Agriculture (USDA), as of 2004 the United States produced 3,900 calories of food every day for each person, including children (Nestle 2006, p. 11; USDA 2009), though we all need far less. It is remarkable, therefore, that even though weight does tend to creep upward as we age and there is an epidemic of obesity, over the course of our adult lives most of us do seem able, without much effort, to keep our weights within a fairly narrow range. Despite the many different foods we eat in the course of a year, individuals usually do not have an extraordinarily different weight from one year to the next. We neither gain much weight nor lose much weight. Mostly, it is the slow creep of additional weight—that pound or two of holiday weight gain—that, as Yanovski and colleagues (2000) have noted, we don't tend to lose.

Most researchers believe that additional weight, whether or not it reaches a level to be considered obesity, results from an energy imbalance—too many calories taken in and not enough expended.

Taubes (2007, p. 293), for example, a journalist who has done extensive research into the history of obesity research, takes issue with this model. To him, a calorie is not necessarily just a calorie, but rather it is the kind of food eaten (particularly carbohydrates) and one's hormone balance (particularly insulin) that determine weight gain. He believes that researchers specialize such that they do not read the journals of other disciplines and that even though they may be doing similar experiments with animals, they reach different conclusions (Taubes 2007, p. 429). For Taubes, "energy intake and energy expenditure are very much dependent variables" (p. 298) so that a change in one will result in a change in the other. He uses the analogy of height: no one would question that height is determined by genetics, rather than just by what we eat (other than in states of severe malnutrition) or how much we exercise. He believes that people who have a weight problem have a constitutional predisposition to accumulate fat (and a compensatory predisposition to eat more calories) whereas those who remain thin "have a constitutional predisposition to resist the accumulation of fat."

Taubes takes the strong (and in our belief, simplistic) position that obesity does not involve any kind of eating or behavioral disorder. Says Taubes (2007, p. 311), "Imagine if diabetologists had perceived ravenous hunger that accompanies uncontrolled diabetes as a behavioral disorder, to be treated by years of psychotherapy or behavioral modification rather than injections of insulin." For Taubes, the regulation of the hormone insulin, as the regulator of fat storage, seems to be the essential key to weight control: humans gain weight "because our insulin remains elevated for longer than nature or evolution intended" (p. 435). And insulin levels remain elevated in predisposed individuals because of the extraordinary amount of carbohydrates, especially refined ones, that we eat today. According to statistics provided by the USDA, in the year 2000, Americans were consuming just under 150 pounds of all caloric sweeteners (including refined sugar and high fructose corn syrup) a year per person (USDA 2005). Interestingly, we are now consuming only 137 pounds of caloric sweeteners per person, per year. Though the USDA does not say, it is possible our drop in consumption is related to greater consumption of nonnutritive sweeteners.

> **THE HOLIDAY CREEP**
>
> Most people gain 1–2 pounds during the holidays but don't tend to lose it afterward, so there is an upward creep in weight.

Compared with those of our evolutionary ancestors, our diets dramatically changed with the advent of agriculture and have gotten progressively worse as civilization and technology have created seemingly endless varieties of carbohydrates for us to consume. For Taubes, it is not fat and cholesterol that are responsible for heart disease, but the excessive carbohydrates, particularly the highly processed, refined ones so prevalent in our diets. Though much of what Taubes says makes sense (and he backs up his theory with an extensive review of the literature over the last 100 years), he may be going too far when he glosses over the major role our cognitive brains play in weight control.

Essentially, we have to eat approximately 3,500 kilocalories above what we expend to increase our weight by 1 pound. A calorie is a measure of energy. When we are referring to food, we customarily drop the prefix *kilo* and just use the word *calorie* (and we do so throughout this book). Katz (2008, p. 54) gives a clear definition: "The calorie is a measure of food energy and represents the heat required to raise the temperature of 1 gram or cubic centimeter of water one degree Celsius at sea level" and a kilocalorie is the amount of heat required to do so for 1 kilogram. So someone who has gained 25 pounds has theoretically eaten 87,500 extra calories that he or she has not expended. And in order to lose a pound in a week, you have to cut your calories by 500 per day (500/day × 7 days = 3,500 calories).

> Theoretically, there are 3,500 calories in a pound of body weight. In order to lose a pound a week, you have to cut your calories by 500 a day. Someone who has gained 25 pounds has eaten 87,500 more calories than he or she has expended.

Katz (2008, p. 55) notes that losing weight is often so much more complicated than just counting the number of calories eaten: genetics, endocrine factors, and even what foods are eaten may "contribute important mitigating influences at any level of calorie consumption." Katz notes (2008, p. 56) that as a *rough estimate*, for a woman with average activity to maintain her ideal weight, she must daily consume in calories 12–14 times her ideal weight, and for a man it is 14–16 times his ideal weight. So if a woman wants to weigh 115 pounds, she should consume between about 1,400 and 1,700 calories daily—not very much, and far below what most people consume.

One of the major problems with calorie counting, though, is that we humans notoriously underestimate how many calories we are eating. Lichtman et al. (1992) have shown that obese people can underreport as much as one-third to one-half of their calorie intake. These researchers studied obese subjects who claimed they could not lose weight consuming 1,200 calories a day (i.e., *diet-resistant* individuals) to assess whether they actually had lower total energy expenditure. In fact, these obese people were not significantly different from control subjects in their energy expenditure. What the study found was that the obese subjects significantly underreported their actual calorie intake and overreported their activity level. But even thin people can underestimate the amounts they eat by 20%. This is called the *eye-mouth gap*, as we have previously mentioned (see Chapter 2, "Obesity in the United States," p. 19) (Lichtman et al. 1992; Tataranni and Ravussin 2002, pp. 48–49). Most people develop "sticker shock" when they realize just how many calories they are actually eating in a day. Recent legislation in New York City to insist that chain restaurants, such as Starbucks, McDonald's, and Kentucky Fried Chicken, list calorie counts next to their menu choices may do much to make people far more aware of how easy it is to pile on additional calories, as have labels that list calorie counts.

The problem, of course, is that most of what we eat at home and in restaurants does not come with calorie counts, so our estimates are often way off.

Furthermore, portion size has had a significant impact on calorie intake. Even when packaging comes with labels, the consumer can be easily deceived if he or she does not read very carefully. A serving size may be far smaller than anticipated. For example, a package with enormous muffins may give the calorie count for only half the muffin as the designated portion, whereas most people will, in fact, eat the entire muffin and assume that is one portion. Over time, portions have become considerably larger. The average size of a serving of french fries at McDonald's has increased dramatically since the 1960s, as have the serving sizes of soft drinks. Brownell (at an October 3, 2008, conference) noted that the "Big Gulp" from 7-Eleven stores has 48 teaspoons of sugar in it! Restaurants are only too happy to "supersize." Sixteen ounces (the medium size, or grande) of a Starbucks Mint Mocha Chip Frappuccino with Chocolate Whipped Cream has 470 calories and 19 grams of fat ("Starbucks beverage details" 2009). This is not coffee: this has become a dessert.

SERVING SIZES	
Pancake:	Compact disc
Apple:	Tennis ball
Fish:	Cell phone
Peanut butter:	Ping-pong ball
Meat:	Deck of cards

Source: Helmering and Hales 2005, adapted from p. 137

Given all these potential hidden sources of calories, how do we, in fact, get rid of calories? There are three major components involved in our daily energy expenditure, sometimes also referred to as our *total energy expenditure* or TEE: 1) our resting metabolic rate (RMR), essentially equivalent to and sometimes referred to as the basal metabolic rate, which is the measurement taken 12 hours after last eating—that is, postabsorptively, so residual thermogenic effects are less relevant; 2) thermogenesis (the amount of energy required related to eating and digestion); and 3) our physical activity.

Tataranni and Ravussin (2002, p. 45) define *resting metabolic rate* as "the energy expended by a subject resting in the fasting state under comfortable ambient conditions." They note that this includes "the cost of maintaining the integrated systems of the body" and our body temperature; for most adults, the RMR is 60%–70% of our daily energy expenditure. Schutz and Jéquier (2004, p. 618) note how difficult it is to consider all the metabolic rates of human organs and tissues noninvasively. The liver, kidneys, brain, and heart have the highest metabolic activity, whereas muscles have a rate 35 times lower than organs such as our hearts or kidneys (p. 618). And interestingly, when considering its weight, adipose tissue is the tissue with the lowest metabolic activity (p. 619). It can account for 4% of the RMR in someone who is not obese, but up to 10% in those who are obese. So it is true that obese people tend to have a higher RMR. As a result, because RMR accounts for so much of the daily energy expenditure, anything that might affect the RMR could potentially have

COMPONENTS OF DAILY ENERGY EXPENDITURE (ALSO CALLED *TOTAL ENERGY EXPENDITURE*)

- Resting metabolic rate (RMR): decreases about 1%–2% per decade as we age, but may decrease less if we exercise; obese individuals have higher RMRs than the nonobese; women have lower RMRs than men; calorie restriction can reduce RMR by 20%

- Diet-induced thermogenesis (hardest to measure): amount of energy required by our organs for eating and digesting; each nutrient (e.g., protein, fat, carbohydrates) processed differently, with protein requiring most energy; affected by size of meals, temperature of food, timing of meals

- Physical activity (most variable): includes fidgeting, posture, even muscle tone; even sedentary people lose 20%–30% of their calories through physical activity

Source: Miller and Wadden 2004; Tataranni and Ravussin 2002

substantial effects on body weight. Though body size does affect RMR, Tataranni and Ravussin (2002, p. 46) also note that RMR can vary up to 20% among people of any body size. Many factors seem to influence it, such as fat-free mass (which includes muscle and nonmuscle); the amount of body fat, especially abdominal; body temperature; age; sex; and even diet composition over the days before the measurement (e.g., how much carbohydrate intake and specifically how much "overfeeding") (Schutz and Jéquier 2004, p. 620).

Twin studies suggest that there is also a genetic component, such that monozygotic twins have more similar RMRs than dizygotic twins. And female hormones have an effect on RMR, hence women can have a lower RMR than men (~3%–10% lower, even after adjustments are made for fat tissue, age, and physical fitness level; Schutz and Jéquier 2004, p. 619). RMR decreases considerably with age, but that may be more a factor of our decrease in muscle mass as we age. According to studies reported by Tataranni and Ravussin (2002, p. 46), RMR decreases less than 1%–2% per decade from age 10 to age 60. It is also suggested that body temperature may be a marker for high or low RMR. And thyroid hormone levels increase our RMR by increasing our sympathetic nervous system response (e.g., with increase in heat production) (Schutz and Jéquier 2004, p. 620).

Miller and Wadden (2004, p. 170) note that RMR is affected by calorie restriction and a rapid reduction in calorie intake can lead to a decrease in the RMR by up to 20%. The authors note that this reduction in the RMR may lead to the dieter's plateau that often occurs despite calorie restriction (p. 170). In times of famine, reduction in RMR with decreased calories was adaptively beneficial, but not so in our time of plenty. Geliebter et al. (1997) studied moderately obese men and women who were assigned to treatment groups of diet plus strength training, diet plus aerobic training, or diet alone. At 8 weeks, all groups lost the same amount of weight

(~9 kilograms), but those who had strength training lost less muscle mass, though all groups had a decrease in their RMRs. Incidentally, those in the two exercise groups had a greater improvement in their mood than those dieting without exercise. Geliebter and his colleagues concluded that strength training helped reduce the typical diet-induced loss of lean muscle but did not prevent a decline in RMR. Said the researchers, "Despite popular opinion and claims made by manufacturers of weight-resistance equipment, no evidence could be found for conservation of RMR when combining diet and exercise" (Geliebter et al. 1997). Miller and Wadden (2004, p. 170) noted that neither strength training nor aerobic exercise could stop the typical decline seen in RMR when calories are restricted. But these authors do believe that aerobic exercise not only may help prevent the typical decline in RMR as we age, but may also help in protecting someone from having age-related weight increase (p. 171). Byrne and Wilmore (2001) investigated the relationship of aerobic exercise and strength (resistance) exercise to RMR in women. They found no significant difference in RMR in those engaging in resistance (strength) training versus aerobic training, but those who were more highly trained tended to have an increase in their RMRs regardless of their mode of training. A small study by Herring et al. (1992) tested highly trained women endurance runners to assess what effects aerobic exercise has on RMR hours after exercise. The researchers found that vigorous exercise (as measured here by treadmill) did boost RMR, but the effect lasted only 15–39 hours. Because RMR is affected by body composition, calorie intake, nutritional status, and even the phase of a woman's menstrual cycle, they kept these potential variables constant. They speculate that catecholamine release (e.g., norepinephrine released from muscle) may be involved in short- and long-term exercise effects.

The second means by which we expend calories is by our processing of the food we eat. This is the thermogenic effect, sometimes referred to as *diet-induced thermogenesis* (Stock 1999); it is the energy generated as heat in the process of food digestion and related processes, as contrasted with other forms of thermogenesis. Stock (1999) makes the point that, evolutionarily, mechanisms of thermogenesis can be seen in very primitive life forms, such as bacteria. In humans, though, thermogenesis also involves maintenance of our body temperature, particularly against cold temperatures. It is responsible for one of our initial reactions to cold, namely shivering. Another aspect of thermogenesis is the production of heat (i.e., the adaptive response of fever) in response to illness. Stock also notes that leptin, the hormone involved in satiety, among other things, involves mechanisms similar to those involved in the production of fever; hence, leptin's role in thermogenesis is even more important than its role in satiety.

Over 24 hours, about 10% (estimates range from 5% to 15%; Tataranni and Ravussin 2002, p. 46) of our calorie expenditure is involved in this processing, including absorption of food and its nutrients as well as glycogen storage. Each nutrient (protein, fat, carbohydrate) is processed differently, so the breakdown of each expends different amounts of calories. Protein breakdown uses the highest amount of energy: 20%–30% of the energy content of protein is expended in the digestive degradation process (e.g., breakdown to amino acids and eventually glucose) (Schutz and Jéquier 2004, p. 622), whereas glucose breakdown expends 8% of its calories and fat ranks lowest at only 2%, making fat the most energy-efficient nutrient. Alcohol (ethanol) also has a thermic effect: 22% of its calories are expended in its breakdown. Says Stock (1999), among the main evolutionary advantages of thermogenesis is that it provides "a mechanism for enriching nutrient-poor diets by disposing of the excess nonessential energy." Unbalanced diets cause "homeostatic waste," though there is apparently considerable variation among humans in response to unbalanced diets (particularly low-protein diets); researchers even believe that a person's response to being overfed an unbalanced diet may be predictive of the person's genetic predisposition to weight gain and that 40% of people have had some degree of increase in diet-induced thermogenesis (Stock 1999). Dulloo and Jacquet (1999) emphasize that researchers do not see much interindividual difference when a balanced diet is used, but unbalanced diets "unmask... [the] diverse range of individual responses." Similarly, not everyone is susceptible to gaining weight on a high-fat diet, though Dulloo and Jacquet (1999) maintain that a challenge with a low-protein diet (3% vs. 20% protein) affords a more discriminating test (a so-called magnifying glass) for the metabolic and genetic predispositions to obesity: overeating a low-protein diet can lead to a "large decrease in energetic efficiency." For humans, optimal efficiency occurs at 12% protein (Stock 1999).

Unlike RMR, thermogenesis is not clearly influenced by female hormones or the menstrual cycle. It is only affected by age in that loss of lean muscle in the elderly does affect it. Thermogenesis is affected, though, by the size our meals, what we eat, the temperature of the food (e.g., drinking a cold liquid uses more energy than drinking a warmer one), the timing of a meal, genetics, and even level of fitness. Thermogenesis has been found to be lower in most obese people, but this may be related to insulin resistance (Schutz and Jéquier 2004, p. 622). Schutz and Jéquier do note that some have questioned whether a thermogenic defect may be involved in the development of obesity, but they discount this possible contribution and support the notion that it is more likely to be a failure to control food intake in the obese: "Thus, the important conclusion is that the concept of 'small eaters' who remain obese with daily energy intake less than 1,800 kcal is certainly wrong" (Schutz and Jéquier 2004, p. 623).

Though thermogenesis is the hardest of the three kinds of energy expenditure to measure, Tataranni and Ravussin (2002, p. 47) do not believe that decreased thermogenesis is responsible for increasing obesity, either. Schutz and Jéquier (2004) also note that both the parasympathetic and sympathetic nervous systems are involved in the thermogenic effect of food processing, and drugs that affect these systems (e.g., the beta-blocker propranolol or the cholinergic blocker atropine) can affect these processes. Van Baak (2008) also emphasizes the role of an activated sympathetic nervous system in diet-induced thermogenesis, though this author notes its role is still not clear. Sympathetic activation (to maintain blood pressure) is most clearly seen after meals rich in carbohydrates. Its role in fat and protein ingestion is still in dispute. Van Baak (2008) believes that when we overconsume food, particularly carbohydrates, we may be causing a gradual downregulation of beta-adrenergically mediated thermogenesis, which may in turn lead to obesity.

Several substances have been found to have properties that increase thermogenesis. Diepvens et al. (2006) have noted that caffeine, ephedrine, capsaicin (the ingredient in red pepper), and green tea, all through different enzyme mechanisms, are agents that may have counteracted decreases in metabolic rate when someone has lost weight. In general, these substances act on the sympathetic nervous system, which has a role in the regulation of fat metabolism (lipolysis) by releasing catecholamines. These authors note studies in which caffeine can reduce food intake, though over time humans may become insensitive to its effects. The combination of ephedrine and caffeine can potentiate the effects of each and can, in fact, lead to weight loss. Recent reports of adverse effects, however, particularly of ephedrine-related cardiovascular changes such as tachycardia, palpitations, and increased blood pressure, have led the U.S. Food and Drug Administration (FDA) to ban ephedra containing products for dieting. Red pepper can lead to a decrease in adipose tissue, but unfortunately, it is not well tolerated (e.g., it is strongly pungent) at doses required for benefit. Green tea definitely stimulates thermogenesis and fat oxidation, though it can increase blood pressure, and may have a role in weight loss for some people.

The third contributor to our daily energy expenditure is the most variable one, physical activity. As expected, there are considerable differences among people in their activity levels. According to Tataranni and Ravussin (2002, p. 47), sedentary adults lose 20%–30% of their calories through physical activity, which can even include things like fidgeting and maintaining posture and muscle tone. For example, in one study by Schulz and Schoeller (1994) in a population of about 300 "healthy adults," some heavier people were shown to be less physically active, but the researchers found "considerable variation in body fatness" even among those people who were sedentary. Tataranni and Ravussin (2002, p. 48) believe that an "inactive lifestyle" may be a contributing factor for obesity, but "Whether a low level of physical activity is a cause or a consequence of obesity" remains to be determined.

The importance of physical activity is covered in Chapter 8 ("Exercise"). Significantly, though, studies such as one by Rosenbaum et al. (2008) have confirmed that physical activity is extraordinarily important in the maintenance of any weight loss long term. Using highly controlled conditions on an inpatient metabolic unit—controlling for food intake and actual diet composition and exercise—these researchers noted that total energy expenditure did decrease after weight loss in both lean and obese subjects, and may even continue to do so indefinitely ("bioenergetic responses to maintenance of a reduced body weight do not wane over time ... beyond those predicted solely on the basis of changes in weight and body composition"), and that this may be a factor in weight regain (Rosenbaum et al. 2008). Because of this tendency for total energy expenditure (and particularly nonresting energy expenditure) to decrease, they noted that those who maintained their weight loss were those who maintained high levels of physical activity. The researchers say that their study confirms the "prolonged persistence of metabolic phenotypes in weight-reduced subjects."

Measuring the daily energy expenditure in these three major categories—RMR, thermogenesis, and physical activity—has provided a challenge for researchers, particularly outside a metabolic chamber. If a metabolic chamber is used in the laboratory, the two major methods are direct calorimetry (measuring total heat loss while the subject is in a confined space), now used mostly in animal experiments, and indirect calorimetry. In indirect calorimetry, the subject's oxygen consumption, carbon dioxide production, and nitrogen excretion are measured with the subject in a respiratory chamber (Tataranni and Ravussin 2002, p. 43). The body usually does not store oxygen or carbon dioxide, and, indirectly, the heat released by the body's chemical processes is calculated. Urinary nitrogen excretion, for example, is a function of protein oxidation.

The third technique for measuring daily energy expenditure is the doubly labeled water technique that uses two stable isotopes and calculates carbon dioxide production. This doubly labeled water technique, which requires samples of urine for the stable isotopes over the course of the measurement (usually 5–20 days), does not require cumbersome monitors and does not limit activity, since the person is not in any respiratory chamber. It is considered "the best and most accurate way of assessing" the energy involved in physical activity (Tataranni and Ravussin 2002, p. 45) It is a noninvasive technique—though expensive and not widely available—so it can be used more easily for pregnant women, children, and the elderly (Tataranni and Ravussin 2002, p. 45).

CARBOHYDRATES

We have cycled from a ubiquitous emphasis on increasing carbohydrate intake during the 1980s to 1990s to a renewed interest in low carbohydrate diets as a means of successful weight control in the first years of the new millennium. The consequences for consumer confidence in scientific research in this area have been catastrophic.

James Stubbs, Stephen Whybrow, and Nik M. Mamat (2008, p. 296)

Pollan (2007) makes the point that we cannot study food out of its context because we never really eat only one thing. In other words, he believes that "a whole food may be more than the sum of its nutrient parts" (Pollan 2007). Nevertheless, we can speak of food as divided into essentially three categories: carbohydrates, fats, and proteins. Pollan speaks of our being in the "age of nutritionism" (Pollan 2008, pp. 18–19): the subject of nutrition has become more of an ideology than a study of nutrition, and food constituents (i.e., macronutrients) seem to be at war with each other, "protein against carbs; carbs against proteins, and then fats; fats against carbs..." (p. 30), where there are always some evil nutrients battling against the good nutrients. Over the years, we have seen how some carbohydrates, like oat bran, have been glorified for a time, only to fall by the wayside; cholesterol, on the other hand, has been demonized, particularly eggs. Today trans fats (appropriately) are in that role. In his book *Fat Land: How Americans Became the Fattest People in the World*, Critser (2003, p. 53) notes how we use science to justify our food choices: "The very notion of self-control was anathema to the new generation of diet books. A diet—even a weight loss diet—was no longer about limits to one's gratification. Instead, the subtext was one of scientific entitlement."

> "Both protein and carbohydrate can be metabolically converted to fat, and there is no evidence that changing the relative proportion of protein, carbohydrate, and fat in the diet without reducing caloric intake will promote weight loss."
>
> Source: Rosenbaum et al. 2008

In the biblical book of Daniel, there is the story of King Nebuchadnezzar of Babylon: it is reported that when the king conquered Jerusalem, he ordered his chief of staff to bring some of the Israelites to serve in his palace:

> They were to be young men who were healthy, good-looking, knowledgeable in all subjects, well-informed, and intelligent....Four Judeans were among the chosen: Daniel, Hananiah, Mischael, and Azariah. The King arranged for them to get a daily allowance of his rich food and wine, but Daniel did not want to defile himself with such a diet and asked...[that] for ten days he and his companions be given only vegetables to eat and water to drink. After ten days, they looked healthier and stronger than the young men who had been eating the King's rich food. (Daniel 1:4–15)

Classification of Carbohydrates

Katz (2008, p. 3) makes the point that carbohydrates, whose main function is to provide a source of energy, supply between 50% and 70% of calories for human populations worldwide; the less developed the country, in general, the higher the percentage of carbohydrates eaten. There are several categories of carbohydrates: sugars, sugar alcohols (polyols), starches (amylopectin, which is rapidly digestible, and amylose, which is less rapidly digestible), and fiber (Wheeler and Pi-Sunyer 2008). Carbohydrates can also be divided into digestible forms (e.g., sugars and, when cooked, starches, such as legumes) and nondigestible forms (e.g., cellulose—dietary fiber from plants).

Typically, sugars are divided into the categories of simple and complex (polysaccharide) forms, though sometimes this division becomes more complicated by the processing of foods. Simple sugars can be monosaccharides, such as glucose, fructose (the sugar in fruit), and galactose, or disaccharides, like sucrose (common table sugar, consisting of one molecule of glucose and one of fructose), lactose (milk sugar, a molecule of galactose and one of glucose), and maltose, two molecules of glucose). In general, simple carbohydrates lead to a much faster rise in blood sugar than complex ones, and a subsequent rise in insulin, the hormone produced by the pancreas.

> ## CLASSIFICATION OF CARBOHYDRATES
>
> Carbohydrates: digestible and nondigestible
>
> Categories: sugars, sugar alcohols, starches, fiber
>
> *Sugars:* 4 cal/g; simple or complex
>
> Simple:
> - Monosaccharides, such as glucose, fructose, galactose
> - Disaccharides, such as sucrose (glucose plus fructose), lactose (galactose plus glucose)
>
> Complex:
> - Polysaccharides
>
> *Sugar alcohols:* 2 cal/g
>
> *Starches:* 4 cal/g; "gel-like carbohydrate molecules" with "glucose sugars linked in chains" (Nestle 2006, p. 319)
>
> *Fiber:* 1.5–2.5 cal/g
>
> **Source: Katz 2008; Nestle 2006**

One of the most popular added simple sugars today is high-fructose corn syrup, an unnatural and inexpensive product made from corn, rather than sugar beets or sugar cane, that is a combination of glucose and varying percentages of fructose (42% when used in canned sweetened fruits, 55% when used in sodas; see "High-Fructose Corn Syrup" section below). Carbohydrates supply 4 calories per gram.

Nestle (2006, p. 313) describes starches as "multiple chains of glucose molecules meshed together in a great jumble—a gel." Potatoes, rice, pasta, bread, and beans are examples of starches.

Sugar alcohols (e.g., maltitol, sorbitol, xylitol, mannitol) have, on average, only 2 calories per gram, as opposed to other carbohydrates that provide 4 calories of energy per gram (fat provides 9 cal/g and protein, ~4 cal/g). Because they do supply some calories, albeit fewer than other carbohydrates, they are still considered nutritive, but they are often used in so-called sugar-free products (see "Nonnutritive Sweeteners" below).

Glycemic Index

Havel (2005) notes that the National Academy of Sciences has recommended a diet that contains between 45% and 65% carbohydrates. (The academy also recom-

NUTRITIVE SUGARS

- Sugars contain 4 calories per gram.

- Glucose is the only sugar that the brain can use as fuel. When our blood glucose level is too low, we can experience coma, seizure, or even death. If the blood glucose level gets too high, glucose is excreted in the urine (diabetes). Chronically high blood glucose levels lead to kidney, eye, and cardiac disease.

- Sucrose is common table sugar. It is a combination of glucose and fructose and is made from sugar cane or sugar beets.

- Fructose is the sugar of natural fresh fruit. In small amounts, it is beneficial. Juices made from pears and apples contain more fructose than glucose and have been found to be a common cause of nonspecific diarrhea in children, whereas children sometimes tolerate the juice of white grapes, which has equal amounts of fructose and glucose. The body, however, is not used to the unnatural mixture used to manufacture inexpensive high-fructose corn syrup, found in sodas, cookies, and other processed goods.

- Lactose is glucose and galactose and is the sugar found in milk. As we age, many develop lactose intolerance, which causes gastrointestinal distress such as gas because of a decrease in the enzyme lactase, used to digest milk.

Source: Katz 2008; Nestle 2006; Valois et al. 2005

mends that 20%–35% of calories come from fat and 10%–35% from protein.) Some simple carbohydrates, though, such as pure glucose and white bread, are processed very quickly by the body. Says Hyman (2006, p. 46), "Eating white bread with pasta is like adding a tablespoon of sugar to a cola." The result is that we become hungry more quickly after eating these foods and experience less satiety, leading to the vicious circle of eating more. This is the concept of the *glycemic index*, a system for classifying foods containing carbohydrates that was established in the early 1980s by Jenkins et al. (1981). Ludwig (2007) considers the glycemic index an "empirical system" for classifying carbohydrates. It essentially eliminates the terms *simple sugar* and *complex carbohydrate* and instead focuses on what happens to glucose levels postprandially. Essentially, when someone eats a high-glycemic diet or even any food, says Ludwig (2007), there develops a cascade of "hormonal events that challenge glucose homeostasis."

Jenkins and colleagues compared all carbohydrates to pure glucose or white bread to assess the body's response, that is, how quickly other carbohydrates are broken down and converted to pure blood glucose after being eaten. Foods that are converted and absorbed more slowly cause less of a rise (or a slower rise) and a slower subsequent fall in blood glucose levels, and hence less of a rise and fall in insulin levels; this is the measure of a food's glycemic index value. Foods with a low glycemic index value therefore are less likely to cause hyperinsulinemia. Pure glucose and white bread have been assigned a glycemic index value of 100. Foods with a lower glycemic index value are often the carbohydrates that have more *fiber* and *water.* As Hyman says (2006, p. 51), "Fiber is like a sponge that soaks up fat and sugar." Ludwig (2002) makes the point that foods can differ by about fivefold in their variations in glycemic index values. The refined starchy foods have a high glycemic index value (>70) and include white potatoes, white rice, and many refined sugars, such as honey. Foods with lower glycemic index values include oatmeal made from steel-cut oats, brown rice, whole grains, sweet potatoes and other nonstarchy vegetables, nuts, and fruits. Low-glycemic foods have a value below 55.

More recently, Salsberg and Ludwig (2007) reported on actual molecular effects of a low-glycemic diet: there was a downregulation of hormone-sensitive lipase, an enzyme involved in the release of fatty acids from fat tissue. The researchers found that mice made deficient in this enzyme did not become obese, either by diet or genetic manipulations. The low-glycemic diet also downregulated transcription factor TCF7L2, the "strongest known genetic predictor of type 2 diabetes" (Salsberg and Ludwig 2007).

Many factors actually determine the glycemic index value of a particular carbohydrate: the amount of food is significant, as is the specific amount of carbohydrate compared to the amount of water or fiber in the food. This is the concept of *glycemic load*, the actual amount of a carbohydrate in a particular food in grams multiplied by the glycemic index value. Weil (2005) makes the point that many dieters avoid foods like carrots or beets because of their high glycemic index but they are missing the point of the importance of glycemic load: because of the water and fiber content, these foods have a much lower glycemic load and hence are perfectly fine to eat except in enormous quantities.

Many other things determine the glycemic value of a food, such as its physical form, particle size, degree of cooking, food processing, and what other foods are eaten with it. For example, steel-cut oats have a low glycemic index value, as noted above, whereas instant oatmeal (the same oats but prepared differently) has a much higher one. And eating protein or fat along with a high-glycemic food may lower its glycemic value, such as when one eats bread with peanut butter. Nestle (2006, pp. 314–315) also notes that the temperature of a food can affect its glycemic value: for example, cold boiled red potatoes have a glycemic index value of 56 (low) whereas the same boiled red potatoes served hot have a high glycemic index value of 89. We also eat foods in combination and in a sequence that can affect how the foods are absorbed. In other words, there are a great many variables involved in assessing the glycemic indices of foods. For example, it is often quite difficult for the typical dieter, outside a laboratory, to factor out how eating a combination meal (i.e., the typical way we eat), with varying temperatures and preparations, as well as different foods (e.g., salad and dressing, baked potato, steak, red wine, and chocolate cake), affects the total glycemic indices and loads. Sometimes, of course, a combination of foods can serve to benefit glucose homeostasis, as for example when someone eats a high-glycemic food such as a bagel with a food like peanut butter (fat, fiber, and protein) (Ludwig 2007). In general, though, calorie for calorie, individual foods with a high glycemic index stimulate more insulin secretion than those with a lower glycemic index (Ludwig 2002). In turn, this may lead to increased insulin resistance.

According to Ebbeling (2007) and her colleagues including Ludwig (2007), some people may also be more sensitive to the effects of the glycemic index because of their own insulin levels. Their study tested the efficacy of two different diets over a period of 18 months—40% carbohydrates and 35% fat versus 55% carbohydrates and 20% fat—paying particular attention to the glycemic load of the carbohydrates eaten. Both study groups were given dietary counseling and nutritional information, as well as motivational phone calls to increase adherence over time. They found that there was a subgroup of people who did much better in losing weight when the diet was specifically tailored to their metabolism: those dieters who had higher levels of insulin secretion initially after a test dose of oral glucose lost more weight and body fat and had lower cholesterol and triglyceride levels when using a low-glycemic diet than when using a low-fat diet. The researchers concluded that the reason some diets work better for some people than others is related to differences among people in their hormonal responses.

Ludwig (2002) believes that even though the importance of the glycemic index remains controversial for some nutritionists, there is a place for a low-glycemic diet in the treatment of diabetes, obesity, and cardiovascular disease and it certainly has no adverse effects. A 12-week study by McMillan-Price and her colleagues (2006) noted that glycemic load may be more important for weight loss in women than in men. The researchers noted that women generally tend to lose weight more slowly and have differences in glucose levels after eating, as well as differences in fat oxidation, compared with men. Their conclusion was that lower dietary glycemic load rather than just consuming fewer calories may lead to a faster rate of loss of fat, particularly in women, at least in the short run.

In a study by Liljeberg et al. (1999) in which breakfast cereals were compared for their glycemic index and load, researchers found that glucose tolerance could be improved in 1 day. The highest satiety level occurred in subjects given a barley cereal for breakfast. The investigators found that a prolonged digestive phase, such as what happens when a meal with low-glycemic foods is given, suppresses the release of fatty acids from the liver for a longer time and leads to improved glucose tolerance in the subsequent meal.

Tables of the glycemic values of foods, though, are not readily available and may be fairly impractical for some dieters, particularly with all the variables a dieter has to consider. And the calculations for glycemic load can be complicated. Wylie-Rosett et al. (2004) make the point that even the ripeness of a fruit can affect its glycemic index, so that, for example, different lists might include values for bananas ranging all the way from 30 to 70. Values for white durum wheat semolina spaghetti can vary from 46 to 65, depending on cooking time. And they found that

Kellogg's All-Bran cereal was listed in Australia as having a glycemic index value of 30—whereas the same cereal in Canada was listed at 51. Nevertheless, individuals who feel they may be particularly sensitive to the effects of some foods with a high glycemic index (i.e., they become hungrier more quickly and find themselves eating more) may find it worthwhile to consider this approach and even have their insulin levels measured.

High-Fructose Corn Syrup (HFCS)

Another problem that researchers (Wylie-Rosett et al. 2004) have found with the glycemic index is that it measures only glucose, whereas many carbohydrates in our diets today have other sugars, particularly HFCS. As mentioned earlier, HFCS is an unnatural and less expensive way to sweeten food than using sucrose; it is a composite of glucose and fructose in varying combinations, sometimes as high as 90% fructose. Whereas sucrose is a disaccharide molecule (a combination of fructose and glucose), HFCS is composed of two monosaccharides—glucose and fructose separately (Soenen and Westerterp-Plantenga 2007). In other words, it is composed of fructose and glucose in the free rather than bound form. Tsanzi et al. (2008) note that although fructose is absorbed more slowly than glucose, the presence of glucose enhances fructose absorption.

Tsanzi et al. (2008) question whether HFCS, as well as other sugars that are overconsumed, may affect mineral balance in bone and even possibly lead to osteo-

---

HIGH-FRUCTOSE CORN SYRUP

- An unnatural mixture of glucose and fructose (typically 42% or 55% fructose)

- Major sweetener for sodas, cookies, cakes because increases shelf life

- Invented in 1970s to get rid of excess U.S. corn supplies

- Too much fructose increases fat (triglycerides) in our blood

- Our bodies, evolutionarily, are not used to such high concentrations of fructose and these high concentrations may lead to an inability of the enzymes in our livers and intestinal tracts to metabolize them completely: we may get diarrhea, bloating, abdominal pain (irritable bowel), and eventually a fatty liver

- Diets very high in fructose impair the normal action of insulin and may promote the development of type 2 diabetes (insulin resistance)

- Long-term high fructose intake can contribute to decreased satiety and increased food intake

- Long-term high fructose consumption may even accelerate the aging process

Source: Critser 2003; Elliott et al. 2002; Gaby 2005; Havel 2005; Wylie-Rosette et al. 2004

porosis. They have reviewed studies and conclude that more research is required. Wylie-Rosett et al. (2004) note, for example, that HFCS produces a pattern of hormone response completely different from the one produced by glucose. They note that insulin is not increased, the satiety hormone leptin is reduced, and ghrelin, the hormone that creates the feeling of hunger, is not suppressed with fructose consumption (thereby often leading to a decreased sense of satiety). Soenen and Westerterp-Plantenga (2007), though, note that fructose can possibly lead to feelings of satiety differently, namely by its pattern of oxidation, an increased thermogenic response, and more rapid metabolism in the liver. They note that through the vagus nerve, the liver signals centrally to the brain to stop meal initiation. Fructose does not cross the blood-brain barrier, so, unlike pure glucose, it cannot be used as a fuel for the brain.

Havel (2005) notes that the National Academy of Sciences recommends that no more than 25% of our total calories come from added sweeteners. Most of the added sweeteners in U.S. diets today come from HFCS. HFCS was invented in the 1970s because of the surplus of corn in the United States (Critser 2003, pp. 10–11). Most of the sweetened sodas we drink (e.g., Coca-Cola, Pepsi) use HFCS. So do most of the packaged bakery goods and even salad dressings we find in our supermarkets. It is remarkable that HFCS has found its way into so many of our processed goods, even in products we think would not contain sugar.

Katz (2008, p. 112) makes the point that one of the dangers of HFCS is that it is so ubiquitously overused: he found that a brand of prepared marinara sauce had more added sugar than chocolate fudge ice cream when matched calorie for calorie. It primes us unnaturally to expect sweet tastes in foods we would not generally expect to be sweet. Our bodies, particularly our livers, though, are just not used to this high influx of fructose in this unnatural mixture. Natural fructose, in small quantities, as occurs in fruits, is healthy, and some nutritionists recommend it as a natural sweetener for people with diabetes because it does not negatively affect glucose levels in the blood. But HFCS is different. Because our capacity to absorb it is limited, it causes, in the short term, diarrhea, bloating, abdominal pain, and gas. However, many researchers, such as Gaby (2005), Havel (2005), and Elliott and colleagues (2002) independently have said they believe the long-term effects are much more dangerous. HFCS has been implicated in the obesity epidemic in this country and worldwide. It may even accelerate the aging process, because its metabolic breakdown produces toxic compounds. Further, it has been implicated in inducing insulin resistance and diabetes and even worsening the effects of the long-term complications of diabetes, such as those involving the kidneys, cardiovascular system, and eyes. Most noteworthy, HFCS has been implicated in leading to much higher levels of triglycerides in the bloodstream, which increase low-density lipoprotein (LDL; harmful cholesterol) levels. It may also lead to a fatty liver, sometimes a precursor to cirrhosis.

According to Wylie-Rosett et al. (2004), who reviewed the extensive literature, fructose can lead to a 3- to 15-fold increase in de novo lipogenesis in the liver, unlike glucose, which leads to hardly any. Furthermore, individuals with type 2 diabetes given fructose along with a high-fiber, high-carbohydrate, and low-fat diet had better glucose levels but actually gained weight. Havel (2005) also emphasizes that the hepatic metabolism of fructose leads to de novo lipogenesis and ultimately to increased triglyceride levels in the blood and heart disease. He believes that both short- and long-term overconsumption of fructose are responsible for promoting unfavorable lipid profiles. He explains that there is a link between lipid metabolism and ultimate insulin resistance: "circulating free fatty acids derived from triglycerides, as well as those synthesized locally, can lead to ectopic fat deposition in liver and skeletal muscle" (Havel 2005) and eventual insulin resistance.

Havel (2005) does note that fructose ingestion can induce glucose intolerance and insulin resistance in rats, though more long-term studies in humans are required. He also recommends further studies to investigate the consumption of large amounts of fructose in combination with a high-fat and high-calorie diet, as is typical of our modern diets, unlike the more controlled situation in the usual nutrition study. He makes the point that obesity has increased in incidence and prevalence in both adults and children during the time that there has been an extraordinary increase in fructose consumption, but notes that some people are more prone to these effects than others, whether biologically or even psychologically (i.e., their relationship to food and dieting) (Havel 2005). Elliott et al. (2002) emphasize that researchers' concerns regarding fructose should apply to HFCS and not to the natural fructose occurring alone in fruits.

As noted earlier, HFCS has been found to inhibit the production of the satiety hormone leptin, depriving the brain of the signal of fullness. That is why, with processed baked goods for example, those who are prone to eat an entire cake can do so and still not be satisfied. Ghrelin levels normally fall after a meal, but when a meal has a high load of HFCS, ghrelin levels do not fall as much. Insulin, leptin, and ghrelin are all involved in our short- and long-term energy balance and food intake. If anything, HFCS keeps giving the wrong signals to the brain.

Melanson et al. (2008) distinguish pure fructose, for which "scientific evidence suggests that high consumption … may be problematic to energy intake regulation," from HFCS, which is more like sucrose. These researchers also support the need for further studies to clarify whether, in fact, HFCS in the short term negatively affects energy balance or increases appetite more than other sweeteners.

Stanhope and Havel (2008) also note that fructose consumption, as opposed to glucose consumption, leads to decreased blood levels of both insulin and leptin. Their concern is that long-term consumption of diets high in fructose might lead to abnormal signaling of energy balance and hence increased intake of calories.

The research on HFCS, though, is confusing at best and overtly contradictory at worst. For example, White (2008), who is a consultant on HFCS and sugar to the food and beverage industry, takes issue with the harmful effects of HFCS. He states emphatically that HFCS has the same sugar composition as other fructose-glucose sweeteners, such as sucrose, honey, or fruit juice concentrates. Furthermore, he believes that the obesity epidemic is not related specifically to added sugars such as HFCS, but rather to our increased consumption of foods with fats, flour, and cereal as well. He also states that all fructose-glucose sweeteners are "metabolized through the same pathways regardless of dietary source" (White 2008).

Research on HFCS is particularly significant because most children today are enormous consumers, particularly in their soda intake. One of the major problems with HFCS-sweetened sodas is that children have become the major consumers of these products. Apovian (2004) notes liquid calories are "a relatively new addition to the human diet" and that a 12-ounce can of sweetened soda contains about 150 calories and 40–50 grams of sweetener.

Malik et al. (2006) conducted a MEDLINE search from 1966 to 2005 for cross-sectional studies of the relationship between sugar-sweetened beverages and weight gain. Their conclusion was that even though more research is required, there was "sufficient evidence" to indicate that a "greater consumption" of sugared beverages should be discouraged when advocating adopting a healthier lifestyle.

A study published in the journal *Circulation* in 2007 by researchers Dhingra and colleagues confirmed that soft drink consumption in middle-aged adults substantially increased their risk of developing a metabolic syndrome—a cluster of abnormalities including increased waist circumference (abdominal obesity), high fasting blood glucose levels, insulin resistance, insulinemia, increased blood pressure, increased triglycerides and other dyslipidemias (see "The Metabolic Syndrome" in Chapter 2). The study included over 6,000 people in their 50s who are all part of the Framingham Heart Study, the long-term study begun in 1948 in Framingham, Massachusetts, to study risks and behavior related to heart disease. This present component of the study, which consisted solely of "white Americans" (as described by the researchers), found that *only one 12-ounce can of soda a day* (e.g., Coke, Pepsi, Sprite) for a year was enough to lead to a significantly higher prevalence of this metabolic syndrome. What confounds and complicates their results, though, is that in addition to sugared sodas, diet sodas, which do not have HFCS in them, were associated with this effect. The result is puzzling, and clearly more research is needed. The researchers speculate that obviously other factors must be involved, including possibly the caramel content of both diet and sugared sodas, as well as other dietary behaviors among those who drink any kind of soda.

> "If daily consumption of liquid sugar (30 to 60 grams a day) can lead either to weight gain or to weight loss, then the discussion needs to shift from human psychology to human dietary behavior."
>
> **Source: Drewnowski and Bellisle 2007**

Drewnowski and Bellisle (2007) reviewed the conflicting literature on liquid calories, weight gain, and satiety, and they note that many of the low-calorie liquid meal replacement shakes have sugar or even HFCS as their principal ingredient, often in the same amount as in sugared soft drinks. And these liquid meal replacements, they say, with sugar contents as high as 36–72 grams of sugar, similar to the amount in 12-ounce cans of soft drinks, have been shown to be effective for some people in weight control. For example, they report that Slim-Fast, the liquid meal replacement, has 36 grams of sugar—providing 144 of its 220 total calories—in its 325-mL portion (just over 11 ounces). Drewnowski and Bellisle (2007) believe that the connection between obesity and sugar consumption, liquid or otherwise, may actually depend on many other factors, including "purpose, context, and mode of use" and even price. They quote studies in which those who tended to consume the most sugar-sweetened soft drinks had other harmful habits: they tended to exercise less and were twice as likely to be smokers. The point is that the situation is very complex and confusing, and we do not yet have the answers. Drewnowski and Bellisle (2007) advise that although psychological and even economic factors must be considered along with physiological ones when studying weight, human dietary behavior is also relevant. They summarize the confusion regarding liquid sugar intake and weight by noting, "the critical issue is not sugar metabolism but the way that sugar is used by the consumer." In other words, "successful weight management requires cognitive control" as well as a "healthy lifestyle" and calorie watching. A television commercial ran in December 2009, sponsored by the New York City Department of Health (www.NYC.gov/health), to emphasize the substantial caloric implications of drinking sugared soft drinks. In this commercial, a young, attractive man drinks from a soda can from which pours, not soda, but truly gross and disgusting globules of yellow fat. The accompanying warning is that drinking one can of soda or other sugared beverages a day can make someone 10 pounds heavier in a year. "Don't drink yourself fat," admonishes this very effective "Pouring on the Pounds" advertisement (which can be viewed on YouTube).

There has been a recent backlash by the Corn Refiners Association, a trade group representing the HFCS business, because some manufacturers have removed HFCS from their products (Vranica 2008). This group is waging an advertisement campaign to try to refute claims that its product is more dangerous than sucrose. Vranica notes that the American Medical Association has called for more research to assess the health effects of HFCS.

One small study of 34 subjects (18 men and 16 women) by Stanhope et al. (2008) has compared the metabolic effects of pure fructose, HFCS, sucrose, and pure glucose over a 24-hour period; researchers found that sucrose and HFCS do not have substantially different metabolic or endocrine effects. They found that the 24-hour postprandial levels of glucose, leptin, and ghrelin were not different when comparing the sweeteners HFCS and sucrose, though insulin levels were slightly higher in those who had eaten sucrose. They also found that fasting plasma levels of triglycerides taken the following morning were increased after both sucrose and HFCS, and men seem to be more sensitive in terms of triglyceride levels in that all four sugars increased their levels, at least transiently. Stanhope et al. (2008) note that studies have been inconsistent regarding whether sugars can cause long-term increases in triglyceride levels.

Levine et al. (2003) make the point, just as Pollan (2007) does, that we cannot really separate carbohydrate, protein, or fat when we are speaking of human diets: for example, people speak of "carbohydrate cravings" when, in fact, they are craving ice cream or candy that is high in both carbohydrates and fats. "This [separating dietary components] works only for the chemist" say the authors (Levine et al. 2003). But carbohydrates, and particularly sucrose, seem to have a special place in our brain reward system. (See "Reward, Cravings, and Addiction [Dopamine, Endocannabinoids]" in Chapter 4, "The Psychology of the Eater.") Studies do support the notion that sucrose may even substitute for drugs of abuse such as opiates and cocaine, by increasing dopamine levels in parts of the brain like the nucleus accumbens (Levine et al. 2003).

Levine et al. (2003) report on studies in which opiate blockers such as naloxone can decrease sucrose intake in rats. These researchers also note that carbohydrate intake may influence energy expenditure and even thermogenesis may be different with sucrose intake, with changes in the brain's neuropeptides such as corticotropin-releasing factor and neuropeptide Y. There is even reason to think that there is a specific glucose-sensing system. Eny et al. (2008) have reported that mice that no longer have the gene for glucose transporter type 2 (*GLUT2*) are not able to control their intake of glucose, "suggesting a potential role for this transporter as a glucose sensor in the brain." These researchers analogize the glucose-sensing system to the beta cells of the pancreas and the release of insulin. They note that the specific genotype (*GLUT2*-null genotype) does not affect intake of fat, protein, or even alcohol. It should not be surprising that specific glucose sensing occurs, inasmuch as glucose is the primary fuel used by the brain. The mechanisms involved are there to prevent hypoglycemia or hyperglycemia and to provide tight control of blood glucose levels.

Eny et al. (2008) describe research in two different human populations—men and women with early type 2 diabetes and young, healthy university students—in whom they found genetic variations of *GLUT2* that led to increased sugar intake in certain people. They hypothesized that *GLUT2*, by sensing glucose levels, contributes to differences in food intake in humans and "may explain individual differences in preference for foods high in sugar" (Eny et al. 2008). Marty et al. (2007) note that one of the important goals of research on weight today is to identify the complex neuronal network involved in glucose sensing; they believe there might be more than just one site involved.

Nonnutritive Sweeteners

One of the problems with our considerably higher intake of sugar over the years is the increased calorie content of foods, particularly soft drinks (liquid calories; e.g., in sodas), as noted above. The American Dietetic Association (2004) notes that nonnutritive sweeteners (providing essentially no calories) can, depending on our diet, lead to 340 fewer calories per day and 1 pound of weight loss in just 9 or 10 days. Mattes and Popkin (2009) call nonnutritive sweeteners "ecologically novel chemosensory signaling compounds" that can affect not only ingestion but also behavior. These researchers acknowledge that although these compounds are not toxic in the short run and do not lead to cancer, "their influence on appetite, feeding, energy balance, and body weight have not been fully characterized." At this point, though, they state that there is no clear evidence that nonnutritive sweeteners change osmotic balance in the body or augment brain signals regarding

---

NONNUTRITIVE SWEETENERS

Synthetic compounds with no caloric value. Most common are:

- Sucralose (Splenda): made from sucrose by adding chlorine atoms(!), it is 600 times sweeter than sucrose (table sugar), is poorly absorbed, and has no effect on insulin levels so can be used by diabetic persons; because it is stable when heated, it can be used in baking and is now found in many bakery goods; advertisements for Splenda say it is made from sugar, but it is clearly not a natural product

- Aspartame (NutraSweet, Equal): sweetener found in diet sodas; about 200 times as sweet as sugar; not heat stable so cannot be used in cooking; does have some effect on insulin levels

---

appetite. Nonnutritive sweeteners do, however, increase our preference for higher levels of sweetness in our foods, but "there is no substantive evidence that inherent liking for sweetness or nonnutritive activation of reward centers is problematic" (Mattes and Popkin 2009).

Over the years, there have been many sugar substitutes, nonnutritive sweeteners (also called *artificial sweeteners*) that provide essentially no calories, or considerably fewer calories than sugar. To date, five artificial sweeteners have been approved for use in the United States: saccharin, aspartame, acesulfame potassium, neotame, and, most recently, sucralose.

Saccharin, a synthetic compound with a bitter aftertaste marketed as Sweet'N Low, is about 500 times sweeter than table sugar (sucrose) and was the first of this group. It is not heat stable so it cannot be used in cooking. There were reports years ago of saccharin as a potential carcinogen, particularly associated with bladder cancer in animals when given in very high quantities, but the FDA subsequently removed it from its list of carcinogenic compounds (Katz 2008, p. 408). There have also been concerns about saccharin use during pregnancy because it can cross the placenta and actually remain in the fetus.

Another synthetic sweetener commonly used is aspartame, marketed as Equal or NutraSweet. It is about 200 times as sweet as table sugar and has been used since the early 1980s. For years, it was used in diet sodas. Aspartame does produce a glycemic response, though a smaller one than glucose (Katz 2008, p. 408). Because, like saccharin, aspartame is not heat stable it cannot be used in cooking. Concerns have been raised about its use during pregnancy, but the FDA has deemed it safe for use during pregnancy (American Dietetic Association 2004). Furthermore, it is contraindicated in persons with phenylketonuria, a rare disease in which a person cannot break down the amino acid phenylalanine, which is produced in the metabolism of aspartame. There have also been questions regarding the long-term safety of aspartame, including questions of high doses causing brain damage (as well as headaches and dizziness; American Dietetic Association 2004), but the most recent position of the FDA (U.S. Food and Drug Administration 2004) is that "[the] FDA has not determined any consistent pattern of symptoms that can be attributed to the use of aspartame, nor is the agency aware of any recent studies that clearly show safety problems."

Most recently, sucralose (marketed as Splenda) was created in the late 1990s. It is 600 times as sweet as table sugar, with virtually no calories because it is mostly not absorbed and is excreted unchanged. It can be used for baking and cooking because it is heat stable. It also does not produce any glycemic response, so people with diabetes can use it (Katz 2008, p. 408). Sucralose is manufactured from sucrose but chlorine is added. Sucralose has become extremely popular as a sugar substitute, and its manufacturers have advertised it as a natural substance "made from sugar." The sugar manufacturers, on the other hand, have begun a crusade to inform the public that sucralose is hardly as natural as table sugar. And manufacturers of other artificial sweeteners, such as Equal, have initiated a lawsuit against the manufacturer of Splenda, contending it is misleading the public (Browning 2007). They contend that Splenda is, in fact, as artificial as the other nonnutritive sweeteners. Browning (2007) reports that $1.5 billion is at stake in the artificial sweetener market. Apparently, the Sugar Association (an organization representing the sugar industry) is also suing the makers of Splenda for misrepresenting its product as natural.

The American Dietetic Association (2004) notes that the FDA has reviewed over 100 studies of sucralose and did not find evidence of carcinogenic, reproductive, or neurological risk for humans. One finding, though, that has appeared in the literature is that sucralose can lead to cecal enlargement, at least in the rat (Grice and Goldsmith 2000). The researchers believe that this does not have pathological significance and has not been seen in human subjects. Abou-Donia et al. (2008) reported that Splenda had adverse effects on the gastrointestinal system in rats: a 12-week administration of Splenda reduced beneficial bacteria in feces; increased fecal pH, which can modify absorption of drugs and nutrients; and had negative effects on the cytochrome P450 enzyme system responsible for metabolism of many drugs. The researchers concluded that Splenda may interfere with drug and nutrient bioavailability and may even lead to multidrug resistance, including resistance to anticancer agents, when used chronically. The researchers also noted that the rats gained weight during the course of the study on this nonnutritive sweetener.

Acesulfame-K is a heat-stable synthetic sweetener that is often used in a combination with other sweeteners. Though it can be used in cooking, it does not add bulk to foods as other sugars can do. Its brand names are Sunnet and Sweet One, and it is 200 times as sweet as sugar (Katz 2008, pp. 408–409) Neotame, made by the NutraSweet Company, is exceptionally sweet and is between 7,000 and 13,000 times sweeter than table sugar. Katz (2008, pp. 408–409) notes it is a derivative of phenylalanine but because of its metabolism, it can be used safely with those people who have the genetic enzyme deficiency that causes the serious brain-damaging disease phenylketonuria.

Another nonnutritive sweetener, considered natural, is stevia. Derived from the leaves of *Stevia rebaudiana*, a South American plant, it is 200–300 times sweeter than table sugar. It can be purchased as a dietary supplement but it has not been approved by the FDA (Katz 2008, p. 409). Rebiana, one of the components of the plant stevia, has no calories or aftertaste and is currently being developed commercially by the Coca-Cola Company and Cargill, Incorporated (Prakash et al. 2008). Another component of stevia is rebaudioside A, which has been tested in humans with type 2 diabetes and found to be well tolerated. Some initial reports suggested that it could have a positive effect on insulin levels and blood pressure in people with type 2 diabetes, but in the first long-term trial (16 weeks) by Maki et al. (2008), conducted at six research sites and involving 122 people, there were no differences in insulin levels or blood pressure levels when subjects were given 1,000 mg of rebaudioside A per day. This dosage is considered about seven times the amount that would normally be consumed. The substance was reasonably well tolerated, though gastroenteritis was reported in some subjects. Maki et al. (2008) note that hemoglobin A_{1c} is the standard accepted measure to assess glycemic control in diabetic patients: a typical red blood cell has a 120-day life cycle, during which glucose binds to the A_{1c} form of hemoglobin. Hemoglobin A_{1c} represents a person's average blood glucose level during those 120 days. Normally, healthy people have 4%–6% levels of hemoglobin A_{1c}, and the American Diabetes Association recommends a level of less than 7% for diabetic patients. Rebaudioside A had no effect on hemoglobin A_{1c} (Maki et al. 2008).

As noted above, sugar alcohols, such as sorbitol, xylitol, maltitol, and mannitol, often used to sweeten chewing gum and often considered

SUGAR ALCOHOLS

- Have 2 calories per gram; used to add texture, bulk, and stabilization to products

- Most are less sweet than sugar: sorbitol, mannitol, D-tagatose, maltitol

- Xylitol is as sweet as sugar

- Several have laxative effect (flatulence, diarrhea) when eaten in great quantities

nonnutritive sweeteners, have about 2 calories per gram (unlike table sugar, at 4 cal/g). They are thought to produce lower glycemic responses (Wheeler and Pi-Sunyer 2008), although Wylie-Rosett and colleagues (2004) report that some of these sugar alcohols, such as maltitol, can produce the same glycemic response as pure glucose and have to be taken into account, particularly when used to sweeten "sugar-free" products. These researchers caution that the *net carbohydrate count*— in which fiber and sugar alcohols are not counted because they are not completely metabolized by the body—is more of a marketing strategy for dieters to promote foods as "low carb" or even "dietetic." And this labeling encourages dieters to eat more of these so-called healthier products, leading, unfortunately, to their consuming more calories. These sugar alcohols are also used as bulking agents to give food texture. They also apparently have less risk of producing dental cavities than sugared products, which can be acidogenic in dental plaque (Lineback and Jones 2003). Katz (2008, p. 409) notes that xylitol, in particular, has antibacterial properties and has been reported to prevent cavities. In excess, though, these sugar alcohols may have a laxative effect and can produce flatulence, diarrhea, and bloating. Other natural substances that are noncaloric and used for bulking agents are fibers such as guar gum, pectin, inulin, and cellulose, as well as polydextrose, maltodextrin, and polysaccharide polyols (American Dietetic Association 2004).

Another issue with nonnutritive sweeteners is the question of whether exposure to noncaloric sweet taste, usually associated with calorie-dense foods, may impair energy regulation. Swithers and Davidson (2008) note that both animals and humans associate tastes, flavors, and textures of food (the *orosensory cues*) with what they call the "postingestive caloric or nutritive consequences of eating." They explain that ingestion of sweet tastes results in many hormonal, metabolic, and thermogenic cephalic-phase reflexes that enable the body to anticipate and prepare for the nutrients. In turn, these reflexes may increase the efficiency of nutrient utilization and even minimize their disturbance to homeostasis. In other words, sweet tastes have always signaled to the body that calories are coming.

Swithers and Davidson (2008) hypothesize that nonnutritive sweeteners may weaken this signal (or *predictive relationship*) and thereby lead to disturbances in control of food intake and, ultimately, weight control. The researchers conducted a series of experiments with rats and found that rats that were fed lower-calorie foods such as yogurt or chocolate-flavored Ensure nutrition drink that had been sweetened with nonnutritive (called *nonpredictive*) sweeteners actually gained more weight (increased fat) than rats that were fed predictive sweetened foods. These rats were less able to compensate for calories later when given a subsequent meal. Say the researchers: "The results demonstrated that, in comparison with rats for which the sweet taste did predict an increase in calories, rats that received the nonpredictive sweet-taste caloric relationship exhibited greater caloric intake, greater body weight gain, increased body adiposity, an impaired ability to compensate for the calories contained in a novel sweet food by eating less during a subsequent test meal, and a smaller increment in core body temperature following consumption of a novel, sweetened high-calorie food" (Swithers and Davidson 2008). They also note, for example, that insulin is generally released preabsorptively when sweet foods are eaten and energy dysregulation in humans has been linked to reduced insulin release, either preabsorptively or with cephalic-phase release. They speculate that the thermogenic response to food is mediated by insulin release. They also note that other researchers have found that the thermogenic effect of food is lessened when meals are given irregularly. In other words, they speculate that when mealtimes are difficult to predict, the usual temporal cues associated with eating are not present and hence thermic reflexes are also lessened.

Along these lines, researchers Frank et al. (2008) note that sucrose seems to activate different human taste pathways than artificial sweeteners do. In their experiments, they compared sucralose with sucrose. Their hypothesis was that a nonnutritive sweetener like sucralose would stimulate taste and reward pathways less than sugar and create an "activated but maybe unsatisfied reward system." In their small study, using functional magnetic resonance imaging, they noted that the brain was able to distinguish the caloric from the noncaloric sweetener. In addition, though, there were variations among subjects in how they rated different levels of sweetness: among women, for some a greater sweetness was less pleasant. In general, higher sucrose concentrations were regarded as syrupy and less pleasant, and the researchers believed this might be a safeguard against consuming too much sugar. They question whether a noncaloric sweetener such as sucralose may activate taste sensation but without this safeguard mechanism, leading to a less satisfying "sweet-tooth" experience. They also believe that sucralose may stimulate the brain reward system faster or more efficiently but "not provide the calories and thus [provide] no natural feedback mechanism of biologic satiety" (Frank et al. 2008).

Fiber

Fiber, the indigestible part of a plant, is classified as a complex carbohydrate. It has 1.5–2.5 calories per gram. Fiber is either soluble (dissolves in water), such as legumes, fruits, and oats, or insoluble, as found in whole grains (e.g., whole or ground seeds of plants such as wheat). Says Hyman (2006, p. 94), "If you can squish bread with your hands you shouldn't eat it. Whole grain bread is very dense and cannot be squished." Both soluble and insoluble fiber may make food seem more filling (increase its satiating effect). Katz (2008, p. 513) makes the point that soluble fiber can delay absorption of glucose and

> **WHAT IS FIBER?**
>
> - Also called *roughage*, it is a carbohydrate mostly found in plants.
>
> - Fiber can be *soluble*, as in dried beans, oat bran, barley, apples, oranges, and potatoes, or *insoluble*, as in whole grains, seeds, nuts, and fruit and vegetable peels.
>
> - Fiber is not easily digested by the body and acts as a sponge soaking up fat and sugar; it is excreted in our stools.

fatty acids in the gastrointestinal tract, so that it lessens the rise in insulin levels after eating and can lower serum lipid levels. As a result, fiber has a role in diabetes control. Examples of soluble fiber are guar gum, psyllium (the major component of the product Metamucil, used to promote bowel regularity and prevent constipation), pectin, and β-glucan. Katz (2008, p. 513) notes that insoluble fiber (e.g., cellulose and lignins) can increase bulk in the feces and can decrease the time food spends in the gastrointestinal system (transit time). One of the reasons that fiber may be so satiating is that it requires chewing and takes longer to eat (Drewnowski and Bellisle 2007). High fiber intake has been reported to reduce the risk of large bowel diseases like cancer and diverticulosis (Katz 2008, p. 513). The Institute of Medicine (2008) recommends a daily intake of at least 25 grams of fiber; Katz (2008, p. 513) notes that up to 38 grams daily is recommended as a guideline for adults. Most Americans get considerably less. There is speculation that primitive humans ate more than 100 grams of fiber each day (Katz 2008, p. 514).

Research by Samra and Anderson (2007) demonstrated that the insoluble fiber in a high-fiber cereal such as Fiber One reduced appetite and actual food intake and improved the postprandial glucose response to a meal served later. They believe the insoluble fiber works in the small intestine because it increases the rate of transit in the small intestine and subsequently reduces the absorption of the starch. Insoluble fiber also increases cholecystokinin, a hormone that increases satiety. The researchers suggest that breakfast cereal with insoluble fiber can therefore have a role in weight loss and control. As Katz said (2008, p. 7), "While sugar added to a whole grain breakfast cereal or to a candy bar is the same in both cases, its metabolic fate is influenced by the company it keeps." Digestible complex carbohydrates have to be broken down (hydrolyzed) in the human gut to simple forms for absorption.

Constipation

As people age, they often report changes in their bowel movements, in that movements can become less frequent and stools can become harder. Patel and Lembo

CONSTIPATION

- Affects 2% to 28% of older people, but up to 50% of nursing home populations; can be intermittent or chronic; usually diagnosed if three or fewer stools a week, but diagnostic criteria can vary, so prevalence depends on definition and demographics

- Can be due to effects of bad eating habits, medications (e.g., antidepressants), aging, and even some medical conditions (e.g., neurological disease, hypothyroidism)

- Stool softeners, which add water to the stool, such as Colace (docusate sodium), can be effective

- Bulk laxatives, such as psyllium (e.g., Metamucil) daily, with additional fiber (bran, some fruits and vegetables) and water, are usually effective

- Stimulant laxatives, which increase intestinal motility and change electrolyte transport, can be effective; when abused (e.g., by those with an eating disorder), they can lead to dangerous, life-threatening electrolyte imbalances

- Older treatments include castor oil and milk of magnesia

Source: Patel and Lembo 2006; Wald 2006

(2006, pp. 221 ff.) note that constipation varies widely in prevalence, depending on its definition and the demographics of the population, and can affect from 2% to 28% of a general population, whereas it can affect up to 50% of a nursing home population. For reasons that are unknown, the symptom is more common in women.

Wald (2006) has reviewed some of the common misconceptions regarding constipation. For example, he notes that daily bowel movements are not necessary or important for health and "toxins" do not need to be emptied from the colon as commonly believed. Says Wald, "a daily bowel movement is not the gold standard for the adult population." Furthermore, Wald notes that chronic constipation does not necessarily result from too little dietary fiber, insufficient fluid intake, or even lack of exercise, although sufficient amounts of all of these are "healthy choices." Wald notes that increased fluid intake, for example, increases the amount of urine produced but does not increase the weight of stool. He also debunks the notion that the chronic use of stimulant laxatives is unsafe or damaging to the colon, nor do these laxatives induce habituation or necessarily lead to physical dependence on them. Of course, if laxatives are abused, as in their excessive use by patients with anorexia nervosa in order to induce weight loss, they can lead to life-threatening electrolyte imbalances.

Constipation may have many different causes, including medications and even neurological disorders. Physicians do not always agree on the definition of constipation, and patients need to clarify what they mean by it as well. One standard diagnosis is three or fewer bowel movements in a week. Constipation can also be either intermittent or chronic. Many medications are constipating, such as the older antidepressant amitriptyline. Sometimes a stool softener, such as Colace (docusate sodium), which acts by allowing water to enter the stool, is sufficient treatment. Dietary fiber, increased water intake, and bulk laxatives, such as psyllium (e.g., Metamucil), used on a daily basis, are also usually effective enough in most people with constipation. Too much fiber, however, can lead to bloating and gas. And because psyllium is a plant husk, some sensitive people may develop acute allergic reactions with tightness in the throat, cough, itching, and even an asthmatic reaction (Patel and Lembo 2006, pp. 221–254; Wald 2006).

WATER

Water is another substance that can make a food seem more satiating. Dehydration is an underlying—though underestimated—culprit, particularly in certain disease states, during strenuous exercise, and in unusually hot climates. Humans, depending on their nutritional and body fat status, can survive without food for weeks or even months at a time if they have water. Askew (2007, p. 1446) has noted that if deprived completely of water, we can live only 6–14 days, depending on the rate of water loss.

The human body has an exquisite homeostatic system for water regulation, involving primarily the kidneys (secretion of renin and angiotensin) and the endocrine system, including the hypothalamus (secretion of antidiuretic hormone and vasopressin). Our body weight is approximately 50%–70% water; even muscles (80%) and the brain (75%) are mostly water, and bones are 25% water (Valtin 2002). We have water within and outside our cells, including in our blood plasma, which is 85% water. Cells can either shrink or swell depending on the water's osmolarity, or specific concentration of salt per liter. Boschmann et al. (2007) describe how extracellular hyperosmolarity leads to cell shrinkage and extracellular hypo-osmolarity leads to cellular swelling. Water drinking can influence this. When body fluids fall below an optimal level (volume depletion), the body enters a toxic state. This causes imbalances in vital electrolytes like sodium and potassium and disturbed brain chemistry. As a result, a variety of signs and symptoms, including dizziness, lethargy, brain swelling, delirium, and even coma and death, can occur.

Drinking water can even lead to increased thermogenesis, that is, an increase in the number of calories used by the body's organs for digestion and absorption. Not all researchers agree, however. But in a small study by Boschmann et al. (2007), researchers found that water drinking increased fat oxidation in nonobese men and carbohydrate oxidation in nonobese women. They noted that obese subjects did not have the same responses to water, that is, they did not have differences in rates of fat and carbohydrate oxidation. Their speculation was that "obese subjects may be less able to switch between carbohydrates and lipid oxidation." The researchers call this phenomenon *metabolic inflexibility*. In general, though, Boschmann et al. (2007) believe that water induces activation of the sympathetic nervous system secondarily to local changes in gastrointestinal organs such as the liver and/or altered activity of the body's sensors (neural osmosensitive receptors) of osmolarity.

How much water do we really need to drink each day? The standard wisdom is that we all require eight 8-ounce glasses of water per day (2 quarts, or 1.9 liters) and that beverages such as soda, juices, coffee, and alcohol do not count. The nutritionist Nestle (2006, p. 401) notes that most people need to drink 2 or more quarts of water per day, or about 1 quart of water for every 1,000 calories we eat, because we lose water when we breathe, sweat, and excrete. Valtin (2002) takes issue with this common admonition. Writing in the journal of the American Physiological Society, Valtin attempted to trace the origin of this recommendation to drink eight glasses of 8 ounces of water a day by performing a comprehensive search of the literature and could not find any scientific validation for it. He acknowledges that some studies have reported that certain conditions, such as bladder cancer, kidney stones, or colorectal cancer or polyps, seem to be less prevalent in those who have a high daily fluid intake, but the correlations may not necessarily be causal and there may be gender differences as well. Negoianu and Goldfarb (2008), supporting Valtin's conclusions, even wonder, "Are people sick because they drink less, or are they drinking less because they are sick?" The evidence is not in. Furthermore, Valtin emphasizes that other liquids, like coffee, juices, soda, and even beer consumed in moderation, "should indeed count" in our daily fluid intake tabulation.

Valtin (2002) also addresses the notion that water—particularly when incorporated into food, as in soups, though not necessarily when drunk along with it—can lead to satiety, but he says it is not clear how long that effect lasts or exactly how much liquid is required. He even takes issue with the commonly held belief that a high fluid intake can relieve constipation, and he debunks the myth that by the time a person is thirsty, he or she is already dehydrated: the body is just too sensitive to subtle changes in plasma osmolarity. He said, "It is hard to imagine that evolutionary development left us with a chronic water deficit that has to be compensated [for] by forcing fluid intake" (Valtin 2002). Ultimately, Valtin concludes that there is no convincing evidence that all healthy adults in temperate climates who are not exercising strenuously require those eight glasses of water daily. He even believes that so much liquid for some people may be dangerous and may lead to hyponatremia (dilution of sodium in the blood) as well as unnecessary exposure to pollutants, and may make people feel guilty for not drinking enough.

Negoianu and Goldfarb (2008) note that people are different in regard to water retention capacities: even the speed with which water is taken in can matter. They note that a large amount of the water drunk in 15 minutes is excreted whereas the same amount over several hours is largely retained. They also note that when water is mixed with a poorly absorbed sugar (e.g., nonnutritive sugars as in diet sodas), it is mostly retained because absorption is slowed from the gut, but water mixed with an easily absorbed sugar is mostly excreted. These researchers conclude that there is "no clear evidence of lack of benefit" from drinking increased amounts of water. "In fact, there is simply a lack of evidence in general" (Negoianu and Goldfarb 2008, p. 2).

But what about bottled water? A very common sight, at least in New York City, is people carrying huge bottles of water with them on the streets, as if they were crossing the Sahara rather than Madison Avenue. Nestle (2006, p. 403) herself admits she cannot decide whether bottled water is any safer than tap water in most parts of the country. She explains that tap water is often not pure but many bottled waters may not be much safer: they may have come into contact with industrial wastes, sewage, and agricultural contaminants, so there may be chemicals as well as harmful bacteria in them. Further, writer Ian Williams, as stated in his 2004 article "Message in a Bottle," thinks that all these plastic bottles are wreaking havoc on the environment. He equates this hype for bottled water to a scheme years ago when a businessman sold "tins of fresh Scottish air" to people in London. Williams debunks the notion of water from melted glaciers being healthful by questioning why people would want to drink water that has been "lying around from the last Ice Age... collecting dioxins, lead, radioactive fallout, polar bear poop and... the occasional dead Inuit or Viking" (Williams 2004).

And writer Jon Mooallem (2007, p. 35) quotes market researcher Michelle Barry: "We believe bottled water has become less about the physical act of hydration and more about being a companion to people. They like to walk around with it and hold it." Mooallem adds, "Each bottle of water is one in a readily available cast of interchangeable security blankets that we can capriciously acquire and toss throughout the day." Of course, that is exactly the opposite of the real intention and purpose of D. W. Winnicott's original concept of the transitional object, or security blanket: it is not interchangeable (even its smell is important), as it represents an extension of the mother (Winnicott 1953).

Nestle's solution (2006, p. 405) is to put a water filter on your tap in the sink. Note that in July 2007 PepsiCo, Inc., admitted that the bottled water it sells under the brand name Aquafina is actually tap water ("Aquafina labels to tell water's source" 2007). The new labels will have *P.W.S.* on them, which stands for "public water source."

ENERGY DENSITY

Both water and fiber contribute to the weight of food. Besides the number of calories in food, some researchers have begun to pay attention to the *energy density* of food—the number of calories in a certain weight of food. Though Americans are used to weighing their food in ounces, our packaging on labels often gives calories in grams (just to confuse us further). It is important to remember that there are 28 grams in an ounce.

Energy density is a concept made popular by Barbara Rolls (2005), who noted that in order to feel full, people are much more likely to eat the same quantity (volume) of food each day than to eat the same number of calories. Her theory is called *volumetrics*. To calculate the energy density of a certain food, divide the number of calories in the food by its weight in grams. The lower the number, the better. For example, nonfat milk and certain fruits and vegetables have a very low energy density because they have a high percentage of water, whereas pretzels and bread have a medium energy density, and cookies, chips, and nuts have a high energy density. By adding water and/or fiber to a food, you can lower its energy density. It is important not to be fooled when packaging notes that a product, such as milk, is only 1% fat: it means its fat content is 1% by weight, and most of the weight is water, so it is always important to check the number of grams of fat to know how many calories are actually from fat.

Soups and stews are often very filling. In one small study in France several years ago, researchers Himaya and Louis-Sylvestre (1998) found that giving both lean and overweight subjects a bowl of chunky soup prior to their main lunch reduced their hunger and hence what else they ate for lunch; in the overweight subjects, it even reduced how much food they ate for dinner. The more water a food naturally contains, the fewer calories per ounce or gram it has, as in fresh fruit, vegetables, and yogurt. B. Rolls et al. (1999) found, though, unfortunately, that drinking water with these foods does not have the same effect of lowering their energy density as when the water is actually part of the food itself. She and her colleagues presented 24 lean subjects with different choices: chicken and rice casserole, chicken and rice casserole with a glass of water, and chicken and rice soup, all of which had exactly the same ingredients. The researchers found that significantly fewer calories were consumed (26% fewer) by subjects who ate the chicken and rice soup than by those who ate the casserole with or without a glass of water on the side.

B. Rolls et al. (1999) acknowledge that sometimes our beliefs about the ability of a food to satisfy us may be a contributing factor; in other words, there is a certain amount of food that is considered to be satiating. Though the researchers found that drinking a large quantity of water with a meal did not decrease the number of calories subsequently eaten, they acknowledge not having data to assess the effect of drinking large quantities of water over a longer time than just at the time of the meal. Further, they note that drink-

> **WHAT IS ENERGY DENSITY?**
>
> - Energy density is the number of calories in a certain weight of food, often given in grams (28 g/oz)
>
> - To calculate energy density, divide the number of calories in a quantity of food by its weight in grams; the lower the number, the better (e.g., nonfat milk and certain fruits and vegetables have very low energy density, 0–0.6, whereas cookies, chips, and nuts have high energy density, 4.0–9.0)
>
> - Water and fiber added to food lower its energy density (e.g., vegetable-based dishes, chunky soups)
>
> - Energy densities:
>   - Fat: 9 cal/g
>   - Protein and carbohydrates: 4 cal/g
>   - Fiber: 2 cal/g
>   - Alcohol: 7 cal/g
>
> **Source: B. Rolls 2005, pp. 17–19**

ing a glass of water involves thirst mechanisms different from hunger mechanisms involved in eating a food containing much water.

Stubbs et al. (2000) take issue with the concept of energy density as the key factor in the regulation of food intake. They feel such a concept is premature and also simplistic. From work with many species, they feel it is "difficult to reconcile [all the data on] nutrient intake with an explanation solely based on dietary energy density." These researchers note that observations about energy density usually are made exclusively in the laboratory in very-short-term studies or are based on cross-sectional examinations of diet records. They believe that energy density may then tend to "assume overriding importance" in these short-term conditions. In other words, they believe that "the apparent tendency for subjects to eat a relatively constant weight of food, when averaged on a daily basis across experimental treatments, may not be the same as saying people eat a constant weight of food from day to day in general." In fact, Stubbs et al. (2000) believe that food intake for most people is not the same from day to day.

Energy-dense foods are often preferred by many people and considered more palatable. Stubbs et al. (2000) define *palatability* of food as "its sensory capacity to stimulate ingestion of that food." Palatability, then, is determined by a food's smell, color, taste, texture, and state as well as by "the sensory capabilities and metabolic state of the subject, and the environment in which the food and subject interact." Furthermore, palatability is not stable but often declines for a food after some of it has been ingested. This is the notion of *sensory-specific satiety* (see Chapter 4, "The Psychology of the Eater"). Stubbs et al. conclude that although both humans and animals do seem to prefer foods with greater energy density, these preferences are not fixed, "so motivation to eat is not necessarily a simple function of weight or volume of food consumed." And they say there is not much evidence that reducing the energy density of someone's diet actually leads to spontaneous weight loss by itself. In conclusion, "replacing one simplistic single-factor model (high fat food makes you fat) with another equally simplistic single-factor model (energy density makes you fat) will not solve the complex problems of current trends in human appetite and energy balance."

PROTEINS

Another major food group besides carbohydrates is proteins. As a rule, humans need a minimum of 65–70 grams of protein per day (Melanson and Dwyer 2002, p. 252). Protein typically has 4 calories per gram, so just under 300 calories a day should be the very minimum that come from protein. A survey done by nutritionist Nestle (2006, p. 143) found that women typically report eating about 70 grams of protein per day whereas men report eating about 100 grams per day. Neither too much protein nor too little is good for humans (as we explain below). A protein deficiency can lead to cardiac, skin, and kidney abnormalities, as well as hair loss, lethargy, fluid and electrolyte imbalances, and exercise intolerance (Melanson and Dwyer 2002, p. 261). Katz (2008, p. 23) makes the point that we need protein in our diets as a source of "essential" amino acids for the synthesis and repair of cells throughout the body. (Amino acids are either *essential*, those that our bodies do not produce naturally and that must therefore come from our diets, or *nonessential*, those that our bodies do produce. Amino acids are even the building blocks for DNA synthesis.) Our protein needs change as we age, and except in pregnant and lactating women, in disease states, during infection, and after surgery—situations in which we have a greater need for protein—we tend to need less protein after adolescence (Katz 2008, p. 25).

Too much protein, though, can be detrimental. Because proteins contain nitrogen, when they are broken down in the body the waste products ammonia and urea are ultimately produced. These products can be toxic if they build up in the body, particularly when the liver or kidneys are not functioning well. Katz (2008, p. 21) emphasizes that protein restriction may be required in persons with hepatic or renal disease.

Many believe that proteins are the most satiating food group and that after a high-protein meal, people usually feel full for a longer time and even eat less later. Blundell and Stubbs (2004, p. 441), however, note that experimentally, all nutrients "have equal power to suppress subsequent energy intake." They note that results have been quite contradictory: some researchers have shown that proteins do suppress hunger to a greater extent, whereas other reports indicate that fats and carbohydrates do; and while some believe fats are the most satisfying, still others say that fat is the least satisfying.

Blundell and Stubbs (2004, pp. 441–442) report on experiments in animals and humans that show that when subjects either have a particular nutrient delivered directly to their stomachs (animals) or swallow the nutrient quickly while wearing noseplugs (humans), fats, carbohydrates, and proteins are all equally satiating. They note that sensory input, particularly taste, may play some role in identifying the nutrient to the subject and that some associative learning may be involved. Blundell and Stubbs (2004, p. 442) further report on experiments in which protein is particularly satiating only when given in large amounts (31%–54% of the meal). They hypothesize that the specific kind of amino acid in the protein may play some role in its satiating effects. Furthermore, they note that energy intake (i.e., number of calories taken in) may be affected by lean body mass. They note when people lose weight, they lose both fat and (sometimes) lean tissue. Afterward they may develop hyperphagia. When they tend to eat and regain the weight, they often gain back much more fat tissue but do not stop gaining weight until the lean tissue is replenished. They speculate that it is the regulation of lean body tissue, "which helps maintain normal physiological function...through oxidation of excess and repletion of deficits in protein intake, [that] may exert some negative feedback effect on longer-term energy intake" (Blundell and Stubbs 2004, p. 443).

In a study by Westerterp-Plantenga et al. (2004), about 150 overweight to moderately obese men and women were placed on a calorie-restricted diet for 4 weeks, after which they were assigned to groups given varying percentages of protein in their diets. Those given the highest amount of protein after weight loss (18% protein intake during maintenance vs. 15%; i.e., 20% more protein in the maintenance phase) regained 50% less body weight, and the weight gained was lean body tissue rather than fat (and hence they had a lower percentage of body fat). In other words, additional protein in the maintenance phase led to a different body composition in those subjects, as well as lower energy efficiency, probably due to higher diet-induced thermogenesis, and increased satiety. Further, the researchers noted that blood levels of leptin, which typically fall with weight loss, increased significantly more slowly in those given additional protein in the maintenance phase.

A more recent article (Clifton et al. 2008) also supports a role for high-protein diets in maintaining weight loss. This study had a 64-week follow-up. Significantly, though, of the original 119 overweight and obese women, 40 withdrew before the end of the study (17 on a high-protein diet and 23 on a high-carbohydrate diet), so only 79 subjects remained at the end. The researchers reported that weight loss was greater in the subjects who consumed a higher-protein diet (both when counting grams of protein and when considering percentage of total calories). Both groups, though, had health benefits such as lowered levels of cholesterol, glucose, insulin, and C-reactive protein (a marker for heart disease).

Dulloo and Jacquet (1999) reanalyzed earlier data to find whether individual responses to variations in protein diets may be markers to "unmask" possible genetic or metabolic differences in susceptibilities to weight gain. There is no question that sometimes different people fed the same number of calories respond differently to the calorie load: some gain weight and others do not gain or gain less. Obviously, many factors are at play. These researchers evaluated their results in terms of thermogenesis. They question why the same person "can apparently dispose of a considerable excess of energy when the diet is low in protein, but [can do so] to a much lesser extent when the dietary protein level is adequate" (Dulloo and Jacquet 1999).

The researchers note that protein deficiency has evolved to be a potent stimulus for thermogenesis, and over the course of evolution this has had survival value in times of nutrient-deficient diets. In other words, the ability to increase diet-induced thermogenesis during such times enabled us to get enough specific nutrients without accumulating excessive fat that might be "a hindrance to optimal locomotion, hunting capabilities, and the ability to fight or flight." Dulloo and Jacquet (1999) theorize that there is not much individual variation in thermogenesis when diets are balanced but that much more variation is found when people are overfed unbalanced diets, particularly low-protein ones. They suggest that a challenge of overfeeding with a low-protein diet, therefore, may serve as a "magnifying glass" to evaluate a particular individual's susceptibility to weight gain.

Many of the diets that recommend high protein intake for weight loss are diets with increased fat intake and carbohydrate restriction. States of hypoglycemia cause metabolic stress because of the brain's need for and sensitivity to levels of glucose specifically. Katz (2008, p. 73) makes the point that extreme carbohydrate restriction has its own problems, some of which are specific to protein and some specific to the carbohydrate restriction itself, such as constipation from lack of any appreciable fiber.

A high intake of protein, on the other hand, with low levels of glucose (i.e., carbohydrate restriction) may, over the course of several hours, cause the formation of ketone bodies and a state of ketosis. Ketones are formed in the liver from the breakdown (oxidization products) of fatty acids. Whereas other tissues can use fatty acids (released by adipose tissue) as fuel, the brain cannot; glucose or its breakdown products are required by the brain for protection from hypoglycemia (Foster and Rubenstein 1983, p. 682).

Foster and McGarry (1983, p. 493) note that amino acids from the breakdown of protein stimulate the release of insulin from the pancreas, but also stimulate the release of glucagon from the liver. Foster and McGarry (1983, p. 493) also note that glucagon is able to prevent hypoglycemia when insulin is stimulated by the dietary intake of protein, when the diet has limited or no carbohydrate intake simultaneously. The state of ketosis can lead to symptoms of bad breath (halitosis) and nausea in the short run (and when given orally, ketone bodies can suppress appetite; Blundell and Stubbs 2004, p. 446). Long-term ketosis can lead to dehydration because ketones may increase sodium and water excretion by the kidneys, and can even lead to kidney stones, as well as osteopenia due to increased excretion of calcium (Katz 2008, p. 73).

FATS

The fat reduction message is now so strong that consumers appear to focus on fat avoidance as a primary nutritional objective while foraging for food in local supermarkets.

Stubbs, Whybrow, and Mamat (2008, p. 305)

Many of the foods that are most palatable to humans (and apparently to rats as well) are those that contain a combination of sugars and fats. Edmund Rolls (2005) notes that the sensation of texture in our mouths seems to be a clue to the presence of fat in our foods. He found that there is even an area in the orbitofrontal cortex that responds to the presence of fat, not only by texture but also by odor (e.g., the odor of cream). He reports that when a subject was fed to the point of satiety with fat, the neurons in that area stopped responding. Interestingly, though, if these neurons were also exposed to the taste of glucose, they began to respond again. Along those lines, Berner et al. (2008) found that they could produce a pattern of binge eating with weight gain in rats that were exposed to a combination of sugar and fat during a restricted time period of 2 hours a day. Rats allowed to binge only on sugar did not increase their weight over time, nor did rats allowed to binge only on fat. The binge eating pattern with weight gain was created by the daily restricted time period (i.e., intermittent exposure) and the excessive exposure to a combination of fat and sugar simultaneously.

Berner et al. (2008) speculate that their rat experiments that created weight gain in the context of "caloric intake dysregulation" could be a model for human binge eaters. Koopmans (2004, p. 412) also notes that high-calorie meals with both fat and carbohydrates predispose people to overeating. He explains that these caloric meals high in fat inhibit the oxidation of the fat: carbohydrate meals release insulin, which in turn, at low levels, inhibits the release of fatty acids. Furthermore, he notes that insulin activates the enzyme lipoprotein lipase, with the effect that some fat goes into adipose tissue, rather than being oxidized and transferred to body tissues as it normally would be. When fat is stored, only 3% of the ingested calories are used; when carbohydrate is converted into fat, 23% of the calories are expended (i.e., when fat is ingested as food, this uses fewer calories than when fat is synthesized from protein or carbohydrate).

The liver also plays a role in fat metabolism by converting carbohydrates into fats, a process called *de novo lipogenesis.* The liver is also involved in the uptake, storage, and release of lipids into the blood; in fatty acid oxidation; and even in the production of ketone bodies during periods of food restriction (Leonhardt and Langhans 2004). Leonhardt and Langhans (2004) make the point that the liver, though only 4% of the body by weight, accounts for 20% of the body's basal energy expenditure and satisfies most of its own energy requirements through the process of fatty acid oxidation.

Schutz (2004) notes that the oxidation of fats and the oxidation of carbohydrates are not mutually exclusive, but rather are related: the more carbohydrates are oxidized, the less fat is oxidized. Carbohydrates can be turned into fat, whereas there is no mechanism for fat to be turned into carbohydrates by the body. When large amounts of carbohydrates are ingested, some of the extra amount of carbohydrates is converted to fat by this process of de novo lipogenesis (as well as by decreased fat oxidation). This has implications clinically in terms of dieting: massive carbohydrate intake (particularly intake of carbohydrates with a high glycemic index) is more likely to make us fat in the context of excessive calorie intake, though not necessarily when we are using all the calories we are eating (Schutz 2004). In other words, as Hellerstein (1999) said, there may be lipogenic and nonlipogenic high-carbohydrate diets. Hellerstein (1999) notes that "surplus" carbohydrates can be stored as glycogen in liver or muscle; converted to fat by de novo lipogenesis in liver (or even adipose tissue); or oxidized to fuel. The most important response, though, to increased carbohydrate is increased storage as glycogen, to be used as fuel later when the body needs it.

Fatty Acids

Fats (*lipids*, as they are referred to scientifically) consist of three fatty acids attached to the sugar alcohol glycerol. This structure is called a *triglyceride* and thus all fats are triglycerides. By convention, if they are solid at room temperature, we refer to them as *fats*. If they are liquid at room temperature, they are called *oils;* oils come from plants (but are also fats). Both fats and oils have 9 calories per gram. Humans need to have two fatty acids, called *essential fatty acids*, in our diets: linoleic acid, also called *omega-6 (ω-6) fatty acid*, and α-linolenic acid, also called *omega-3 (ω-3) fatty acid* (Nestle 2006, p. 395). Incidentally, olive oil (oleic oil) contains ω-9 fatty acid, but this type is not considered essential because our bodies can manufacture it. Linoleic, α-linolenic, and oleic fatty acids are all considered "heart healthy."

Nestle believes that most American diets contain about 10 times more ω-6 than ω-3 fatty acids, but she notes that many researchers actually recommend a ratio of about 6:1 for ω-6 to ω-3. Flaxseed oil consists of more than 50% ω-3 fatty acids, as do walnuts. The ω-3 fatty acids can be found in fish (particularly salmon, mackerel, sardines, and scallops; Katz 2008, p. 19), chicken, and eggs, and even in leafy vegetables (Nestle 2006, p. 531). The ω-6 fatty acids are mostly found in vegetable oils, such as safflower oil (consisting of 75% ω-6), corn oil (>50%), and soybean oil (~50%) (Nestle 2006, p. 395). Even sunflower oil contains ω-6 fatty acids (Katz 2008, p. 131).

Research by Westerterp-Plantenga et al. (2004) has shown that some people (as well as rats) are more sensitive to the taste of linoleic acid than others. Those who are more sensitive to it, whom he calls *tasters*, are likely to eat less fat than nontasters. He reported that in one study of over 200 people, about 46% were linoleic acid tasters. They were more apt to stop eating a fatty food (e.g., ice cream with linoleic acid added) based on satiety rather than pleasantness. Westerterp-Plantenga notes that conjugated linoleic acid may have a role for some people in preventing fat regain after weight loss (though apparently not in losing fat during weight loss) because it lowers lipoprotein lipase activity so that less fat is taken up by adipocytes.

Along the lines of Westerterp-Plantenga et al.'s research, Cooling and Blundell (1998) reported their findings from a small study indicating that those who consume more fat in their diets are different from those who typically consume less fat. They noted that those who consumed more fat were more likely to have higher levels of hunger prior to eating, seemed less sensitive to the amount of fat in a food, and were more likely to "passively over-consume" high fat. They also noted that those who ate more fat were more likely to eat a uniform weight of food, whereas those who consumed less fat were more likely to eat different weights of food (when given different diets) but a more consistent amount of calories. The researchers believe two distinct phenotypes were involved.

Fatty acids can be divided into different categories depending on their *saturation*, the number of hydrogen atoms that are part of their structure. Nestle (2006, p. 392) emphasizes that all fats and oils are mixtures of saturated, monounsaturated, and polyunsaturated fatty acids, but the predominant proportion determines how we classify them. Examples of saturated fatty acid fats are butter, meat, cheese, and certain oils like coconut and palm oils. Dietary intake of saturated fatty acids has been associated with an increased risk of heart disease. Trans–fatty acids have been found to be particularly dangerous to humans: these are "abnormal" fatty acids (Nestle 2006, p. 530) produced artificially by hydrogenation. They were initially introduced because they have a long shelf life and, until recently, were used extensively in processed baked goods found in the supermarket. Margarine in stick form is another example of a trans fat. Katz (2008, p. 131) notes that tub margarine has a lower level of trans fat than the stick form. Says Hyman (2006, p. 38), "Put a tub of margarine on the counter and see that no bug will go near it." In some areas of the country, like New York, trans fats have been banned from foods. As Katz remarks, "Dietary fats that reliably extend the shelf life of food products tend to shorten the shelf lives of the people consuming these products" (Katz 2008, p. 131). (As Katz notes, conventional recommendations are that fat intake in our diet should be not more than 30% of our total calories, with saturated fat no more than 10%.)

Fatty acids that are unsaturated (not fully hydrogenated, or partially hydrogenated) tend to be liquid at room temperature. Unsaturated oils tend to become rancid over time. Unsaturated fatty acids can be further divided into monounsaturated fatty acids (they have one point where there is no hydrogen atom; e.g., olive, canola, and peanut oils) and polyunsaturated fatty acids (they have two or more points where there are no hydrogen atoms; e.g., corn, soy, and safflower oils). Sesame oil is a mixture of half monounsaturated and half polyunsaturated fatty acids. Unsaturated fatty acids in the diet seem to be associated with better cardiac health. Monounsaturated fatty acids are typical of the so-called Mediterranean diet, characterized by the use of olive oil along with fresh vegetables, fruits, and seafood.

Fat Substitutes

As noted earlier, fat adds texture (also called *mouthfeel* or *mouthsense*; see also Chapter 4, "The Psychology of the Eater") to food, but because fats have been vilified over the years, researchers have developed fat substitutes. Katz (2008, p. 410) notes that though fat substitutes may be effective at reducing fat intake, they do not necessarily lead to reduced calorie intake, because people may tend to compensate for their reduced fat intake. Several substances have been used as fat substitutes, including starches, cellulose, pectin, and polydextrose, among others (Katz 2008, p. 411). These products can have from no calories to about 4 calories per gram.

Sucrose polyester is the product olestra, used most commonly in snack foods like potato chips. Olestra is made from fatty acids that are esterified into sucrose, but it has no calories and can apparently be used in any food that requires fat. It can be made from either unsaturated fatty acids or saturated fatty acids: when it is made from unsaturated fatty acids, it remains liquid at room temperature, and when it is made from saturated fatty acids, it is solid at room temperature (Eldridge et al. 2002). Olestra is not digestible by the human body. It does, however, decrease the absorption of the fat-soluble vitamins, A, D, E, and K. Products containing olestra now have these fat-soluble vitamins added. Serum carotinoid levels are also somewhat decreased but without apparent negative clinical effects, such as macular pigment changes (Neuhouser et al. 2006). Initially, olestra received bad publicity because of its gastrointestinal side effects, and consumer groups even criticized the FDA for approving it for use in foods (Neuhouser et al. 2006). Subsequent studies have found fewer problems with gastrointestinal effects. Eldridge et al. (2002) note that olestra does produce stool softening but no diarrhea when consumed at 20–40 grams per day. These researchers note that it acts more like dietary fiber by adding bulk, unlike the nonnutritive sugar sorbitol, which does cause diarrhea. These researchers believe that olestra can play a role in low-fat dieting by increasing the palatability of foods and increasing long-term compliance with a low-fat regimen.

Lipoproteins and Cholesterol

Cholesterol is a "soft, fatlike substance" (DeBakey et al. 1996, pp. 19–20) found exclusively in animals, so there is no need for vegetable oils to advertise that they contain

"No cholesterol." Of course, they don't have cholesterol; nor do any other plants, seeds, or nuts. Cholesterol, though, is found in every cell in the body. Cholesterol is not required in the diet because the body manufactures its own supply, mostly in the liver. Dietary cholesterol, though, comes from meat, poultry, egg yolks, fish, and dairy products. DeBakey et al. (1996, p. 19) note that the designations of various kinds of cholesterol refer to how cholesterol is "packaged" for transport. Lipoproteins are protein vessels that carry the various forms of cholesterol; they also carry triglycerides (which are found in both animals and plants). There are five kinds of lipoproteins, dependent on their densities. LDL (low-density lipoprotein) is harmful to the body and is commonly referred to as bad cholesterol; HDL (high-density lipoprotein), commonly called good cholesterol, is considered beneficial because it is thought to carry excess cholesterol away from cells (and away from clogging up our arterial walls—atherosclerosis) (DeBakey et al. 1996, p. 20). Intermediate-density lipoproteins tend to carry triglycerides; VLDLs are very-low-density lipoproteins, which also carry triglycerides. Chylomicrons are the largest lipoproteins and the most dense, and they also carry triglycerides. When people are watching their cholesterol levels, they look at their total cholesterol and their LDL levels. Medication aimed at reducing cholesterol is usually aimed at reducing LDL. A total cholesterol level of less than 200 mg/dL (and, really, below 160 mg/dL) is considered most desirable, and an LDL below 100 mg/dL is ideal. HDL levels should be greater than 40 mg/dL at a minimum, and closer to 60 mg/dL ideally (DeBakey et al. 1996, p. 21).

Triglyceride levels should be less than 150 mg/dL (MDConsult 2007). Katz (2008, p. 15) notes that all tissues in the body can synthesize cholesterol. The medications used to lower cholesterol levels, the statins, work by interfering with the enzyme 3-hydroxy-3-methylglutaryl (HMG)–coenzyme A reductase, which is the rate-limiting step in cholesterol synthesis. The recommended maximum intake of cholesterol in our diets is approximately 300 mg daily. For many years now, the public has been warned against eating eggs because the yolk has so much cholesterol. Nestle (2006, p. 253) notes that one and one-half eggs supply that maximum recommended daily amount of cholesterol, while a small beef hamburger has 100 mg and 8 ounces of whole milk has 25 mg.

Kritchevsky (2004) notes that the recommendation to avoid eggs stemmed from observations that dietary cholesterol increases cholesterol levels in our blood and that increased blood cholesterol levels have been associated with heart disease. In reviewing the literature, however, he found no association between egg consumption and blood cholesterol levels. Kritchevsky reports on several studies, including one study with over 12,000 men (Multiple Factor Intervention Trial or MFIT; Tillotson et al. 1997) and another study of 20,000 men (Third National Health and Nutrition Examination Survey or NHANES III; Song and Kerver 2000). In the Multiple Factor Intervention Trial, men with cholesterol levels lower than 200 mg/dL actually consumed more eggs than men with higher cholesterol levels; data from NHANES III showed that those eating one egg or less per week had higher cholesterol levels than those eating four or more eggs per week. Hu et al. (1999) studied over 37,000 men for 14 years and over 80,000 women for 8 years and found there was no increased risk of cardiovascular disease in those men eating more than seven eggs a week compared with those eating less than one egg weekly.

In addition to dietary intake of cholesterol, another 800 mg of cholesterol is synthesized endogenously daily by the body (Katz (2008, p. 16). Although cholesterol has acquired a bad name in the lay press, it should be noted that cholesterol has important functions in the body, such as in production of the sex hormones testosterone and estrogen, and in cell membrane structure. Benarroch (2008) notes that the human brain contains about 25% of the total cholesterol in our bodies, although our brains are only 2% of our bodies by weight. Cholesterol is the major component of the nerve cell's myelin sheath and has a role in the development of the brain as well as in communication between nerve cells. Furthermore, Benarroch notes, the cholesterol in our brains is "largely independent" of our diets and of that made in the liver because the rest of the body's cholesterol does not cross the blood-brain barrier. Cholesterol is essential for normal neuronal functioning: the nerve cell (the astrocyte) secretes cholesterol that is bound to apolipoprotein E (apoE), both important for synaptic functioning in the brain. Brain diseases like Huntington disease and even Alzheimer disease involve "abnormal CNS cholesterol homeostasis" (Benarroch 2008), and levels of apoE have become a marker for Alzheimer disease.

- Diet must be high enough in protein to provide essential amino acids, the building blocks for protein, and high enough in carbohydrates to maintain blood glucose levels: in general, a diet should have ≥65–70 grams of protein a day and 50–100 grams of carbohydrates.

- Once a diet contains enough protein and carbohydrates, variations in protein, fat, and carbohydrate intake have relatively less effect on metabolism than actual calorie count.

Source: Melanson and Dwyer 2002

REFERENCES

Abou-Donia MB, El-Masry EM, Abdel-Rahman AA, et al: Splenda alters gut microflora and increases intestinal p-glycoprotein and cytochrome p-450 in male rats. J Toxicol Environ Health A 71:1415–1429, 2008

American Dietetic Association: Position of the American Dietetic Association: Use of nutritive and nonnutritive sweeteners. J Am Diet Assoc 104:255–275, 2004

Apovian CM: Sugar-sweetened soft drinks, obesity, and type 2 diabetes. JAMA 292:978–979, 2004

Aquafina labels to tell water's source—the tap: Pepsi agrees to change as industry comes under increased criticism. Associated Press, Food Inc.—MSNBC.com. July 27, 2007. Available at: http://www.msnbc.msn.com/id/19985269/. Accessed October 25, 2009

Askew EW: Nutrition, malnutrition, and starvation, in Wilderness Medicine, 5th Edition. Edited by Auerbach PS. St Louis, MO, Mosby, 2007, pp 1445–1463

Benarroch EE: Brain cholesterol metabolism and neurologic disease: clinical implications of neuroscience research. Neurology 71:1368–1373, 2008

Berner LA, Avena NM, Hoebel BG: Bingeing, self-restriction, and increased body weight in rats with limited access to a sweet-fat diet. Obesity (Silver Spring) 16:1998–2002, 2008

Blundell JE, Stubbs J: Diet composition and the control of food intake in humans, in Handbook of Obesity: Etiology and Pathophysiology, 2nd Edition. Edited by Bray GA, Bouchard C. New York, Marcel Dekker, 2004, pp 427–460

Boschmann M, Steiniger J, Franke G, et al: Water drinking induces thermogenesis through osmosensitive mechanisms. J Clin Endocrinol Metab 92:3334–3337, 2007

Brownell K: The Obesity Crisis: Psychiatry Weighs In. Speech delivered at Yale University, Anlyan Center for Medical Research and Education, October 3, 2008

Browning L: See you in court, sweetie: makers of Splenda and Equal parse the phrase "made from sugar." The New York Times, Business section, April 6, 2007

Byrne HK, Wilmore JH: The relationship of mode and intensity of training on resting metabolic rate in women. Int J Sport Nutr Exerc Metab 11:1–14, 2001

Clifton PM, Keogh JB, Noakes M: Long-term effects of a high-protein weight-loss diet. Am J Clin Nutr 87:23–29, 2008

Cooling J, Blundell J: Are high-fat and low-fat consumers distinct phenotypes? Differences in the subjective and behavioural response to energy and nutrient challenges. Eur J Clin Nutr 52:193–201, 1998

Critser G: Fat Land: How Americans Became the Fattest People in the World. Boston, MA, Houghton Mifflin, 2003

DeBakey ME, Gotto AM Jr, Scott LW, et al: The New Living Heart Diet (completely revised and updated). New York, Simon and Schuster, 1996

Dhingra R, Sullivan L, Jacques PF, et al: Soft drink consumption and risk of developing cardiometabolic risk factors and the metabolic syndrome in middle-aged adults in the community. Circulation 116:480–488, 2007

Diepvens K, Westerterp KR, Westerterp-Plantenga MS: Obesity and thermogenesis related to the consumption of caffeine, ephedrine, capsaicin, and green tea. Am J Physiol Regul Integr Comp Physiol 292:R77–R85, 2006

Drewnowski A, Bellisle F: Liquid calories, sugar, and body weight. Am J Clin Nutr 85:651–661, 2007

Dulloo AG, Jacquet J: Low-protein overfeeding: a tool to unmask susceptibility to obesity in humans. Int J Obes Relat Metab Disord 23:1118–1121, 1999

Ebbeling CB, Leidig MM, Feldman HA, et al: Effects of a low-glycemic load vs low-fat diet in obese young adults: a randomized trial. JAMA 297:2092–2102, 2007

Eldridge AL, Cooper DA, Peters JG: A role for olestra in body weight management. Obes Rev 3:17–25, 2002

Elliott SS, Keim NL, Stern JS, et al: Fructose, weight gain, and the insulin resistance syndrome. Am J Clin Nutr 76:911–922, 2002

Eny KM, Wolever TM, Fontaine-Bisson B, et al: Genetic variant in the glucose transporter type 2 is associated with higher intakes of sugars in two distinct populations. Physiol Genomics 33:355–360, 2008

Foster DW, McGarry JD: Intermediary metabolism of carbohydrates, lipids, and proteins, in Harrison's Principles of Internal Medicine, 10th Edition. Edited by Petersdorf RG et al. New York, McGraw-Hill, 1983, pp 490–495

Foster DW, Rubenstein H: Hypoglycemia, insulinoma, and other hormone-secreting tumors of the pancreas, in Harrison's Principles of Internal Medicine, 10th Edition. Edited by Petersdorf RG et al. New York, McGraw-Hill, 1983, pp 682–689

Frank GK, Oberndorfer TA, Simmons AN, et al: Sucrose activates human taste pathways differently from artificial sweetener. Neuroimage 39:1550–1569, 2008

Gaby AR: Adverse effects of dietary fructose. Altern Med Rev 10:294–306, 2005

Geliebter A, Maher MM, Gerace L, et al: Effects of strength or aerobic training on body composition, resting metabolic rate, and peak oxygen consumption in obese dieting subjects. Am J Clin Nutr 66:557–563, 1997

Glassner B: The Gospel of Food: Everything You Think You Know About Food Is Wrong. New York, HarperCollins, 2007

Grice HC, Goldsmith LA: Sucralose—an overview of the toxicity data. Food Chem Toxicol 38 (suppl 2):1–6, 2000

Havel PJ: Dietary fructose: implications for dysregulation of energy homeostasis and lipid/carbohydrate metabolism. Nutr Rev 63:133–157, 2005

Hellerstein MK: De novo lipogenesis in humans: metabolic and regulatory aspects. Eur J Clin Nutr 53:S53–S65, 1999

Helmering DW, Hales D: Think Thin, Be Thin: 101 Psychological Ways to Lose Weight. New York, Broadway Books, 2005, pp 139–140

Herring JL, Molé PA, Meredith CN, et al: Effect of suspending exercise training on resting metabolic rate in women. Med Sci Sports Exerc 24:59–65, 1992

Himaya A, Louis-Sylvestre J: The effect of soup on satiation. Appetite 30:199–210, 1998

Hirsch J: Obesity: matter over mind? The Dana Foundation. January 1, 2003. Available at: http://www.dana.org/news/cerebrum/detail.aspx?id=2908. Accessed July 6, 2009.

Hu FB, Stampfer MJ, Rimm EB, et al: A prospective study of egg consumption and risk of cardiovascular disease in men and women. JAMA 281:1387–1394, 1999

Hyman M: Ultrametabolism: The Simple Plan for Automatic Weight Loss. New York, Scribner, 2006

Institute of Medicine of the National Academies: Dietary Reference Intakes for Energy, Carbohydrate, Fiber, Fat, Fatty Acids, Cholesterol, Protein, and Amino Acids. Washington DC, National Academies Press, 2008

Jenkins DJA, Wolever TMS, Taylor RH, et al: Glycemic Index of Foods: a physiological basis for carbohydrate exchange. Am J Clin Nutr 34:362–366, 1981

Katz DL: Nutrition in Clinical Practice: A Comprehensive, Evidence-Based Manual for the Practitioner, 2nd Edition. Philadelphia, PA, Wolter Kluwers Health/Lippincott Williams & Wilkins, 2008

Koopmans HS: Experimental studies on the control of food intake, in Handbook of Obesity: Etiology and Pathophysiology, 2nd Edition. Edited by Bray GA, Bouchard C. New York, Marcel Dekker, 2004, pp 373–425

Kritchevsky SB: A review of scientific research and recommendations regarding eggs. J Am Coll Nutr 23:596S–600S, 2004

Leonhardt M, Langhans W: Fatty acid oxidation and control of food intake. Physiol Behav 83:645–651, 2004

Levine AS, Kotz CM, Gosnell BA: Sugars: hedonic aspects, neuroregulation, and energy balance. Am J Clin Nutr 78:834S–842S, 2003

Lichtman SW, Pisarska K, Berman ER, et al: Discrepancy between self-reported and actual caloric intake and exercise in obese subjects. N Engl J Med 327:1893–1898, 1992

Liljeberg HG, Akerberg AK, Björck IM: Effect of the glycemic index and content of indigestible carbohydrates of cereal-based breakfast meals on glucose tolerance at lunch in healthy subjects. Am J Clin Nutr 69:647–655, 1999

Lineback DR, Jones JM: Sugars and Health Workshop: summary and conclusions. Am J Clin Nutr 78:893S–897S, 2003

Ludwig DS: The glycemic index: physiological mechanisms relating to obesity, diabetes, and cardiovascular disease. JAMA 287:2414–2423, 2002

Ludwig DS: Clinical update: the low-glycaemic-index diet. Lancet 369:890–892, 2007

Maki KC, Curry LL, Reeves MS, et al: Chronic consumption of rebaudioside A, a steviol glycoside, in men and women with type 2 diabetes mellitus. Food Chem Toxicol 46 (suppl 7):S47–S53, 2008

Malik VS, Schulze MB, Hu FB: Intake of sugar-sweetened beverages and weight gain: a systematic review. Am J Clin Nutr 84:274–288, 2006

Marty N, Dallaporta M, Thorens B: Brain glucose sensing, counterregulation, and energy homeostasis. Physiology (Bethesda) 22:241–251, 2007

Mattes RD, Popkin BM: Nonnutritive sweetener consumption in humans: effects on appetite and food intake and their putative mechanisms. Am J Clin Nutr 89:1–14, 2009

McMillan-Price J, Petocz P, Atkinson F, et al: Comparison of 4 diets of varying glycemic load on weight loss and cardiovascular risk reduction in overweight and obese young adults: a randomized controlled trial. Arch Intern Med 166:1466–1475, 2006

MDConsult: What are cholesterol, other lipids, and lipoproteins? MDConsult: Cholesterol, Other Lipids, and Lipoproteins: Patient Education. Available at: http://www.mdconsult.com/das/patient/body/71726979–3/589305645/10041/9468.html. Accessed April 22, 2007

Melanson K, Dwyer J: Popular diets for treatment of overweight and obesity, in Handbook of Obesity Treatment. Edited by Wadden TA, Stunkard AJ. New York, Guilford, 2002, pp 249–282

Melanson KJ, Angelopoulos TJ, Nguyen V, et al: High-fructose corn syrup, energy intake, and appetite regulation. Am J Clin Nutr 86 (6 suppl):1738S–1744S, 2008

Miller WC, Wadden TA: Exercise as a treatment for obesity, in Handbook of Obesity: Clinical Applications, 2nd Edition. Edited by Bray GA, Bouchard C. New York, Marcel Dekker, 2004, pp 169–183

Mooallem J: The unintended consequences of hyperhydration. The New York Times Magazine, May 27, 2007, pp 30–35

Negoianu D, Goldfarb S: Just add water. J Am Soc Nephrol 19:1041–1043, 2008

Nestle M: What to Eat. New York, North Point Press, 2006

Neuhouser ML, Rock CL, Kristal AR, et al: Olestra is associated with slight reductions in serum carotenoids but does not markedly influence serum fat-soluble vitamin concentrations. Am J Clin Nutr 83:624–631, 2006

Patel SM, Lembo AJ: Constipation, in Sleisenger and Fordtran's Gastrointestinal and Liver Disease: Pathophysiology, Diagnosis, Management, 8th Edition. Edited by Feldman M, Friedman LS, Brandt LJ. Philadelphia, PA, WB Saunders, 2006, pp 221–254

Pollan M: Unhappy meals: thirty years of nutritional science has made Americans sicker, fatter and less well nourished: a plea for a return to plain old food. The New York Times Magazine, January 28, 2007, pp 40–47, 65, 67, 69

Pollan M: In Defense of Food: An Eater's Manifesto. New York, Penguin, 2008

Prakash I, DuBois GE, Clos JF, et al: Development of rebiana, a natural, non-caloric sweetener. Food Chem Toxicol 46 (suppl 7):S75–S82, 2008

Rolls B: The Volumetrics Eating Plan: Techniques and Recipes for Feeling Full on Fewer Calories. New York, HarperCollins, 2005

Rolls BJ, Bell EA, Thorwart ML: Water incorporated into a food but not served with a food decreases energy intake in lean women. Am J Clin Nutr 70:448–455, 1999

Rolls ET: Taste, olfactory, and food texture processing in the brain, and the control of food intake. Physiol Behav 85:45–56, 2005

Rosenbaum M, Hirsch J, Gallagher DA, et al: Long-term persistence of adaptive thermogenesis in subjects who have maintained a reduced body weight. Am J Clin Nutr 88:906–912, 2008

Salsberg SL, Ludwig DS: Putting your genes on a diet: the molecular effects of carbohydrate. Am J Clin Nutr 85:1169–1170, 2007

Samra RA, Anderson GH: Insoluble cereal fiber reduces appetite and short-term food intake and glycemic response to food consumed 75 min later by healthy men. Am J Clin Nutr 86:972–979, 2007

Schulz LO, Schoeller DA: A compilation of total daily energy expenditures and body weights in healthy adults. Am J Clin Nutr 60:676–681, 1994

Schutz Y: Dietary fat, lipogenesis and energy balance. Physiol Behav 83:557–564, 2004

Schutz Y, Jéquier E: Resting energy expenditure, thermic effect of food, and total energy expenditure, in Handbook of Obesity: Etiology and Pathophysiology, 2nd Edition. Edited by Bray GA, Bouchard C. New York, Marcel Dekker, 2004, pp 615–653

Soenen S, Westerterp-Plantenga MS: No differences in satiety or energy intake after high-fructose corn syrup, sucrose, or milk preloads. Am J Clin Nutr 86:1586–1594, 2007

Song WO, Kerver JM: Nutritional contribution of eggs to American diets. J Am Coll Nutr 19:525S–531S, 2000 [NHANES III study population]

Stanhope KL, Havel PJ: Endocrine and metabolic effects of consuming beverages sweetened with fructose, glucose, sucrose, or high-fructose corn syrup. Am J Clin Nutr 88(suppl):1733S–1737S, 2008

Stanhope KL, Griffen SC, Bair BR, et al: Twenty-four-hour endocrine and metabolic profiles following consumption of high-fructose corn syrup-, sucrose-, fructose-, and glucose-sweetened beverages with meals. Am J Clin Nutr 87:1194–1203, 2008

Starbucks beverage details: Mint Mocha Chip Frappuccino blended coffee with Chocolate Whipped Cream. Nutrition facts table. Available at: http://www.starbucks.com/retail/nutrition_beverage_detail.asp?selProducts={FC397D06-2F23-4602-89D9-D1E323361021}&x=11&y=12&strAction=GETDEFAULT. Accessed August 8, 2009.

Stock MJ: Gluttony and thermogenesis revisited. Int J Obes Relat Metab Disord 23:1105–1117, 1999

Stubbs J, Ferres S, Horgan G: Foods: effects on energy intake. Crit Rev Food Sci Nutr 40:481–515, 2000

Stubbs J, Whybrow S, Mamat NM: Macronutrients, feeding behavior and weight control in humans (Chapter 16), in Appetite and Food Intake: Behavioral and Physiological Considerations. Edited by Harris RBS, Mattes RD. Boca Raton, FL, CRC Press, 2008, pp 295–322

Swithers SE, Davidson TL: A role for sweet taste: calorie predictive relations in energy regulation by rats. Behav Neurosci 122:161–173, 2008

Tataranni PA, Ravussin E: Energy metabolism and obesity, in Handbook of Obesity Treatment. Edited by Wadden TA, Stunkard AJ. New York, Guilford, 2002, pp 42–72

Taubes G: Good Calories, Bad Calories: Challenging the Conventional Wisdom on Diet, Weight Control, and Disease. New York, Alfred A Knopf, 2007

Tillotson JL, Bartsch GE, Gorder D, et al: Food group and nutrient intakes at baseline in the Multiple Risk Factor Intervention Trial. Am J. Clin Nutr 65 (1 suppl):228S–257S, 1997

Tsanzi E, Fitch CW, Tou JC: Effect of consuming different caloric sweeteners on bone health and possible mechanisms. Nutr Rev 66:301–309, 2008

U.S. Department of Agriculture: Sweetener consumption in the United States: distribution by demographic and product characteristics. Electronic Outlook Report from the Economic Research Service, August 2005 (Publ No SSS-243-01). Available at: http://www.ers.usda.gov/Publications/SSS/aug05/sss24301/sss24301.pdf. Accessed October 25, 2009.

U.S. Department of Agriculture: Food availability (per dapita) data system. Economic Research Service (updated March 2009). Available at: http://www.ers.usda.gov/data/food-consumption. Accessed October 25, 2009.

U.S. Food and Drug Administration: Food allergies rare but risky. FDA Consumer. May 1994 (updated December 2004). Available at: http://vm.cfsan.fda.gov/~dms/wh-alrg1.html. Accessed August 8, 2009.

Valois S, Costa-Ribeiro H Jr, Mattos A, et al: Controlled, double-blind randomized clinical trial to evaluate the impact of fruit juice consumption on the evolution of infants with acute diarrhea. Nutr J 4(Aug):23, 2005

Valtin H: "Drink at least eight glasses of water a day." Really? Is there scientific evidence for "8 x 8"? Am J Physiol Regul Integr Comp Physiol 283:R993–R1004, 2002

van Baak MA: Meal-induced activation of the sympathetic nervous system and its cardiovascular and thermogenic effects in man. Physiol Behav 94:178–186, 2008

Vranica S: High fructose corn syrup mixes it up: sweetener advocate, soured by obesity links, targets moms in ads. The Wall Street Journal, Media and Marketing section, June 23, 2008

Wald A: Constipation in the primary care setting: current concepts and misconceptions. Am J Med 119: 736–739, 2006

Weil A: Healthy Aging: A Lifelong Guide to Your Well-Being. New York, Anchor Books, 2005

Westerterp-Plantenga MS: Fat intake and energy balance effects. Physiol Behav 83:579–585, 2004

Westerterp-Plantenga MS, Lejeune MP, Nijs I, et al: High protein intake sustains weight maintenance after body weight loss in humans. Int J Obes Relat Metab Disord 28:57–64, 2004

Wheeler ML, Pi-Sunyer FX: Carbohydrate issues: type and amount. J Am Diet Assoc 108 (suppl 1):S34–S39, 2008

White JS: Straight talk about high-fructose corn syrup: what it is and what it ain't. Am J Clin Nutr 88:1716S–1721S, 2008

Williams I: Message in a bottle. IR magazine. September 2004. Available at: http://www .thecrossbordergroup.com/ir_archive/pages/944/September+2004.stm?article_ id=5785. Accessed July 13, 2007.

Winnicott DW: Transitional objects are transitional phenomena; a study of the first not-me possession. Int J Psychoanal 34:89–97, 1953

Wylie-Rosett J, Segal-Isaacson CJ, Segal-Isaacson A: Carbohydrates and increases in obesity: does the type of carbohydrate make a difference? Obes Res 12:124S–129S, 2004

Yanovski JA, Yanovski SZ, Sovik KN, et al: A prospective study of holiday weight gain. N Engl J Med 342:861–867, 2000

4

THE PSYCHOLOGY
OF THE EATER

We like fries not in spite of the fact they are unhealthy, but because of it.

Malcolm Gladwell, "The Trouble With Fries" (2001)

OBESITY AS A BRAIN DISORDER

Not only do those of us watching our weight have to contend with bodies seemingly wired to gain weight as we age, and even to regain any lost weight, we also have brains and minds that seem predisposed to sabotage us at any moment. Malcolm Gladwell's comment (2001) is indicative of the psychologically complicated and contrary relationship humans have with food and diet. Most people, and particularly those with a weight problem, have had the experience of feeling they want to eat something that they know is unhealthy or of having an inability to control their food intake despite a strong desire to do so. Judith Beck (2008, p. 16) calls that rebellious voice the "inner saboteur." As Sindelar (2008) so aptly says, we humans "do not always make rational decisions, especially with regard to health habits," such as abuse of drugs, alcohol, and food. In other words, we do not eat just for calories or sustenance; we also eat for pleasure (Zheng and Berthoud 2007). And we have what Zheng and Berthoud (2008) call a *metabolic brain*, as well as a cognitive and emotional one. For humans, eating has evolved into a complex, highly elaborate behavior with not only personal meaning but also social, psychological, and cultural dimensions (Alonso-Alonso and Pascual-Leone 2007).

> When it comes to eating, the unattended metabolic brain overrides the cognitive and emotional brain.

An editorial in the *American Journal of Psychiatry* (Volkow and O'Brien 2007) even suggested we consider obesity a brain disorder, just as we consider substance abuse a disorder. And the Strategic Plan for NIH Obesity Research from the National Institutes of Health (Spiegel and Alving

101

2005; Spiegel et al. 2005) emphasized the importance of collaborative efforts among researchers studying the brain and reward circuits and those studying the genetic and metabolic aspects of the control of food intake. Spiegel et al. (2005) even went so far as to say that brain imaging will become the "cornerstone of efforts to understand the biology of human eating behavior."

In many ways, though, we are no different from rats, in that if you present rats just with more variety in the flavors of their food (unrelated to a preference or favorite flavor), even satiated rats will eat more and gain weight (Treit et al. 1983). The investigators concluded that the cessation of eating is partially controlled by a flavor-specific inhibition that builds up slowly. They suggested that this may have had adaptive significance, in that a sensitivity to a variety of flavors may increase the likelihood that a balanced range of nutrients are eaten. Unfortunately, with our smorgasbord of choices, humans get much more than a balance of nutrients.

Further, if you give rats larger portions, they will eat more: rats with access to five bottles of sucrose ate considerably more than those given access to one bottle, and gained significant weight over time (Tordoff 2002). Tordoff called this "obesity by choice"—not unlike human availability-based overconsumption due to the vast number of choices in the modern supermarket. And if you give rats a large choice of highly palatable foods rich in additional fat and sugar, they eat beyond satiety. By the tenth day of a 60-day experiment, weight gain in the enriched group was significantly greater than in the control group and continued to be so throughout the experiment, although not all rats gained the same amount of weight (Sclafani and Springer 1976).

What makes the integration of the biological with the psychological so much more complex in humans than in animals like rats is that there are so many aspects involved in food intake. Berthoud (2007) makes the point that the human cortex has evolved such that major parts of our brain, such as the prefrontal cortex, amygdala, and orbitofrontal cortex, involve mechanisms that enhance our ability to survive, such as the drive to find a food source. He also notes that one of the first steps is distinguishing harmful from beneficial food, which, of course, also often involves cognitive processes like memory and learning. So, just as it was important for primitive humans to remember where they found their last food source, people in our civilization "remember the location of their favorite restaurants very well and do not forget the secret drawer where that chocolate is hidden" (Berthoud 2007).

We also tend to remember previous experiences with food, and more so if an experience was particularly pleasurable or disgusting (Zheng and Berthoud 2008). Most people, for example, can remember that four-star restaurant meal years ago, as well as a particular food elsewhere that made them vomit 10 years earlier. And we have such good abilities to imagine and visualize food that just thinking about eating a food can produce physiological responses like increased saliva, gastric acid, and even insulin secretion (Berthoud 2007). Different parts of our brain are involved in wanting a food (i.e., involving motivation) as distinguished from the psychological state of liking (i.e., involving pleasurable effect). For example, Berthoud (2007) notes that the mesolimbic dopaminergic system is not involved in the liking of a pleasurable stimulus, but it is crucially involved in getting us to obtain something we want. (See also the "Reward, Cravings, and Addiction" section later in this chapter.)

Hirschmann and Munter (1988, p. 104), along those same lines, speak of mouth hunger as distinguished from stomach hunger. They define *stomach hunger* as physiological hunger, or hunger that satisfies our need to eat. We might even call it *metabolic hunger*. Stomach hunger leads to a sense of fullness and satisfaction. *Mouth hunger*, on the other hand, is psychological hunger, hunger that has nothing to do with sustenance. It often develops suddenly and is not related to time. It is the hunger that is often specifically a taste for something and "summons you to the refrigerator as soon as you sit down to work" and it is the hunger that makes you continue to eat something because part of you wants to, long after you are full (Hirschmann and Munter 1988, pp. 104 ff.). Incidentally, humans are very sensitive to what is called *mouthsense*, a term referring to the texture of food and related to the integration of perceptions of flavor (involving taste and smell) with oral sensations (Rozin 1982). Mouthsense is what makes the addition of fat important in many foods. The term *mouthfeel* (Pivk et al, 2008), which seems to be synonymous with *mouthsense*, is used more recently in the scientific literature to describe our human capacity to be exquisitely sensitive to sensations of different levels of fat in the oral cavity. For example, Pivk et al. (2008) note how their experimental subjects could detect a thickness difference of 25 μm in their perceptions of lipid deposited directly (to avoid visual cues) on their subjects' tongues. Our cognitive abilities to discriminate certain aspects of fat so precisely has obvious ramifications: as a result, we may be disappointed (a peculiarly human emotion) if our usual "mouthfeel" for a particular fatty food is different because its fat content has been altered (e.g., as in low-fat products.)

- *Stomach hunger*—metabolic hunger—seeks sustenance.

- *Mouth hunger*—psychological hunger—seeks satisfaction.

Mouth hunger is most often the hunger that develops from or leads to remorse, anxiety, or even a depressed mood. It is also the hunger that one sees during stress, and particularly chronic stress.

For many years now, researchers have been attempting to locate exactly where in the human brain our preoccupation with eating and food resides. Many neurological disorders may result in abnormal eating habits. For example, the Klüver-Bucy syndrome results in emotional placidity, hypersexuality, and hyperorality in which patients indiscriminately mouth anything. Originally described in monkeys after experimental ablation of the bilateral temporal lobes, including the amygdala, this syndrome can be seen in humans as well as when there is bilateral temporal lobe damage secondary to infections like herpes simplex encephalitis or head injury, or even after status epilepticus (Moore and Jefferson 2004, p. 304). Mesulam (2000,

p. 57) describes behavioral changes in patients with this syndrome: indiscriminate, inappropriate initiation of sexual activity and a seeming visual inability to distinguish edible from inedible substances such that these patients will put anything in their mouths. Moore and Jefferson (2004, p. 203) further note that these patients even eat toilet paper or drink their own urine and display "a remarkable gluttony" (i.e., "hyperoral behavior"). Pick disease is a degenerative neurological disease, with temporal and frontal lobe involvement, characterized by personality changes, disinhibition, dementia, and hyperorality (Mesulam 2000, pp. 497–498). And pica, a syndrome seen in iron deficiency states, is characterized by a "morbid craving" for bizarre substances such as clay, laundry starch, or cigarette ashes (Regard and Landis 1997).

More than 10 years ago, Regard and Landis (1997) reported on a group of neurologically impaired patients who developed what they called the *gourmand syndrome*, a fascinating constellation of symptoms including a new, passionate preoccupation with food (altered eating habits that included a preference for fine dining) in the context of no previous history of eating disorder, psychiatric illness, or metabolic disturbance. Their 36 patients had decreased impulse control and emotional lability, and all had evidence (on computed tomography scan) of focal brain damage, mostly involving the right anterior corticolimbic areas. The damage was brought on by a variety of lesions, including tumors, vascular infarctions or malformations, or trauma.

More recently, with the use of positron emission tomography (PET) scans, researchers have examined the relationship of the brain to food intake. For example, Gautier et al. (2000), in a small sample of 11 obese men and 11 lean men, found significantly increased regional cerebral blood flow in the prefrontal cortex of the obese. According to Zheng and Berthoud (2008), the right prefrontal cortex is involved in keeping "reward-generating mechanisms in check," such that when there is damage to this area we have a general disregard for possible adverse consequences of our actions. Gautier et al. (2000) speculate that hypothalamic responses to satiation are attenuated in the obese; they suggest that lean and obese men have different brain responses to eating in areas of the brain involved in inhibition of behavior and emotion (e.g., prefrontal and limbic/paralimbic regions).

DelParigi et al. (2007) used PET scans and magnetic resonance imaging (MRI) scans of the brain to assess the brain's response to a meal in a small group of successful women dieters (whose body mass index values had decreased from ≥ 35 kg/m^2 to 25 kg/m^2) compared with a group of nondieting overweight women. The researchers found that the dorsal prefrontal cortex, the area involved in conscious experience and inhibition of emotions, as well as the dorsal striatum, was particularly activated in successful dieters compared with nondieters. Furthermore, the orbitofrontal cortex (involved in immediate reward) was significantly more activated in the nondieters. Lesions in this area have been associated with eating disorders, gambling, and other behaviors in which choice is involved (Padoa-Schioppa and Assad 2008). DelParigi et al. (2007) speculate that this interconnected circuit may function as a means of inhibiting food reward. In other words, the dieters may be able to keep in mind the expectation of the great reward (activation of the dorsal striatum) in continuing their dieting rather than succumb to the immediate reward of eating.

Rolls and McCabe (2007) found that there are actually differences, as evidenced in functional MRI scans in certain areas of the brain—including the medial orbito-frontal cortex but, interestingly, not the taste centers—between those who consider themselves chocolate cravers and those who do not. The areas of the brain involved are those related to visual cues (e.g., the pleasant sight of the chocolate) and their impact on cravings.

Alonso-Alonso and Pascual-Leone (2007) support the notion that obesity is actually a right brain disorder. They, like others, cite research suggesting that the right prefrontal cortex is involved and note that the very obese have difficulty with decision making. They distinguish *reflective eating* (involving a cognitive dimension, with consideration of social expectations and long-term goals regarding health) from *reflexive eating* (a phylogenetically older model involving reward and motivation dimensions).

Alonso-Alonso and Pascual-Leone's (2007) article, published in the *Journal of the American Medical Association*, drew some criticism. Bachman and Histon (2007), for example, took issue with the authors' suggestion that obesity is a right brain disorder, as evidenced by the facts that some obese individuals seem less embarrassed by their weight than others and that some have difficulty making decisions (and hence are less able to commit to a diet). Said Bach-

> • *Reflexive eating* functions within the paradigm of immediacy of reward and motivation.
>
> • *Reflective eating* functions within the paradigm of long-term health and social consequences.

man and Histon (2007), "Before adding the stigma of 'brain-damaged' to the high physical and social burden obese persons already bear," they would like to see more compelling data (Bachman and Histon 2007).

The brain research connection to obesity, to date, remains highly speculative, but as Spiegel and colleagues suggest, it may become at least one building block, if not the cornerstone, in understanding the science behind obesity (Spiegel and Alving 2005; Spiegel et al. 2005). For example, there is no question that weight control involves not only internal physiological processes but also those involving perceptions from the external world. Our higher cognitive processes are very much involved in our food intake. But all levels of our neuroanatomy are involved. Tataranni and Pannacciulli (2008, p. 273) summarize the different areas of our brain involved in integrating these highly complex behaviors, namely: "physiological responses mainly represented in the brain stem and hypothalamus, more complex motivational and affective responses represented in the amygdala, striatum, and insula, and higher cognitive control represented in the prefrontal cortex." Scott (2008, pp. 114–115) suggests that taste is the "chemical gatekeeper" for the body in determining a food's nutritional or harmful value. But then input is sent to the gut to mediate reflexes of the gastrointestinal system, to the hindbrain that controls those reflexes that lead to ingesting or rejecting a food, to the thalamus and cortex of the insula for the cognitive aspects of taste appreciation, and to the orbitofrontal cortex and ventral forebrain that are involved in those strong hedonic responses that incorporate sight, smell, and texture to give intense enjoyment or even intense revulsion.

HOMEOSTASIS, ALLOSTASIS, STRESS, AND THE HPA AXIS

The psychology of the eater must also take into account the concept of *stress*—although stress, of course, is not just seen in humans but can be inferred by certain signs in every living organism. It was in the mid 1930s that an Austrian-born physician, Hans Selye, first wrote of a typical "syndrome produced by diverse nocuous agents," such as temperature changes (e.g., exposure to cold), excessive exercise, surgical injury, or drugs, that produced what he considered a classic response that was independent of the actual agent itself (Selye 1936/1998). Selye called this syndrome the *general adaptation syndrome* and explained that it reflects a generalized effort of an organism to adapt to the new situation, that is, a stressor. He divided the organism's response into three stages: 1) the general alarm reaction, 2) the stage of resistance, and 3) the stage of exhaustion and death (when the stress is severe enough). Over the years, the word *stress* has entered common parlance and its connotation has become very different from Selye's original concept. Though Selye defined *stress* as "the nonspecific response of the body to any demand" and defined a *stressor* as an "agent that produces stress at any time," he emphasized that stress responses are patterned and highly specific in their manifestations but nonspecific in their causes (Selye 1985). Selye also made a point of noting that stress did not have to be negative, undesirable, or pathological (i.e., *distress*). It could, in fact, be positive, that is, agreeable or healthy (i.e., *eustress*), such as when someone feels good after challenging, creative work (Selye 1985).

Selye also noted that different individuals may react differently to the same stress, depending on endogenous factors (e.g., genetic predisposition, age, or sex) and exogenous factors (e.g., exposure to social issues, environment, or drugs). Though Selye believed that psychological stressors are particularly important in humans, he also believed that stress reactions could occur in animals and plants lacking a nervous system. He felt that stress is the "salt of life" (Selye 1976) and that, as such, it is impossible, and not even advantageous, to eliminate stress from human life. For Selye, the challenge was to contain stress and channel it into feelings of accomplishment and mastery.

Even after 40 years of research in the field, Selye admitted that he did not know much about the nature of what he called the "first mediator," that is, the signal that carries the message of stress from the area of the body directly affected by the stress to the parts of the brain that regulate homeostatic reactions (the hypothalamus and pituitary gland) (Selye 1976). He did, however, appreciate the finely tuned elaborate feedback system that has evolved in humans and other organisms to reestablish homeostasis, and he was well aware of the differences between acute stress and chronic stress, and even the role of inflammation in both acute and chronic stress reactions.

It was Walter Cannon in the 1920s who first proposed the word *homeostasis* to describe the specific mechanisms characteristic of living organisms that are used, as Moore-Ede (1986) says, to "preserve internal equilibriums in the face of an inconstant world." And Cannon chose the word *homeo*, from the Greek meaning "similar" as opposed to *homo*, meaning "same," says Moore-Ede, "to admit some variation and to avoid the implication of fixed and rigid constancy." Moore-Ede, though, differentiates Cannon's "reactive" homeostasis, "corrective actions in response to a change which has already occurred," from his new concept of "predictive" homeostasis, "corrective responses initiated in anticipation of a predictably timed challenge." Moore-Ede speaks of our "environmental cycles," such as our day and our year as "extremely predictable." Some examples of the body's anticipatory changes are variations in our plasma cortisol and core body temperature hours before we awaken. Though Moore-Ede wrote his article in the 1980s, years before the discovery of the hormone ghrelin, he clearly anticipated the fact that levels of this hormone rise before we eat our meals. (For more on circadian rhythms, see Chapter 9 in this volume.) Incidentally, Power and Schulkin (2009, p. 173) speak of the "paradox of eating" as "both necessary for homeostasis and a threat to homeostasis at the same time."

Over the years, we have come to know more about the complex role of the many critical mediators involved between stressors and the human body in its attempt to maintain its homeostasis, that is, its balance or equilibrium. McEwen (2002) notes that *homeostasis* technically applies to systems that are truly essential for life and are part of the body's internal milieu, such as pH balance and body temperature. He defines *stress* as the physiological and behavioral responses that occur when an individual's homeostasis is actually threatened or perceived as threatened.

McEwen emphasizes that the types of perceived stress that cause considerable upheaval for the body and are some of the most powerful for humans are psychological and experiential stresses, such as those involving novelty, withholding of a reward, or anticipation of punishment (even more so than the punishment itself). He calls the adaptive, physiological coping responses of the body (e.g., variations in blood pressure) that maintain homeostasis in the presence of stressors *allostasis*, which he defines as "achieving stability through change." In other words, accord-

STRESS AND THE HPA AXIS

- The body reacts to stress in a complicated feedback system involving parts of the brain (hypothalamus and pituitary gland) and the adrenal glands, called the *HPA axis*. Whether a stress is physical or psychological the body responds the same way, with increased secretion of the hormones ACTH and cortisol, and increased heart rate and blood pressure.

- When the HPA axis is activated frequently by stress, with increased cortisol secretion, researchers have found visceral obesity, hypertension, increased lipids in the blood, and insulin resistance.

Source: Traustadóttir et al. 2005

ing to McEwen (2002), allostasis is the "process that keeps the organism alive and functioning." Power and Schulkin (2009, p. 328), with an evolutionary perspective in mind, note that animals achieve "evolutionary success" not by maintaining stability but rather by "maintaining viability." As such, these authors define "homeostasis" as "achieving viability through resistance to change (stability)" and "allostasis" as "achieving viability through change" itself. Not only is the hypothalamic-pituitary-adrenal (HPA) axis involved, this process of adaptation also involves the immune system, the autonomic nervous system, and the brain. In the short run, the many hormones and neurotransmitters produced by the body in response to stress are protective and can lead to the typical fight-or-flight reaction. For example, glucocorticoids, produced by the adrenal glands in response to stress, can regulate behaviors, such as increasing one's appetite for food and even food-seeking behavior to replenish energy reserves after fending off a predator. This response to stress is supposed to be time limited or transient (Kyrou and Tsigos 2007). But when the allostatic systems (e.g., the glucocorticoid system) remain turned on, through repeated challenges to the body, the body can develop what McEwen calls "wear and tear" or *allostatic load*. Allostatic load is "the price the tissue or organ pays for an overactive or inefficiently managed" response, says McEwen (2002). Psychological stress and sleep deprivation, for example, may lead to chronically elevated levels of glucocorticoids and, in turn, to pathological behavioral responses such as overeating, alcohol or drug abuse, or smoking, as well as excessive anxiety and worry. Eventually, these pathological responses (i.e., chronic wear and tear on the body) create their own problems, which can be manifested by higher insulin levels and insulin resistance, the accumulation of dangerous abdominal (visceral) fat, the loss of minerals in bone, and the atrophy of brain cells in the hippocampus that are responsible for some forms of memory, among other disturbances.

Corticotropin-releasing hormone (CRH), produced in the hypothalamus, is the hormone that coordinates the stress response, but arginine vasopressin (AVP) in the hypothalamus is also involved (Kyrou and Tsigos 2007). Both AVP, synergistically, and CRH, more directly, are involved in stimulating the secretion of adrenocorticotropic hormone (ACTH) by the pituitary. In turn, ACTH stimulates secretion of the glucocorticoids (cortisol in humans) by the adrenal cortex. This hormonal cascade, simplistically described, is the HPA axis—and its exact functioning is crucial as one of the major responses to stress. Likewise, it is involved in an elaborate feedback system to turn off the stress response. According to García-Bueno et al. (2008), the most specific function of the glucocorticoids in the hippocampus is this feedback inhibition of the HPA axis at the end of the stress. When humans are not stressed, both AVP and CRH are secreted in a circadian pattern, with a low for cortisol blood levels occurring around midnight and a peak between 6 A.M. and 8 A.M. This diurnal pattern can be disturbed by stress, changes in lighting, and even feeding schedules, and disturbed cortisol secretion is one of the factors involved in the feeling of discomfort known as jet lag.

The HPA axis is not the only pathway involved in the stress reaction. The autonomic nervous system (sympathetic and parasympathetic) is also involved by its secretion of a whole range of neurotransmitters—including serotonin, acetylcholine, and the catecholamines epinephrine, norepinephrine, and dopamine—that actually set in motion the HPA hormonal cascade (García-Bueno et al. 2008). The sympathetic and parasympathetic components innervate the major systems of the body, such as the cardiovascular, respiratory, gastrointestinal, renal, and endocrine systems, and are responsible for the control of the peripheral signs of anxiety (e.g., tachycardia and breathlessness) as well as increased blood pressure and a shifting of blood from digestive processes to the muscles.

Furthermore, the mesocorticolimbic system, which is responsible for the secretion of dopamine, is also involved in the stress reaction. It aids in our cognitive responses, such as anticipating, recognizing, and even remembering danger, and is involved in motivation and reward phenomena. Many other hormones are also involved (particularly those that regulate food intake—e.g., leptin, insulin, and neuropeptide Y), and stress, particularly when chronic, is now clearly linked to severe metabolic disturbances, such as the metabolic syndrome with its cluster of abnormalities including increased waist circumference (abdominal obesity), abnormal fasting blood glucose levels, insulin resistance, insulinemia, increased blood pressure, and abnormal triglycerides and other dyslipidemias.

Experiments by Kuo and her colleagues (2007) have also demonstrated that stress in mice exacerbates diet-induced obesity, specifically by activating the hormone neuropeptide Y, found in adipose tissue, which causes animals and humans to eat. They concluded that stress is not just in the mind and that stress, combined with a diet high in fat and sugar, can lead to gross obesity and the serious metabolic disturbances that accompany it. Dallman et al. (2006) note that with chronic stress in rats, corticosterone (analogous to cortisol in humans) acts in the brain in an excitatory rather than inhibitory way, and the researchers believe that the presence and quantity of circulating insulin is essential in modulating the effects of increased corticosterone. In other words, insulin, in the presence of corticosterone, lessens the catabolic effects of the glucocorticoids and hence increases visceral fat accumulation; when insulin secretion is reduced or absent, as in type 1 diabetes, fat accumulation decreases. Both starvation and restricted feeding produce increases in glucocorticoid levels prior to obtaining food and decreases in glucocorticoid levels after food ingestion (Pecoraro et al. 2006).

Another aspect of the stress response is the simultaneous release of chemical mediators called cytokines, which signal the presence of infection or inflammation, including inflammation of the brain (neuron inflammation) and activation of the immune system (García-Bueno et al. 2008). Cytokines are produced by different kinds of cells, such as macrophages and lymphocytes in the periphery and astrocytes in the brain. Researchers are only beginning to appreciate their importance physiologically, and García-Bueno et al. (2008) believe that a study of cytokine release is crucial to an understanding of the impact of stress on the brain, because inflammation can have effects on mood and memory and even on the life of a cell. Cytokines are divided into two types: one type includes interferon-γ, tumor necrosis factor-α, and interleukin-2, whereas the other includes the interleukins 4, 5, 6, and 10. Interestingly, levels of certain proinflammatory cytokines have been found to be elevated in the blood of depressed patients; levels of others are elevated in patients with bipolar disorder; and it is speculated that cytokines may be responsible for "depressive-like behaviors" sometimes seen during stress (García-Bueno et al. 2008).

Chronic stress, with its hyperactivation of the HPA axis, has also been implicated in psychological depression (Kyrou and Tsigos 2007). De Kloet (2004) summarizes studies that indicate that at least half of depressed patients have an abnormal circadian rhythm for cortisol secretion along with hyperactivity of the sympathetic nervous system, and increased secretion of cortisol is sometimes the hallmark of severe depression with psychotic features.

Pecoraro et al. (2006) describe experiments that showed that animals subjected to repeated stresses can develop two different forms of adaptation: *habituation*, in which repeated exposure diminishes the effect of the stress, or *facilitation* (sensitization), in which repeated exposure intensifies the reaction to the stress. Pecoraro et al. (2006) believe that the paraventricular thalamus may be involved in whether a stress reaction leads to habituation or facilitation. They also note that novel stimuli in a chronically stressed animal were more apt to produce facilitated responses.

• Desensitization (*habituation*) to chronic stress is a healthy adaptation, diminishing the effect of stress.

• Sensitization (*facilitation*) to chronic stress is an unhealthy reaction, intensifying the effect of stress.

There have also been experiments with animals and humans that have demonstrated changed eating patterns when subjects are under stress. Ulrich-Lai et al. (2007) report that humans under stress tend to increase their consumption of foods high in sugar and/or fat, the so-called comfort foods. They found that rats under conditions of both acute stress and chronic variable stress, although they might decrease their food intake in general, tended to gravitate toward comfort foods if given the opportunity and consumed up to 40% of their daily calories in sucrose. The researchers concluded that, particularly for acute stress, a sucrose drink may serve to dampen the stress response—but it did not do so for chronic stress, indicating that responses to acute and chronic stress may be under the control of different mechanisms. Dallman et al. (2005), in studying rats, also reported that comfort foods (those high in fat or sugar or both) dampened the stress reaction in research animals by reducing both the autonomic and the HPA responses generally seen with chronic stress. They further noted that although acute stress increased dopamine secretion, chronic stress inhibited it. Their speculation is that there is an interplay between the negative effects of the chronic stressors and the positive effects of the comfort foods in that these foods not only inhibit the HPA responses but also inhibit dopamine secretion.

Pecoraro et al. (2006) report on their own studies with rats that showed that although they reduced their total food intake when under stress, they ate proportionately more sugar and lard, that is, high-energy foods. The investigators explain that this type of diet makes sense in a hostile environment, as energy-dense foods can both maximize calorie intake and minimize hostile encounters. In other words, according to Pecoraro et al. (2006), their animal model with rats predicts that "repeated stressors call forth defensive behaviors" that are not compatible with feeding: stressed rats are less likely to go out foraging for food, and hence energy-dense food enables them to get a high caloric intake without exposing themselves as much to the dangers of a hostile environment. In a study of stress involving social hierarchy among rats (Tamashiro et al. 2006), the researchers found that subordinate rats lost weight due to hypophagia, but when they were no longer stressed, they gained the weight back as visceral fat (and were classified as obese by the researchers) and their levels of leptin and insulin remained elevated. The researchers concluded that chronic social stress resulted in long-term physiological changes in these rats and they related these changes to what happens in humans under stress in our society.

> Acute stress increases dopamine secretion, whereas chronic stress decreases it; comfort foods (high fat, high sugar) dampen these stress reactions in both conditions.

Gibson (2006) has focused on the complex emotional influences on food choice in humans. He notes that many things can affect how we feel about a meal, including how different it is from our usual meals (e.g., too much, less healthy). Sensory, psychological, and physiological pathways may be involved, and he noted that our mood can be altered by any number of things, such as by a particular food, a particular combination of foods, the social context in which food is eaten, our cognitive expectations, our psychological distractions, or changes in appetite. In general, perceived stress may make some more likely to reduce their food intake, whereas others, particularly those considered "emotional eaters," may increase their food intake and often favor foods high in fat and sugar, such as chocolate. Earlier studies by Polivy and Herman (1999) made the point that distress suppresses eating in those who are not dieting but increases eating in those who are chronic dieters (restrained eaters). Their theory is that dieters use overeating in order to distract themselves from distress in other areas of their lives that they cannot control. In other words, they can then attribute their distress to their eating patterns rather than to other areas of their lives.

Oliver and Wardle (1999) surveyed 212 students to investigate the effects of perceived stress on their eating patterns and found dieting status predicted which students would restrict their eating and which would eat more. Most respondents reported that stress did, in fact, affect their eating. All respondents tended to eat more snack types of foods and fewer meal-type foods like meat, fish, and vegetables. But those who tended to be restrained eaters (i.e., dieters) were more likely to report eating more when stressed than those who were not restrained eaters. Wardle et al. (2000) also reported that work stress, as measured by the number of hours of work in a department store (i.e., in a community setting, not laboratory research), led to greater calorie intake, particularly of fat and sugar, in those employees who were normally restrained eaters (dieters). Interestingly, these then-hyperphagic employees experienced a heightening of stress as a result of their eating pattern rather than a lessening of stress. The investigators thought that this pattern might be related to the phenomenon of disinhibition—the tendency of the dieters to put aside their usual cognitive inhibitions in the context of other, more pressing demands—rather than an attempt by these eaters to manage their stress through eating.

Weinstock (2008) notes that stress in a pregnant mother can have far-reaching effects on the developing fetus. This effect, because there are no direct neural connections between mother and fetus, must, says Weinstock, be mediated by the stress hormones such as CRH and cortisol, as well as by alterations in the blood flow to the placenta. Weinstock believes that the human fetal brain is greatly at risk for pathological development, including possible future behavioral disorders (e.g., attention problems and learning difficulties) as well as anxiety and depression, if maternal stress is present during critical stages of development. Mastorci et al. (2009) came to similar conclusions in studying prenatally stressed rats and believe that even though prenatal stress does not necessarily affect a structure or a function, it very much affects the animals' subsequent resilience and makes them more susceptible to pathophysiological outcomes.

> Because there is no neural connection between mother and fetus, the stress hormones of the mother are what predispose the fetal brain to potentially pathophysiological outcomes.

PERSONALITY, TEMPERAMENT, AND CHARACTER

> *"Personality" is one of the most abstract words in our language, and like any abstract word suffering from excessive use, its connotative significance is very broad, its denotative significance negligible.*
>
> Allport 1937, p. 25

> *Character is personality evaluated, and personality is character devaluated.*
>
> Allport 1937, p. 52

Personality is an umbrella term that incorporates temperament, character, and self-awareness (psyche). As such, it is an individual's distinctive manner of behaving, feeling, and thinking. Gordon Allport (1937, pp 24–54) defined *personality* as a unique, dynamic (i.e., evolving), organized system within an individual that determines his or her specific way of interacting with and adapting to the environment. And DSM-IV-TR defines *personality traits* as "enduring patterns of perceiving, relating to, and thinking about oneself and the environment" (American Psychiatric Association 2000, p. 686).

    Temperament.   Temperament is the most heritable aspect of personality; it is relatively stable over time, and is even somewhat correlated with adolescent and adult behavior. It can be defined as the body's automatic predisposition to respond to physical stimuli in a particular way. Allport (1937, p. 54) defined temperament as the "characteristic phenomena of an individual's nature," including fluctuations in mood, strength and speed of reactions, and susceptibility to "emotional stimulation." For Allport, temperament was "dependent upon constitutional make-up, and therefore largely hereditary in origin." Chess and Thomas (1986, p. 4) thought of temperament as the "how" of behavior, as differentiated from the "what" (e.g., content), the "why" (motivation), and the "how well." Back in the 1950s, they initiated a long-term study of infants and found nine categories of temperament that could be seen very early in an infant's life (pp. 273–278): 1) *activity level*; 2) *rhythmicity* (regularity), as in sleeping or eating patterns, for example; 3) *approach-withdrawal* response to a new stimulus; 4) *adaptability* to new situations; 5) *threshold of response* (i.e., what level intensity does infant respond to?); 6) *intensity or energy level of reaction*; 7) *quality of mood*; 8) *distractibility*; and 9) *attention span and persistence*. From these nine categories, the researchers found that, in general, infants and children fell into three major categories: 40% had an "easy" temperament (positive, regular, adaptable); 10% were "difficult" (irregular, negative, not adaptable); and 15% were "slow to warm up" (initially negative but slowly adaptable) (p. 279). But not all children fit into the Chess and Thomas categories. The researchers also emphasized that temperament is only one aspect of a person and should not be used exclusively (Chess and Thomas 1986, pp. 4–5) to categorize the person. Many factors, particularly the interaction of the person with the environment over time, may be involved in an evaluation of a person's behavior. In fact, not all of the children in their long-term study maintained the same temperament over time.

Cloninger and Svrakic (2009, pp. 2198–2199), who call temperament the "emotional core of personality," have divided traits of temperament into four major categories with their corresponding emotions: 1) harm avoidance (fear); 2) novelty seeking (anger); 3) reward dependence (attachment); and 4) persistence (ambition). Each category has major advantages and disadvantages. For example, those who fit the harm avoidance group may be shy, fearful, and pessimistic; likewise, they may also be adaptively cautious and able to plan ahead. These categories are not completely exclusive; individuals may fit into more than one. Cloninger and Svrakic (2009, pp. 2199–2201) report, for example, that those who are high in harm avoidance as well as novelty-seeking traits may have cycles of approach-avoidance, such as in binge eating cycles. They note that these four dimensions have been found to be universal in that they are seen in all ethnicities, all cultural groups, and even all political systems. And they are also seen in other mammals.

Temperament is most associated with procedural memory, that is, memory based on association or behavior conditioning. There are psychobiological correlates of Cloninger and Svrakic's four categories (2009, pp. 2199–2203); for example, functional MRI and PET scans indicate differences in specific brain volumes for individuals in the different groups, and they may even have different levels of neurotransmitters in circulation, such as plasma levels of γ-aminobutyric acid (GABA). A study by Beaver et al. (2006) reported that there is a network of interconnected brain regions involved in aspects of food rewards; persons high in the trait of reward dependence experienced more food cravings and were more likely to be overweight or have eating disorders. The researchers found that individual differences in reward sensitivity were highly correlated with activation of the frontostriatal-amygdalar-midbrain network when healthy subjects were shown pictures of foods like chocolate cake and pizza. They concluded that there is "consid-

- *Temperament* is primarily biological and represents the *how* of a person's pattern of perceiving, relating, and behaving.

- *Character* is the developmental outcome of the interaction between the person's temperament and his or her environment; it is the *who* of a person—the self identity.

- *Psyche* is a person's self-awareness of his or her personal memories; it is the *what* of a person.

- *Personality* is the umbrella term that incorporates temperament, character, and psyche.

erable personality-linked variability" in response to food cues that correlates with neural pathway activation.

Van Laere et al. (2009) have used the Cloninger and Svrakic model of personality (Cloninger and Svrakic 2009, pp. 2198–2204) to evaluate the PET scans of 47 healthy people. They found that those with personality high in novelty-seeking traits (e.g., impulsive, thrill seeking, *overeating*, substance abusing, and irritable) had low availability of type 1 cannabinoid receptors, primarily in the amygdala region, a region related to fear. In other words, the researchers speculate that those with novelty-seeking personalities may be more emotional and impulsive secondary to disrupted emotional learning and an inability to make use of memories of problematic (i.e., aversive) situations.

Character.   Character involves semantic memory, that is, declarative memory or memory involving cognitive functions like abstraction and reasoning. As such, one would not speak of character in regard to other animals. Cloninger and Svrakic (2009, p. 2204–2206) note that character is one's mental "self-government," and they have identified three distinct adaptive character traits: self-directedness, cooperativeness, and self-transcendency. Character develops over time and its development is very much dependent on an interaction of one's biological temperament with the people in one's environment, particularly one's parents. Psychoanalyst Francis Baudry (1983, 1989), who defined *character* as a recurrent, stable, and consistent cluster of traits and attitudes, reviewed the complicated evolution of Sigmund Freud's thinking in regard to character, starting from Freud's 1905 paper on sexuality (Freud 1906 [1905]/1953). For Freud, character derived from the interaction of one's biological constitution with one's libidinal drives (e.g., oral, anal, phallic-oedipal); identifications with parents; superego formation; fantasy life; and defense mechanisms. Baudry (1989) makes the point that character really reflects one's sense of identity. He admits he is not sure when one can talk of character formation beginning, though it is probably after the oedipal period (i.e., after age 4 or 5). The psychobiological model of character underscores the conscious nature of character formation whereas the psychoanalytic model focuses more on the unconscious realm (Cloninger and Svrakic 2009, pp. 2205–2206).

Psyche.   The third aspect of personality is the psyche, a person's consciousness or self-awareness, which, as Cloninger and Svrakic point out (2009, pp. 2206–2208), is unique to humans. It involves episodic memory, that is, recollection, or memory involving "recall of events in a context that gives personal meaning to the when and where of life experiences" (p. 2206). The authors also note that it is memory involving a conscious state of awareness of one's past, present, and future. They explain that when mental health professionals think of treatment, they must consider whether they are focusing on temperament, character, or psyche (pp. 2208–2210). For example, medications and behavior conditioning may target the biology of temperament, whereas long-term cognitive or psychodynamic treatment may target issues related to conflicts involving one's character.

We have noted that personality traits tend to fall into several different categories, using psychological parlance, though there is considerable overlap among categories. When a behavior pattern or way of relating is inflexible and maladaptive, then mental health professionals speak of an actual personality disorder. There are many ways that common personality traits may influence all aspects of life, including dieting, exercise, and even sex:

- If you have *paranoid traits,* you may be suspicious of any diet and not believe that any can work for you, or you may question the number of calories or other ingredients listed on a package—or whether a restaurant really left out the butter when you asked them to; you are more apt to accuse others about your weight gain and may even wonder if someone tampered with your scale; you may lie awake at night thinking of the injustices done to you that day; you may be excessively jealous and accuse your partner of infidelity unfairly.

- If you have *antisocial traits*, you are more likely to cheat on your diet, tamper with your scale, and misrepresent how much you weigh, eat, or exercise, even to your physician; you may abuse drugs or alcohol, and you may be more likely to abuse sleeping medications and develop an addiction; you may sabotage someone else's diet without much regard to their welfare; you are not a faithful type and may "love them and leave them" without much intimacy.

- If you have *histrionic traits,* you are more likely to exaggerate how well or how badly you have done in an all-or-none fashion: "I ate all day and didn't stop" or "I exercised for hours!" or "I didn't sleep a wink last night"; calorie counting and exact measuring are not for you. You may also be particularly focused on how people notice the weight you lost and their reactions; you may be overly stylish and seductive in your exercise attire, and you may be more interested in socializing than exercising; you are seductive but may actually be afraid of sex and intimacy.

- If you have *borderline traits*, you may be most likely to sabotage your dieting efforts impulsively by bingeing (and purging), abusing substances like alcohol, or even abusing diet medications in an effort to curb your eating; you may also become addicted to sleep medications; you may idealize or devalue your physicians, trainers, and other care providers, as well as your partner; you may also shop impulsively and you may feel particularly empty afterward. You alternate between being clingy and pushing your partner away; you may also be demanding and hypersexual with your partner or even promiscuous with many partners.

- If you have *narcissistic traits,* you may be more likely to feel your diet is the best one and others are worthless; you must have the "best" trainer or "best" physician; you need people to admire your efforts, and you are smug and condescending toward others who fail; your own self-esteem plummets, though, if you fail in your efforts; you may also have a "why me?" attitude about your weight problem ("Why do I have to watch what I eat when others don't?"). Sexually, you are not particularly sensitive to or empathic toward your partner.

- If you have *avoidant traits*, you may tend to hide and be even more inhibited if you gain weight; you are less likely to want to exercise in a gym or with a trainer, but rather to do so alone; Weight Watchers or Overeaters Anonymous is definitely not for you; you crave being with others but are too shy to do so without much coaxing; you may avoid intimacy and sex unless you know your partner really loves you.

- If you have *dependent traits*, you may want to have your eating plan, calorie count, and exercise all determined by someone else; you are easily influenced by others and may try the latest fad diet if an expert recommends it. You are in their hands and don't want to have to make any decisions—everyone else is the authority; you may thrive on specific diet plans that include prepackaged food, and may like to work with a trainer who organizes your exercise. You always want to be in a relationship: you may have trouble ending a relationship without having someone else, and you may be too self-sacrificing in order to keep a relationship. You sleep best when you are with someone.

- If you have *obsessive-compulsive traits*, you may want to follow a diet and exercise program to the letter. You may write down everything you eat and take to keeping an accurate food diary, but for you, it is all or none; you may get easily discouraged if you eat more than you want or exercise less than you feel you should. And you feel particularly guilty if you misrepresent how much you have eaten or how much you weigh. You take easily to counting calories, measuring portions, or counting miles on the treadmill exactly; you have the most accurate balance scale available, though you may complain about its cost; you feel most comfortable with schedules and always feel somewhat pressured by time—sleeping and sex may be on a fairly rigid schedule as well. You probably write down your dreams, but may be kept up at night thinking of all the things you need to do tomorrow.

PSYCHOLOGICAL DEFENSE MECHANISMS

Defense mechanisms are human psychological (mental) processes that occur automatically—that is, out of conscious awareness—in all of us. They serve to protect us from or help us cope with perceived dangers and painful thoughts or emotions. In that sense, defense mechanisms are our means of adaptation, or as Harvard psychiatrist George Vaillant (1992, p. 45) says, they help us "restore our psychological homeostasis." They are our way of involuntarily "coping with sudden changes [in our] external or internal milieu" (Vaillant 1992, p. 44). Freud, who thought they were part of ego functions, was the first to study the defense mechanisms systematically. In fact, Vaillant believes that the concept of defense mechanisms was one of Freud's most original contributions to the field (Vaillant 1992, p. 3).

SOME DEFENSE MECHANISMS ON EATING

- *Repression:* inability to remember physicians' or dietitians' advice

- *Displacement:* blaming others for one's weight problems—spouse, restaurants, etc.

- *Denial:* inability to accept the reality (e.g., believing dry cleaning is shrinking one's pants)

- *Projection:* attributing undesirable ideas to the external world (the scale is faulty)

- *Rationalization:* talking oneself out of something (I'm too busy to exercise; I have too slow a metabolism; I cannot resist chocolate)

- *Intellectualization:* trying to master the subject intellectually (If you diet you may live a few years longer? Well, it may *feel* like that....)

The concept of defense is central to psychoanalytic theory and clinical practice. Vaillant (1992) believes that any clinical formulation of a patient should include a focus on the patient's primary mechanisms of defense. Psychoanalyst Robert Waelder (1951), as stated in his paper on paranoid ideas, believed that a patient's defense mechanisms essentially determine the patient's pathology. And DSM-IV-TR includes (for further study) a proposed "defensive functioning scale" (American Psychiatric Association 2000, pp. 807–813) in which a clinician would list up to seven specific defenses, including those observed during the evaluation and those typical of the patient's recent functioning. In this scale, defenses are arranged functionally, with the highest adaptive level, such as use of humor or sublimation, listed first and "defensive dysregulation," such as psychotic denial or distortion, listed last.

Vaillant (1992, p. 4) notes that over the years, Freud delineated 17 different mechanisms. Initially, Freud considered repression, the unconscious withholding from consciousness of an idea or feeling that causes anxiety; it is the first defense he encountered clinically, the "most venerated and most central weapon in the defense arsenal" (Siegal 1969). Siegal notes that repression is actually present to some degree in all defense mechanisms ("in all defending, something...is kept from consciousness"). According to Vaillant (1992, p. 4), Freud thought of defense mechanisms as having five significant properties: 1) they are a way of managing biological instincts and affects; 2) they occur unconsciously; 3) they are discrete from one another, though several often operate together; 4) they are not fixed but rather are dynamic and reversible; and 5) they can be adaptive as well as pathological.

Many theoreticians since Freud have studied defense mechanisms. Each theorist has his or her own list of them, and many, including Freud, have attempted to categorize them according to level of pathology. Freud's daughter Anna Freud, a child analyst, wrote her book *The Ego and the Mechanisms of Defense* (A. Freud 1966) as an eightieth birthday present for her father and looked at defense mechanisms developmentally. Waelder (1951) requested an "alphabet of defense mechanisms." Bibring et al. (1961), who delineated 24 basic (first-order) and 15 complex (second-order) defense mechanisms, called for a "catalogue of defenses." Otto Kernberg focuses on the hierarchical nature of defense mechanisms, particularly in regard to patients with borderline conditions, and has noted the importance of categorizing defenses along a continuum, with defense mechanisms like splitting, primitive idealization, projective identification, and psychotic denial regarded as particularly pathological and primitive (Clarkin et al. 2006, pp. 16–19; Kernberg 1983, pp. 25–34). Charles Brenner (1981), on the other hand, believed that the entire concept of defense mechanisms was wrong and outdated and felt there are no special ego functions that are exclusively mechanisms of defense. Brenner felt that "whatever ensues in mental life that results in the diminution of unpleasurable affects...belongs under the heading of defense" (Brenner 1981). He felt that defenses could be identified only by their function or consequence, namely, to ward off some impulse, displeasure, or anxiety, and that "all aspects of ego functioning are all-purpose." He also felt that denial, in the sense of negating something, is part of every defense and he did not agree that a person's defense "repertory" is necessarily limited or characteristic.

Vaillant (1992, p. 130), though, in disagreement with Brenner, has sought to study defense mechanisms more systematically by means of a questionnaire he devised. He has divided defenses into categories of narcissistic, immature, neurotic, and mature, and has been able to correlate them with the notion of mental health. He acknowledges, though, that they are extremely difficult to study because the "whole concept of mechanisms of defense is metaphorical.... We will never be able to measure defenses in milligrams per cubic centimeter" (Vaillant 1992, p. 41). He further notes that they cannot be directly visualized, and it is only through a patient's resistances and symptoms that defense mechanisms become apparent at all. As Siegal (1969) has said, mental processes can be " 'seen' only by inference." Siegal also cautions against the typical confusion of using the term *defense* interchangeably with *defense mechanism*, thereby "confusing mental contents with mental processes." Furthermore, because defense mechanisms rarely occur in isolation, defining a single defense becomes reductionistic (Vaillant 1992, p. 50).

Siegal (1969) points out that the defense mechanism of reaction formation—in which a person who has aggressive wishes toward a person behaves unusually pleasantly toward that person, for example—really involves a constellation of mechanisms, including repression (pushing an idea out of consciousness), displacement (substituting one affect for another), and reversal of the original wish. Ultimately, Vaillant (1992, p. 145) notes, his own studies could not find a clear relationship between a patient's defense style as measured by his questionnaire and a patient's diagnosis (as then diagnosed by DSM-III [American Psychiatric Association 1980]). Forty years ago Siegal said, "We may some day be talking about chemistry, electricity, and neurophysiology when we are trying to describe functions and structures underlying behavior and those special processes we call defense mechanisms" (Siegal 1969). All these years later, despite functional MRI and other technology, we have yet to locate ego functions and defense mechanisms specifically.

Nevertheless, because most theoreticians do believe that people tend to use the same few defense mechanisms repeatedly—"rounding up the usual suspects," as it were—those helping patients with their weight may find a study of defense mechanisms helpful in understanding unconscious patterns of behavior. Here are examples involving some of the most common defense mechanisms:

- With *repression*, a person is unable to remember something unpleasant; *examples:* forgetting you were ever told by your physician that you should not drink alcohol with the medication you are taking or that diabetes can lead to serious kidney, cardiac, or eye disorders.
- With *displacement*, there is a transfer or redirecting of intense ideas or feelings from one person onto a substitute, stand-in person or object; *examples:* angrily blaming your weight problem on your parents instead of your poor eating habits; complaining about the hospital food instead complaining about your illness and that you have to be hospitalized; being afraid of needles instead of being fearful of learning the outcome of a medical procedure.
- With *denial*, there is an inability to accept something painful or unpleasant, or, when severe, even a failure to see some reality; *examples:* believing the dry cleaner is shrinking your clothes rather than that you are gaining weight; ignoring a lump in your breast rather than going to see a physician; refusing to accept that a loved one is dying, despite evidence to the contrary.
- With *reaction formation*, some painful idea is replaced in the consciousness with its opposite; *examples:* being extremely solicitous toward someone you really hate; being a crusader against smoking when you were a smoker; having a "holier than thou" attitude, as in "the lady doth protest too much."
- With *regression*, a person resorts to an earlier, more primitive functioning; *examples:* having a full-blown temper tantrum when you need blood drawn for a procedure; crying when you hear bad news about your health; yelling at your doctor's nurse for having to wait for an appointment; adamantly refusing to follow doctor's orders initially, despite your need to do so.
- With *projection*, a painful impulse or idea is attributed to the external world; *examples:* you don't hate someone, it's that that person hates you; imbuing some inanimate object with human attributes, such as "The scale hates me" or "We can trick the fat into vanishing by varying our exercises."
- With *isolation*, there is a splitting off of a painful feeling from the ideas attached to it; *examples:* thinking of eating something harmful to you without the appropriate emotional feeling; discussing your serious illness matter-of-factly, without much accompanying affect, as if you were discussing the weather.

- With *identification*, a person behaves like or takes on the attributes of someone else admired or respected; *example:* beginning to dress and behave like your parents, physician, trainer, or therapist.
- With *identification with the aggressor,* a person takes on the characteristics of someone who has caused pain or suffering: *examples:* abusing a child when you yourself were abused as a child; reprimanding your child for eating too much when you were reprimanded by your parents for the same behavior.
- With *rationalization*, one essentially talks oneself out of something by reasoning; *examples:* saying you can just eat a little (and truly believing it at the moment) when you know that has never worked before; saying you are too busy to exercise or that you can't lose weight because you have a "slow metabolism" rather than because you are eating too much.
- With *intellectualization,* one controls feelings and impulses by thinking about them instead of experiencing them; handling your anxiety and discomfort by trying to master the subject; *examples:* you have been told that you have diabetes and the metabolic syndrome and you read everything there is on the Internet in an attempt to know more than your physicians; discussing your symptoms abstractly as if you were talking about someone else.
- With *undoing*, there is an action and then a reversal of that action; often seen in obsessive-compulsive symptoms, like turning off and on the gas jets; *examples:* you lose weight and then gain it back; you exercise and then eat voraciously afterward, taking in as many calories as you just worked off.
- With *sublimation*, one of the highest-level defense mechanisms (i.e., one of the healthiest), there is a transforming of sexual or aggressive impulses or conflicts into something creative and more socially acceptable; *examples:* becoming a medical researcher when you were overweight as a child; writing a book about dieting when you have your own conflicts about eating.
- With *humor,* also one of the highest-level defense mechanisms, a person is able to experience a painful emotion and look directly at it without the anxiety and discomfort normally associated with the emotion; *example:* the gallows humor of being able to laugh at one's impending death or, as your father's coffin is being lowered into the ground and gets stuck for a moment on one of the pulleys, laughing with your brother, knowing that your father, who was particularly known for his impatience, would be cursing away at the workers' incompetence.

THE PSYCHOLOGY OF TEMPTATION AND SELF-CONTROL

Some experiments done years ago by Shoda and his colleagues (1990) found that preschoolers (mean age, 4 years, 4 months) who were able to resist an impulse and delay gratification did significantly better in school and even had higher SAT scores when they were adolescents. Initially, the researchers presented the children with the possibility of a reward, such as a marshmallow, pretzel, or colored poker chip, but told the children that they would get twice as much if they could delay taking the first one (for 15–20 minutes) until the researcher returned from an errand. They noted that it was particularly difficult for some preschoolers to resist when they could actually see the reward, when the rewards were, in the researchers' words, exposed rather than obscured. (Think how difficult it is for most adults to resist dessert when the dessert tray is actually brought to the table.) This is the *marshmallow test* that Daniel Goleman wrote about in his book *Emotional Intelligence* (Goleman 1995, pp. 80–82). For Goleman, delaying an impulse is the "essence of emotional self-regulation" and has far-reaching implications.

> Temptation is "the desire to behave in a certain way that is expected to be regretted at a later time."
>
> **Source: Magen and Gross 2007**

The researchers (Shoda et al. 1990) were cautious in interpreting the connection between preschool impulse control and adolescent behavior. They acknowledge that many other factors, such as child-rearing practices or the stability of the families involved, may be responsible, though they do feel that "the qualities that underlie effective self-imposed delay [in gratification] in preschoolers may be crucial ingredients…[for] intelligent social behavior" (Shoda et al. 1990). Though they also acknowledge that postponing gratification is not always the wise or adaptive choice, they believe that children who can postpone it when they want to at least have the "freedom to make that choice."

That freedom to choose is what differentiates us from animals and is directly related to an understanding of weight control in humans. Psychologist Roy Baumeister, who has written extensively on self-control, explains that self-control "allows humans to stop what they are doing in the middle…[to] override responses that are already in progress" (Baumeister 2005, p. 310). It is what gives us the capacity for flexibility in our responses, unlike most other species, which have "predictable and stereotyped behavior." Temptation as defined by Magen and Gross (2007) is "the desire to behave in a certain way that is expected to be regretted at a later time." In other words, a particular behavior will bring *certain*, rather than probable, regret.

> Obesity may involve lack of intrinsic and extrinsic motivations.

Baumeister (2005, p. 163) notes that human motivations can be divided essentially into two kinds: intrinsic motivation, where someone wants something for its own sake (to satisfy one's own needs), and extrinsic motivation, where someone wants something as a means to something else (where there may be a desire to gain a reward or avoid a punishment). Because of our ability to "form complex chains of associations and [foresee] distant outcomes" (p. 311), humans are capable of being motivated by something in the future—something that does not have an intrinsic, immediate result, but rather may have a later payoff. His examples include voting in an election, recycling trash, and obeying the speed limit. Baumeister (2005, p. 164) believes that extrinsic motivation "in its full fledged form" (i.e., not just conditioned responses) may be unique to humans. And Vohs and Baumeister (2004, p. 3) go as far as to say that nearly every major personal and social problem (including addictions, obesity, debt, and procrastination) in society may involve some kind of difficulty with self-regulation.

Self-regulation is the broader term—as differentiated from *self-control*, which deals only with conscious, more deliberate processes—incorporating both conscious and nonconscious (i.e., automatic) efforts by humans to regulate thoughts, feelings, attention, emotions, impulses, or appetites (Baumeister and Vohs 2004, p. 2). It involves areas of our brain such as the prefrontal cortex that are involved with executive functions (or, in Sigmund Freud's vocabulary, *ego functions* such as working memory, attention, and decision making) as well as connections to the limbic (emotional circuits) and motor areas of the brain (Banfield et al. 2004, pp. 62, 68).

THE PSYCHOLOGY OF TEMPTATION

- Do not confuse truly irresistible impulses (breathing, sleeping) with resistible ones (eating, shopping); take care of your emotional distresses (anxiety, depression), which cause breakdowns in self-control that make you more apt to eat unhealthy foods or seek immediate gratification.

- Selectively use self-control: self-control is weakest among those who have already performed acts of self-control; self-control is stronger in the morning and may wane with each decision you have to make.

- Regulate your sleep: sleep restores self-control.

Source: Baumeister 2002

One question that has puzzled researchers is why self-control fails. Baumeister (2002) makes the point that few impulses are in reality irresistible, even though many of us have had thoughts like "I just couldn't resist" in situations involving shopping, sex, or food. Irresistible impulses, on the other hand, are physical needs such as breathing, sleeping, or urinating. As Baumeister says, "Even the gun to the head will not prevent" these acts from eventually occurring, no matter how much a person wants to resist. In other words, most other impulses (including crimes such as murder, which "never seem to be committed in the presence of an armed police officer") can, in fact, actually be controlled when it is to the advantage of the person to do so (Baumeister 2002). Baumeister considers most other so-called irresistible impulses mere "rationalizations."

But self-control does fail. For Baumeister (2002), effective self-control involves having standards (i.e., goals, norms, ideals), some kind of monitoring system, and the capacity to modify one's behavior. People get into trouble, for example, when they have conflicting goals or ambivalent attitudes toward something. Sparks and his colleagues (2001) note that people can have ambivalent attitudes, including *cognitive* ambivalence ("mixed beliefs"), *affective* ambivalence ("torn feelings"), or both.

For example, they showed how subjects' conflicting attitudes (ambivalence) toward consuming foods like meat or chocolate (e.g., "chocolate is delicious" vs. "chocolate is fattening") interfered with their intentions to eat or restrict these foods.

Self-control, that is, resistance to temptation, is also easier for some than for others, for reasons that are complex (including genetic, neuroanatomical, and environmental influences) and not completely understood. What we do know is that self-control for most people is a finite quantity. In other words, it can be depleted by fatigue, stress, time of day, substance use such as alcohol use, and even the number of times it is called into effect. This is the *strength model* of self-control (Baumeister 2002). So, for example, when a person's self-control is depleted for one reason or another, the person is more likely to be impulsive. An example of this is the dieter who resists temptations all day, and perhaps even makes sensible choices all through dinner (exerting self-control several times in regard to choices), but is depleted by the end of the meal and cannot resist the dessert. Schmeichel and Baumeister (2004, p. 95) also noted that resisting something tempting to eat is depleting only when that person is dieting—when the person has the goal of restricting calories or consumption of a specific food. Baumeister (2002) makes the point that people are more likely to make impulsive purchases at the mall or in the grocery line at the end of a long day of shopping, and they often make purchases to make themselves feel better. Says Baumeister (2002), "sad or distressed shoppers may show an increase in purchases of snack foods, music CDs, and flashy clothes, but much less change in their purchases of light bulbs, toilet paper, or oven cleaners." Sleep, incidentally, can replenish our self-control.

SELF-CONTROL AND STRESS

- Sad or distressed shoppers are more likely to purchase snack foods, flashy clothes, or CDs than light bulbs, toilet paper, or oven cleaners.

- Likewise, sad or distressed diners are more likely to order chocolate cake and ice cream than extra salad with dressing on the side.

Source: Baumeister 2002

Monitoring one's behavior is a crucial element in maintaining self-control, and one we will return to specifically in regard to maintaining weight loss (see Chapter 10, "Diet and Weight"). First of all, one has to remember what one has done, whether it is spending too much money or eating too many calories. Higgs (2008) reports that people will eat less if they are reminded of what they have already eaten, and she even notes that both laboratory animals and people with hippocampal lesions who cannot remember having eaten will eat another entire meal immediately thereafter.

Brian Wansink, in his book *Mindless Eating*, notes that people eat less when their dirty plates (e.g., bones of eaten chicken wings) are left around (Wansink 2006, pp. 37–40); he found when people were given a bowl of soup that was secretly being filled (so that it would never get empty), they had no idea of how much they were eating and ate considerably more soup than they would have had they seen the bowl emptying. John Tierney, a reporter for the *New York Times*, in reporting on functional MRI studies of the brain (Knutson et al. 2007), spoke of his own "lazy" insula, the area of the brain that is supposed to light up "when you smell something bad, see a disgusting picture, or anticipate a painful shock" (Tierney 2007). His insula, instead of lighting up when he saw a price that was too high, was "particularly stoic" and so did not protect him sufficiently to prevent him from overspending. For those who have trouble controlling their spending, having an automatic picture of their credit card bills appear every time they have the temptation to buy something that they do not need—to "jump start" the insula—may be enough to deter them. That is also why monitoring food intake with food diaries can help prevent overeating.

Studies by Knoch and Fehr (2007) also report on areas of the brain that seem to control temptation. Say the authors, "Based on the results of these studies, we dare to claim that the capacity to resist temptation depends on the activity level of the right prefrontal cortex" (Knoch and Fehr 2007). In a bold move, as it were to "jump start" our insulas, New York City, in December 2008, became the first city in the nation not only to ban toxic trans fats from all restaurants, but also to require fast food chain restaurants to post their foods' calories on their menus in large type easily visible to patrons—providing a kind of sticker shock. And an article in *New York* magazine listed the calorie count for the average nine-course meal, which costs around $250 (without wine) for one person at the four-star New York restaurant Per Se. It tallied over 1,230 calories; with wine and some extras, the calorie count rose to over 2,400 calories and over 100 grams of fat—more than the recommended amount for an entire day's worth of calories! The author of the article, Charles Stuart Platkin (2007), noted that a person who weighs 155 pounds would have to walk the entire New York City marathon (26 miles) plus an additional 5 miles to work off all those calories.

Experiments by Shiv and his colleagues involving consumer studies have shown many of us often make emotional, mindless, and impulsive decisions rather than cognitive, mindful ones when we are shopping, particularly if the choices are right in front of us (as opposed to photographs of items) and particularly if we are distracted (Shiv and Fedorikhin 1999). We are, for example, more apt to buy on impulse if there is a particularly attractive display or music in the background. Even a shorter check-out line makes us more impulsive because we have less time to reconsider impulsive purchases. These researchers found that some people are just more impulsive than those whom they call the "prudents," who are more apt to think about their choices and the consequences.

Impulsive decisions are often associated with a positive response to a product that has negative consequences (e.g., buying chocolate cake, which tastes delicious but is fattening and unhealthy). The authors raise the question, "Why do we continue to observe consumers who, for example, know more about the importance of nutrition than ever before and yet struggle with their efforts to control their weights and cholesterol levels?" (Shiv and Fedorikhin 1999). They say that one aspect is that many consumers rationalize their behavior immediately after an impulsive behavior, "resulting in the view that the behavior was appropriate, but after a period of time they may experience pangs of guilt, leading to attempts at self control." They also note that consumers often make decisions "mindlessly," that is, without giving enough cognitive thought to their underlying feelings. But asking their subjects to wait before making a choice made some people reconsider, whereas it made others feel more deprived and yield more quickly to temptation (Shiv and Fedorikhin 1999).

Another aspect to temptation is the temporal element involved. Magen and Gross (2007) explain that yielding to temptation brings immediate gratification, whereas resisting it may bring immediate discomfort but delayed gratification. They note people often value less (devalue, or discount) something that will take place in the future, and this may be part of why people procrastinate, fail to maintain a diet, or do not exercise regularly. It may also be a part of why people do not give up smoking: they can discount the possibility that they will get cancer some time in the future.

The researchers (Magen and Gross 2007) recommend a "cognitive reconstrual" process of obtaining self-control. This is a process of empowering people to resist temptation by having them think more positively about their short-term goals and aligning them with long-term goals to reduce the discrepancy between short- and long-term consequences. It is a cognitive effort to make the temptation less tempting. Resisting temptation can then be seen more positively, as an important test of willpower rather than as a deprivation. The authors do appreciate that this reshaping has a potential liability because when someone fails to resist temptation, the person may develop lower self-esteem and other negative feelings.

> Resisting temptation can be seen as an important test of willpower rather than as a deprivation.

Kivetz and Keinan (2006) take a different tack altogether. They have studied how time can make people wistful about some of their previous decisions in which they exerted self-control. They interviewed former college students about their winter break plans of 40 years earlier and compared them with present-day college students' plans. They noted that "with the passage of time, choices of virtue over vice [work over pleasure] evoke increasing regret" (Kivetz and Keinan (2006). In other words, "while yielding to temptation generates [regret about indulgences] in the short run," it has the opposite effect in the long term. Kivetz and Keinan (2006) explain that people have "indulgence guilt" in the short term that diminishes over time.

Yielding to temptation in the short term and regretting it afterward is one thing, but actually changing a behavioral pattern is something different; this gets to the heart of weight control. Studies have shown (Rothman et al. 2004, p. 133) that people initiate a change in behavior when they have confidence in their ability to change that behavior. In other words, they must first have the expectation of a favorable outcome. This is the notion of *self-efficacy* (Rothman et al. 2004, pp. 140–141), and one's mindset is crucial. The authors also note that people tend to be more successful when some of their goals can be met immediately (p. 137). So, for example, losing those few pounds initially can be very reinforcing for the dieter, as when someone giving up smoking notices the riddance of the foul cigarette smell that permeates one's surroundings. They also explain that anything that undermines a person's ability to be optimistic about the outcome (e.g., a sabotaging partner or a generally pessimistic personality) will likely interfere with this vulnerable initial phase (p. 136). This phase is also particularly susceptible to the "what the hell" effect, the all-or-nothing attitude that dieters sometimes have, whereby if they eat something they should not, they then give up completely; Herman and Polivy (2004, p. 498) call this the "perverse logic of the dieter." Rogers and Smit (2000) speak of the diet boundary that some dieters cross when they have eaten more calories than intended, then find themselves going from normally restrained eating to unrestrained eating.

If one can get beyond the initial phase, the next is the maintenance phase, where the new behavior, such as watching one's weight or giving up smoking, is continually being reassessed (Rothman et al. 2004, p. 138). Maintaining the new behavior takes less conscious effort; people are not actively struggling, and they can stay in the maintenance phase indefinitely. People in this phase are more concerned with whether the behavior continues to have value to them. The last transition is to the phase in which the new behavior is a habit. Here people no longer need to reassure themselves that they can maintain the behavior and no longer need to evaluate the behavior's value. Once in the habit stage, people continue the behavior "until an event of sufficient magnitude causes them to reconsider it" (p. 138).

Another aspect of self-regulation is the significance of other people with whom we have relationships. It is human nature that our own goals can be triggered by watching the behavior of those important to us. This is called *goal contagion* (Fitzsimons and Bargh 2004, p. 158), and it has been found to occur automatically, without conscious awareness. Further, we are also influenced to adopt for ourselves the goals that a significant person may have for us. In other words, a person's social network may be a contributing element in the obesity epidemic. Christakis and Fowler (2007), for example, conducted a long-term study with 32 years of follow-up (as part of the Framingham Heart Study) involving over 12,000 people; they found that a person had a 57% greater chance of becoming obese (as measured by body mass index) if that person had a friend who also became obese in the same time frame. And those who had the closest friendships with each other were more of an influence on each other than those whose friendships were more one-sided: with mutually valued friendships, one had a 171% chance of becoming obese if the friend was. In other words, the researchers found there were "discernible clusters of obese people at all time points" across this longitudinal study.

Among pairs of adult siblings in the same study, if one became obese, there was a 40% greater chance that the other would become obese; among spouses, if one spouse became obese, there was a 37% greater chance the other spouse would become obese in that time. Apparently, changes in neighbors' weights did not necessarily affect the likelihood of someone else in the same locale becoming obese, so environmental issues did not seem to be significant here, and smoking status did not confound the results. Notably, people of the same sex seemed to have a somewhat greater influence on one's chances of becoming obese than did people of the opposite sex. The authors' conclusion was that social distance seems more important than physical or geographical distance in obesity trends.

A more recent study by The and Gordon-Larsen (2009) confirmed that those sharing a "household environment" are more apt to become obese, and the longer the pair is together, the more likely obesity will occur in both men and women. When these couples were in relationships for longer than 2 years, they were more likely to be inactive and sedentary as well. (See Chapter 12, "Pharmacological and Surgical Treatments," for another reference to "social distance" and its relationship to obesity.)

Another tactic used for self-regulation and motivation is that of financial incentives. Volpp et al. (2009) found that those who were paid were much more likely to give up smoking over the course of a year of follow-up than those who were only given information regarding the harmful effects of smoking. Financial incentives, though, work only when the reward is valuable enough to someone. Volpp et al (2009) speculate that when a reward doesn't work as effectively, it may be that the particular incentive was not significant enough for the person. Certainly this mode of external self-regulation is the basis for the popular television show *The Biggest Loser,* in which both fame and fortune, as well as competition with others (and possibly humiliation and embarrassment), motivate contestants to lose substantial amounts of weight over time.

Finally, self-regulation can be maintained when we have our own "cognitive set point," as first delineated by Booth in the late 1970s (Booth 1978; Rogers and Smit 2000). This involves our deliberate control of eating, and it involves how we perceive our own shape, size, and weight, perceptions often based on the norms of our society. When we notice a change in the way our clothes are fitting or a change in our weight on a scale, we realize we have deviated from our cognitive set point. Though this point can shift over time one way or another, most of us have had the feeling that there is a number on the scale we dare not cross.

REWARD, CRAVINGS, AND ADDICTION (DOPAMINE, ENDOCANNABINOIDS)

Morton et al. (2006) have noted how very complicated is our decision to eat something: cognitive, visual, and olfactory cues help us determine whether the food could even be potentially toxic. After all, infants will mouth anything (food and nonfood) throughout the first year of life; Sigmund Freud even called the first year of life the oral phase. Unconsciously, even before the first bite is taken, our minds, bodies, and brains make extraordinary calculations to maintain our homeostasis, involving both "food-seeking behavior (important for meal initiation) and satiety perception (important for meal termination)" (Morton et al. 2006). And all this takes place at every meal. Morton et al. (2006) believe that the lateral hypothalamus is the area of the brain that may be responsible for integrating energy homeostasis, satiety, and reward aspects of food with the motor-related activities that are required, such as obtaining food and eating it. Berthoud (2007) emphasizes that involvement of large areas of the nervous system in the obtaining of food was a major survival mechanism in both humans and animals. He believes the neocortex (including the orbitofrontal, cingular, and insular areas), the older limbic cortex (hippocampus and amygdala), the striatum (nucleus accumbens, ventral pallidum), the hypothalamus (lateral, perifornical areas), and the ventral midbrain (ventral tegmental area) are all involved.

Berridge and Robinson (2003) describe three psychological components to reward: 1) learning about relationships among stimuli and the consequences of actions; 2) pleasure ("hedonic consequences"); and 3) motivation to learn about and to act on this knowledge. Zheng and Berthoud (2008), on the other hand, believe *reward* is a "fuzzy psychological construct" that is "neurologically ill-defined."

Pelchat (2002) makes the point that food cravings, which are extremely common (almost everyone has them now and then), involve not only an intense desire to eat but also a specificity for a particular food, and this is what differentiates food cravings from general hunger. In a sense, then, food cravings can be evolutionarily beneficial because they may lead to interest in and a search for a variety of foods, and hence to a greater tendency to meet nutritional requirements. Pelchat (2002) also notes that there is a difference between liking a food and craving it: one can like a food without craving it, and of course, one can crave a food without even being hungry. Wise (2006) further differentiates wanting a food from liking it in animals as well as humans: *wanting* is the state of mind before taking in a reward, whereas *liking* is that state "once the reward has been earned and sensed"; he further notes, as does Berthoud (2007), that dopamine is important for wanting but not for liking. Berridge and Robinson (2003) note that wanting is motivational and that it "transforms mere sensory information about rewards and their cues (sights, sounds, and smells) into attractive, desired, riveting incentives." In other words, wanting "refers to a conscious or subjective desire" and is considered "incentive salience." Berthoud speculates that wanting and liking evolved separately: wanting may have evolved early as "an elementary form of stimulus-guided goal direction" (e.g., for food or sex; Berthoud 2007); liking, on the other hand, may have evolved as a means of facilitating "comparison and choice among competing rewards that have incommensurate 'likes' (e.g., food, sex, and shelter)."

Grigson (2002) summarizes the overlapping relationship between substance abuse and "natural rewards" like water, food, or sucrose. Opiates can increase one's

> There is a high correlation between a preference for drugs and a preference for sweets.
>
> **Grigson 2002**

responsiveness to food, and one's intake of food can increase the release of endogenous opiates. Endogenous opioids are β-endorphin, enkephalin, and dynorphin (Cota et al. 2006). There is a high correlation between a preference for drugs and a preference for sweets (Grigson 2002). Further, restricting one's food consumption can lead to increased cravings and even increased self-administration of drugs, and a sensitization-like response (an increase in the response to the stimulus) can develop when there is repeated exposure to drugs or food. And cravings for food and drugs can be conditioned by certain cues. In humans, cravings for food, even when the person is not hungry, can increase when food-related cues such as smell or visual imagery are present.

Grigson (2002) makes the point that naturally motivated behaviors such as food or water intake or having sex share a common reward circuit and that "[although] each motivated behavior has its own internal mechanism for satiety…the common reward substrate, itself…has no means for 'satiety.'" Grigson explains that this re-

> Contrary to common belief, those with an immediate strong impulse to eat or to take drugs are not simultaneously interested in sex.

ward circuit evolutionarily is then "prepared for continuous activation" as the "animal seamlessly switches from one motivated behavior to another." Unfortunately, this does not serve an animal (including humans) with an addiction well, although one motivated behavior may interfere with another (e.g., those with an immediate strong impulse to eat or take drugs are not simultaneously interested in sex). Kelley and Berridge (2002) point out that our brains evolved to respond to natural rewards like food or sex that were important from an evolutionary perspective for survival and reproduction. But addiction remains ill defined, partly because we do not completely understand why only some of those exposed to certain substances like drugs actually develop an addiction (Baler and Volkow 2006).

Essentially, addiction is a process involving uncontrollable, compulsive seeking and use of a substance or substances despite negative health and social consequences. According to Baler and Volkow (2006), addiction involves at least four different and interrelated neurological circuits, all involving dopamine: 1) *reward* circuits (located in the nucleus accumbens, ventral pallidum, and hypothalamus); 2) *motivation and/or drive* circuits (located in the orbitofrontal cortex); 3) *memory and learning* circuits (located in the amygdala and hippocampus); and 4) *cognitive control* circuits (located in the prefrontal cortex and dorsal anterior cingulate gyrus). Other neurotransmitters, such as glutamate, may also be involved in the reward system. Kelley and Berridge (2002) believe that drugs of abuse act on dopamine and glutamate synapses and cause changes at the cellular and molecular levels: these changes, in turn, may be responsible for "abnormal information processing and behavior, resulting in poor decision making, loss of control, and the compulsivity that characterizes addiction." Kalivas and Volkow (2005) note that drugs that block glutamate release in animals prevent drug seeking. Further, it has been demonstrated that there are differences in male and female responses to substances of abuse in rodents and humans. Lynch et al. (2002) report on studies that indicate that females are more vulnerable to the reinforcing effects of stimulants, for example, and that the effects of these stimulants vary with different phases of the menstrual cycle. The researchers speculate that estrogen may be involved and also note that dopamine transmission varies with the menstrual cycle. They note that male and female rats actually have different densities of dopamine receptors in the striatum and nucleus accumbens areas of the brain.

Warren and Gold (2007) have found, in agreement with others, that there is an inverse relationship between use of drugs and overeating, possibly because drugs, alcohol, and food compete for the same reward areas in the brain. They even suggest that overeating may be protective against developing a drug addiction.

One of the other characteristics of addiction is that those afflicted tend to relapse. As Kalivas and Volkow (2005) observe, "The cardinal behavioral feature of drug addiction is continued vulnerability to relapse after years of drug abstinence." A review by Brownell et al. (1986) notes that some studies quote relapse rates as high as 90%. Almost half of these relapses occurred during periods of stress. The authors differentiate *lapse*, a single event, from *relapse*, a process involving a recurrence of symptoms after a time when there was an improvement: "The individual's response to these lapses determines whether relapse has occurred" (Brownell et al. 1986). They found that lapses were more likely to be associated with environmental factors, whereas relapses were more likely to occur when the individual was experiencing negative emotions or stress. In discussing potential treatment strategies, Kalivas and Volkow (2005) note that medications can target one of three potential routes: decreasing the motivational value of the drug; increasing the importance or strength (salience) of nondrug reinforcers; or inhibiting conditioned responses to things in the environment that alert someone to the availability of a drug.

Volkow and Wise (2005) note that not all addictive substances are equally addictive: animals given unlimited access to intravenous cocaine or amphetamine will take these drugs "to the point of death," but this is not so with nicotine. Likewise, not all foods have the same potential to generate what can be considered addiction, and there is a genetic component to one's proclivity to develop an addiction. Volkow and Wise (2005) also note that the regulation of food intake, which involves central and peripheral signals, is more complex than drug intake because drug intake seems to involve predominantly central effects. And food intake is, of course, also more problematic because food is essential for our survival. Whereas we can recommend complete abstinence for drug or alcohol addictions, we obviously cannot do the same for those with food addictions. The relevant notion is *priming*, in which once a person has had a taste of something, it is harder to stop (just like the alcoholic with one drink) than if the person has not tasted the substance at all. Weight specialist

Stephen Gullo (1995, pp. 105–107) was thinking along those lines when he said, "Where there can be no moderation, there must be elimination." Both addictive drugs and foods similarly involve reward, motivation, and decision making, and the neurotransmitter dopamine is directly involved (Volkow and Wise 2005).

Higher-function cognitive processes as well as the more primitive ones are factors in our control of food intake. We have vast capacities to appreciate subtle differences in individual tastes, as well as tastes in combination: we have taste neurons for sweet, bitter, salty, and sour, as well as *umami*, considered to be the flavor of protein. We also can appreciate the texture, temperature, smell, and visual appearance of food. These are the so-called orosensory factors that are all involved in our decisions to eat something. And our brains are so complex that we activate different areas when we are processing an odor emanating from something edible like chocolate or nonedible like roses (Chapelot and Louis-Sylvestre 2008, pp. 134–135). Edmund Rolls (2006) makes the point that we can identify a food's taste and intensity separately from the food's palatability or pleasantness; this ability enables us "to represent what a taste is, and to learn about it, even when we are not hungry." And we can appreciate a food's flavor, which is a combination of taste and smell. We also have the capacity for *sensory-specific satiety:* foods we have eaten to satiety are less pleasant than a new food presented. This is the buffet syndrome, in which we can eat tremendously more food when presented with a large variety of foods. Olszewski and Levine (2007) call it the "dessert effect" and note that it has been seen in animals as well: when a palatable food was presented to rats even after they had eaten to satiation, they ate more. Opioids increase this effect and opioid antagonists like naltrexone and naloxone block it. Experiments have shown that naloxone can reduce the intake of foods with sugar and fat in binge eaters (Drewnowski et al. 1995). The researchers speculate that the food reward system was affected; only intake of palatable foods (sugary, high-fat foods) was affected, not the total amount of food consumed. As a result, they suggest that opiate antagonists may be more helpful for reducing the length and size of a binge eating episode than for long-term control of body weight. Cota et al. (2006) also reported that opioids increased the length of a meal (meal maintenance) rather than the initiation of a meal, and that naloxone brought on satiety in animals more quickly but did not stop them from initiating a meal. In other words, naloxone decreased calorie intake only after the animals had eaten considerable amounts of food.

Another system involved in food intake is the endogenous system of cannabinoids (the active ingredients in marijuana); cannabinoids have been found throughout the central nervous system and may be involved in affecting (i.e., modulating) the release of neurotransmitters like dopamine, glutamate, norepinephrine, GABA, and serotonin on a kind of demand basis (Cota et al. 2006). Five endocannabinoids have been isolated. Research grew out of anecdotal reports that marijuana induces hyperphagia, particularly for sugared, fatty foods. The antiobesity medication rimonabant counters the effects of the endocannabinoid system and increases satiety; it is used in Europe but has not been approved by the U.S. Food and Drug Administration because it can cause depression. Cota et al. (2006) suggest that the treatment of obesity may lie in the synergistic combined use of both opioid and cannabinoid antagonists because "individuals eat for many reasons and one drug effect may not be sufficient."

Levine et al. (2003) note that sugar seems to have an important relationship to the opioid reward system. These researchers make the point that sugar intake involves brain functions pertaining not only to feeding (and energy homeostasis) but also to reward circuits, and they believe there is a complex relationship between the meso-limbic dopaminergic system and the opioid system in regard to sugar. Human infants respond to sugar, unlike bitter substances such as quinine, with tongue protrusion and smiles, reactions clearly indicating they like it (Kelley and Berridge 2002). Inter-estingly, these reactions (e.g., different facial expressions and tongue protrusions for bitter vs. sugar) can be seen in many species, as for example chimpanzees, monkeys, rats, and mice, as well as humans (Berridge and Robinson 2003).

Intermittent exposure to sugar, but not continuous exposure (i.e., not ad libi-tum), in rats can lead to an opiate-like withdrawal syndrome with anxiety and in-creased levels of acetylcholine, which has been implicated in satiety, reflecting "the negative effects of being reward-deprived" (Avena et al. 2008). Colantuoni et al. (2002) found similar results: intermittent bingeing on sugar caused dependency, as manifested by a physical and biochemical withdrawal syndrome. This withdrawal syndrome was produced either by sugar deprivation or by a naloxone-induced physical withdrawal; it included anxiety, teeth chattering, forepaw tremor, and head shakes. When naloxone was used, the sugar-treated rats had a rise in acetylcholine levels and a decrease in dopamine levels, a pattern of imbalance typical of intermit-tent morphine–naloxone use. Avena (2007) noted that this kind of imbalance may also play a role in the reinforcing bingeing-purging behavior of bulimic patients; she noted that purging drastically reduced acetylcholine release, which in turn re-inforced the purging (i.e., dopamine without acetylcholine release) and mimicked a drug abuse paradigm rather than a normal eating paradigm. Avena (2007) also found evidence for the *gateway effect*, in that rats intermittently exposed to sugar were more apt to have a greater intake of alcohol. Olszewski and Levine (2007) make the point that opioid receptor blockade did not affect the initiation of a meal but only affected the continuation of eating once it had started; this is understood to mean that this blockade affected the reward-related aspects of feeding rather than the actual biological drive to eat.

Not all people, though, are equally sensitive to reward, whether it be drugs or food. Tiggemann and Kemps (2005) studied food cravings by surveying a sample of undergraduate students. They note that chocolate is the most craved substance in many cultures (though they report on another study that found that vegetable dishes apparently are in Egypt). In their research, Tiggemann and Kemps (2005) noted that the vividness of a visual image, even more than a subject's hunger, was most related to the intensity of a craving. They suggest that visuospatial processing techniques, therefore, might be helpful in reducing craving imagery in those with particularly intense cravings and resultant eating disorders. A study by Beaver et al. (2006) using functional MRI found that those high in the reward sensitivity trait, as measured by the Behavioral Activation Scale, were more apt to have increased activity in the frontostriatal-amygdalar-midbrain areas—areas with high concentrations of dopamine and opioids—when shown only visual images (not even the actual foods) of palatable foods like chocolate cake, ice cream, or pizza. The researchers believe their study "provides the necessary data to bridge the gap between human behavioral findings and comparative neurobiology[,] demonstrating a powerful role for this network in motivating food selection"; that is, it provides "a mechanism for translating reward drive into increased vulnerability" for some people with compulsive eating (Beaver et al. 2006). And Rolls (2006) emphasizes that we are much more sensitive to the sensory factors of a food (e.g., its appearance, texture, flavor, and shape) than we are to its metabolic properties (whether it contains protein, fat, or carbohydrates).

Rolls also differentiates sensory-specific satiety from *alliesthesia*, which is a change in our perception of a food's pleasantness because of internal signals such as a full stomach or blood glucose levels. In fact, Rolls describes experiments that showed that chewed food does not even have to be swallowed for sensory-specific satiety to occur. He notes another study in which feeding to satiety with unsweetened cream (high in fat) *alone* decreased the responses of the neurons involved, but once glucose was added, the neuron response was no longer decreased and subjects then ate more (the satiety response was overridden, as it were). Rolls (2005) notes that cognitively, humans can be influenced by the color or other aspects of the visual presentation of a food (or wine) and that these factors can influence our perception of its flavor. But he also presents experiments that showed how we can be influenced even by a food's description. In experiments using isovaleric acid with cheddar cheese flavor, subjects were asked to rate the pleasantness of the odor when it was labeled as either body odor or cheddar cheese (de Araujo et al. 2005). Subjects rated the "body odor" as significantly more unpleasant even though it was the same substance. Rolls' conclusion is that "cognitive factors can have profound effects on our responses to the hedonic and sensory properties of food" (Rolls 2005).

Mela (2006) distinguishes liking a food, that is, the anticipation of getting pleasure from eating a food (its palatability or its "hedonic value") from desire (wanting a food now or in the near future) and from preference (comparison and selection of food from alternatives). Mela notes that we humans are able to choose one food over another on the basis of extrinsic factors, such as brand, cost, convenience, and even health. And amazingly (and so differently from other species), we are even capable of choosing "less desired food alternatives" when we consider these extrinsic factors like health or the wish to engage in "restrained eating" (Mela 2006). Along those lines, Friedman (2008, pp. 12–13) distinguishes regulatory eating (i.e., "homeostatic" or relating to the internal environment) from nonregulatory eating (associated with external factors like palatability, variety, or even availability, but also with cognitive and cultural features such as learning, cravings, and even the timing of meals). And Chapelot and Louis-Sylvestre (2008, p. 135) further emphasize that even palatability is "highly idiosyncratic and not fixed over the lifecycle."

Lowe and Butryn (2007), in their discussion of "restrained eaters," differentiate the very human ability to eat "less than one wants, rather than less than one needs." Eaters who do so are then in a state of "relative" deprivation rather than "absolute" deprivation. Lowe and Butryn (2007) suggest that eating palatable foods may be "anxiolytic" for humans and that when we cease eating these foods we increase our stress levels, and thus we "hasten a return to eating them" and develop those typically human patterns of "emotional eating."

REFERENCES

Allport G: Personality: A Psychological Interpretation. London, Constable, 1937

Alonso-Alonso M, Pascual-Leone A: The right brain hypothesis for obesity. JAMA 297:1819–1822, 2007

American Psychiatric Association: Diagnostic and Statistical Manual of Mental Disorders, 3rd Edition. Washington, DC, American Psychiatric Association, 1980

American Psychiatric Association: Diagnostic and Statistical Manual of Mental Disorders, 4th Edition, Text Revision. Washington, DC, American Psychiatric Association, 2000

Avena NM: Examining the addictive-like properties of binge eating using an animal model of sugar dependence. Exp Clin Psychopharmacol 15:481–491, 2007

Avena NM, Bocarsly ME, Rada P, et al: After daily bingeing on a sucrose solution, food deprivation induces anxiety and accumbens dopamine/acetylcholine imbalance. Physiol Behav 94:309–315, 2008

Bachman KH, Histon TM: Obesity and the right brain (letter). JAMA 298:738, 2007

Baler RD, Volkow ND: Drug addiction: the neurobiology of disrupted self-control. Trends Mol Med 12:559–566, 2006

Banfield JF, Wyland CL, Macrae CN, et al: The cognitive neuroscience of self-regulation, in Handbook of Self-Regulation: Research, Theory, and Applications. Edited by Baumeister RF, Vohs KD. New York, Guilford, 2004, pp 62–83

Baudry F: The evolution of the concept of character in Freud's writings. J Am Psychoanal Assoc 31:3–31, 1983

Baudry F: Character, character type, and character organization. J Am Psychoanal Assoc 37:655–686, 1989

Baumeister RF: Yielding to temptation: self-control failure, impulsive purchasing, and consumer behavior. J Consum Res 28:670–676, 2002

Baumeister RF: The Cultural Animal: Human Nature, Meaning, and Social Life. New York, Oxford University Press, 2005

Beaver JD, Lawrence AD, van Ditzhuijzen J, et al: Individual differences in reward drive predict neural responses to images of food. J Neurosci 26:5160–5166, 2006

Beck JS: The Complete Beck Diet for Life. Birmingham, AL, Oxmoor House, 2008

Berridge KC, Robinson TE: Parsing reward. Trends Neurosci 26:507–513, 2003

Berthoud HR: Interactions between the "cognitive" and "metabolic" brain in the control of food intake. Physiol Behav 91:486–498, 2007

Bibring GL, Dwyer TF, Huntington DS, et al: A study of the psychological processes in pregnancy and of the earliest mother-child relationship—II: methodological considerations. Psychoanal Study Child 16:25–72, 1961

Booth DA: Acquired behavior controlling energy intake and output. Psychiatr Clin North Am 1:545–579, 1978

Brenner C: Defense and defense mechanisms. Psychoanal Q 50:557–569, 1981

Brownell KD, Marlatt GA, Lichtenstein E, et al: Understanding and preventing relapse. Am Psychol 41:765–782, 1986

Chapelot D, Louis-Sylvestre J: The role of orosensory factors in eating behavior as observed in humans, in Appetite and Food Intake: Behavioral and Physiological Considerations. Edited by Harris RBS, Mattes RD. Boca Raton, FL, CRC Press, 2008, pp 133–161

Chess S, Thomas A: Temperament in Clinical Practice. New York, Guilford, 1986

Christakis NA, Fowler JH: The spread of obesity in a large social network over 32 years. N Engl J Med 357:370–379, 2007

Clarkin JF, Yeomans FE, Kernberg OF: Psychotherapy for Borderline Personality: Focusing on Object Relations. Washington, DC, American Psychiatric Publishing, 2006

Cloninger CR, Svrakic DM: Personality disorders, in Kaplan and Sadock's Comprehensive Textbook of Psychiatry, 9th Edition, Vol II. Edited by Sadock B, Sadock V, Ruiz P. Philadelphia, PA, Lippincott Williams & Wilkins/Wolters Kluwer, 2009, pp 2197–2240

Colantuoni C, Rada P, McCarthy J, et al: Evidence that intermittent, excessive sugar intake causes endogenous opioid dependence. Obes Res 10:478–488, 2002

Cota D, Tschöp MH, Horvath TL, et al: Cannabinoids, opioids and eating behavior: the molecular face of hedonism? Brain Res Rev 51:85–107, 2006

Dallman MF, Pecoraro NC, la Fleur SE: Chronic stress and comfort foods: self-medication and abdominal obesity. Brain Behav Immun 19:275–280, 2005

Dallman MF, Pecoraro NC, La Fleur SE, et al: Glucocorticoids, chronic stress, and obesity. Prog Brain Res 153:75–105, 2006

de Araujo IE, Rolls ET, Velazco MI, et al: Cognitive modulation of olfactory processing. Neuron 46:671–679, 2005

De Kloet ER: Hormones and the stressed brain. Ann N Y Acad Sci 1018:1–15, 2004

DelParigi A, Chen K, Salbe AD, et al: Successful dieters have increased neural activity in cortical areas involved in the control of behavior. Int J Obes (Lond) 31:440–448, 2007

Drewnowski A, Krahn DD, Demitrack MA, et al: Naloxone, an opiate blocker, reduces the consumption of sweet high-fat foods in obese and lean female binge eaters. Am J Clin Nutr 61:1206–1212, 1995

Fitzsimons GM, Bargh JA: Automatic self-regulation, in Handbook of Self-Regulation: Research, Theory, and Applications. Edited by Baumeister RF, Vohs KD. New York, Guilford, 2004, pp 151–170

Freud A: The Ego and the Mechanisms of Defense: The Writings of Anna Freud, Vol 2. New York, International Universities Press, 1966

Freud S: My views on the part played by sexuality in the aetiology of the neuroses (1906 [1905]), in The Standard Edition of the Complete Psychological Works of Sigmund Freud, Vol 7. Translated and edited by Strachey J. London, Hogarth Press, 1953

Friedman MI: Food intake: control, regulation and the illusion of dysregulation, in Appetite and Food Intake: Behavioral and Physiological Considerations. Edited by Harris RBS, Mattes RD. Boca Raton, FL, CRC Press, 2008, pp 1–20

García-Bueno B, Caso JR, Leza JC: Stress as a neuroinflammatory condition in brain: damaging and protective mechanisms. Neurosci Biobehav Rev 32:1136–1151, 2008

Gautier JF, Chen K, Salbe AD, et al: Differential brain responses to satiation in obese and lean men. Diabetes 49:838–846, 2000

Gibson EL: Emotional influences on food choice: sensory, physiological and psychological pathways. Physiol Behav 89:53–61, 2006

Gladwell M: The trouble with fries: fast food is killing us: can it be fixed? The New Yorker, March 5, 2001, pp 52–57

Goleman D: Emotional Intelligence: Why It Can Matter More Than IQ. New York, Bantam Books, 1995

Grigson PS: Like drugs for chocolate: separate rewards modulated by common mechanisms? Physiol Behav 76:389–395, 2002

Gullo SP: Thin Tastes Better: Control Your Food Triggers and Lose Weight Without Feeling Deprived. New York, Carol Southern Books, 1995

Herman CP, Polivy J: The self-regulation of eating: theoretical and practical problems, in Handbook of Self-Regulation: Research, Theory, and Applications. Edited by Baumeister RF, Vohs KD. New York, Guilford, 2004, pp 492–508

Higgs S: Cognitive influences on food intake: the effects of manipulating memory for recent eating. Physiol Behav 94:734–739, 2008

Hirschmann JR, Munter CH: Overcoming Overeating. New York, Fawcett, 1988

Kalivas PW, Volkow ND: The neural basis of addiction: a pathology of motivation and choice. Am J Psychiatry 162:1403–1413, 2005

Kelley AE, Berridge KC: The neuroscience of natural rewards. J Neurosci 22:3306–3311, 2002

Kernberg OF: Borderline Conditions and Pathological Narcissism. New York, Jason Aronson, 1983

Kivetz R, Keinan A: Repenting hyperopia: an analysis of self-control regrets. J Consum Res 33:273–282, 2006

Knoch D, Fehr E: Resisting the power of temptations: the right prefrontal cortex and self-control. Ann N Y Acad Sci 1104:123–134, 2007

Knutson B, Rick S, Wimmer GE, et al: Neural predictors of purchases. Neuron 53:147–156, 2007

Kuo LE, Kitlinska JB, Tilan JU, et al: Neuropeptide Y acts directly in the periphery on fat tissue and mediates stress-induced obesity and metabolic syndrome. Nat Med 13:803–811, 2007

Kyrou I, Tsigos C: Stress mechanisms and metabolic complications. Horm Metab Res 39:430–438, 2007

Levine AS, Kotz CM, Gosnell BA: Sugars: hedonic aspects, neuroregulation, and energy balance. Am J Clin Nutr 78:834S–842S, 2003

Lowe MR, Butryn ML: Hedonic hunger: a new dimension of appetite? Physiol Behav 91:432–439, 2007

Lynch WJ, Roth ME, Carroll ME: Biological basis of sex differences in drug abuse: preclinical and clinical studies. Psychopharmacology (Berl) 164:121–137, 2002

Magen E, Gross JJ: Harnessing the need for immediate gratification: cognitive reconstrual modulates the reward value of temptations. Emotion 7:415–428, 2007

Mastorci F, Vincentini M, Viltart O, et al: Long-term effects of prenatal stress: changes in adult cardiovascular regulation and sensitivity to stress. Neurosci Biobehav Rev 33:191–203, 2009

McEwen BS: Sex, stress and the hippocampus: allostasis, allostatic load and the aging process. Neurobiol Aging 23:921–939, 2002

Mela DJ: Eating for pleasure or just wanting to eat? Reconsidering sensory hedonic responses as a driver of obesity. Appetite 47:10–17, 2006

Mesulam M-M: Aging, Alzheimer's disease, and dementia: clinical and neurobiological perspectives, in Principles of Behavioral Cognitive Neurology, 2nd Edition. Edited by Mesulam M-M. New York, Oxford University Press, 2000a, pp 439–522

Mesulam M-M: Behavioral neuroanatomy: large-scale networks, association cortex, frontal syndromes, the limbic system, and hemispheric specializations, in Principles of Behavioral Cognitive Neurology, 2nd Edition. Edited by Mesulam M-M. New York, Oxford University Press, 2000b, pp 1–120

Moore DP, Jefferson JW: Kluver-Bucy syndrome, in Handbook of Medical Psychiatry, 2nd Edition. Philadelphia, PA, Elsevier/Mosby, 2004, pp 303–304

Moore-Ede MC: Physiology of the circadian timing system: predictive versus reactive homeostasis. Am J Physiol RegulIntegrComp Physiol 250:R737–R752, 1986

Morton GJ, Cummings DE, Baskin DG, et al: Central nervous system control of food intake and body weight. Nature 443:289–295, 2006

Oliver G, Wardle J: Perceived effects of stress on food choice. Physiol Behav 66:511–515, 1999

Olszewski PK, Levine AS: Central opioids and consumption of sweet tastants: when reward outweighs homeostasis. Physiol Behav 91:506–512, 2007

Padoa-Schioppa C, Assad JA: The representation of economic value in the orbitofrontal cortex is invariant for changes of menu. Nat Neurosci 11:95–102, 2008

Pecoraro N, Dallman MF, Warne JP, et al: From Malthus to motive: how the HPA axis engineers the phenotype, yoking needs to wants. Prog Neurobiol 79:247–340, 2006

Pelchat ML: Of human bondage: food craving, obsession, compulsion, and addiction. Physiol Behav 76:347–352, 2002

Pivk U, Godinot N, Keller C, et al: Lipid deposition on the tongue after oral processing of medium-chain triglycerides and impact on the perception of mouthfeel. J Agric Food Chem 56:1058–1064, 2008

Platkin CS: Per Se, per calorie. New York magazine, May 7, 2007, p 62

Polivy J, Herman CP: Distress and eating: why do dieters overeat? Int J Eat Disord 26:153–164, 1999

Power ML, Schulkin J: The Evolution of Obesity. Baltimore, MD, Johns Hopkins University Press, 2009

Regard M, Landis T: "Gourmand syndrome": eating passion associated with right anterior lesions. Neurology 48:1185–1190, 1997

Rogers PJ, Smit HJ: Food craving and food "addiction": a critical review of the evidence from a biopsychosocial perspective. Pharmacol Biochem Behav 66:3–14, 2000

Rolls ET: Taste, olfactory, and food texture processing in the brain, and the control of food intake. Physiol Behav 85:45–56, 2005

Rolls ET: Brain mechanisms underlying flavour and appetite. Philos Trans R Soc Lond B Biol Sci 361:1123–1136, 2006

Rolls ET, McCabe C: Enhanced affective brain representations of chocolate in cravers vs. non-cravers. Eur J Neurosci 26:1067–1076, 2007

Rothman AJ, Baldwin AS, Hertel AW: Self-regulation and behavior change: disentangling behavioral initiation and behavioral maintenance, in Handbook of Self-Regulation: Research, Theory, and Applications. Edited by Baumeister RF, Vohs KD. New York, Guilford, 2004, pp 130–148

Rozin P: Taste-smell confusions and the duality of the olfactory sense. Percept Psychophys 31:397–401, 1982

Schmeichel BJ, Baumeister RF: Self-regulatory strength, in Handbook of Self-Regulation: Research, Theory, and Applications. Edited by Baumeister RF, Vohs KD. New York, Guilford, 2004, pp 84–98

Sclafani A, Springer D: Dietary obesity in adult rats: similarities to hypothalamic and human obesity syndromes. Physiol Behav 17:461–471, 1976

Scott TR: Orosensory control of feeding, in Appetite and Food Intake: Behavioral and Physiological Considerations. Edited by Harris RBS, Mattes RD. Boca Raton, FL, CRC Press, 2008, pp 113–132

Selye H: Forty years of stress research: principal remaining problems and misconceptions. Can Med Assoc J 115:53–56, 1976

Selye H: The nature of stress. Basal Facts 1985; 7:3–11, 1985

Selye H: A syndrome produced by diverse nocuous agents: 1936. J Neuropsychiatry Clin Neurosci 10:230–231, 1998

Shiv B, Fedorikhin A: Heart and mind in conflict: the interplay of affect and cognition in consumer decision making. J Consum Res 26:278–292, 1999

Shoda Y, Mischel W, Peake PK: Predicting adolescent cognitive and self-regulatory competencies from preschool delay of gratification: identifying diagnostic conditions. Dev Psychol 26:978–986, 1990

Siegal RS: What are defense mechanisms? J Am Psychoanal Assoc 17:785–807, 1969

Sindelar JL: Paying for performance: the power of incentives over habits (editorial). Health Econ 17:449–451, 2008

Sparks P, Conner M, James R, et al: Ambivalence about health-related behaviours: an exploration in the domain of food choice. Br J Health Psychol 6:53–68, 2001

Spiegel AM, Alving BM: Executive summary of the Strategic Plan for National Institutes of Health Obesity Research. Am J Clin Nutr 82 (1 suppl):211S–214S, 2005

Spiegel A, Nabel E, Volkow N, et al: Obesity on the brain. Nat Neurosci 8:552–553, 2005

Tamashiro KL, Hegeman MA, Sakali RR: Chronic social stress in a changing dietary environment. Physiol Behav 89:536–542, 2006

Tataranni PA. Pannacciulli N: Conscious and unconscious regulation of feeding behaviors in humans: lessons from neuroimaging studies in normal weight and obese subjects, in Appetite and Food Intake: Behavioral and Physiological Considerations. Edited by Harris RBS, Mattes RD. Boca Raton, FL, CRC Press, 2008, pp 267–282

The NS, Gordon-Larsen P: Entry into romantic partnership is associated with obesity. Obesity 17:1441–1447, 2009

Tierney J: The voices in my head say 'Buy it!' Why argue? The New York Times, January 16, 2007, Science section, p F1

Tiggemann M, Kemps E: The phenomenology of food cravings: the role of mental imagery. Appetite 45:305–313, 2005

Tordoff MG: Obesity by choice: the powerful influence of nutrient availability on nutrient intake. Am J Physiol Regul Integr Comp Physiol 51:R1536–R1539, 2002

Traustadóttir T, Bosch PR, Matt KS: The HPA axis response to stress in women: effects of aging and fitness. Psychoneuroendocrinology 30:392–402, 2005

Treit D, Spetch ML, Deutsch JA: Variety in the flavor of food enhances eating in the rat: a controlled demonstration. Physiol Behav 30:207–211, 1983

Ulrich-Lai YM, Ostrander MM, Thomas IM, et al: Daily limited access to sweetened drink attenuates hypothalamic-pituitary-adrenocortical axis stress responses. Endocrinology 148:1823–1834, 2007

Vaillant GE: Ego Mechanisms of Defense: A Guide for Clinicians and Researchers. Washington, DC, American Psychiatric Press, 1992

Van Laere K, Goffin K, Bormans G, et al: Relationship of type 1 cannabinoid receptor availability in the human brain to novelty-seeking temperament. Arch Gen Psychiatry 66:196–204, 2009

Vohs KD, Baumeister RF: Understanding self-regulation: an introduction, in Handbook of Self-Regulation: Research, Theory, and Applications. New York, Guilford 2004, pp 1–12

Volkow ND, O'Brien CP: Issues for DSM-V: should obesity be included as a brain disorder? (editorial) Am J Psychiatry 164:708–710, 2007

Volkow ND, Wise RA: How can drug addiction help us understand obesity? Nat Neurosci 8:555–560, 2005

Volpp KG, Troxel AB, Pauly MV, et al: A randomized, controlled trial of financial incentives for smoking cessation. N Engl J Med 360:699–709, 2009

Waelder R: The structure of paranoid ideas—a critical survey of various theories. Int J Psychoanal 32:167–177, 1951

Wansink B: Mindless Eating: Why We Eat More Than We Think. New York, Bantam, 2006

Wardle J, Steptoe A, Oliver G, et al: Stress, dietary restraint and food intake. J Psychosom Res 48:195–202, 2000

Warren MW, Gold MS: The relationship between obesity and drug use (letter). Am J Psychiatry 164:1268; author reply 1268–1269, 2007

Weinstock M: The long-term behavioural consequences of prenatal stress. Neurosci Biobehav Rev 32:1073–1086, 2008

Wise RA: Role of brain dopamine in food reward and reinforcement. Philos Trans R Soc Lond B Biol Sci 361:1149–1158, 2006

Zheng H, Berthoud HR: Eating for pleasure or calories. Curr Opin Pharmacol 7:607–612, 2007

Zheng H, Berthoud HR: Neural systems controlling the drive to eat: mind versus metabolism. Physiology (Bethesda) 23:75–83, 2008

5

THE METABOLIC COMPLEXITIES OF WEIGHT CONTROL

There can be considerable ambiguity about the degree of volition in the timing, frequency, location, and circumstances of any particular act of eating or exercise. In the moment, snacking may appear to be altogether subject to conscious control; in the aggregate, however, such behavior assumes a certain biological inevitability.

William Ira Bennett, "Beyond Overeating" (1995)

GENERAL CONSIDERATIONS

Most researchers in the field of obesity would acknowledge the impact of our "toxic" environment on weight control. In other words, the extraordinary availability of a seemingly infinite array of palatable, often processed, highly caloric foods rich in sugar and fat has made dieting much more difficult than ever before (see Chapter 10, "Diet and Weight"). Furthermore, particularly in the United States, we have become an increasingly sedentary society: computers, remote controls, escalators, automobiles, televisions, and other technological advances have enabled us to utilize fewer of the calories we ingest daily. But, as we have previously mentioned, researchers also appreciate the enormous contribution of genetics in this equation: up to 70% heritability has been found for body mass index (BMI) values (O'Rahilly and Farooqi 2006) (see "Genetics and Obesity" section in Chapter 2, "Obesity in the United States"). And these two elements—the toxic environment and genetics—are not mutually exclusive. Mark (2008) notes how genetic factors promote either sensitivity or resistance to weight gain in the midst of our environment and enable us to understand why some people do manage to keep their weights in check whereas others, exposed to the same environment, fail miserably.

A classic study by Bouchard et al. (1990) illustrates this point: the researchers overfed 12 pairs of monozygotic male twins an extra 1,000 calories a day (4.2 mega-joules) for 84 days in a tightly supervised setting. They found that even though the twins were all given the same diet and were sedentary, some twin pairs gained more weight than other pairs, with a range of 4.3–13.3 kilo-grams and an average of 8.1 kilograms. They also found considerable variation between pairs (a threefold dif-ference), and not much within pairs, in where fat ac-cumulated on their bodies: some twin pairs were more apt to accumulate fat on the trunk, others in the abdominal area, and others in both places. The researchers concluded that there are strong genetic components involved in weight gain, even when individuals are exposed to the same toxic environment.

> Genetic factors promote either sensitivity or resistance to obesity.

The genetics of an individual, though, works through many systems in the body, including the brain and the endocrine system. Researcher Barry Levin, who has said, "The drive to regain lies mainly in the brain" (Levin 2004), calls this drive a *metabolic strategy* that predisposes some individuals to become heavier, and remain heavier, than others (Levin 2006).

Even prenatal and postnatal exposures can influence a person's subsequent metabolism. Waterland and Garza (1999) spoke of "meta-bolic imprinting" to designate the important role that nutrition during the perinatal time period has for the future health and weight of a person. Using an analogy from studies on

> Nutritional exposure during the perinatal time period leaves its metabolic imprint—a kind of "endocrinological memory"—on the child.
>
> Source: Waterland and Garza 1999

imprinting by Konrad Lorenz, these researchers believe that there is a critical win-dow of nutritional exposure that has profound and persistent effects, that a kind of "endocrinological memory" is established (Waterland and Garza 1999). They note that during the course of development pre- and postnatally, the body's organs enlarge by either hypertrophy (increasing a cell's size) or hyperplasia (increasing the number of cells). It makes sense that nutritional exposure, either in utero or postnatally, could affect these processes as well as those involved in metabolic dif-ferentiation, such as those involved in establishing patterns of enzyme or hormone regulation. For example, both severe undernutrition and severe overnutrition of the mother during her pregnancy and in the postnatal period can lead to obesity and metabolic irregularities, such as insulin resistance, later in life. Bray and Champagne (2005) note that famine conditions during World War II in the Netherlands affected the postnatal weights of infants exposed to the famine in utero. But even infants born small for their gestational ages may be more apt to develop abdominal obesity and diabetes later in life. In a large population sample (640 men and 886 women) in India, where there were serial records of height and weight and BMI over a period of years, for example, Bhargava et al. (2004) found that infants who had weighed 2.25 kg or below at full-term birth and continued to have lower body weight for the first 2 years of life were more likely to have impaired glucose tolerance or diabetes in adulthood than those who weighed more than 3.5 kg. Low-birth-weight infants, whether they developed type 2 diabetes or not, were also more apt to have what these researchers called "adiposity rebound," that is, accelerated weight gain after the age of 12. The researchers' conclusion was there is "an association between thinness in infancy and the presence of impaired glucose tolerance or diabetes in young adulthood" (Bhargava et al, 2004).

THE SET POINT

Back in the mid 1970s, Keesey (1978) proposed the concept of *set point*. Keesey acknowledged that the concept of set point is usually designated for physical systems with values that do not fluctuate much more than 10%. For example, body temperature is fairly constant for most people, whereas body weights can vary enormously between two different people. The hypothesis, though, was that one's weight does remain seemingly regulated within a fairly narrow range. For example, the weight of a 60-year-old person is usually only a few pounds more than the same person's at age 30 years—that is, our weight gain over time is usually modest

> We all have our weight-related *set point*, an "adipostatic" physiological resistance to losing weight and maintaining the loss should it occur.

(Keesey and Hirvonen 1997). An individual's weight, though it fluctuates, tends to hover around a certain point. In other words, we have a kind of "stability and precision" in our body weight, though there is extraordinary variation within the population (Keesey 1978).

What Keesey (1978) proposed is that just as we "defend" our body temperature, we also "defend" our body weights to a large extent. Our set point can be raised or lowered by certain situations (e.g., diet or experimental lesions in animal studies). For example, genetically engineered obese rats (Zucker fatty rats), with an elevated set point, stubbornly resisted weight change, and rats with lesions in their lateral hypothalamus, with a lowered set point, also maintained their lower body weight. In both cases, Keesey believes there were metabolic adjustments involving both energy expenditure and calorie intake—"a coordinated pattern of compensatory intake and expenditure adjustments" (Keesey 1978, p. 539). However, when the rats were fed a high-fat diet for 6 months, both the size and number of fat cells increased; when these rats were returned to their normal food their fat cells shrank, but the increase in fat cell numbers was apparently irreversible (Keesey and Hirvonen 1997).

According to Keesey and Hirvonen (1997) human and animal obesity is an example of a physiologically elevated set point, either genetically or nutritionally based, and there is a physiological resistance to losing weight and maintaining that weight loss. Sometimes the reduction in metabolic rate after weight loss is an even larger percentage than the weight loss itself.

There was speculation that there is some control mechanism, set at a predetermined level by a feedback system (Harris 1990), that regulates just how much weight we will accumulate—a kind of "adipostat" in our brain (Bennett 1995). Early experiments demonstrated that lesions to the ventromedial hypothalamus led to changes in body weight, with hyperphagia; hence this area was considered a satiety center. Hirsch (2003) noted that rats subjected to these experiments ate so voraciously after surgery that they would rupture their stomachs. But the situation became more complicated when researchers realized that these lesions resulted in other behavioral changes such as aggressive behavior, as well as metabolic changes such as increased insulin secretion. Furthermore, when researchers also created lesions in the vagus nerve, some of these effects were reversed (Harris 1990). Ultimately, most researchers came to believe that the notion of one set point area is just too simplistic to explain weight control. Bennett (1995) says, "It is almost certainly not confined to the hypothalamus." And Levin (2004), for example, believes there is not one set point "localized in one precise place." If there is a hypothetical set point, though, he believes it is "regulated by genetic, gender, perinatal, developmental, dietary, environmental, neural, and psychosocial factors."

THE SET POINT

- Still theoretical and not localized to one place in the brain

- What regulates fat accumulation in humans is very complicated and determined by "genetic, gender, perinatal, developmental, dietary, environmental, neural, and psychosocial factors"

Source: Levin 2004

Wirtshafter and Davis (1977) have questioned the concept of set point and raised the question, "if body weight is regulated by an internal set point mechanism...why is it so singularly ineffective in the face of altered dietary palatability?" They prefer the term *settling point*—a point related to intake in and expenditure—where body weight "settles." Levitsky (2002) more recently suggested a "settling zone," since our bodies don't have a fixed "point" but rather a "range or zone of body weight" that depends on the environment.

The problem of weight regain in humans makes the concept of set point an appealing one. The idea is that the body, once it loses weight, seeks to regain the lost weight; that adaptive metabolic changes in the body occur and "a homeostatic feedback system" leads us back to a preset weight (Weinsier et al. 2000). Weinsier et al. (2000) reviewed the literature and noted equivocal findings regarding whether a person's resting metabolic rate actually changes with weight loss. With their own experiments in a clinical research center with a group of 24 overweight, postmenopausal women (and a control group of 24 women who had never been overweight), they found that with calorie restriction (800 cal/day: 64% carbohydrates, 14%–20% fat, and 16%–22% protein), there was a *transient* state of slower metabolism (resting metabolic rate fell 6%) and even hypothyroidism, but that this normalized when calorie intake was no longer restricted, in what they called "energy-balanced conditions." At 4-year follow-up, the weight-reduced, previously overweight women, with the exception of 16%, had gained back much of their weight: initial weight loss averaged 13 kilograms and weight regain at 4 years was more than 9 kilograms. Weinsier and colleagues noted that previous researchers may have been misled by not establishing energy-balanced conditions after their subjects lost weight prior to taking their measurements. They concluded that adaptive metabolic changes were *not* responsible for the fact that subjects do tend to regain weight over time. They noted that even after months of calorie restriction, resting metabolic rates returned to normal once calorie intake was no longer restricted. They did caution that their study might have produced different results had the population of women not been so homogeneous and had they lost much more weight initially (Weinsier et al. 2000).

MacLean et al. (2004) studied the same issue with obesity-prone rats. Because rats are not affected by human motivations such as peer pressure or the concept of an ideal physique, these researchers noted they could study metabolic issues and environmental stresses without those contaminating factors. They found that there was a "metabolic propensity" for their rats to regain weight after weight loss with calorie restriction. They noted that their rats had increased appetite and "persistent suppression" of their resting metabolic rate: a 10% weight loss in their rats produced a 15% suppression of this rate. In other words, they had "enhanced metabolic efficiency," which persisted for up to 16 weeks when their weights were maintained. Only when the rats were no longer calorie restricted and had regained their lost weight (even on a low-fat diet) did their metabolic rate return to its original level. In other words, the change in metabolic efficiency did not resolve immediately. MacLean et al. (2004) note, "With prolonged weight maintenance, the potential energy imbalance becomes more profound as metabolic rate remains suppressed in the face of increasing appetite." These researchers hypothesized that their data may be applicable to humans, in whom the tendency to regain lost weight is well known. But they also note that results of studies with human subjects may be inconsistent because human motivation and behavioral changes complicate the picture: "Given the difficulties in controlling or even standardizing human motivation and behavior, it is not surprising that resting energy expenditure does not always predict weight regain in weight-reduced subjects." MacLean et al. believe it is "reassuring" that humans are, in fact, able to counteract their metabolic tendency to regain weight by various means such as changes in their behavior (e.g., consciously changing eating habits, exercising more, taking weight-reducing medications), and they believe exercise may be critical in preventing weight regain in the context of metabolic changes.

MacLean et al. (2006) confirmed their earlier findings, again in rodents, and do believe this model is applicable to humans. Compensatory metabolic changes (e.g., higher levels of the hormones leptin and insulin, which may persist; persistent suppression of fat oxidation) occurred after weight reduction and promoted rapid and efficient weight regain. And there was considerable "pressure" to regain early in the relapse process such that even "short-term lapses in maintenance strategies can have profound consequences" (MacLean et al. 2006). Furthermore, increases in adipose tissue occurred, by increases in the number of fat cells, such that these little fat cells facilitated even greater fat accumulation over time. And an energy imbalance—"a drive to consume while suppressing energy expenditure"—not only developed but continued and became more profound during the period of weight maintenance such that weight "drift[ed] back upwards." MacLean et al. (2006) also noted that a high-fat diet may make the process of weight regain even worse.

> "The clear pathological hallmark of [obesity] is enlargement of [white] fat cells."
>
> Source: Bray 2004

ADIPOSE TISSUE

The metabolic complexities of weight control and maintenance involve many of our major organ systems, particularly the brain, the endocrine system, and the entire gastrointestinal system (e.g., stomach, pancreas, bowel, liver). Adipose tissue, long thought to be just inert storage tissue or a support to protect other organs, is actually one of our body's largest endocrine organs. We have both white adipose tissue (the most prevalent and "the main energy reservoir in mammals") and brown adipose tissue (specifically for heat production) (Trayhurn 2007).

Brown Adipose Tissue

For years, researchers thought that brown adipose tissue was found predominantly only in human infants and was responsible for their being able to regulate their body temperature without shivering. The assumption was that human brown adipose tissue remains only in "vestigial amounts" as we age (unlike in animals like rodents, for example, which keep their brown fat). Nedergaard et al. (2007) explained that nuclear medicine scans, using fluorodeoxyglucose (FDG; a substance that marks glucose uptake, indicating metabolically active tissue) as an indication for tumors, unexpectedly showed an unusual symmetrical pattern of uptake—mostly in the neck and shoulder (supraclavicular) areas—that was originally thought to be simply due to tense muscles in anxious patients. Only with the advent of higher-resolution imaging, with combined positron emission tomography and computed tomography (PET-CT) scans with glucose uptake markers, were researchers able to discern that this tissue was, indeed, metabolically active brown adipose tissue. It is speculated that brown adipose tissue has a thermogenic role and also some role in "actively clearing glucose from the circulation" (Nedergaard et al. 2007). Furthermore, brown adipose tissue becomes more active when a human is in a cold environment, such as being in a cold room for a nuclear medicine scan. If the patient is kept warm, the brown fat does not show up on imaging (as evidenced by glucose uptake). And norepinephrine, released from our sympathetic nervous system, controls thermogenesis. Significantly, the beta-blocker propranolol decreases glucose uptake, and hence thermogenesis, in brown fat. And interestingly, brown adipose tissue is seen quite readily in patients with pheochromocytomas, tumors that secrete norepinephrine.

More recently, Wallberg-Henriksson and Zierath (2009) have speculated that brown adipose tissue actually protects against obesity by regulating thermogenesis through the action of thyroid hormones and β-adrenergic stimulation. The process occurs through a protein uncoupling process involving mitochondria, which are plentiful in brown fat. The rich vascular supply gives brown adipose tissue its brown color. There is also some speculation that brown fat may be sensitive to specific nutrients (e.g., one gene regulator may be a lipid sensor) as well as temperature. Brown fat may play a role in energy homeostasis and specifically in energy dissipation rather than formation of fat cells, and there may be a "metabolic brake" process involved in brown fat that might one day, when manipulated genetically or pharmacologically, lead to therapeutic treatments for obesity (Pan et al. 2009). Virtanen et al. (2009) took tissue biopsies from several adult humans who were healthy and actually confirmed "the presence of substantial amounts of metabolically active brown adipose tissue." Their speculation is that brown adipose tissue "has the potential to contribute substantially to energy expenditure."

Finally, Cypess et al. (2009) analyzed PET-CT scans, also using the glucose uptake marker FDG, of more than 1,900 men and women. They confirmed that brown adipose tissue is most commonly located in the cervical and supraclavicular areas and is present in a "substantial percentage" of adults. They found it most frequently in subjects who were younger, had lower BMI values, were not using beta-blockers, and had never smoked cigarettes. Furthermore, brown adipose tissue was more commonly seen in women than men. Cypess et al. (2009) speculate that brown adipose tissue may protect against age-related obesity and may also be a factor in weight gain that is seen in those taking beta-blockers. How this preliminary research into the function of brown fat in human adults will affect clinical practice and the treatment of obesity remains to be seen. At this point, though, this knowledge merely demonstrates once again the extraordinary complexity of the metabolic and genetic processes involved in obesity.

White Adipose Tissue

Although the functions of brown adipose tissue in humans are just beginning to be elucidated, we have a much better understanding of white adipose tissue. One component of white adipose tissue is adipocytes; these fat-filled cells secrete more than 100 factors, including fatty acids, estrogen (in postmenopausal women), prostaglandins, and tumor necrosis factor alpha (TNF-α).

One of the substances secreted by fat cells, as well as by muscle and other cells, is interleukin-6 (IL-6). Adipose tissue, and particularly visceral adipose tissue, accounts for about one-third of the IL-6 circulating in our bodies (Esposito et al. 2006). IL-6 levels are associated with decreased insulin sensitivity and are even predictive of the development of type 2 diabetes and coronary artery disease. There are large quanti- ties of IL-6 in atherosclerotic plaques, and IL-6 increases levels of free fatty acids circulating in our bodies.

> Adipose tissue is responsible for one-third of the body's interleukin-6—the substance associated with decreased insulin sensitivity and the development of type 2 diabetes.

As noted above, another factor secreted by white adipose tissue is TNF-α. This is one of the markers associated with chronic low-grade inflammation in the body, and it has been associated with both insulin resistance and hypertension in humans (Esposito et al. 2006). According to Esposito et al. (2006), it is speculated to be able to induce production of IL-6 as well as C-reactive protein, another nonspecific marker of vascular inflammation (e.g., atherosclerosis) in the body. Although C-reactive protein is not directly produced by white adipose tissue, it is affected by factors like IL-6, which white adipose tissue does produce.

Two other factors produced by white adipose tissue (i.e., *adipokines*) are adiponectin and leptin. Adiponectin modulates insulin sensitivity and anti-inflammatory responses, and adiponectin levels are lower in obese individuals than in nonobese individuals. Leptin modulates appetite and energy homeostasis, and leptin levels are usually higher in obese individuals (Trayhurn 2007). White adipose tissue also produces many other peptides and proteins, some of which have unknown clinical importance and even unknown functions (Hauner 2004). This type of adipose tissue is also believed to be involved in the immune response, particularly acutely, and even may be involved in acute sepsis (Halberg et al. 2008). Halberg et al. note, for example, that the metabolic syndrome may involve chronic low-grade inflammation that may develop in fat tissue. According to Trayhurn (2007), this inflammatory state plays a key causal role in the development of type 2 diabetes, hypertension, atherosclerosis, and hyperlipidemia (i.e., the metabolic syndrome). Hauner (2004) describes white adipose tissue as a "multifunctional organ" that maintains extensive communication "with both neighboring and [distant] organs."

White adipose tissue consists of preadipocytes that do not contain lipid but have the capability to become lipid-filled adipocytes; endothelial cells; nerve fibers; and macrophages (cells involved in inflammation). Interestingly, these preadipocytes also have the potential, like stem cells, to become other cells types (e.g., muscle cells) (Hauner 2004). Adipose cells require an extensive blood supply and the adipocyte secretes factors that help create neovascularization. When white adipose tissue loses its blood supply—for example, because of medication—there can be a loss of fat tissue. It has even been suggested that drugs that inhibit angiogenesis might be used against obesity (Halberg et al. 2008). White adipose tissue is different morphologically depending on whether it is found subcutaneously or intra-abdominally: intra-abdominal fat is much more metabolically active, with a richer blood and sympathetic nerve supply. And those who are overweight or obese with an accumulation of white adipose tissue abdominally—the so-called apple shape—are more apt to develop metabolic disturbances such as the metabolic syndrome (hyperlipidemia, hypertension, insulin insensitivity, and eventually type 2 diabetes), although the exact nature of the mechanism is not fully understood. We do know that fatty acid blood levels are high in persons with abdominal obesity. This state leads to inhibition of the uptake and oxidation of glucose by muscles, which in turn leads the pancreas to produce more insulin until its beta cells cannot keep up with the demand (i.e., the state of insulin resistance). Because visceral fat is less sensitive to insulin than subcutaneous fat is, it is more likely to release free fatty acids into the bloodstream. In this situation, free fatty acids then accumulate in organs like the liver (by way of the portal vein) and muscle, and even the pancreas (so-called ectopic fat storage) (Snijder et al. 2006).

We have about 30 billion fat cells in our bodies; the very obese, according to Hirsch (2003), can have 75 billion, with twice as much fat packed into each cell. When someone loses weight, his or her fat cells shrink but do not change in number. When someone gains a great deal of weight, fat cells can increase in number. Obese people have fat cells that are more than twice the diameter of those in thin people (Hauner 2004). Halberg et al. (2008) note that white adipose tissue has the plasticity, as a person becomes obese, to adjust to extensive "remodeling and expansion" as its cells increase in size and number, coping with the need to provide more storage for fat. They further note that sometimes local inflammation can occur when the "extracellular matrix" interferes with this expansion, and they believe that this is reflective of "a systemic dysregulation of metabolism" (Halberg et al. 2008).

> The average person has about 30 billion fat cells; obese persons may have as many as 75 billion, with twice as much fat packed into each cell.

Unger (2003) sees white adipose tissue as essentially protective of other, lean tissues through its storage of fat. When fat spills over into other tissues, as it does in obesity, these so-called ectopic lipids cause damage to the other tissues. In the case of the heart, for example, Unger reports that those with a BMI value greater than 30 kg/m² may have lipotoxic cardiomyopathy—triglyceride deposits that result in impaired cardiac functioning such as impaired contraction. He facetiously calls these ectopic fat deposits "weapons of lean body mass destruction" (Unger 2003).

> When someone gains weight, fat cells may increase both in number and in size to store more fat.

Obesity (i.e., increased white adipose tissue) is also associated with inflammation and metabolic disturbances, and essentially "a number of perturbations that alter adipose tissue homeostasis" (Qi et al. 2009). Qi et al. report there is a protein activated in adipose tissue in obesity—cAMP response element–binding protein, or CREB protein—that actually promotes insulin resistance in mice. Their speculation is that large increases in adipose tissue create pockets of microhypoxia that result in inflammation and an accumulation of macrophages, ultimately leading to insulin resistance in the liver and muscle and an increase in free fatty acids in the circulation (Qi et al. 2009). When CREB protein is inhibited experimentally, even obese mice (with genetic or diet-induced obesity) do not develop insulin resistance. These researchers are hopeful that targeting this CREB system may ultimately lead to therapies for insulin resistance.

SATIETY

There are many physiological processes involved in how the body prepares itself for the ingestion, digestion, and metabolism of our food. These anticipatory responses are called *cephalic-phase* responses, and they can be physical (e.g., the motility of our gastrointestinal system), secretory (e.g., enzymes and hormones), or even metabolic (e.g., process of thermogenesis) (Power and Schulkin 2009, pp. 208-209).

But how does the body prepare itself, as it were, to stop the ingestion of food? Elmquist et al. (1999) described the earlier (and "inherently crude") lesions produced experimentally in the 1940s that established the crucial role of parts of the hypothalamus as a satiety/feeding center. In this "dual center model" (Elmquist et al. 1999), researchers found that lesions to the lateral hypothalamus produced decreased eating (hypophagia), profound loss of weight, and even eventual death by starvation, whereas lesions of the ventromedial area of the hypothalamus produced hyperphagia and massive obesity. The ventromedial area, then, became known as the *satiety center*.

Zhang et al. (1994) summarized two of the older theories involved in regulating the "feedback loop" of food intake: the lipostatic theory maintained that the amount of fat in the body, as somehow sensed by the hypothalamus and the central nervous system, was crucial for food intake and energy regulation, whereas the glucostatic theory emphasized the importance of blood glucose levels. The answer, though, is extraordinarily more complex than those earlier theories and may include a cascade of mechanical (e.g., distention of the stomach) and chemical (e.g., hormonal secretions) processes. Our higher cortical functioning, such as the conscious wish to stop eating or to eat less (Friedman 2004), may be involved. The concept of satiety is also implicated, however, and Smith (1998a, p. 3) points out that satiation involves, for the most part, an unconscious physiological process. Morton et al. (2006) define *satiation* as the process whereby the "drive to eat decreases as food is ingested." Blundell and Stubbs (2004, p. 433) note that satiation functions essentially to "monitor the biological value of foods," and they make a distinction between intrameal satiety (what brings a particular meal to an end) and postingestive, or intermeal, satiety (what inhibits eating between meals), and even the length of the interval between meals. In other words, separate physiological processes are involved in short-term satiation (from one meal) and long-term satiation (involving food intake for the entire day or longer) (Koopmans 2004, p. 386). Power and Schulkin (2009, pp. 188–189) distinguish "satiation" from "satiety." Satiation regulates short-term eating and refers to the processes that stop a particular eating episode, whereas satiety regulates the frequency of eating (i.e., the number of meals) or the time between one meal and another..

Smith notes that the process of satiation begins to occur preabsorptively (Smith 1998a, p. 4), that is, before nutrients are even absorbed in the blood. This process acts as the body's safety measure to ensure that we maintain energy homeostasis and do not take in more food than the body is able to handle at one time. This is in contrast, for example, to those rats with lesions in their medial hypothalamus that would literally eat until their stomachs ruptured if not prevented (Hirsch 2003; see earlier section "The Set Point"). The

- *Intrameal satiation* (what brings a particular meal to an end) is related to the body's energy homeostasis.

- *Intermeal satiety* (what inhibits eating between meals) is related to nonhomeostatic mechanisms.

Source: Blundell and Stubbs 2004

body is constantly making adjustments on a meal-to-meal basis to account for variations in meal size and/or frequency (Morton et al. 2006). Unfortunately, though, our cognitive functions (including the rewarding aspects of food, such as wanting or liking a food; see Chapter 4, "The Psychology of the Eater") can overwhelm these homeostatic regulatory systems, and we then overeat (Berthoud 2004, 2007). But even rats can be seduced to eat more when foods are made more palatable to them by being made more flavorful (Olszewski and Levine 2007). *Sensory-specific satiety* is defined as a temporary loss of interest (and pleasure) in a *particular* food after eating it when confronted with different foods that have not been tasted yet (Havermans et al.

If you eat only one kind of food at a meal, sensory-specific satiety will have you stop eating before energy homeostasis acts on your appetite.

2009). These researchers noted that sensory-specific satiety involves not only a decrease in wanting more of the previously eaten food but also even a decrease in liking that food.

Throughout the years, most researchers have focused on total food intake rather than the discrete, biological unit of eating that for most mammals, including humans, is the meal. G. J. Schwartz (2004) notes that meals are "distinct temporal units." He divides the process into signals that initiate food intake, those that maintain feeding, and those that involve stopping a meal, and also notes the importance of visual, olfactory, and taste sensations in initiating eating. The vagus nerve is one crucial component in a feedback system determining meal size. In fact, severing the vagus nerve can result in both increased meal size and longer meal duration (G. J. Schwartz 2004). Koopmans (2004, p. 377) notes that animals usually require from

5 to 30 minutes to finish a meal. Humans do, of course, demonstrate considerable variation in how long meals take—from minutes to hours. Geary (2005) points out that when animals are studied, variables such as the environment in which they are kept can affect meal patterns, and notes also that researchers do not all agree on the definition of a meal. Nevertheless, says Geary (2005), "a neuroscience of eating that does not include behavior [such as looking at the meal] will sooner or later come to a dead end before reaching its goal." And Koopmans (2004, p. 373) notes that the brain must mediate this process inasmuch as eating is a behavior. The meal, however, does become the unit through which satiety is measured, although palatability, type of diet, and even how recently the animal was fed ("level of deprivation") factor into meal size (Davis 1998, p. 71).

What actually controls meal size? In other words, how does satiety develop? Smith (1998b, p. 10) notes that Pavlov did some of the early, classic experiments with dogs with what he called *fictional feeding* and what we now call *sham feeding*, in which ingested food did not reach the stomach but drained out of an esophageal fistula he had artificially created. Pavlov found that dogs continued to eat considerably more than usual and that this procedure seemed to interfere with their satiation (i.e., the more they ate, the less they seemed to be satiated). Later experiments by other researchers, such as by Young and colleagues (1974), used rats in which gastric fistulas were created that also produced overeating in the animals. This research suggested that, at least for short-term satiation, food in the stomach, that is, gastric distention, is important. In other words, Young et al. (1974) felt it was "decisive evidence" that food in the mouth (i.e., oropharyngeal stimuli) does not elicit satiety (at least in the rat) when that ingested food is prevented from accumulating in the stomach and moving to the small intestine. The small intestine may also be an important factor in regulating satiety. Koopmans (2004, p. 387), though, notes that a short-term "intestinal satiety signal" has not yet been conclusively demonstrated during normal feeding. He explains that often studies of the small intestine involve delivering food nonphysiologically. Research in which the intestines of one rat are crossed with another, though, does demonstrate that the small intestine is involved in monitoring *daily* food intake rather than intake at one specific meal (Koopmans 2004, p. 387). He further notes that "the gut is the largest endocrine system in our body" (p. 388) and many hormones are secreted by our gastrointestinal system, including cholecystokinin (CCK), gastrin, and neuropeptide Y, among others. Koopmans believes that research supports the view that "a complex combination of neural and hormonal signals" is actually involved in producing satiety and that focusing on one aspect in this complex system may be misleading (Koopmans 2004, p. 396).

Wolfgang and Lane (2006) have suggested that malonyl coenzyme A (malonyl CoA), an intermediate in the synthesis of fatty acids, may be one of the signaling molecules for satiety in the hypothalamus. In other words, they speculate that malonyl-CoA is a "mediator of energy expenditure" and that fluctuations in its levels may act to inhibit eating. When malonyl CoA levels increase, an animal decreases its food intake, and malonyl CoA levels in the hypothalamus fall when an animal's food is restricted and rise again after feeding.

G. J. Schwartz et al. (2008) demonstrated experimentally that dietary fat, but not protein or carbohydrates, in the duodenum of rodents leads to satiety. What happens is that the presence of fat in the small intestine stimulates activation of a lipid messenger, oleoylethanolamide (OEA), which in turn activates a receptor speculated to be involved in the processes of absorption, storage, and utilization of fat ingested in the diet (peroxisome proliferator–activated receptor alpha, or PPAR-α). This process, also involving the vagus nerve, leads to a lengthening of the time between meals. In other words, the speculation is that OEA leads to satiety when dietary fat is consumed, and that this process is localized to the small intestine and is considered postingestive, not involving the actual orosensory processes. The unsaturated dietary fat oleic acid (found in cocoa butter and olive oil) is a precursor to OEA, but there seems to be a feedback system involved in that prolonged exposure to dietary oleic acid can lead to decreases in OEA production, at least in rodents. G. J. Schwartz et al. (2008) suggest that obesity might be treated eventually by either nutritional or pharmacological attention to this OEA process.

The process of satiation, particularly on a molecular level, is an extraordinarily complex one, and in many ways our knowledge about it is in its infancy. For example, Blouet et al. (2008) has shown in rodents that an enzyme that is involved in protein synthesis and growth and proliferation of cells, S6 kinase, may also be involved in the process of satiety and energy balance as a "nutrient-sensing" enzyme in the mediobasal region of the hypothalamus.

HORMONES OF FOOD INTAKE

Gastrin

Schubert (2008) describes the stomach as an "active reservoir" that "stores, grinds, and slowly dispenses" partially digested food to the small intestine, where it will be further digested and absorbed. The stomach secretes hydrochloric acid that is required for the digestion of protein and prevention of "bacterial overgrowth," as well as for the absorption of iron, calcium, and other substances. Of course, when there is too much acid, we can get poor digestion and even the formation of stomach ulcers. As a result, says Schubert, the secretion of gastric acid must be "precisely regulated." This regulation is actually quite complicated and involves a "highly coordinated" interaction of the brain, stomach, and intestine. Gastrin, which actually acts by releasing histamine, is a hormone that is secreted by cells in the antrum of the stomach, and its function is to stimulate acid secretion during ingestion of food. Likewise, there are hormonal mechanisms in the small intestine that function to inhibit acid secretion. Schubert notes that the "intestinal factor or factors" involved in inhibiting acid secretion are called "enterogastrones." The peptide "prime candidates" that may be involved in this inhibitory system include cholecystokinin (CCK) and glucagon-like peptide 1 (GLP-1, described later in this chapter) and may also involve the vagal nerve pathways.

Leptin

Leptin is a protein secreted primarily by adipose tissue and was only discovered in the early 1990s (Friedman 2009), when it was found to be involved in the regulation of food intake, as well as in the expenditure of energy by increasing thermogenesis (Matarese et al. 2008). Leptin takes its name from the Greek word *leptos*, meaning thin (Flier and Maratos-Flier 2007). It is one of the hormones of satiety, and researchers believe that its physiological function is to indicate starvation when its levels are low (Otero et al. 2005). Leibel (2002) notes that leptin evolutionarily is found in vertebrates and

> Leptin is an inhibitor of food intake.

may have been "co-opted" to ensure that sexual maturation and pregnancy occur only when there are sufficient fuel stores for the development of a fetus. Bray (2007) notes that leptin reduces food intake by decreasing levels of neuropeptide Y, one of the most powerful orexigenics (substances that stimulate eating), and by increasing levels of α–melanocyte-stimulating hormone (α-MSH), a potent inhibitor of eating. Zhang and Scarpace (2006) believe that α-MSH agents may eventually be used to treat obesity. Lago et al. (2008) note that leptin, which can cross the blood-brain barrier and activate hypothalamic receptors, also increases levels of cocaine- and amphetamine-regulated transcript (CART) and pro-opiomelanocortin (POMC),

LEPTIN

- A hormone mostly secreted by adipose (fat) tissue that serves as a signal involved in the regulation of appetite and energy balance—a "satiety hormone"
- Has a diurnal variation, with levels much higher in the middle of the night, possibly to control appetite while we are sleeping
- Has a role in the onset of puberty (may be essential for sexual maturation and fertility)
- Levels are higher in obese people (state of *leptin resistance*, analogous to insulin resistance)
- Levels are higher in infants, children, and pregnant women
- Speculation that leptin may have some role in enhancing alcohol consumption (i.e., craving for alcohol)
- Plays a key role in an adaptive response to starvation

Source: Friedman 2009; Kiefer et al. 2005

both of which decrease food intake. (See "Neuropeptide Y" and "Other Neurochemical Mechanisms Involved in Eating" later in this chapter.)

Zhang et al. (1994) report that leptin was actually discovered in Jeffrey Friedman's lab at Rockefeller University during the investigation of autosomal recessive genes for obesity in mice. One of these mutations is called the *obese mutation* (Ob), and it was found years earlier to produce massive obesity and hormonal abnormalities (even type 2 diabetes) in these animals (Zhang et al. 1994). Furthermore, this gene, after being cloned and sequenced, apparently encoded for the protein leptin. Leptin now seemed to provide the missing "putative" (Friedman 2009) biochemical "satiety factor" that had been hypothesized years earlier in mice experiments linking the blood circulation of obese mice with normal mice ("parabiosis") (Coleman 1978). Said Coleman (1978), about his own research, "These experiments suggest that the obese mouse is unable to produce sufficient satiety factor to regulate its food consumption." Mice with this Ob mutation are, in fact, leptin-deficient and develop hyperphagia, with massive obesity, hyperinsulinemia, insulin resistance, and other hormonal abnormalities, including infertility and temperature dysregulation. (Coleman 1978; Zhang et al. 1994) (Figure 5–1). Significantly, injections of exogenous leptin can reverse these alterations (Friedman 2009).

A genetic leptin deficiency (extremely rare in humans) results in extreme hyperphagia, endocrine abnormalities (e.g., thyroid and gonad dysfunction), and even morbid obesity beginning in childhood. This rare condition can be treated with injections of leptin, as in the Ob mutation mice, which result in major weight loss and no further hyperphagia. Leibel (2002) notes that the typical discomfort of dieting very much resembles the leptin-deficient state in humans or animals, with hunger and lower energy expenditure.

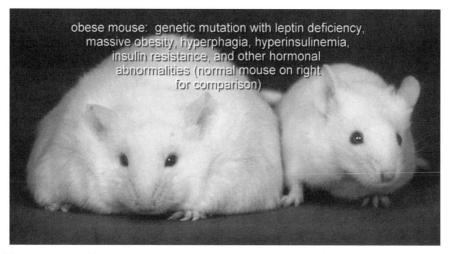

Figure 5–1. Obese mouse.

Source. Photo by Benjamin Cummings. Used with permission.

When leptin was first discovered, scientists thought they had found a major biochemical key to obesity. However, leptin is much more than an inhibitor of food intake and, unfortunately, the situation is very complicated. For one thing, the overwhelming majority of those who are overweight or obese have no leptin deficiency. In fact, most have higher than average leptin levels, and some researchers believe such individuals have the condition of leptin resistance, analogous to insulin resistance (in which insulin is present in high but ineffective levels) as seen in diabetes. Friedman (2004) notes that only about 5%–10% of obese people (as well as some lean people with type 2 diabetes) have low leptin levels. Zhang and Scarpace believe that leptin resistance is "both a consequence and one cause of obesity" (Zhang and Scarpace 2006). In other words, becoming obese for many leads to leptin resistance, which then leads to a worsening of the obesity in an "ever-escalating" cycle. Unger believes that everyone who lives long enough will eventually become leptin deficient (Unger 2003). Leptin levels do fall during dieting, and they are low in states of anorexia nervosa and malnutrition. Rosenbaum et al. (2005) believe that one of the major functions of leptin is "to defend—not reduce—body fat" and that it does this by "food-seeking and decreasing energy expenditures when fat stores are insufficient." In other words, it seems to signal the brain about the amount of fat stores in the body (Bray 2007). Incidentally, leptin levels fall after liposuction, the cosmetic removal of fat from the body, even though many researchers do not believe that liposuction significantly improves the metabolic abnormalities typically seen in obesity (Klein et al. 2004) (see Chapter 12, "Pharmacological and Surgical Treatments for Overweight and Obesity"). Unger (2003) notes that leptin levels are lower in visceral adipose cells than in subcutaneous fat cells.

Leptin seems to have many other roles in the body. Blood leptin levels are higher in infants and children, and pregnant women have higher leptin levels than nonpregnant women (Ostlund et al. 1996). Further, leptin is found in breast milk and may play a role in reducing the risk of childhood obesity in infants who are breast-fed. Owen and colleagues (2006) note there is a lower incidence of type 2 diabetes in those adults who had been breast-fed babies, although they note that the social class and weight of the mother, as well as an infant's low birth weight, may influence whether a mother chooses to breast-feed and whether there is a subsequent risk of type 2 diabetes. Leptin levels in the blood increase during childhood, and higher levels, such as in obese children, are associated with an earlier onset of puberty. Leptin seems essential for sexual maturation and fertility, according to Harris (2000), who also notes that leptin levels triple during puberty in nonobese girls and that there is a prepubertal surge in leptin in nonobese boys, which declines with puberty. And leptin levels are generally higher in women than men. Leptin levels in the blood also have a diurnal variation, with levels being up to 40% higher in the middle of the night, and this pattern can shift with a time-zone shift in the

> Breast-feeding may reduce the risk of childhood obesity; breast milk contains leptin.

timing of meals. Eating, though, does not lead to immediate changes in leptin levels (Schoeller et al. 1997). Insulin secretion, in some reports, has been inhibited by leptin, and leptin levels are very low in patients with uncontrolled diabetes and compromised beta cells in the pancreas (Harris 2000). Harris also makes the point that studies regarding leptin secretion may produce conflicting results because experimental (i.e., pharmacological) conditions may differ from those physiologically produced in the body. There is the suggestion by Gomez et al. (2009), for example, that leptin may be able to enhance insulin sensitivity, and they propose that leptin may have a major role in glucose control itself. In other words, disordered leptin function in the pancreas may be responsible for the obesity associated with diabetes, and leptin may eventually be used as one treatment modality in controlling type 2 diabetes.

Leptin levels have been reported to be elevated in autoimmune disorders, including multiple sclerosis and rheumatoid arthritis (Otero et al. 2005, 2006), and Matarese et al. (2008) believe that leptin may be the missing link relating the body's immune response to metabolic functioning and nutrition. These researchers have found that, at least in mice, starvation lowers leptin levels and can significantly improve the entire symptomatic course of experimental autoimmune encephalitis, an experimental disease model for multiple sclerosis. Whether this has applicability to humans remains to be seen. There have been reports, though, that symptoms of rheumatoid arthritis in humans can be improved by fasting (Otero et al. 2005, 2006). Leptin levels also increase during infection and inflammation (Otero et al. 2005, 2006), and Lago et al. note that leptin levels in the blood are elevated in acute ulcerative colitis, at least in males, and that leptin has an important role in intestinal inflammation (Lago et al. 2008). These researchers also speculate that osteoarthritis, more common in women, may be related to higher levels of leptin in adult women than men. Lago et al. (2008) further note that leptin acts centrally (by crossing the blood-brain barrier) to control food intake, but acts peripherally when it is involved in inflammatory processes.

Weigle et al. (2003) studied leptin levels in the context of dietary manipulations. These researchers varied the percentage of fat in diets given to human subjects, as well as varying calorie-restricted versus nonrestricted conditions. For 2 weeks subjects were given either a diet of 15% fat and 65% carbohydrates or a comparison diet with the same number of calories (2,000) but with 35% fat (i.e., a typical American diet). Then for 12 weeks the subjects were given the 15%-fat diet, with no calorie restrictions. Subjects lost approximately 4 kilograms of weight after 12 weeks. The researchers speculated that a diet lower in fat (but not calorie restricted; individuals could eat ad libitum) would produce weight loss in their subjects, without increasing hunger, by either increasing circulating leptin levels or else increasing the brain's sensitivity to leptin. Normally, calorie restriction leads to loss of body fat and decreased leptin levels, but also to increased levels of ghrelin and a subsequent increase in hunger. In fact, the researchers found that after 12 weeks on the 15%-fat,

high-carbohydrate, unrestricted-calorie diet, their subjects reduced their food intake naturally and lost weight without a subsequent rise in leptin levels. They believe
that because these lower leptin levels did not cause an increase in appetite, their
subjects had developed an increase in leptin sensitivity, and that this was due to the
lower amount of fat in their diets rather than the fact they had lost weight. Weigle
et al. (2003) also found that this low-fat, high-carbohydrate, unrestricted-calorie
regimen did not increase levels of ghrelin, the hormone that normally increases
hunger, and they speculate that the lower levels of ghrelin may have been related to
the enhanced leptin sensitivity.

In a small inpatient study using functional magnetic resonance imaging (MRI)
scans, Rosenbaum et al. (2008) noted that leptin injections in subjects who had
lost weight could reverse the increased activity in areas of the brain in response to
visual food cues. They noted that the weight-reduced state should be considered a
state of "relative leptin insufficiency." They believe that this weight-reduced state
leads to changes in the brain that involve "emotional and cognitive control of food
intake as well as integration of motor planning" (Rosenbaum et al. 2008), and that
these changes in turn predispose people who have lost weight to regain their weight.
In other words, these researchers speculate that with weight loss, people have increased sensory responses to food and decreased control of eating, both of which
seem to be responsive to leptin injections. Their subjects, given exogenous leptin
after their weight loss, seemed less hungry and more satiated. Rosenbaum et al.
(2008) postulate that leptin, rather than a weight loss medication per se, might be
better used as a weight maintenance medication following weight loss.

Further, Kiefer et al. (2005) have also shown that increased leptin blood levels
are associated with relapse to alcohol use in alcoholics who have been detoxified.
These researchers note that leptin must have a much wider range of effects than just
affecting weight because leptin receptors (there are at least six different leptin receptors; Lago et al. 2008) are found not just in areas typically associated with weight
regulation, but also in the cerebellum, cortex, hippocampus, and thalamus, for example. They found that leptin levels are significantly greater at the beginning of alcohol withdrawal and also are associated with reports of cravings for alcohol in
alcoholics. They note that leptin levels decrease
during treatment with anticraving medications
such as acamprosate and naltrexone, and speculate that leptin may have mediating effects
with these medications.

> Leptin levels are higher in the
> obese. In contrast, adiponectin
> levels are significantly lower.

Friedman (2009), in looking back on the 14 years since his lab discovered leptin,
summarizes its importance by noting, "Finally there is a powerful biological basis
for obesity, a fact that is (correctly) changing the public perception about this medical condition." In other words, the discovery of leptin confirmed the presence of a
"homeostatic system" regulating weight. Friedman emphasizes that leptin plays "a
key role in the adaptive response to starvation" by its effect on many physiologi-

cal systems in our body. As a result, leptin has a key function in communicating changes in our nutritional states. Friedman believes that while it is true that obese people consume more and get less exercise, the underlying (and not yet fully answered) question is, "Why do the obese eat more and exercise less?" For Friedman, it is "less about conscious choices…and more about their biological makeup."

Adiponectin

Adiponectin, discovered in the 1990s, is an amino acid protein hormone that is secreted in adipose tissue but found circulating in blood. Díez and Iglesias (2003) note that the levels of adiponectin found in plasma are three times the levels of most other hormones. These researchers also note that, in contrast to levels of leptin, which are higher in obese people, levels of adiponectin are significantly lower in the obese. In other words, adiponectin levels are negatively correlated, they say, with BMI values and the actual amount of body fat. Furthermore, levels are lower in people who have insulin resistance, that is, those with high levels of insulin and abnormal glucose tolerance test results (Kraemer and Castracane 2007). At least in animals, administration of adiponectin is known to enhance the action of insulin, and it has been found to lower circulating levels of glucose (Havel 2004). Circulating levels are also lower in people with a visceral fat distribution (the so-called apple shape) (Havel 2004). Furthermore, adiponectin levels are lower in patients with coronary artery disease. Those with high levels of triglycerides and low levels of HDL (high-density lipoprotein or "good") cholesterol, both risk factors for atherosclerosis, have lower levels of adiponectin (Díez and Iglesias 2003). In fact, these researchers speculate that adiponectin may have protective as well as anti-inflammatory roles in the body.

Adiponectin levels, like leptin levels, are higher in women than in men (Díez and Iglesias 2003). Havel (2004) notes, however, that this sex difference may be due to differences in adipocyte size and body shape, given that women are more likely to have the pear-shaped body with smaller and more numerous fat cells. Levels have been reported to be much higher (2.5 times higher) in those undergoing kidney dialysis and "moderately" higher in female patients with anorexia nervosa (Díez and Iglesias 2003). After gastric bypass surgery, adiponectin levels that were previously low normalize; researchers found

> People with low adiponectin levels have high (but ineffective) levels of insulin (insulin resistance) and abnormal glucose tolerance test results.

that patients who had the lowest presurgical levels of adiponectin were the ones to lose the most weight after bypass surgery (Havel 2004). Calorie restriction, in general, has been reported to produce higher levels (Fernández-Real et al. 2005). Fernández-Real et al. also note that adiponectin levels seem to be sensitive to the intake of different kinds of fatty acids in our diets ("[the] proportion of fatty acids in plasma mirror the dietary fat composition"), and that, for example, greater intake of the essential fatty acid omega-3 leads to higher levels of adiponectin circulating in the blood. They also note that adiponectin promotes greater fatty acid oxidation and hence decreased fat, particularly in muscle. Havel (2004) notes that adiponectin seems to be involved in the metabolic regulation of both carbohydrates and fats.

Studies have been done to examine the relationship of exercise to certain hormone levels, including adiponectin levels, because both exercise and increased adiponectin levels can lead to greater insulin sensitivity. Kraemer and Castracane (2007) note that exercise affects the metabolism of carbohydrates and lipids differently. When we exercise at a higher intensity, we utilize (oxidize) carbohydrates more, and when we exercise at a low to moderate intensity, we are more likely to oxidize fat (by stimulating the adipocyte hormone–sensitive lipase enzyme).

> When we exercise at a low to moderate intensity, we oxidize fat by stimulating the adipocyte hormone–sensitive lipase enzyme.

This cycle also involves reduced insulin levels and increases in glucagon levels in the blood. Kraemer and Castracane (2007) report that short-term moderate or even strenuous exercise did not affect adiponectin levels in either men or women.

Studies of chronic exercise (longer than 2 months) in obese men and women, as well as those with type 2 diabetes and those who have undergone gastric bypass surgery, have demonstrated that adiponectin levels increase in the context of improved fitness, greater insulin sensitivity, and actual weight loss. Kraemer and Castracane (2007) speculate, though, that it may not be the exercise per se but rather the weight loss that is responsible for increasing the adiponectin levels.

Adiponectin levels have a diurnal variation: they are significantly lower in the evening than during the day, with the nadir in the very early morning and peak in the late morning (Gavrila et al. 2003). They reach their lowest level 2 hours after cortisol, so there may be some relationship. In other words, Gavrila et al. report that serum adiponectin and cortisol have "similar but not overlapping diurnal variations." They also speculate that since adiponectin increases insulin sensitivity and cortisol decreases insulin sensitivity, "the nocturnal cortisol decline" may indirectly determine "compensatory" changes in adiponectin with the effect of keeping "the degree of insulin resistance stable." They are not in phase with the diurnal variation of leptin. Levels of adiponectin do not change with intake of food (Gavrila et al. 2003).

Williams et al. (2008) report that adiponectin levels, though, are about 20% higher in women who habitually consume four or more cups of caffeinated coffee daily compared with those who drink decaffeinated coffee or tea. The researchers also confirm that these people who drink caffeinated coffee also have less insulin resistance, lower levels of type 2 diabetes, and lower levels of the inflammation marker C-reactive protein, and they speculate that the higher adiponectin levels may be contributory. These results were not found in those who drank decaffeinated coffee or tea, though it was not common for those who were drinkers of decaffeinated coffee to drink four or more cups.

Ghrelin

Ghrelin is an amino acid peptide, related to growth hormone, that is secreted primarily in the stomach but is found throughout the gastrointestinal system and even in the hypothalamus and amygdala, among other sites (Jayasena and Bloom 2008). It was discovered in the late 1990s and stimulates appetite. In rats, at least, ghrelin has also been found to be involved in sleep regulation (Szentirmai et al. 2006). Its pattern is that levels typically rise before meals, as much as twofold (Cummings et al. 2001) (and hence may be involved in triggering eating), and fall after eating; in normal-weight individuals, the level of the fall (i.e., the postprandial suppression) is directly related to the number of calories consumed (le Roux et al. 2005). In rodents, peripheral injections of ghrelin increased not only initiation of meals, but also sniffing, foraging for food, and hoarding of food—in other words, appetitive behaviors involved in "the animals' motivation to seek out food and initiate feeding" (Cummings 2006).

> Ghrelin, produced mainly in the stomach, is an appetite-stimulating hormone.

Experiments by Malik et al. (2008) demonstrated that when ghrelin was administered intravenously to healthy volunteers, functional MRI scans showed that areas in the brain such as the amygdala, orbitofrontal cortex, striatum, and parts of the insula were more responsive. These are areas involved in the "incentive value of food cues" (Malik et al. 2008), areas in the brain involved with reward and motivation and appetitive behavior. The insula, for example, seemed responsive to pictures of food and even things like restaurant menus. Malik et al. (2008) also note that appetitive responses involve attention and anticipation of pleasure, as well as motivation to eat, actual consumption of food, and memory for food-related cues. These researchers note that feeding in response to triggers, such as the actual presence of food or the anticipation of enjoying eating, is called hedonic and nonhomeostatic. In other words, it can occur when the person is not necessarily hungry—that is, in the "absence of nutritional or caloric deficiency"—and involves the reward and motivational centers (mesolimbic areas) of the brain. Nonhomeostatic feeding can be contrasted with homeostatic feeding that is mediated by the hypothalamus and regulates energy balance.

> Ghrelin may be responsible for hedonic/nonhomeostatic eating behavior.

Cummings (2006) also reports that ghrelin levels rose before eating in normal-weight humans when they initiated their meals voluntarily "in the absence of cues related to time and food." Fasting ghrelin levels are higher in patients with anorexia nervosa and malnutrition, and when patients with these conditions gained weight their ghrelin levels fell (Erdmann et al. 2003). Overweight and obese subjects with binge eating disorder (without purging) were found to have lower ghrelin levels before eating, and the levels declined only slightly after eating (Geliebter et al. 2005).

When obese people lose weight, their ghrelin levels increase (Druce et al. 2004), and this is thought to contribute to increased hunger and the potential for people to regain their lost weight (Havel et al. 2004). Ghrelin levels rise with age, and this may contribute to weight gain as we age (Cummings et al. 2001). Ghrelin levels are extremely high (and do not fall after eating) in people with Prader-Willi syndrome, a rare (1 in 10,000 to 16,000 births) genetic disorder characterized by obesity, hypogonadism, growth hormone deficiency, cognitive impairment, and hyperphagia (DelParigi et al. 2002). Cummings (2006) reports that ghrelin levels decrease with long-standing infection and chronic gastritis due to *Helicobacter pylori.*

Significantly, patients who have lost weight after gastric bypass surgery maintain markedly lower levels of ghrelin. They do not demonstrate the typical meal-related fluctuations seen with ghrelin, nor do they have its normal diurnal variation, and they report less hunger between meals. This lower ghrelin level postsurgery may be one factor in why this surgery is so successful in weight loss maintenance (Cummings et al. 2002).

Normally, ghrelin exhibits diurnal variations, with lowest values between 9 and 10 A.M. and peak levels between midnight and 2 A.M. This pattern is in phase with that of leptin; both leptin and ghrelin rise throughout the day, and leptin is also synchronized to mealtimes (Cummings et al. 2001). Insulin levels are reciprocal to ghrelin levels, such that insulin levels rise after eating.

Le Roux et al. (2005b) report that ghrelin levels (and particularly the lower levels of ghrelin seen after eating) may be sensitive to the type of food eaten—whether fat, carbohydrate, or protein—though the results have not been consistent. For example, some studies have shown that in people of normal weight, meals with more fat increase ghrelin levels, whereas others have shown that a meal high in fat (versus carbohydrates) produces some degree of fall in ghrelin levels (le Roux et al. 2005b). Erdmann et al. (2003) found in their study of healthy, normal-weight volunteers that a meal high in fat decreased ghrelin levels, with lowest levels 3 hours after eating; a meal high in carbohydrates (either liquid or solid food) also decreased ghrelin but within a different time period, that is, within 1 hour; a high-protein meal, on the other hand, increased ghrelin levels. In other words, meals rich in carbohydrates decrease ghrelin levels more powerfully than those rich in fats. Blom et al. (2006), on the other hand, found that ghrelin levels decreased more in healthy men after a high-protein breakfast (Blom et al. call protein the most satiating of nutrients) than after a high-carbohydrate breakfast. Protein, because it cannot be stored in the body, is metabolized more quickly and has a greater thermogenic effect than carbohydrates or fats. Also, Blom et al. (2006) note that protein may tend to stimulate secretion of other peptides, such as the gut peptides CCK and glucagon-like peptide 1 (GLP-1), both of which increase feeling full and slow gastric emptying. These researchers found that the breakfast high in protein did slow food from leaving the stomach. Blom et al. (2006) do note that results from other studies may be conflicting because not only protein, but the specific type of protein used (with different amino acid structures; e.g., whey vs. casein), may factor into the results. They note further that although protein intake in their study did lead to a decrease in ghrelin blood levels, their subjects did not report differences in a subjective sense of fullness (i.e., satiety) or even subsequent calorie intake.

Le Roux et al. (2005b) conducted a series of experiments comparing normal-weight people to obese people, varying the amount of fat and calories (up to 3,000 calories per meal) in different meals. They found that obese people actually have lower fasting levels of ghrelin and that their levels of ghrelin do not fall as much as levels do in normal-weight individuals after eating. They speculate that this reduced suppression after eating in obese people may interfere with their feelings of satiety. In other words, it just takes more calories for an obese person to feel full. For example, even a meal of 3,000 calories sup-

> Even a meal of 3,000 calories can suppress ghrelin levels less in obese individuals than a meal of 1,000 calories does in normal-weight individuals.
>
> **Source: le Roux et al. 2005b**

pressed ghrelin levels less in their obese subjects than a meal of 1,000 calories did in normal-weight subjects (le Roux et al. 2005b). In these experiments, the meals were a combination of protein, fat, and carbohydrates, with increasingly more fat added as the calories increased. Le Roux et al. (2005b) note that ghrelin may work by increasing both neuropeptide Y and agouti-related protein in the hypothalamus, and these are both potent stimulators of hunger.

But exactly how ghrelin exerts its effect is not clear. Jayasena and Bloom (2008) note that understanding the mechanism involved may help us develop treatments for obesity. The arcuate nucleus of the hypothalamus, where the blood-brain barrier is weak, seems to be involved in receiving ghrelin signals, and the vagus nerve may mediate its actions in the brain stem (Jayasena and Bloom 2008).

Ghrelin levels do not seem to be affected by short-term exercise such as running or cycling at moderate to high levels, even though exercise does increase levels of growth hormone, which is structurally related to ghrelin (Kraemer and Castracane 2007). Long-term exercise does produce increases in ghrelin levels when there is weight loss (Kraemer and Castracane 2007).

Teff et al. (2004) examined the effects of fructose consumption as contrasted with glucose consumption on circulating hormones, including ghrelin, insulin, and leptin levels. In a study of normal-weight women, these researchers found that circulating levels of ghrelin did not fall as much after fructose consumption as after glucose consumption. They speculate that because leptin, insulin, and ghrelin all function as major regulators of long-term energy balance, any changes in these patterns may lead to changes in calorie intake and even weight gain. For example, they found that fructose ingestion not only led to higher triglyceride levels than glucose ingestion but also lower insulin and leptin levels and higher ghrelin levels. In other words, compared with glucose, fructose behaves "more like fat" when consumed in a mixed meal (with carbohydrates, protein, and fat) and leads to "substantially smaller" postprandial levels of glucose and insulin, "attenuated" leptin levels, and a "relative elevation" of ghrelin after eating. Teff et al. (2004) suggest that fructose's failure to suppress ghrelin levels, in combination with a reduced insulin and leptin response, may be responsible for the typical decreased satiety and increased calorie intake when fructose consumption is a regular part of one's diet. Fructose consumption, of course, has increased dramatically in the American diet, particularly because of the high-fructose corn syrup found in sodas and hundreds of other products in American supermarkets, including processed soups; this is in addition to the fructose consumed as part of table sugar, sucrose. (See also "Carbohydrates" in Chapter 3, "Food: The Basic Principles of Calories.")

Leidy and Williams (2006) studied ghrelin levels in nonobese women over the course of 24 hours that included three meals and a snack. They found that ghrelin levels were related not only to the number of calories ingested in a specific meal, but also to the calories accumulated prior to the next meal. These researchers note, as have other researchers, that ghrelin levels were directly related to calorie intake—the more calories consumed, the more ghrelin levels fell after eating—but they also note that the sum of calories consumed for breakfast and lunch was negatively correlated with the subsequent ghrelin peak prior to dinner. That is, the dinner peak was greater and consistent with the fact that ghrelin levels tend to rise throughout the day, though they fall after each meal. They do note that Americans tend to eat more of their food at dinner and the higher ghrelin peak prior to dinner may be related to an insufficient number of calories during the day. In other words, ghrelin was not only an energy sensor but also a modulator of energy balance in the course of a day. There is even the suggestion that medications that antagonize the effect of ghrelin may have a role eventually in the control of type 2 diabetes (Gomez et al. 2009).

> Insulin and leptin working as convergent signals are responsible for energy homeostasis.

And there may be some connection between ghrelin secretion and the vagus nerve: when the vagus nerve had been transected in patients who had had esophageal or gastric surgery, (and had lost their appetites), exogenous ghrelin did not result in any increased meal intake (le Roux et al. 2005a). These researchers speculate that an intact vagus nerve "may be required for exogenous ghrelin to increase appetite and food intake in man." What role manipulations of the vagus nerve could potentially have on ghrelin and appetite control remains to be seen.

Insulin, Amylin, and Glucagon

Insulin is a hormone secreted by the beta cells of the pancreas. Initially it was assumed, because of its size, that insulin could not cross the blood-brain barrier. Insulin, essentially, lowers blood glucose levels as it increases glucose uptake in peripheral tissues (Woods et al. 2006). Because insulin does not regulate glucose use by the brain, it was thought that the brain was not particularly insulin sensitive (M. W. Schwartz et al. 2005). It is now known that insulin does enter the brain and although the brain is "insulin-independent" (with respect to glucose use) it is very much involved in receiving the metabolic signaling of hormones like insulin and leptin (M. W. Schwartz and Porte 2005). Schwartz and Porte, in fact, believe in a neurocentric model by which abnormal neuronal signaling of hormones such as leptin and insulin links abnormal glucose metabolism with obesity. There are insulin receptors in many areas of the brain, and insulin sensing is very much responsible for control of food intake as well as energy homeostasis (Woods et al. 2006). Significantly, experiments with rats have shown that when insulin levels are high, carbohydrates are preferred, whereas when insulin levels are low, fat is the preferred source of calories (Woods et al. 2006).

Though insulin has a direct effect on metabolic functioning, particularly the regulation of glucose, Mantzoros and Serdy (2008) note that it "directly or indirectly affects the function of virtually every tissue in the body." They note that glucose can be obtained from the absorption of food we eat; from the breakdown of glycogen, the storage form of glucose; or from the process of gluconeogenesis, that is, the synthesis of glucose from the metabolism of carbohydrates, fats, or proteins. They also explain that insulin can inhibit the breakdown of glycogen and inhibit gluconeogenesis. It also can increase the transport of glucose into adipose tissue (but mostly into skeletal muscle); can increase the breakdown of glucose in fat and muscle; and can stimulate the synthesis of glycogen, mostly in the liver. In other words, insulin acts

INSULIN

- A hormone synthesized and secreted by cells in the pancreas
  - Type 1 diabetes: usually diagnosed in childhood; pancreas not able to synthesize insulin (i.e., insulin deficiency)
  - Type 2 diabetes: most commonly diagnosed in adulthood but, with the recent epidemic of childhood obesity, now being seen in children and adolescents; insulin is produced but an insensitivity to the effects of insulin (i.e., insulin resistance) develops

- A powerful regulator of metabolic function: directly or indirectly, affects the function of virtually every tissue in the body

- Has major effects on glucose, including increasing glucose uptake by fat and muscle

- With increased insulin secretion, more storage of triglycerides in fat cells

- Normal insulin secretion and action are essential for normal growth and growth regulation, but there is also evidence that abnormally high insulin levels may contribute to the development of colorectal, ovarian, and breast cancers

Source: Mantzoros and Serdy 2008

as the "coordinator" of glucose and free fatty acids, the fuels of the body, in order to meet the various demands of the body such as eating, fasting, or exercise (Mantzoros and Serdy 2008). After eating, for example, insulin secretion increases and this in turn facilitates the storage of triglycerides in fat cells. When there is prolonged fasting or uncontrolled type 1 diabetes, conditions in which insulin levels are low, there is an increase in fat mobilization and an increase in free fatty acids to the liver. The liver, in turn, metabolizes these free fatty acids into ketone bodies, which can be used as fuel, particularly by skeletal muscle and the heart.

Power and Schulkin (2009, p. 158) summarize the two main ways energy is stored in our bodies: in the form of glycogen (the storage form of glucose) in our liver and muscles and in the fat of adipose tissue. Only in extremes (e.g., major energy expenditure or starvation conditions) does the body break down protein from muscle.

M. W. Schwartz et al. (2000) make the point that fat deposition requires the presence of insulin, and those with type 1 diabetes (insulin deficiency) typically have increased intake of food (diabetic hyperphagia) but do not gain weight. Here the extra calories are seen in the increased blood glucose levels and ultimately in the urine (hence the name diabetes mellitus, or "sweet urine"). On the other hand, in those with high but ineffective insulin levels (i.e., insulin resistance, type 2 diabetes), weight gain and even obesity develop (Havel 2005). Cherian and Santoro (2006) note that obesity can be divided into two types: *hypertrophic obesity*, with increase in fat cell size, and *hyperplastic obesity*, with increase in fat cell number. They also note that people can have one of these as a dominant type or both as a mixture. They report on studies that indicate that the size of the fat cells in abdominal (visceral) obesity more likely predicts a state of insulin resistance rather than the actual percentage of body fat in an individual. They explain that larger fat cells are more resistant to insulin and "more susceptible to the effects of hormones that cause lipolysis" (Cherian and Santoro 2006). They make the point that people with enlarged adipocytes develop insulin resistance because these fat cells, when they enlarge too much, can no longer maintain cellular homeostasis. These hypertrophied fat cells also secrete TNF-α, which also interferes with insulin. The result is that insulin no longer has its antilipolytic effect and triglycerides "spill over" into the circulation (i.e., serum triglyceride levels increase). Eventually, a fatty liver can develop. These researchers further speculate that the procedure of liposuction, by removing subcutaneous fat tissue, reduces the number of fat cells available for storage and may even predispose individuals to insulin resistance and the full metabolic syndrome. In other words, this procedure predisposes someone to "saturation of the residual fat depot," which, they believe, is the most important factor involved in the development of insulin resistance.

There has been controversy in the literature about the value of liposuction in improving the metabolic profile of overweight

> Liposuction, by removing subcutaneous fat tissue, reduces the number of fat cells available for storage and may predispose a person to insulin resistance.

or obese individuals. Snijder et al. (2005), for example, note that removing visceral fat may help improve a person's metabolic disturbances, but removing subcutaneous fat, as in the common cosmetic procedure of liposuction, seems to do little to help with a person's abnormal metabolic profile (see Chapter 12, "Pharmacological and Surgical Treatments for Overweight and Obesity").

Woods et al. (2006) emphasize that insulin levels in the blood reflect both circulating energy (i.e., glucose) and stored energy (i.e., adipose tissue.) And leptin and insulin work as "convergent signals" in the brain to regulate energy and glucose homeostasis. They also note, though, that insulin levels correlate better with visceral fat (and hence the metabolic syndrome) whereas leptin levels correlate better with subcutaneous fat, which is not as dangerous. Because men are apt to have more visceral fat, insulin is a "more relevant adiposity signal" in men and leptin is a more relevant signal in women (Woods et al. 2006).

Havel (2005), though, makes the point that although insulin stimulates the synthesis and storage of fat, insulin itself does not cause weight gain and obesity, and diets that emphasize avoiding foods that stimulate insulin (low-carbohydrate diets or, more specifically, the low glycemic index craze) do not necessarily lead to weight loss. He differentiates the natural state of insulin secretion in response to meals (a rapid increase in insulin levels, with return to baseline) as opposed to the abnormal state of chronic increased insulin secretion secondary to insulin resistance and beta cell disorder. Havel (2005) also emphasizes that fructose does not create the same kind of normal insulin response that glucose does. Because fructose does not cross the blood-brain barrier, it is more likely to lead to dysregulation of food intake when excessive fructose is consumed.

Chaput et al. (2008), including researcher Ludwig, studied individual physiological differences in insulin secretion when subjects were exposed to high- and low-fat diets over a period of 6 years. They found these differences may contribute to differences in some individuals' sensitivities to the effects of foods with higher glycemic index values. These researchers believe there is a unique physiological phenotype that is more sensitive to foods with a high glycemic index

> People with a particular phenotype may be more susceptible to carbohydrates with a high glycemic index value and may be more susceptible to large weight gain.

value or high *glycemic load* (i.e., the glycemic index value times the actual amount of carbohydrate in a food; see "Glycemic Index" section in Chapter 3, "Food: The Basic Principles of Calories"). In other words, people with this particular phenotype may be more susceptible to "especially great weight gain" with high-glycemic foods. Their study examined the results of insulin levels at 30 minutes (insulin-30 levels; a time marker they believe is a "good measure of insulin secretion in humans"), when their subjects were given oral glucose tolerance tests. They found that a subgroup of individuals who had a high level of insulin secretion at 30 minutes lost substantially more weight when given a diet with a low glycemic load, as compared with a diet low in fat. The same subgroup gained considerably more weight when exposed to a low-fat diet (but with more high-glycemic carbohydrates). They found that those subjects who had the highest insulin-30 levels and lowest amount of dietary fat gained 1.8 kilograms more than those in the highest insulin-30 and highest dietary fat group, and 4.5 kilograms more than those in the lowest insulin-30 group and lowest dietary fat group over the 6 years of the study. This was a "novel diet-phenotype interaction." They speculated that the use of insulin levels taken at 30 minutes can be used as one screening device by clinicians to help in "individualizing dietary prescriptions."

There is a recent suggestion that high insulin levels and high estradiol levels are two independent risk factors for postmenopausal breast cancer. Gunter et al. (2009) studied over 800 women with breast cancer, but not diabetes (and over 800 women as control subjects). All of the study subjects are enrolled in the Women's Health Initiative observational study, which includes over 93,000 postmenopausal women at 40 clinical centers. Researchers found that increased fasting insulin levels (i.e., hyperinsulinemia) were associated with a significantly greater risk of breast cancer (2.4 times higher), but only among those who had never used hormone replacement therapy. The relationship apparently did not hold for those who had used exogenous hormones, but this finding may have been "obscured" by high levels of estrogen in those who were taking hormone replacement therapy.

Amylin is a peptide hormone also secreted after meals, along with insulin, by the beta cells of the pancreas. According to Woods et al. (2006), insulin and amylin are cosecreted in a fixed ratio, but obesity, type 1 diabetes, and pancreatic cancer may result in more amylin being secreted relative to insulin. Amylin inhibits the stomach from emptying, as well as inhibiting gastric acid and glucagon secretion. It has the capacity to reduce food intake and meal size (Cummings and Overduin 2007). In fact, amylin is secreted in proportion to food intake and can be considered a hormone of satiety (Bloom et al. 2008). But Woods et al. (2006) make the point that amylin has characteristics of both insulin and glucagon: Like insulin, it functions as an adiposity signal; like glucagon, it functions as a satiety signal. During fasting, amylin levels are low, but they increase with meals. Amylin levels are also highly correlated with body fat (Woods et al. 2006). Amylin does cross the blood-brain barrier and works directly on certain areas of the brain, and is considered a neuroendocrine hormone (Hollander et al. 2004). Rushing et al. (2000) believe that amylin is not just a short-term satiety signal but may function in the long-term control of energy balance as well.

There is a synthetic version of amylin called *pramlintide* that is used to treat diabetes but that, as Hollander et al. (2004) point out, also has the capacity to cause clinically meaningful weight loss over time. These researchers note that such weight loss has occurred in studies in which overweight or obese patients with type 2 diabetes were actually discouraged from altering their diet or exercise level, and the weight loss was not believed to result from the transient nausea this medication can cause. Furthermore, these patients, and particularly very obese ones, were able to decrease their daily insulin requirements.

Glucagon is a hormone secreted by the alpha cells of the pancreas that decreases food intake; that is, it acts as a satiety signal. Glucagon is the "hormone of starvation," and levels of glucagon do increase when someone fasts (Koopmans 2004, p. 390).

Woods et al. (2006) note that glucagon and insulin work in opposite ways metabolically. Glucagon mainly stimulates glucose production either by breaking down glycogen or by producing more glucose (gluconeogenesis) in the liver, particularly during the fasting condition or when the body has an increased need for glucose. Glucagon secretion, though, unlike that of insulin or amylin, is not related to the amount of fat in the body and is not an adiposity signal (Woods et al. 2006). Woods et al. note that within 1 minute of eating, glucagon levels rise briefly, but Koopmans (2004, p. 390) notes that glucagon levels fall immediately after a meal of pure carbohydrates whereas insulin and amylin levels rise. Most other meals stimulate glucagon secretion, but a high-protein meal stimulates its secretion the most (Woods et al. 2006). Koopmans (2004, p. 390) further notes that if there is protein or fat intake, though, glucagon levels can stay elevated and even increase slowly, but these levels can also decrease after a mixed meal. Glucagon seems to work directly on the liver to inhibit food intake. It acts centrally as well and branches of the vagus nerve are also known to be involved (Leibowitz and Hoebel 2004, p. 327) because severing the vagus nerve blocks its effect (Koopmans 2004, p. 390).

Cholecystokinin

Cholecystokinin is a hormone produced primarily in the duodenum and jejunum parts of the small intestine, but also in the brain. CCK was the first hormone that was found to be associated with satiation, back in the 1970s; that is, it decreases meal size. It is secreted primarily in response to fats, but also in response to proteins. Severing of the vagus nerve can decrease the effects of CCK, and CCK most likely signals the brain directly and indirectly (Cummings and Overduin 2007). Cummings and Overduin note that CCK is involved in short-term satiation, acutely shortening mealtime, rather than long-term control. Interestingly, CCK has been implicated in the reward aspects of food. It is speculated that CCK seems to potentiate the effects of dopamine when they are released together in the nucleus accumbens, although it may inhibit the release of dopamine in the hypothalamus. It has been shown to "devalue the incentive properties of food" in experiments with animals (Leibowitz and Hoebel 2004, p. 329).

Sharkey (2006) notes that CCK that is released in the proximal small intestine may possibly alter the release of leptin. They have reported that *H. pylori*, the bacterium found in the stomach that has been directly associated with gastric ulcers, changes levels of gastrin, leptin, and CCK. When an individual is successfully treated for *H. pylori* infection, that person often experiences an increase in appetite and changes in levels of ghrelin. Jayasena and Bloom (2008) note that CCK stimulates the pancreas and the gallbladder, as well as inhibiting the emptying of the stomach (by constricting the pyloric sphincter) (Leibowitz and Hoebel 2004, p. 328) and increasing intestinal movement. In fact, it is probably the synergistic combination of

H. pylori changes levels of gastrin, leptin, and cholecystokinin, reducing a person's appetite.

CCK with a distended stomach that contributes to the sense of satiety (Cupples 2005). Powley and Phillips (2004) note that, in general, gastric satiety occurs from distention (mechanical or volumetric) whereas intestinal satiety comes from nutrients in the diet. As noted above, Schubert (2008) believes that CCK is also involved in the inhibition of stomach acid secretion.

Burton-Freeman et al. (2002) report that CCK release is affected not only by the amount of fat in a meal but also by the amount of fiber (e.g., viscous polysaccharides, such as barley or beans), at least in women. In a small study, these researchers found that the women in their study reported a greater sense of satiety (and had higher CCK levels) when the fat or fiber content of their breakfast meals was increased from a low-fat, low-fiber meal. Interestingly, though, in men, a breakfast with either high or low fiber content, but each low in fat, was more satiating than a low-fiber, high-fat meal. Increasing the fat and fiber also reduced the insulin response to a meal. Burton-Freeman et al. (2002), therefore, believe that foods that increase the release of CCK may lead to not only increased satiety but also improved glucose control and may be especially useful for individuals with type 2 diabetes.

Neuropeptide Y

Neuropeptide Y is one of the most prevalent peptides throughout the brain (including the hypothalamus) and even the sympathetic nervous system. It stimulates feeding behavior and weight gain. According to Leibowitz and Hoebel (2004, p. 311), it is particularly responsive to times of increased metabolic requirements or states of insufficient calorie intake. In other words, neuropeptide Y helps to maintain energy

Neuropeptide Y is an appetite-stimulating hormone and may be involved in the weight gain associated with stress.

homeostasis, and especially intake of carbohydrate (the "preferred dietary nutrient" [p. 311]), in the context of increased levels of stress. Leibowitz and Hoebel (2004, p. 312) further note that neuropeptide Y stimulation leads to decreased sympathetic nervous system activity, increased parasympathetic nervous system activity, and decreased thermogenesis and energy expenditure. Further, it stimulates fat synthesis by diverting glucose from muscle. Neuropeptide Y is also involved with the hypothalamic-pituitary-adrenal (HPA) axis, the secretion of cortisol, and the circadian rhythms involved in eating. In that sense, neuropeptide Y can be considered to function as a neurotransmitter (Krysiak et al. 1999). Notably, both insulin and leptin, which decrease food intake, inhibit neuropeptide Y, and fasting increases its levels. Obesity reduces neuropeptide Y levels, particularly when the obesity is produced by a high-fat, high-calorie diet (Leibowitz and Hoebel 2004, p. 313).

Kuo et al. (2007) note that many stressors, particularly those that are chronic, lead to the release of neuropeptide Y from sympathetic nerves in humans as well as rodents. These researchers speculate that neuropeptide Y may be involved in the weight gain associated with stress and increased calorie intake, or what they call "stress-induced augmentation of diet-induced obesity." For example, they note that neuropeptide Y stimulates the proliferation of the endothelial cells and the precursors of fat cells (preadipocytes). In their study, they exposed rats to 2 weeks of cold temperatures (a stressor for the rats) in combination with a diet high in fat and sugar. They found that neuropeptide Y levels increased as well as levels of corticosterone, the hormone of stress. Furthermore, the rats developed abdominal obesity within 2 weeks and a full-blown metabolic-like syndrome after 3 months' exposure. They note that there is a common genetic mutation, particularly in Northern Europeans, associated with atherosclerosis, obesity, and diabetic retinopathy, whereby levels of neuropeptide Y increase substantially in the context of exposure to stress. Their speculation is that people with this genetic mutation are particularly vulnerable to diet-induced obesity and even a metabolic syndrome, with glucose intolerance, hyperlipidemia, and increased levels of insulin.

Kuo et al. (2007) further note that researchers have not identified the specific cells responsible for the increased neuropeptide Y production in adipose tissue. They do note, however, that production of resistin, an inflammatory *adipokine*—that is, a hormone produced by fat cells—is increased by both stress and neuropeptide Y, and this substance has been associated with metabolic disturbances. These researchers believe that medications that target neuropeptide Y (neuropeptide Y antagonists) might one day be used for "fat remodeling," in other words, pharmacological lipolysis. Their conclusion is that stress is not just in the mind, but rather can lead to pathological changes in both weight and metabolism by means of the neuropeptide Y pathway. Prod'homme et al. (2006) suggest that neuropeptide Y also has a role in "fine-tuning" immune responses in the body. They believe neuropeptide Y inhibits activation of T cells and that an excess of neuropeptide Y may be involved in reducing "immune surveillance" such that the body becomes more vulnerable to cancers and infections. They further note that neuropeptide Y levels have been found to be increased in patients with asthma and those with systemic lupus erythematosus, both chronic diseases of inflammation.

Other Neurochemical Mechanisms Involved in Eating

Galanin, like neuropeptide Y, stimulates eating. It has cell bodies in the hypothalamus (Leibowitz and Hoebel 2004, p. 303). Leibowitz and Hoebel (p. 313) note that galanin, like neuropeptide Y, inhibits sympathetic nervous system activity and decreases energy expenditure, but it is different from neuropeptide Y in many ways. For example, it has no particular impact on carbohydrate or fat metabolism. Furthermore, unlike neuropeptide Y, it increases gastric acid secretion but suppresses release of both insulin and cortisol. Galanin's circadian rhythm is different from that of neuropeptide Y: in animal experiments with rats, it was found to peak during the middle of a feeding cycle, when there is greater fat absorption (p. 314). Further, galanin levels are higher with a higher proportion of body fat and are higher with higher fat consumption, whereas neuropeptide Y levels are lower in proportion to fat consumption and total body fat. Also, it has been noted that obese women have significantly higher levels of galanin than men have (p. 314).

Agouti-related protein "colocalizes" with neuropeptide Y and stimulates eating even more powerfully than neuropeptide Y. Just like neuropeptide Y, it increases insulin levels and is stimulated during fasting (when there is a negative energy balance) and when leptin levels are low. Furthermore, it functions as an antagonist to α-MSH, a satiety hormone (see "Leptin" above), and its precursor, POMC, which is itself a precursor to β-endorphin. α-MSH "colocalizes" with CART, another satiety hormone (Leibowitz and Hoebel 2004, pp. 314–315).

The **orexins** (orexin A and orexin B), also referred to as **hypocretins,** are found throughout the brain but are mostly produced in the lateral hypothalamus (Boutrel and de Lecea 2008). They also stimulate feeding. But these neuropeptides seem to be involved in many different functions, including energy balance, the sleep-wake cycle, and even autonomic functions like increasing blood pressure (Leibowitz and Hoebel 2004, p. 316). It is even believed that a disorder of the orexin system is responsible for the condition of narcolepsy, a disease characterized by sudden attacks of daytime sleepiness and cataplexy (Boutrel and de Lecea 2008). Leibowitz and Hoebel (2004, p. 316) further note that injections of orexins in animals have led to increased grooming, motor activity, and vigilance and arousal. Boutrel and de Lecea (2008) believe that orexins are involved, as well, in brain reward systems and in addictive behavior, including cocaine sensitization and the potential for relapse after an abstinent period. They speculate that the orexin system functions as a kind of alarm signal for an organism and even suggest that the orexins might be used eventually in treating drug cravings and states of relapse.

Orexin levels do not increase or decrease in response to changes in leptin levels that occur, for example, with obesity (Leibowitz and Hoebel 2004, p. 315). Leibowitz and Hoebel note, though, that orexin levels seem to be responsive to changes in glucose levels and may increase feeding behavior specifically when glucose levels are low. (See Chapter 9, "Circadian Rhythms, Sleep, and Weight," for more on orexins.)

MCH (melanin-concentrating hormone), found in the lateral hypothalamus, also stimulates food intake but not as powerfully as neuropeptide Y or even agouti-related protein. Its levels are decreased by leptin, increased with leptin deficiency, and increased with fasting. And just as with the orexins, MCH levels are higher in cases of hypoglycemia induced by insulin (Leibowitz and Hoebel 2004, pp. 316–317).

POMC (pro-opiomelanocortin) is a protein synthesized in the brain, including the anterior pituitary, where it becomes adrenocorticotropic hormone, and the arcuate nucleus, where it is processed to α-MSH and β-lipoprotein (which itself becomes β-endorphin) (Leibowitz and Hoebel 2004, p. 321). This protein as α-MSH works to decrease food intake and body weight. Leibowitz and Hoebel (2004, p. 322) note that leptin interacts with this melanocortin system, either by increasing levels of α-MSH or by decreasing its antagonist, agouti-related protein. Furthermore, the melanocortin system, which restricts eating, acts in opposite balance (antagonistically) to neuropeptide Y, which increases eating.

CART (cocaine- and amphetamine-regulated transcript) is a peptide found in the brain, primarily in areas of the hypothalamus, that decreases food intake and works antagonistically with neuropeptide Y. CART secretion is stimulated by leptin and is lowered by leptin deficiency. Leibowitz and Hoebel (2004, pp. 323–324) note that researchers believe CART is involved in body fat distribution and even metabolic abnormalities.

GLP-1 (glucagon-like peptide 1) is a peptide produced primarily in the gastrointestinal tract, but also in the brain, from a precursor to glucagon and secreted in response to meals containing fat and carbohydrates. Its main function is the control of blood glucose levels by stimulating the secretion of insulin, as well as by inhibiting the secretion of glucagon, resulting in decreased production of glucose by the liver. Furthermore, according to Leibowitz and Hoebel (2004, p. 327), GLP-1 decreases gastric acid secretion and slows emptying of the stomach. Primarily, though, it can decrease food intake chronically and works as a satiety signal, mostly when a meal is high in carbohydrates.

Peptide tyrosine-tyrosine (also known as PYY, where *Y* abbreviates *tyrosine*) is a polypeptide hormone found in the distal part of the intestine and released into our circulation after we eat. The amount of PYY released depends on how many calories we eat, and it inhibits stomach, pancreatic, and intestinal secretions, as well as the motility of our gastrointestinal tract. It is speculated that PYY also has a role in the changes in appetite seen in patients who are critically ill (e.g., intensive care patients); levels of PYY seem to be elevated in those patients, along with levels of CCK, whereas ghrelin levels seem to be lowered (Vincent and le Roux 2008). Furthermore, high PYY levels may contribute to food intake restriction in patients with anorexia nervosa, and there has been reported "blunting" of PYY levels in those who engage in binge eating. And people who have undergone bariatric surgery for obesity have increased levels of both PYY and GLP-1. High protein intake, interestingly enough, produces the highest levels of PYY and the most satiating effect in both normalweight and obese people. A nasal spray of PYY is being developed to suppress food intake (Vincent and le Roux 2008).

Nesfatin-1 is a new biochemical marker that has been found in the hypothalamus in the same area where orexins and MCH are found. Fort et al. (2008) speculate that nesfatin-1 is involved in food regulation (i.e., decreased food intake initially and weight loss over time) and may counterbalance the appetite-enhancing effects of MCH, as well as having a role in regulating sleep-wake cycles, motor activity, stress, and mood.

CONCLUSION

As we can see from the above (and only partial) list of neurochemical substances that are involved in eating, in addition to the major hormones discussed earlier, the regulation of food intake in humans is an extraordinarily complicated process that researchers have only begun to understand. It is quite beyond the scope of this book to provide a more detailed discussion of all the metabolic complexities involved, and we refer the curious reader who wants more information about the pathophysiology of obesity to the extraordinary textbook edited by George Bray and Claude Bouchard (2004), *Handbook of Obesity: Etiology and Pathophysiology* (see the "Selected Readings and Web Sites" appendix).

The system of food regulation is an intricate, coordinated system of checks and balances involving the central nervous system, the sympathetic and parasympathetic nervous systems, the endocrine system, including adipose tissue, and the entire gastrointestinal system, among others. All of these systems must function in concert in order to maintain our homeostasis—our energy balance—both in the short term (during a meal and throughout the course of a day) and over weeks, months, and years in an ever-changing and challenging internal milieu. (For more on diurnal variations in hormone levels, see Chapter 9, "Circadian Rhythms, Sleep, and Weight.")

REFERENCES

Bennett WI: Beyond overeating. N Engl J Med 332:673–674, 1995

Berthoud HR: Neural control of appetite: cross-talk between homeostatic and non-homeostatic systems. Appetite 43:315–317, 2004

Berthoud HR: Interactions between the "cognitive" and "metabolic" brain in the control of food intake. Physiol Behav 91:486–498, 2007

Bhargava SK, Sachdev HS, Fall CHD, et al: Relations of serial changes in childhood body mass index to impaired glucose tolerance in young adulthood. N Engl J Med 350:865–875, 2004

Blom WA, Lluch A, Stafleu A, et al: Effect of a high-protein breakfast on the postprandial ghrelin response. Am J Clin Nutr 83:211–220, 2006

Bloom SR, Kuhajda FP, Laher I, et al: The obesity epidemic: pharmacological challenges. Mol Interv 8:82–98, 2008

Blouet C, Ono H, Schwartz GJ: Mediobasal hypothalamic p70 S6 kinase 1 modulates the control of energy homeostasis. Cell Metab 8:459–467, 2008

Blundell JE, Stubbs J: Diet composition and the control of food intake in humans, in Handbook of Obesity: Etiology and Pathophysiology, 2nd Edition. Edited by Bray G, Bouchard C. New York, Marcel Dekker, 2004, pp 427–460

Bouchard C, Tremblay A, Després JP, et al: The response to long-term overfeeding in identical twins. N Engl J Med 322:1477–1482, 1990

Bouchard C, Tremblay A, Després JP, et al: Overfeeding in identical twins: 5-year postoverfeeding results. Metabolism 45:1042–1050, 1996

Boutrel B, de Lecea L: Addiction and arousal: the hypocretin connection. Physiol Behav 93:947–951, 2008

Bray GA: Obesity is a chronic, relapsing neurochemical disease. Int J Obes Relat Metab Disord 28:34–38, 2004

Bray GA, Champagne CM: Beyond energy balance: there is more to obesity than kilocalories. J Am Diet Assoc 105 (suppl 1):S17–S23, 2005

Burton-Freeman B, Davis PA, Schneeman BO: Plasma cholecystokinin is associated with subjective measures of satiety in women. Am J Clin Nutr 76:659–667, 2002

Chaput JP, Tremblay J, Rimm EB, et al: A novel interaction between dietary composition and insulin secretion: effects on weight gain in the Quebec Family Study. Am J Clin Nutr 87:303–309, 2008

Cherian MA, Santoro TJ: The role of saturation of fat depots in the pathogenesis of insulin resistance. Med Hypotheses 66:763–768, 2006

Coleman DL: Obese and diabetes: two mutant genes causing diabetes-obesity syndromes in mice. Diabetologia 14:141–148, 1978

Cummings DE: Ghrelin and the short- and long-term regulation of appetite and body weight. Physiol Behav 89:71–84, 2006

Cummings DE, Overduin J: Gastrointestinal regulation of food intake. J Clin Invest 117:13–23, 2007

Cummings DE, Purnell JQ, Frayo RS, et al: A preprandial rise in plasma ghrelin levels suggests a role in meal initiation in humans. Diabetes 50:1714–1719, 2001

Cummings DE, Weigle DS, Frayo RS, et al: Plasma ghrelin levels after diet-induced weight loss or gastric bypass surgery. N Engl J Med 346:1623–1630, 2002

Cupples WA: Physiological regulation of food intake. Am J Physiol Regul Integr Comp Physiol 288:R1438–R1443, 2005

Cypess AM, Lehman S, Williams G, et al: Identification and importance of brown adipose tissue in adult humans. N Engl J Med 360:1509–1517, 2009

Davis JD: Measuring satiety: from meal size to the microstructure of ingestive behavior, in Satiation: From Gut to Brain. Edited by Smith GP. New York, Oxford University Press, 1998, pp 71–96

DelParigi A, Tschöp M, Heiman ML, et al: High circulating ghrelin: a potential cause for hyperphagia and obesity in Prader-Willi syndrome. J Clin Endocrinol Metab 87:5461–5464, 2002

Díez JJ, Iglesias P: The role of the novel adipocyte-derived hormone adiponectin in human disease. Eur J Endocrinol 148:293–300, 2003

Druce MR, Small CJ, Bloom SR: Minireview: gut peptides regulating satiety. Endocrinology145:2660–2665, 2004

Elmquist JK, Elias CF, Saper CB: From lesions to leptin: hypothalamic control of food intake and body weight. Neuron 22:221–232, 1999

Erdmann J, Lippl F, Schusdziarra V: Differential effect of protein and fat on plasma ghrelin levels in man. Regul Pept 116:101–107, 2003

Esposito K, Giugliano G, Scuderi N, et al: Role of adipokines in the obesity-inflammation relationship: the effect of fat removal. Plast Reconstr Surg 118:1048–1057, 2006

Fernández-Real JM, Vendrell J, Ricart W: Circulating adiponectin and plasma fatty acid profile. Clin Chem 51:603–609, 2005

Flier JS, Maratos-Flier E: What fuels fat. Sci Am 297:72–81, 2007

Fort P, Salvert D, Hanriot L, et al: The satiety molecule nesfatin-1 is co-expressed with melanin concentrating hormone in tuberal hypothalamic neurons of the rat. Neuroscience 155:174–181, 2008

Friedman JM: Modern science versus the stigma of obesity. Nat Med 10:563–569, 2004

Friedman JM: Leptin at 14 y of age: an ongoing story. Am J Clin Nutr 89(suppl):973S–979S, 2009

Gavrila A, Peng CK, Chan JL, et al: Diurnal and ultradian dynamics of serum adiponectin in healthy men: comparison with leptin, circulating soluble leptin receptor, and cortisol patterns. J Clin Endocrinol Metab 88:2838–2843, 2003

Geary N: A new way of looking at eating. Am J Physiol Regul Integr Comp Physiol 288:R1444–R1446, 2005

Geliebter A, Gluck ME, Hashim SA: Plasma ghrelin concentrations are lower in binge-eating disorder. J Nutr 135:1326–1330, 2005

Gómez R, Lago F, Gómez-Reino JJ, et al: Novel factors as therapeutic targets to treat diabetes: focus on leptin and ghrelin. Expert Opin. Ther Targets 13:583–591, 2009

Gunter MJ, Hoover DR, Yu H, et al: Insulin, insulin-like growth factor-I, and risk of breast cancer in postmenopausal women. J Natl Cancer Inst 101:48–60, 2009

Halberg N, Wernstedt-Asterholm I, Scherer PE: The adipocyte as an endocrine cell. Endocrinol Metab Clin North Am 37:753–768, 2008

Harris RB: Role of set-point theory in regulation of body weight. FASEB J 4:3310–3318, 1990

Harris RB: Leptin—much more than a satiety signal. Annu Rev Nutr 20:45–75, 2000

Hauner H: The new concept of adipose tissue function. Physiol Behav 83:653–658, 2004

Havel PJ: Update on adipocyte hormones: regulation of energy balance and carbohydrate/lipid metabolism. Diabetes 53 (suppl 1):S143–S151, 2004

Havel PJ: Dietary fructose: implications for dysregulation of energy homeostasis and lipid/carbohydrate metabolism. Nutr Rev 63:133–157, 2005

Havermans RC, Janssen T, Giesen JC, et al: Food liking, food wanting, and sensory-specific satiety. Appetite 52:222–225, 2009

Hirsch J: Obesity: matter over mind? The Dana Foundation. January 1, 2003. Available at: http://www.dana.org/news/cerebrum/detail.aspx?id=2908. Accessed July 6, 2009

Hollander P, Maggs DG, Ruggles JA, et al: Effect of pramlintide on weight in overweight and obese insulin-treated type 2 diabetes patients. Obes Res 12:661–668, 2004

Jayasena CN, Bloom SR: Role of gut hormones in obesity. Endocrinol Metab Clin North Am 37:769–787, 2008

Keesey RE: Set-points and body weight regulation: biological constants or "set-points." Psychiatr Clin North Am 1:523–543, 1978

Keesey RE, Hirvonen MD: Body weight set-points: determination and adjustment. J Nutr 127:1875S–1883S, 1997

Kiefer F, Jahn H, Otte C, et al: Increasing leptin precedes craving and relapse during pharmacological abstinence maintenance treatment of alcoholism. J Psychiatr Res 39:545–551, 2005

Klein S, Fontana L, YoungVL, et al: Absence of an effect of liposuction on insulin action and risk factors for coronary heart disease. N Engl J Med 350:2549–2557, 2004

Koopmans HS: Experimental studies on the control of food intake, in Handbook of Obesity: Etiology and Pathophysiology, 2nd Edition. Edited by Bray GA, Bouchard C. New York, Marcel Dekker, 2004, pp 373–425

Kraemer RR, Castracane VD: Exercise and humoral mediators of peripheral energy balance: ghrelin and adiponectin. Exp Biol Med (Maywood) 232:184–194, 2007

Krysiak R, Obuchowicz E, Herman ZS: Interactions between the neuropeptide Y system and the hypothalamic-pituitary-adrenal axis. Eur J Endocrinol 140:130–136, 1999

Kuo LE, Kitlinska JB, Tilan JU, et al: Neuropeptide Y acts directly in the periphery on fat tissue and mediates stress-induced obesity and metabolic syndrome. Nat Med 13:803–811, 2007

Lago R, Gómez R, Lago F, et al: Leptin beyond body weight regulation—current concepts concerning its role in immune function and inflammation. Cell Immunol 252:139–145, 2008

Leibel RL: The role of leptin in the control of body weight. Nutr Rev 60:S15–S19, 2002

Leibowitz SF, Hoebel BG: Behavioral neuroscience and obesity, in Handbook of Obesity: Etiology and Pathophysiology, 2nd Edition. Edited by Bray GA, Bouchard C. New York, Marcel Dekker, 2004, pp 301–371

Leidy HJ, Williams NI: Meal energy content is related to features of meal-related ghrelin profiles across a typical day of eating in non-obese premenopausal women. Horm Metab Res 38:317–322, 2006

le Roux CW, Neary NM, Halsey TJ, et al: Ghrelin does not stimulate food intake in patients with surgical procedures involving vagotomy. J Clin Endocrinol Metab 90:4521–4524, 2005a

le Roux CW, Patterson M, Vincent RP, et al: Postprandial plasma ghrelin is suppressed proportional to meal calorie content in normal-weight but not obese subjects. J Clin Endocrin Metab 90:1068–1071, 2005b

Levin BE: The drive to regain is mainly in the brain. Am J Physiol Regul Integr Comp Physiol 287:R1297–R1300, 2004

Levin BE: Metabolic imprinting: critical impact of the perinatal environment on the regulation of energy homeostasis. Philos Trans R Soc Lond B Biol Sci 361:1107–1121, 2006

Levitsky DA: Putting behavior back into feeding behavior: a tribute to George Collier. Appetite 38:143–148, 2002

MacLean PS, Higgins JA, Johnson GC, et al: Enhanced metabolic efficiency contributes to weight regain after weight loss in obesity-prone rats. Am J Physiol Regul Integr Comp Physiol 287:R1306–R1315, 2004

MacLean PS, Higgins JA, Jackman MR, et al: Peripheral metabolic responses to prolonged weight reduction that promote rapid, efficient regain in obesity-prone rats. Am J Physiol Regul Integr Comp Physiol 290:R1577–R1588, 2006

Malik S, McGlone F, Bedrossian D, et al: Ghrelin modulates brain activity in areas that control appetitive behavior. Cell Metab 7:400–409, 2008

Mantzoros C, Serdy S: Insulin action. UpToDate, Edition 16.2, Reprint. 2008. Available at: http://www.uptodate.com. Accessed July 17, 2009.

Mark AL: Dietary therapy for obesity: an emperor with no clothes. Hypertension 51:1426–1434, 2008

Matarese G, Procaccini C, De Rosa V: The intricate interface between immune and metabolic regulation: a role for leptin in the pathogenesis of multiple sclerosis? J Leukoc Biol 84:893–899, 2008

Morton GJ, Cummings DE, Baskin DG, et al: Central nervous system control of food intake and body weight. Nature 443:289–295, 2006

Nedergaard J, Bengstsson T, Cannon B: Unexpected evidence for active brown adipose tissue in adult humans. Am J Physiol Endocrinol Metab 293:E444–E452, 2007

Olszewski PK, Levine AS: Central opioids and consumption of sweet tastants: when reward outweighs homeostasis. Physiol Behav 91:506–512, 2007

O'Rahilly S, Farooqi IS: Genetics of obesity. Philos Trans R Soc Lond B Biol Sci 361:1095–1105, 2006

Ostlund RE Jr, Yang JW, Klein S, et al: Relation between plasma leptin concentration and body fat, gender, diet, age, and metabolic covariates. J Clin Endocrinol Metab 81:3909–3913, 1996

Otero M, Lago R, Lago F, et al: Leptin, from fat to inflammation: old questions and new insights. FEBS Lett 579:295–301, 2005

Otero M, Lago R, Gómez R, et al: Leptin: a metabolic hormone that functions like a proinflammatory adipokine. Drug News Perspect 19:21–26, 2006

Owen CG, Martin RM, Whincup PH, et al: Does breastfeeding influence risk of type 2 diabetes in later life? A quantitative analysis of published evidence. Am J Clin Nutr 84:1043–1054, 2006

Pan D, Fujimoto M, Lopes A, et al: Twist-1 is a PPARδ-inducible, negative-feedback regulator of PGC-1α in brown fat metabolism. Cell 137:73–86, 2009

Power ML, Schulkin J: The Evolution of Obesity. Baltimore, MD, Johns Hopkins University Press, 2009

Powley TL, Phillips RJ: Gastric satiation is volumetric, intestinal satiation is nutritive. Physiol Behav 82:69–74, 2004

Prod'homme T, Weber MS, Steinman L, et al: A neuropeptide in immune-mediated inflammation, Y? Trends Immunol 27:164–167, 2006

Qi L, Saberi M, Zmuda E, et al: Adipocyte CREB promotes insulin resistance in obesity. Cell Metab 9:277–286, 2009

Rosenbaum M, Goldsmith R, Bloomfield D, et al: Low-dose leptin reverses skeletal muscle, autonomic, and neuroendocrine adaptations to maintenance of reduced weight. J Clin Invest 115:3579–3586, 2005

Rosenbaum M, Sy M, Pavlovich K, et al: Leptin reverses weight loss-induced changes in regional neural activity responses to visual food stimuli. J Clin Invest 118:2583–2591, 2008

Rushing PA, Hagan MM, Seeley RJ, et al: Amylin: a novel action in the brain to reduce body weight. Endocrinology 141:850–853, 2000

Schoeller DA, Cella LK, Sinha MK, et al: Entrainment of the diurnal rhythm of plasma leptin to meal timing. J Clin Invest 100:1882–1887, 1997

Schubert ML: Hormonal regulation of gastric acid secretion. Curr Gastroenterol Rep 10:523–527, 2008

Schwartz GJ: Biology of eating behavior in obesity. Obes Res 12 (suppl 2):102S–106S, 2004

Schwartz GJ, Fu J, Astarita G, et al: The lipid messenger OEA links dietary fat intake to satiety. Cell Metab 8:281–288, 2008

Schwartz MW, Porte D Jr: Diabetes, obesity, and the brain. Science 307:375–379, 2005

Schwartz MW, Woods SC, Porte D Jr, et al: Central nervous system control of food intake. Nature 404:661–671, 2000

Sharkey KA: From fat to full: peripheral and central mechanisms controlling food intake and energy balance: view from the chair. Obesity (Silver Spring) 14 (suppl 5):239S–241S, 2006

Smith GP: Introduction, in Satiation: From Gut to Brain. Edited by Smith GP. New York, Oxford University Press, 1998a, pp 3–9

Smith GP: Pregastric and gastric satiety, in Satiation: From Gut to Brain. Edited by Smith GP. New York, Oxford University Press, 1998b, pp 10–39

Snijder MB, Visser M, Dekker JM, et al; Health ABC Study: Low subcutaneous thigh fat is a risk factor for unfavourable glucose and lipid levels, independently of high abdominal fat. Diabetologia 48:301–308, 2005

Snijder MB, van Dam RM, Visser M, et al: What aspects of body fat are particularly hazardous and how do we measure them? Int J Epidemiol 35:83–92, 2006

Szentirmai E, Hajdu I, Obal F Jr, et al: Ghrelin-induced sleep responses in ad libitum fed and food-restricted rats. Brain Res 1088:131–140, 2006

Teff KL, Elliott SS, Tschöp M, et al: Dietary fructose reduces circulating insulin and leptin, attenuates postprandial suppression of ghrelin, and increases triglycerides in women. J Clin Endocrinol Metab 89:2963–2972, 2004

Trayhurn P: Adipocyte biology. Obes Rev 8 (suppl 1):41–44, 2007

Unger RH: Minireview: weapons of lean body mass destruction: the role of ectopic lipids in the metabolic syndrome. Endocrinology 144:5159–5165, 2003

Vincent RP, le Roux CW: The satiety hormone peptide YY as a regulator of appetite. J Clin Pathol 61:548–552, 2008

Virtanen KA, Lidell ME, Orva J, et al: Functional brown adipose tissue in healthy adults. N Engl J Med 360:1518–1525, 2009

Wallberg-Henriksson H, Zierath JR: A new twist on brown fat metabolism. Cell 137:22–24, 2009

Waterland RA, Garza C: Potential mechanisms of metabolic imprinting that lead to chronic disease. Am J Clin Nutr 69:179–197, 1999

Weigle DS, Cummings DE, Newby PD, et al: Roles of leptin and ghrelin in the loss of body weight caused by a low fat, high carbohydrate diet. J Clin Endocrinol Metab 88:1577–1586, 2003

Weinsier RL, Nagy TR, Hunter GR, et al: Do adaptive changes in metabolic rate favor weight regain in weight-reduced individuals? An examination of the set-point theory. Am J Clin Nutr 72:1088–1094, 2000

Williams CJ, Fargnoli JL, Hwang JJ, et al: Coffee consumption is associated with higher plasma adiponectin concentrations in women with or without type 2 diabetes: a prospective cohort study. Diabetes Care 31:504–508, 2008

Wirtshafter D, Davis JD: Set points, settling points, and the control of body weight. Physiol Behav 19:75–78, 1977

Wolfgang MJ, Lane MD: Control of energy homeostasis: role of enzymes and intermediates of fatty acid metabolism in the central nervous system. Annu Rev Nutr 26:23–44, 2006

Woods SC, Lutz TA, Geary N, et al: Pancreatic signals controlling food intake; insulin, glucagon and amylin. Philos Trans R Soc Lond B Biol Sci 361:1219–1235, 2006

Young RC, Gibbs J, Antin J, et al: Absence of satiety during sham feeding in the rat. J Comp Physiol Psychol. 87:795–800, 1974

Zhang Y, Scarpace PJ: The role of leptin in leptin resistance and obesity. Physiol Behav 88:249–256, 2006

Zhang Y, Proenca R, Maffei M, et al: Positional cloning of the mouse obese gene and its human homologue. Nature 372:425–432, 1994

6

PSYCHIATRIC DISORDERS AND WEIGHT

It has long been recognized that emotional factors are closely related to obesity, but recently our conception of this relationship has undergone a radical change. Early studies viewed emotional disturbances as causes of obesity, but recent research suggests that these disturbances are more likely to be consequences of obesity.

Thomas A. Wadden and Albert J. Stunkard (1985)

CAUSE OR CONSEQUENCE?

Many studies across the years have examined the connection between weight disorders (primarily excessive weight) and psychiatric disorders. The results of these studies, however, have been confusing, inconsistent, and even contradictory. As Wadden and Stunkard (1985) note, one of the major issues has been causality. Does excessive weight cause psychiatric disorders or do psychiatric disorders cause excessive weight? In the third decade after the publication of Wadden and Stunkard's 1985 paper, we can say the answer is still not necessarily a straightforward one.

Psychiatrist Albert Stunkard and his colleagues (1998) emphasize that it should not be surprising that those with weight problems would have psychological difficulties. After all, as they point out, "prejudice and discrimination [i.e., the behavioral enactment of prejudice] plague the lives of the obese" (Stunkard et al. 1998; see also "Discrimination Against the Obese" in Chapter 2, "Obesity in the United States"). This prejudice was documented as early as the twelfth century in Japan, where a scroll seems to indicate that men are laughing at an obese woman who has to be carried by two other women. In Europe, the prejudice was seen even earlier, with Paul, whose letter to the Philippians (3:18–19) speaks of "the enemies of the cross of Christ, whose end is destruction, whose god is their belly." There was evidence in Christianity in the third century (Tertullian), the fifth century (Augustine), and the seventh century (Gregory I), all leading to considering gluttony as one of the seven deadly sins (Stunkard et al. 1998). Hieronymus Bosch, in the fifteenth century, painted the obese in his own version of the seven deadly sins (*The Table of Wisdom*), and in the sixteenth century Shakespeare wrote of Falstaff as "fat-kidneyed" and having "fat guts" and a "huge hill of fat," among several other derogatory epithets. Not only does obesity have moral implications, said Wadden and Stunkard (1985), it is also an "aesthetic crime"—namely, "it is ugly."

Straus (1966) notes that there are many factors in our society and around the world that influence our own attitudes regarding problem eating, or the "excessive consumption of food," as he calls it. He emphasizes that specifically in American society, attitudes regarding problem eating are characterized "by inconsistency, by ambiguity, and by discontinuity" (Straus 1966). For example, though consumption of food seems to be part of every social activity, different subcultures in American society "vary markedly in their degree of food orientation." Furthermore, through-out the developmental life cycle, we view eating differently. For example, pregnancy has been seen as a chance to eat for two, and a good mother has been considered "one whose baby eats well and gains weight rapidly" (Straus 1966). During child-hood, many heard the idea that wasting food was actually sinful. But by adolescence we are supposed to adopt the American ideal of being slender. Straus (1966) makes the point that society ignores the needs of the obese: seats in theaters, airplanes, buses, and elsewhere are too narrow for them, as are most chairs and even turn-stiles; at every turn, the fat woman or man is made to feel different and is made aware of the fact that she or he doesn't really "fit." It is no wonder that obesity might be seen as a predisposing factor for psychiatric disorders.

Psychiatrist Mallay Occhiogrosso (2008, pp. 265–276) has pointed out the ex-traordinarily complicated relationship of psychiatry to issues regarding eating, and particularly to overeating, seen in the past 150 years: overeating has never been studied systematically or even clearly delineated as either behavioral or psychologi-cal. Recently, though, there has been an explosive interest in the subject of overeat-ing and a focus on "medicalizing" the subject (p. 266).

Occhiogrosso examined changes in psychiatrists' views by reviewing articles published in the *American Journal of Psychiatry* since its inception in the mid 1800s. At that time psychiatrists, who ran the asylums, were mostly concerned with feed-ing their patients healthy food and dealing with patients who might refuse food. When psychiatrists in the mid 1800s did encounter gluttony, they saw it as sinful, such that "inculcating more temperate and restrained eating habits in these pa-tients would be equivalent to advancing them morally" (Occhiogrosso 2008, p. 269). Somewhat later, Occhiogrosso reports, temperance in diet was seen as a crucial foundation to good mental health, whereas overindulgence was linked to criminal-ity. By the early twentieth century, with the influence of Freud, psychiatry spoke of the *oral character* and *excessive oral fixations* in those who overeat. Significantly, though, it was not until the 1970s and even 1980s that separate eating disorders such as anorexia nervosa and bulimia nervosa were delineated (and a separate Eating Disorders section appeared in the *Diagnostic and Statistical Manual of Mental Disorders*). Even now in the twenty-first century, some psychiatrists still question the validity of binge eating disorder and the night eating syndrome. Summing up the work of Hilde Bruch in the 1950s more than 50 years later, Occhiogrosso points out that "psychiatrists and the medical community at large are not much closer to definitive answers about the biological and psychological underpinnings of overeating, but it is not for lack of trying" (Occhiogrosso 2008, p. 274).

EXCESSIVE WEIGHT AND COMORBID PSYCHIATRIC SYMPTOMS

Even though there were often "recurring themes" in the lives of obese people, Stunkard (1959) could not find "psychological characteristics" in those who were obese that could "consistently distinguish them" from those who were not obese, whether one considered basic personality structure, basic psychodynamic conflict, or an increased intensity of certain basic drives.

Back in the early 1960s, Stunkard and his colleagues (Weinberg et al. 1961) conducted a small controlled study of 18 obese men in which they assessed personality traits to see whether there were commonalities among the men. In other words, did these obese men have a distinctive personality? The subjects, ages 19–60, were given psychological tests including the Thematic Apperception Test, the Draw-a-Man Test, and some of the subtests of the Wechsler-Bellevue Intelligence Scale. Initially the researchers speculated that obese men were more anxious and "neurotically disturbed," "more intellectually conforming," and "more feminine in their interests" than those who were not obese. What they found instead was that psychological testing did not reveal any specific differences between their obese subjects and those who were not obese. However, the researchers did not define obesity and acknowledged that their results might not be completely generalizable to other populations of obese subjects studied differently. Stunkard (personal communication, October 9, 2009) acknowledged that before the standardization of body weight classifications through the use of body mass index (BMI), definitions of obesity were considerably less precise ("overweight" and "percent overweight") and actually changed "every five years." Some of the research from the 1970s, for example, such as Herman and Mack's study on restrained eating (1975), noted a rough division of subjects into "normal" and "obese," where "obese" was more than 15% overweight. It is not clear exactly when BMI became one of the standard measurements. In other words, we could not find mention of how BMI went from historical obscurity when it was first used by statistician Adolphe Quételet in the mid nineteenth century to its widespread use, albeit with its own set of problems, as a measurement today.

Obesity is now considered to be present at BMI values $\geq$30 kg/m^2; as we have noted, Keys et al. (1972) seem to be the first to use the term *body mass index*. (For more discussion of BMI and the subclasses of obesity, see Chapter 2.) Significantly, even though the original study by Stunkard and colleagues (Weinberg et al. 1961) was such a small one, it has been often quoted in the literature throughout the years as evidence that there is not a specific personality typical of the obese.

Another early study, by Crisp and McGuiness (1976), actually called "Jolly Fat…," studied a "representative sample" of over 300 middle-aged men and 400 middle-aged women in the suburban London area. These researchers used a version of the Quételet index (BMI measurements) and measured skinfold thickness on the triceps and subscapular skin. Surprisingly, this study found that obese men and women were less likely to be anxious or depressed than nonobese individuals, and the researchers even questioned, "Is the chemistry of obesity or overeating incompatible with anxiety and depression?" (Crisp and McGuiness 1976). They wondered whether the periodic overeating of the obese was somehow protective against "the experience and display of anxiety and depression." They did acknowledge, however, that other studies contradicted their results and that it is possible that their subjects were less likely to reveal their symptoms to others by the questionnaire method their study employed. Stunkard and Messick (1985) make the same point in their classic paper describing their eating questionnaire to measure dietary restraint, namely, that patients, in an attempt to appear "socially desirable," may distort how much they actually engage or don't engage in dietary restraint.

In an earlier paper, Stunkard (1959) had delineated three variables he found worthwhile when considering eating patterns: the "presence (or absence) of expressions of self-condemnation" in the context of a "deviant" eating pattern; the "degree of personal meaning or symbolic representation" a person attaches to a particular eating pattern; and a person's assessment of his or her own level of stress due to an eating pattern. Stunkard and Messick (1985), deriving some of their questions from earlier research by Herman and Mack (1976), among others, on "restrained eating," devised the 51-question "Three-Factor Eating Questionnaire." A version of this questionnaire is still in use today (Stunkard, personal communication, October 9, 2009). Stunkard and Messick (1985) found that "three stable factors" emerged: "cognitive restraint of eating, disinhibition, and hunger." Most significantly, they found that differences in their patients' responses could have therapeutic implications: those who scored high on cognitive restraint "might be especially responsive" to information regarding calories or nutrition and behavioral strategies; those who scored high on disinhibition (e.g., those with an alcohol problem as well) might benefit from support groups that focus on anxiety, depression, or even loneliness. And those who are high scorers on hunger might do well with the long-term use of appetite suppressant medications.

Wadden and Stunkard (1985) acknowledged that even though there was not much evidence for increased psychopathology in most obese people, there had been many reports of "significant psychopathology," such as mild depression, hypochondriasis, and impulsivity, in those who are "severely" (i.e., 75% or more) overweight. Wadden and Stunkard (1985) took issue with some of the previous studies, arguing that they had not had appropriate control groups; they stated that many of the early studies indicating more severe psychopathology in the obese were poorly done, some without any control groups at all, and did not take into consideration that increased levels of depression and anxiety are not uncommon "in

> Obesity is heterogeneous with respect to psychopathology and personality.

those seeking medical care, regardless of body weight" (Wadden and Stunkard 1985). Furthermore, those obese patients who did seek treatment were more likely to be symptomatic with anxiety or depression, as well as more likely to have experienced body image issues and even be binge eating, than those who did not seek treatment. In fact, even though Wadden and Stunkard believed that obese patients might have "mild levels of psychopathology," this level was "no greater than that of other patients presenting for medical and surgical procedures." It is possible that those who were overweight experienced adverse effects not measured by standard assessments. For example, the researchers did believe that disparagement of body image (where the obese think of their bodies as "grotesque" and "loathsome" and have an overwhelming preoccupation with their weight) is one form of psychopathology that is specific to the obese. We now know, of course, that body image disparagement may be seen as part of the larger category we now call *body dysmorphic disorder*, which can occur in those who are not obese, can involve any part of the body, and can include anorexia nervosa, which involves severe body image disparagement and even severe distortions (see section on body image and body dysmorphic disorder later in this chapter).

In the mid 1990s, Friedman and Brownell (1995) reviewed previous studies in an attempt to understand the relationship of obesity to psychological disturbances. Their focus, unlike reports from earlier studies, was on the issue that obesity "is strikingly heterogeneous with respect to etiology, effects of excess weight on medical variables, and response to various treatments." In other words, "the effects of being obese vary across individuals." Their specific aim was to determine why some obese people suffer psychologically because of their obesity and others do not. Like Wadden and Stunkard, these authors emphasized the importance of prejudice: given that society not only condemns the obese for their appearance, but blames them for it, it makes sense that this bias would have negative psychological consequences. In their article, they lump together "excess body weight and body fat" as a broad definition of obesity and use *overweight, excess weight,* and *increased body fat* interchangeably. Ultimately, their review found that in obese individuals who actually presented for treatment there was a higher prevalence of psychopathology, and they found that those presenting for treatment were nearly all females. Their speculation was that even though the prevalence of obesity in men and women was identical, women seemed to experience more distress in our society from the stigma of obesity, particularly in body image disturbances, low self-esteem, and pessimism. They also found that the greater the level of obesity, the more psychological suffering. In their article, they distinguished *body image disparagement* from *body image distortion*, but found both to be higher in the obese, particularly in women. They noted that body image dissatisfaction, though not perfectly correlated with distortion, "is probably related to it."

There is, though, a subset of those with obesity who are binge eaters, and Friedman and Brownell (1995) found that those with this symptom are more apt to have psychopathology. Binge eaters who were not obese were not as likely to have increased psychopathology. Further, weight cyclers (not clearly defined, other than persons having "repeated cycles of weight loss and gain") were more likely to have increased psychopathology and also to be at risk for binge eating disorder. Friedman and Brownell concluded back in 1995 that further studies were indicated to assess who among the obese are more likely to experience psychological problems.

Although those who deal with the obese, particularly obese women, should consider the possibility of depression in these patients, they should not "mistakenly conclude that most obese females have significant psychological problems; they do not" (Wadden et al. 2002, p. 148). Health care professionals would be stereotyping these patients to think that most of them, men and women, have depression, anxiety, or other psychiatric disorders. "Personality is as diverse in obese individuals as it is in those of average weight," observe Wadden et al. (2002, p. 148). Body image dissatisfaction, though, is a more significant problem and is seen more commonly in women, as reflected in these women's overwhelming preoccupation with their weight, negative statements about themselves, actual avoidance of social situations, and camouflaging of areas of the body with which they are dissatisfied (p. 152). Dissatisfaction with body image, apparently even after bariatric surgery (p. 159), is also more likely to occur in those patients who have been obese since childhood or adolescence, when body image is "crystallizing."

More recent studies have also attempted to grapple with the relationship of obesity to psychiatric disorders. Simon et al. (2006) evaluated the relationship between obesity and mood, anxiety, and substance abuse disorders in over 9,000 respondents to a national U.S. survey conducted between 2001 and 2003. (Participants completed an in-person interview, including assessment of a range of mental disorders, but heights and weights were self-reported.) There were "significant positive associations" between obesity and major depression, bipolar disorder, and panic disorder or agoraphobia, but a lower risk of substance use disorder, in their sample, which was considered representative of U.S. households. There were no differences between obese men and women in the rates of psychiatric disorders, which contrasts with many other studies in which rates have been significantly higher in women. Their findings did not indicate a causal direction or even a specific mechanism for a negative association between substance use and obesity. Their conclusion was that obesity is "meaningfully" (i.e., modestly) associated with mood and anxiety disorders, but there are variations according to race and social class. Typically, the effect of the stigma of being overweight or obese is greater (and hence more likely to lead to anxiety or depressive disorders) in groups that characteristically have lower obesity rates, such as those with higher levels of education or in a higher socioeconomic class. This had also been

> The prevalence of obesity is identical in men and women, but women seem to experience more distress from its stigma.

found in a much earlier study in mid-Manhattan over 40 years ago, where obesity was more likely to be associated with depression in those of higher socioeconomic status (Moore et al. 1962). So, for example, Simon et al. (2006) found a stronger association between obesity and mood disorders in younger respondents, in non-Hispanic whites, and in those with higher levels of education. Even though nearly one-quarter of cases of obesity seemed associated with a mood disorder, the researchers could not demonstrate a causal direction. Further, about one-fifth of the cases of mood disorder were related to obesity, but again, the researchers were not able to make a causal connection.

A study by Pickering et al. (2007) examined the relationship of overweight, obesity, and extreme obesity (as defined by BMI values ≥ 40, but with self-reported weights and heights) in men and women with psychiatric Axis I and Axis II diagnoses. Their population was the 2001–2002 National Epidemiologic Survey on Alcohol and Related Conditions (NESARC), a representative population of the United States involving over 40,000 people, with a response rate of 81%. Here rates of overweight, obesity, and extreme obesity were highest in those individuals who had never married, as well as among those who were separated, divorced, or widowed. Obesity, then, does not just affect one's medical status, but may have far-reaching consequences, such as changes in economic or marital status. Furthermore, again it was seen that the lower the socioeconomic and educational status, the more likely individuals (especially women) were to be overweight, obese, or extremely obese. At least in women, obesity seemed related to the depressive component of bipolar illness, and particularly to atypical symptoms of depression such as increased sleeping and increased eating. In this study, there was no association of alcohol, drug, or nicotine abuse or dependence with states of obesity. Further, overweight men had more evidence of panic disorder, whereas specific and more severe phobias were more likely to be seen in overweight and obese women, often brought on by traumatic stresses. Women who were overweight and those with extreme obesity had higher levels of antisocial personality disorder, and those women with extreme obesity also had higher rates of avoidant personality disorder.

Petry et al. (2008), using the same large representative population (NESARC, with >40,000 respondents from 2001–2002 and self-reports of height and weight), and controlling for effects of medication, found that there were higher rates of specific mood disorders (e.g., major depression, dysthymia, and manic disorder) in those with obesity and extreme obesity. Those who were moderately overweight had higher rates of generalized anxiety, panic disorder (without agoraphobia), and specific phobia, and those with obesity and extreme obesity were more likely to have anxiety disorders. In this study, unlike the Pickering study, the researchers did find evidence of a higher risk of lifetime alcohol abuse in those with higher BMI values. The researchers caution that they cannot imply causality regarding the higher prevalence of mood, anxiety, or personality disorders, but they do believe that 10%–20% of those with obesity have "a current mood and/or anxiety disorder and about 18% of those obese have some kind of personality disorder." Those with extreme obesity had almost a 25% chance of having at least one personality disorder. In this study, eating disorders and psychotic disorders were not assessed.

Mather et al. (2008) examined the relationship between different categories of abnormal body weight and personality disorders. These researchers also used the large 2001–2002 NESARC population with self-reported heights and weights. They found that those with extreme obesity (BMI > 40) were more likely to have avoidant or antisocial personality disorders, but there was a gender factor. Those women with "higher than normal" weight had greater odds of having paranoid, antisocial, and avoidant personality disorders, whereas overweight men had lower rates of personality disorders. The prevalence of personality disorders in the general U.S. population is about 15% (the most frequent is obsessive-compulsive disorder) and almost 6% have two personality disorders.

Van den Bree et al. (2006) examined the relationship of personality styles to eating behavior and people's attitudes toward food in an attempt to understand why people in the United States fail to follow accepted dietary recommendations. The researchers' speculation was that psychological factors may be involved, particularly when one considers that 95% of U.S. adults appreciate the need for "balance, variety, and moderation as keys to healthy eating" (van den Bree et al. 2006). In other words, having nutritional information, just as with information about medication prescriptions, is often not enough to induce people to comply. In the mid 1990s, over 600 persons in a population-based study were questioned, with follow-up a year later (van den Bree et al. 2006). The investigators found that different personality styles did contribute to different attitudes and behaviors toward eating. Those who had hostility and low levels of cooperativeness as well as being prone to anxiety (high harm avoidance) were more apt to continue eating even after feeling full. On the other hand, those who had sociability (high reward dependence), rigidity, and reflectiveness (i.e., low levels of novelty-seeking behavior) demonstrated more cognitive control over eating. Those who had low persistence were more likely to consume snacks and alcohol. Furthermore, those who had low self-directedness (were immature and irresponsible), low reward dependence (were "cold and aloof"), and low self-transcendence (were "self-conscious and self-gratifying") were more apt to be "susceptible to hunger." Demographic variables including age and marital status should be considered as well, as should lifestyle variables (e.g., exercise, smoking, alcohol consumption) and personality variables. Even after considering these other factors, there was a significant association between low novelty seeking and healthy eating and between lower persistence and more frequent snacking and alcohol use.

Sullivan et al. (2007) assessed personality characteristics and their relationship to weight and weight loss. Obese subjects (as defined by a BMI level > 35 kg/m²) in a community scored higher in novelty seeking, lower in persistence, and lower in self-directedness than nonobese subjects. Further, the researchers found that those who were able to lose weight after 22 weeks of behavioral therapy scored lower in novelty seeking than those who were not successful in weight loss. This study, as had the earlier one by van den Bree et al. (2006), used the Temperament and Character Inventory, which measures seven dimensions of personality: novelty seeking, reward dependence, harm avoidance, persistence, self-directedness, self-transcendence, and cooperativeness. Obese people who did enroll in a weight loss program had a higher level of reward dependence and cooperativeness than those who did not enroll. Specific personality characteristics, in fact, may help identify those most likely to succeed at weight loss. Those who are higher in novelty-seeking behavior are more apt to be "thrill seekers" who are easily bored and hence likely to be impulsive, and may use overeating to overcome their boredom. Environmental factors, hence, can influence the expression of personality. The connection of novelty seeking and obesity was a significant one that seemed related to a "strong appetitive drive" in obese individuals in this study. Reward dependence (i.e., a need for social approval), on the other hand, was strongly associated with treatment-seeking behavior and diet success.

McLaren et al. (2008) examined the relationship between BMI values and mental health in a study of over 5,000 adults in a general but "socioeconomically advantaged" population in Alberta, Canada. They found a diversity of patterns in their population regarding body weight and mental health. Previous studies had not uniformly supported a particular relationship between body weight and mental health either, and this had led to "limited, diverse, and sometimes contradictory patterns" (McLaren et al. 2008). These authors acknowledge that several different causal relationships have been proposed to explain abnormal weight either leading to psychiatric symptoms or following from psychiatric symptoms. For example, there may be common genetic, hormonal, or neurotransmitter connections (a *biophysiological model*) such as when abnormal weight leads to metabolic abnormalities that, in turn, lead to mood disturbances. Another proposed path is the *sociobehavioral/ environmental model*, such as when stress or mood disturbance leads to changes in eating or physical activity, or when dieting per se leads to psychiatric symptoms, or even when weight discrimination leads to stress. Any association between abnormal body weight and psychiatric disorders is heterogeneous, involving factors "at the cellular, intrapsychic, behavioral, and social levels" (McLaren et al. 2008). Compared with older studies (e.g., Crisp and McGuiness 1976), more recent literature is more likely to report on significant connections between weight and psychiatric symptoms, possibly due to improved methodologies or possibly because these symptoms are more commonly seen now. McLaren et al. (2008) summarize the situation, though, by noting, "While the physical health correlates and consequences of obesity are fairly well established, the same cannot be said of the association between atypical body weight and mental health." In McLaren et al.'s (2008) Canadian study, substance use disorder was more commonly seen in younger obese men than older ones; mood disorders were more commonly seen in obese women than in normal-weight women; and there was "marginal support" for a higher prevalence of anxiety disorders in obese women than in obese men. It is notable that in their study 2.8% of the subjects were underweight and 44% were normal weight, with 34.8% overweight and 18.2% obese (McLaren et al. 2008).

Baumeister and Härter (2008) also noted discrepancies in findings and heterogeneous results in several recent studies examining the connection between obesity and mental disorders. Some of the discrepancies may be due to methodological issues, such as the type of control group used. For example, Baumeister and Härter (2008) suggested comparing obesity and the presence of other somatic diseases. These researchers believe that the connection between obesity and psychiatric disorder is "rather small," but they argue for "improved recognition and treatment of mental disorders" in patients who may have one or more somatic illnesses. Petry and her colleagues disagree with Baumeister and Härter about using a control group that is of normal weight and is screened for other diseases (see author reply in Baumeister and Härter 2008; Petry et al. 2008): not everyone thinks of obesity as a disease. For example, not all obese or overweight people have somatic disorders other than the presence of an abnormal BMI value.

Willemen et al. (2008), using data from the United Kingdom from 1987 to 2002, addressed the relationship of baseline risk of psychiatric as well as cardiovascular illness in diabetic patients who later started to use antiobesity medications ($n > 500$) and those who did not ($n > 3,000$). In this study, all of the subjects had either type 1 or type 2 diabetes mellitus. The antiobesity medications fluramine or fenfluramine (both of which were eventually withdrawn from the market because of potentially deadly pulmonary hypertension and cardiac disease) and orlistat were used here. In the year prior to beginning medication, those who did later take medication were more likely to have had a higher BMI value, to have been younger, and to have been female. Most importantly, though, those who eventually began medication were more likely to have had anxiety or depression in the year prior to beginning antiobesity medication and were also somewhat more likely to have had cardiovascular disease. In fact, over 19% (vs. only 10% of control subjects) had been prescribed antidepressant medication in that previous year. Those taking antiobesity medications may be more psychiatrically vulnerable to begin with and this may be independent of any effects of the antiobesity medications. It is certainly worth noting the importance of being "very careful in interpreting the benefits and risks" of any antiobesity medication, particularly when prescribing them to those with psychiatric morbidity, as well as in evaluating causality "when a possible drug-induced problem occurs" (Willemen et al. 2008).

Most of the studies evaluating the relationship of psychiatric illness to weight have been cross-sectional. Hasler et al. (2004) examined the hypothesis that being overweight is associated with psychiatric comorbidity, particularly atypical depression, binge eating, and aggression. The cross-sectional design of other studies may be responsible for some of the inconsistent results reported over the years. For example, acute psychiatric symptoms, in particular, may lead to transient weight changes and hence "disguise" any of the long-term connections between psychiatric conditions and BMI values. Hasler et al.

> Most of the studies evaluating the relationship of psychiatric disorders to weight have been cross-sectional; this may be responsible for some of the inconsistent results reported by different researchers.

(2004) instead conducted a prospective study of a community sample of almost 600 young adults in the Zurich, Switzerland, area for 20 years. Over the 20 years, more than 60% of the subjects continued to participate, though only 47% of this group was available for all six follow-up interviews. One of the most interesting findings was that "being overweight turned out to be remarkably stable over the 20 years" (Hasler et al. 2004). One other finding from this study, unlike results of cross-sectional studies, was that being obese (having a BMI value of > 30) was not associated with greater psychopathology than was being merely overweight (BMI > 25). There was also a strong connection

> Being overweight is a remarkably stable condition.

between atypical depression (with symptoms of overeating and hypersomnia) and being overweight, and between binge eating and being overweight (and with weight gain from age 20 to age 40). Hypomanic symptoms, particularly disinhibition, were related to increased weight in males, but not females. Both aggressive and antisocial behaviors were seen more commonly in those who were overweight, but there was a strong negative association between generalized anxiety disorder and being overweight. Here the use of antidepressants was not connected to being overweight; nor was drug or alcohol use. However, the researchers noted limitations of their long-term study: a single age cohort (ages 20–40 only) was used; over the course of the study there was an attrition rate of 38%; and, as in most of the studies in this field, heights and weights were self-reported.

Roberts et al. (2003) examined the relationship between obesity and depression over the course of 5 years, from 1994 to 1999, to assess whether each is a risk factor for the other. This was a two-wave study from Alameda County, California, that involved more than 2,000 people age 50 and older. Researchers have studied the physical and psychological health of people in this county for 30 years. In this particular study, the researchers noted there were four possible hypotheses: 1) that obesity increases the risk of depression; 2) that depression increases the risk of obesity; 3) that there exists a reciprocal relationship, such that each group is at a higher risk for the other condition; and 4) that there is no relationship between obesity and depression. There was evidence only for the first hypothesis: having obesity initially (with a BMI value of >30) was associated with an increased risk of having depression 5 years later, but having depression initially did not necessarily increase the presence of obesity 5 years later. Depression, in general, is not associated with obesity, because many of those who become depressed actually lose weight (though not those with symptoms of atypical depression). Depression in this study was associated with social isolation, poor social support, being older, being female, and having less than a complete high school education. One of the major limitations of the study was that it consisted of only two waves of measurements, which may "capture only a small interval in the lives" of the subjects. Furthermore, the BMI data, as in most studies in this field, were based on self-reports. Another limitation was that the study did not include information on subjects' use of psychotropic medications. The conclusion, though, was that there are multiple dimensions, including psychological stigma, involved in the obesity-depression connection. As found in other studies, "the less common, less normal, and less acceptable it is to be overweight in a group, the greater would be its psychological impact" (Roberts et al. 2003).

> Having obesity (BMI >30) was associated with an increased risk of depression 5 years later, but having depression initially did not necessarily increase the presence of obesity 5 years later.
>
> Source: Roberts et al. 2003

McElroy et al. (2004) evaluated the major studies of obesity in people with mood disorders, as well as those of mood disorders in people with obesity, during the years 1966–2003. They concluded that the two conditions are heterogeneous and separate, but nevertheless may be related. In other words, there are forms of obesity and mood disorders that are "pathogenically related," as well as forms that are not. They note, of course, that for 50 years researchers have been questioning the relationship of obesity with mood disorders. Further, iatrogenic factors, such as the use of medications that may cause weight changes or mood changes, may be involved. In the most "methodologically sound" *clinical* studies, there has been a positive relationship in both men and women between obesity (especially when severe) and both bipolar disorder and major depressive disorder. In *community* studies, though, there has been a positive relationship between obesity and major depressive disorder in women but inconsistent results in men (possibly due to methodological differences among the studies). The studies have shown that depressive symptoms may produce weight gain in some (particularly with atypical "reversed neurovegetative features") and weight loss in others, and cross-sectional data may not demonstrate this (McElroy et al. 2004). Further, there may be different patterns dependent on the ages of those studied. Overweight and obesity are commonly seen clinically in those who present for treatment for mood disorders (particularly when there has been childhood-onset major depression or bipolar disorder). Community studies have indicated that most obese people do not have a mood disorder, though particular mood disorders, such as atypical depression in adults in general, are associated with weight gain as well as with being overweight or obese. Obesity in females is associated with major depressive disorder, but specifically abdominal obesity (and the metabolic syndrome) is associated with depression in both males and females. Treatment guidelines for mood disorders typically do not address the issue of obesity, and obese patients may need to be managed differently from nonobese patients. Likewise, obese individuals who present for weight loss may also have to be treated differently if they have concomitant mood disorders. Studies of mood disorders tend not to include body weight as a factor, and studies of obesity tend not to factor in mood disorders.

- Major depression causes weight loss.

- Atypical depression may cause weight gain in some people and weight loss in others.

Atlantis and Baker (2008) conducted a systematic review, examining epidemiological studies, to assess whether obesity causes depression. They looked in detail at 24 studies (of >4,000 considered "potentially relevant"), four of which were prospective studies and 20 of which were cross-sectional studies (only 10 of which were conducted in the United States). Few high-quality prospective cohort studies have been conducted. Because most studies have been cross-sectional, solid conclusions for causality cannot be determined. Prospective studies have consistently suggested that obesity seems to increase the odds for developing depressive symptoms. But there is a discrepancy in the cross-sectional data: in the United States, for example, most studies have supported the connection between obesity and depression in women but not in men, whereas in non-U.S. populations, most cross-sectional studies have failed to find this connection. In some people with obesity, bodily pain, such as in the knee joint, may be a factor linked to depression.

An intriguing new theory linking depression and obesity is the so-called *leptin hypothesis of depression*. Lu (2007) suggests that the hormone leptin can actually have antidepressant efficacy in animal studies. He reports that leptin may also have a role in regulating the hypothalamic-pituitary-adrenal (HPA) axis and that lower leptin levels have been found in depressed people who have attempted suicide. He further speculates that leptin resistance, so common in obesity, may be responsible for the higher rate of depression in those who are obese. Lu also suggests that leptin may eventually have therapeutic efficacy in treating depression. (See also "Hormones of Food Intake" in Chapter 5, "The Metabolic Complexities of Weight Control.")

Whether there is a hormonal link connecting obesity and depression remains to be seen, but most researchers would accept that psychosocial factors may also be involved. For example, issues like negative stereotyping of the obese, negative body image, and negative feelings of self-efficacy may all contribute to the development of depressive symptomatology. And it is sometimes the *perception* of being over-weight rather than obesity itself that may lead to greater psychological distress, all of which is, of course, reinforced by a culture's ideals of body weight as portrayed in the media. Is it possible, for example, that we see more connection to depressive symptomatology, particularly in women, here in the United States than elsewhere because of the media's incessant message of needing to be thin to a degree that is impossible for most people? Atlantis and Ball (2008) conducted a study to investi-gate whether a person's actual weight, as opposed to his or her perceptions of weight, is independently associated with "nonspecific psychological distress." Obesity, did, in fact, "significantly increase the odds of psychological distress," but so did one's weight perception and misperception, and these perceptions and misperceptions may be even more important with some people than others. Inconsistencies among the re-sults of other studies involving obesity and psychological mor-bidity may be due to the fact that other studies have not taken into account subjects' *perceptions* of their weights. When a person's perceived weight deviated from the ideals of society, he or she was much more likely to have

CONTRIBUTORS TO DEPRESSION IN OVERWEIGHT INDIVIDUALS (ESPECIALLY WOMEN)

- Bodily pain (e.g., in joints)
- Self-perceived negative body image
- Bulimia nervosa
- Social and sexual rejections
- Other psychological distresses

psychological distress. Atlantis and Ball (2008) concluded that this lends support for a psychosocial rather than a typical biological explanation, such as theorizing a dysregulation of the HPA axis. Because this study was cross-sectional, the investiga-tors could not determine causality. In other words, it is not clear whether psycho-logical distress caused weight misperceptions or whether weight misperceptions caused psychological distress. As in other studies, the BMI data came from self-reports.

DIETING AND PSYCHOLOGICAL SYMPTOMS

Dieting, defined by Wadden et al. 2002 (p. 154) as "the intentional and sustained restriction of caloric intake for the purpose of reducing body weight or changing body shape," itself may be stressful and cause psychological symptomatology. Hilde Bruch (1952) was one of the first to describe untoward reactions to dieting when she noted psychotic states (where preoccupation with weight assumed a "delusional character") occurring in some females in late adolescence who had been "reducing." Success or failure in achieving weight loss may depend on the meaning of the loss to the patient, and particularly in emotionally disturbed obese people the weight loss can have an "irrational meaning." Bruch found that the overweight "do not represent a homogeneous group." Even though she was writing more than 50 years ago, she noted that weight reduction had already become "big business" and the object of commercial exploitation. Bruch was fairly pessimistic in that she said it was only someone "exceptionally well-integrated" or someone "very obsessive" who could follow a diet. The great appeal, she said, of the then-current reducing methods was that "most people are more ready to accept an extraordinary situation than just a slight voluntary change of an established habit" (Bruch 1952).

Stunkard (1957) wrote of "dieting depression," in which he described his study of 100 patients who had come to a nutrition clinic for dieting. Of the 72 people who had dieted previously, more than half of them reported physical symptoms such as nervousness, anxiety, restlessness, and irritability. And in a group of 25 obese people, so-called dieting depression developed, characterized by intense anxiety and prolonged depression with crying spells, sleep disturbances, difficulty working, and even thoughts of suicide—even though there had often been initial elation when the decision to diet was made. Stunkard's conclusion was that this high incidence of symptoms during the course of dieting indicated that, at least for some obese people, dieting may actually be dangerous. Stunkard (1957), in this early article, emphasized the particular "vulnerability" of those who are obese "during attempts at weight reduction" and added, "It is important for the physician dealing with obese patients to bear in mind the relative ineffectiveness of current measures of treatment, the suffering and hazards they entail, and the remarkably poor results of long-term follow-up."

In a large review article, Stunkard and Rush (1974) revisited the connection between dieting and depression. They found that patients who had been obese since childhood were considerably more vulnerable to the stresses of dieting, as manifested by increased anxiety, depression, pessimism, and apathy. And the longer these individuals remained on a calorie-restricted diet, the more they became hostile and aggressive. Significantly, the age at onset of obesity was probably the "most distinctive factor in vulnerability" in these people (Stunkard and Rush 1974). Further, dieters who had severe calorie restriction, rather than short-term fasting (<2 weeks), tended to have more emotional difficulty: in short-term fasting, hunger declined, but with the introduction into the diet of even a small amount of carbohydrates, hunger reappeared. It seems that dieting with caloric restriction may be more stressful—and more uncomfortable—than actual fasting. Fasting for more than 2 weeks, though, may lead to a "dramatic rise in emotional disturbance," including increased aggression, mood fluctuations, anxiety, depression, and even almost psychotic reactions. Likewise, outpatient treatment seemed to be more stressful than inpatient treatment. In previously reported studies that had demonstrated the positive effects of dieting, there had often been a very high dropout rate, from 20% to as high as 80% in some studies. Dropping out of a dieting program may actually be "a highly adaptive method of coping with impending complications" for those who are "biologically vulnerable" (Stunkard and Rush 1974).

Smoller et al. (1987) performed a critical review, including 35 empirical studies, of the relationship of dieting and depression almost 15 years after their 1970s review. They found discrepancies among the studies, with some reporting positive changes in the mood of their dieters and others finding negative effects. The authors observed that "Like the parable of the blind man and the elephant, there may be multiple truths in the description of emotional processes" (Smoller et al. 1987). What they did note, though, is that the "single best predictor of the nature of the mood changes" was the method by which the mood changes had been measured. For example, there were "benign" mood changes when the assessment was conducted with "objective, fixed-alternative" choices, but when the questions were open-ended, the researchers found patients had "adverse" moods. Furthermore, Smoller and colleagues found that group and behavioral treatment, as well as short-term fasts on an inpatient service, were not associated with "emotional complications." According to their own research study, another factor that may determine whether there are beneficial or adverse reactions is the frequency of assessment; that is, weekly or even daily assessments of mood, rather than assessment only before and after treatment, may increase the possibility of finding adverse reactions (Wadden et al. 1986). Much more recently, others have also reported that dieting causes depression and even binge eating, but Wadden et al. (2002, p. 154) believe these reports are "without merit."

DIETING DYSPHORIA

Dieting dysphoria (shifts in mood that are not necessarily as severe as depression) may depend on a number of factors:

- Initial failure in losing weight

- Inability to maintain the diet

- Other reasons for dieting besides being overweight

- Present-time orientation

- Being surrounded by people who do not have to diet

- Having certain maladaptive personality traits (e.g., low frustration tolerance; experiencing dieting as punishment or deprivation)

Many of the early studies had been based on patients who had been referred for psychiatric treatment (certainly that was the case with the sample in Bruch's 1952 study) and hence would more likely have psychological issues not related to weight loss. Some patients, although not experiencing actual depression, can experience shifts in mood during the dieting process (Wadden et al. 2002, p. 155)— what we might call "dieting dysphoria." There are many factors that may predispose people to dieting dysphoria, including how successful at dieting they are initially (i.e., how easily they can lose some weight as a reinforcement to lose more weight); how easily they are able to maintain their diet over the long term; and even whose idea the diet was (e.g., whether it was begun for medical reasons). People who are negatively predisposed by nature may feel a diet offers considerable restriction and deprivation. Those who have difficulty visualizing the future may have more difficulty with long-term goals, particularly if they reach weight plateaus, and may become easily frustrated. Further, dysphoria may be more common in those who are surrounded by people who do not have to diet or who sabotage their efforts and encourage cheating. Lowe and Levine (2005), in reviewing the literature, summarize the potential negative psychological effects of dieting: it produces a "vulnerability to emotional eating" and creates difficulties regulating eating in those who are "restrained eaters"; it produces "untoward emotional reactions" in those who are obese and do lose weight; it is "psychologically unhealthy," particularly for women, inasmuch as it "promotes unrealistic expectations" about just how much body weight and shape can actually change; and it even can produce cognitive difficulties in processing information when dieters are so preoccupied with food.

THE PSYCHOLOGY OF WEIGHT CYCLING

What about the effect of weight cycling on the psychological state of the dieter? *Weight cycling*, or *yo-yo dieting*, as we have discussed earlier (see "Other Medical Consequences of Obesity" in Chapter 2, "Obesity in the United States"), has never been officially defined in any standard way. For example, no one specifies how much weight needs to have been regained, nor how many times weight cycling needs to have occurred, nor during what period of time. It may mean different things to different people, but as used here the term essentially refers to regaining weight unintentionally after having lost weight intentionally by dieting. Of course, many conditions can lead to intentional weight cycling, including the normal gain and loss of weight during and after pregnancy or an actor's deliberate loss or gain of weight in preparation for a role in a film (e.g., Robert De Niro's famous weight gain when he played the boxer Jake La Motta for the last part of Martin Scorsese's *Raging Bull*).

Foster et al. (1996) studied the psychological effects of weight cycling in 48 obese women in a long-term study covering 58 months. During the first 6 months of the study, each woman lost more than 21 kilograms (by severe calorie restriction), but by 58 months, some were nearly 11 kilograms heavier than their baseline weight and 81% had regained at least three-quarters of the weight they had lost. The majority had had two cycles of weight loss and regain by the end of the study. Those who dieted during the follow-up phase did so only when their weight had exceeded their initial weight. Cognitive factors may play a role in the decision to diet again, but it was not clear what really made these subjects start to diet again. Despite the significant weight gain over time, and contrary to the expectations of the researchers, these women reported decreased binge eating and hunger, more control over eating, and even improved mood. Unfortunately, though, "weight regain remains the most common long-term outcome of obesity treatment" (Foster et al. 1996).

Both cross-sectional and longitudinal studies have demonstrated that weight cycling does not necessarily lead to depression but that weight regain may have a "moderately to very negative effect" on how people feel about their appearance, their self-esteem, or their self-confidence (Wadden et al. 2002). Wadden et al. (2002) also note that weight cycling "may affect dimensions of personal experience that simply are not assessed by standard depression scales" (p. 162).

BODY IMAGE, FAT ACCEPTANCE, AND BODY DYSMORPHIC DISORDER

In our culture, with its focus on appearance, inevitably many people will have difficulties and even perceptual distortions regarding their body image. German researchers Hewig et al. (2008) speak of the drive for thinness that leads to lowered self-esteem, depression, and body image distortions. There are two aspects to body image: the perceived size and shape—that is, the mental image one has of one's body—and the emotional aspect of feelings and beliefs about it. There can be perceptual distortions (i.e., the inability to accurately assess its size or shape) and body dissatisfaction (i.e., actual negative feelings about it). Hewig et al. (2008) speculate that body image distortion is associated with "deviant attention" to certain areas of the body to the exclusion of others. In fact, in a study of university students, those who had the so-called drive for thinness had an attentional bias when they looked at photos of male and female models, focusing longer and more often on the waist, hips, legs, and arms, and looking less often at the head and face (and hence missing potentially important social cues). It is possible that eye scan studies may even be used clinically to ascertain who might be at risk for an eating disorder (Hewig et al. 2008).

> **BODY IMAGE AND WEIGHT LOSS**
>
> • The primary reason given by patients for wanting to lose weight—the reason that patients say is most important—is *appearance*, rather than health.
>
> • This is true even among the most severely obese with serious obesity-related diseases, such as diabetes or hypertension, who are going for bariatric surgery.
>
> Source: Sarwer amd Thompson 2002, p. 451

Years ago, Stunkard and Mendelson (1967) studied disturbances in body image in a group of over 70 randomly selected obese people from medical and psychiatric clinics in the Philadelphia area. For the purposes of their study, they divided body image disturbances "rather arbitrarily" into three categories: views of the self, general self-consciousness, and particular self-consciousness in regard to the opposite sex. Body image disturbances were not present in all obese people, and some, in fact, viewed their obesity in a "thoroughly realistic manner." Body image disturbances tended to persist for years, although their intensity may fluctuate widely, and even weight loss did not alter the disturbed perceptions. The person's age at onset of obesity (i.e., obesity during childhood or adolescence) was one of the most important predisposing factors, but the presence of an emotional disturbance (not specified in their research) and a critical evaluation of the obesity by others in early years may also factor into the development of a body image disorder. Once such a disorder had developed, it made no difference what other qualities the person possessed (e.g., talent, wealth, intelligence): that person's weight became his or her overriding concern and it was through the lens of body weight that the person viewed the world. One extreme is the starving person with anorexia nervosa who believes that she or he (mostly women are affected) is fat. By custom, though, those with anorexia are in a separate category because this distortion in body image is part of the diagnosis itself.

The National Association for the Advancement of Fat Acceptance (NAAFA), originally called the National Association to Aid Fat Americans, began in 1969 as a nonprofit human rights organization that "speaks out against discrimination based on body size" (Saguy and Riley 2005). As such, it offers workshops and support groups to improve the quality of life for those who are obese, and it acts as a "national legal clearinghouse" for those lawyers who advocate against size discrimination. According to Saguy and Riley (2005), NAAFA also functions as a social network for its members. They note that the fat acceptance movement rejects the word *obese* because it "pathologizes heavier weights" but has reclaimed the word *fat*, just as gay activists have claimed the word *queer*. It believes that fatness, analogous to racial, ethnic, or sexual preference diversity, is "a form of body diversity that should be tolerated and respected." Saguy and Riley (2005) report that some fat acceptance advocates refer to those who conduct scientific research in the field of obesity as the "obesity mafia" and accuse those researchers of benefiting financially from their connections to diet or pharmaceutical companies.

The fat acceptance movement frames obesity differently from those who believe in the "personal behavior theory of illness," where obesity is due to "risky behavior," that is, unhealthy lifestyle choices (Saguy and Riley 2005). Those in this movement believe that someone can be healthy at any size and the health concerns regarding obesity are exaggerated. Though there is a subgroup of obese people who have "metabolically benign obesity" (Stefan et al. 2008), as we have mentioned, there is overwhelming evidence that obesity leads to considerable deleterious medical consequences for every organ system, and even small amounts of weight loss can have substantial health benefits (see Chapter 2, "Obesity in the United States"). And we hope we have made it abundantly clear that obesity, particularly morbid (Class 3) obesity, is multidimensional and not simply a matter of unhealthy lifestyle choices.

McKinley (2004) examined how 128 obese women who supported the fat acceptance movement viewed their own body experience. They were interested in how these women viewed their bodies as an outside observer (body surveillance); whether they felt they were "bad" if they did not conform to cultural standards (body shame); and whether they felt they could control their appearance (appearance control beliefs), all part of "objectified body consciousness." McKinley (2004) found that personal body ideals of these women were more important than their body size, and those who actually advocated for social change tended to have greater self-esteem and self-acceptance than those who wanted only personal change.

Body image disorders do not always have to involve preoccupation with a person's weight. Related to body image disorders is the newer category of *body dysmorphic disorder*, a severe disorder in which a person has a "distressing preoccupation" with an imagined or slight defect in appearance. This may involve any part of the body. Phillips (1991) calls it "the distress of imagined ugliness." Commonly, there is comorbidity with other psychiatric disorders, such as major depression, obsessive-compulsive disorder, social phobia, or even substance use disorders. There are more similarities than differences between obsessive-compulsive disorder, for example, and body dysmorphic disorder, even though body dysmorphic disorder is now classified as a somatoform disorder and obsessive-compulsive disorder is classified as an anxiety disorder. Some believe body dysmorphic disorder should be classified as an anxiety disorder (Phillips et al. 2007). Those with body dysmorphic disorder, though, have poorer psychosocial functioning—having few friends and avoiding social situations—and poorer academic and occupational functioning than those with an anxiety disorder. The disorder can be incapacitating. About 80% of those with this disorder have suicidal

WHAT IS BODY DYSMORPHIC DISORDER?

- Excessive concern and preoccupation with a defect in appearance: the defect can be real or imagined and can involve any part of the body (e.g., thighs, breasts, genitals, facial features, or other)

- This preoccupation causes significant distress or impairment in relationships or work; no amount of reassurance helps; may lead to social isolation; considerable time is spent *checking* the defect

- In cosmetic surgical practices, from 6% to 15% of patients requesting procedures present with this disorder

Source: Buescher and Buescher 2006; DSM-IV-TR, p. 510

ideation and almost 30% have actually attempted suicide, a considerably higher percentage than in those with obsessive-compulsive disorder (19%) (Phillips et al. 2007). Nearly 40% of individuals with body dysmorphic disorder can actually be delusional in their fixed belief that there is something wrong with their appearance, and almost half have a history of a psychiatric hospitalization. The disorder often goes undiagnosed (and those who have it may not even mention it spontaneously because of their embarrassment), though the prevalence rate has been estimated at up to 2.4%. Both men and women can have the disorder, but women seem to be affected more commonly. Women may be unhappy with their breasts, hips, or face, for example. Often, a minor flaw is seen as a major imperfection. Those affected may spend hours each day checking their so-called deformities, attempting to hide them. They may also spend hours looking at themselves in the mirror, or, on the contrary, they may avoid mirrors altogether. It has been estimated that of the millions of people who request cosmetic procedures, about 10% have body dysmorphic disorder (Buescher and Buescher 2006), but the range can be up to 15% (DSM-IV-TR; American Psychiatric Association 2000). It is important for professionals to diagnose this condition, because no cosmetic or dermatological procedure will alleviate the person's pain, and patient dissatisfaction may even lead to violence against the plastic surgeon or dermatologist (Phillips et al. 2008). The patient's expectations of such procedures are often totally unrealistic. Both cognitive-behavioral therapy and medication with serotonin reuptake inhibitors (e.g., fluoxetine 60 mg), as well as augmentation with other medications, including possibly an atypical antipsychotic, may be helpful for some patients.

CERTAIN PSYCHIATRIC ILLNESSES AND COMORBID ABNORMAL WEIGHT

Depression

Major depression, which affects 8% of men and 15% of women, is a recurring disorder: more than half of those who recover from an episode will relapse within 6 months if not given maintenance antidepressant medication, and of those who never get treatment, 15% will commit suicide (Gold and Chrousos 2002). Essentially, there are two main subtypes of major depression, *melancholic depression* and *atypical depression*. Psychological stress may be responsible for precipitating major depression and may affect its severity and course, and stress and depression may both lead to similar states, such as less flexibility in cognitive and emotional responses, abnormalities in arousal, and disturbances in neuroendocrine and autonomic functioning. Mediators of the stress response are hyperactive in melancholic depression and hypoactive ("downregulated") in atypical depression. These two subtypes are essentially opposites. Individuals with melancholic depression have anxiety, insomnia, and loss of appetite (and subsequent weight loss), as well as a diurnal variation (feeling worse at the beginning of the day), with dread of the future and a sense of worthlessness. Conversely, those with atypical depression experience lethargy, fatigue, hypersomnia, and increased eating (with weight gain), as well as a sense of emptiness, a sense of disconnectedness, and diurnal variation, feeling worse later in the day. The majority of those with major depression, however, do not necessarily conform to these classifications: less than 30% have pure melancholic depression and another 30% have atypical depression (Gold and Chrousos 2002).

Both cortisol and norepinephrine secretion are increased in melancholic depression, and this hypersecretion may be responsible for the state of hyperarousal and anxiety found in these patients. Cortisol secretion during acute stress is adaptive, but chronic cortisol secretion is toxic to the body: excessive anxiety, insulin resistance, and visceral fat deposition may result, and even potentially osteoporosis, decreased immune response, and loss of muscle (sarcopenia). There is speculation that major depression, in general, is associated with less activity in cortical brain areas and greater activity in paralimbic subcortical areas (e.g., the amygdala): pa-

> Chronic cortisol secretion in depression may result in visceral fat deposition and insulin resistance.

tients with melancholia may have left-sided defects, whereas patients with atypical depression may have right-sided lesions (Gold and Chrousos 2002).

Stunkard et al. (2003) addressed the question of the relationship between depression and being overweight or obese. One issue that complicates a discussion of the relationship is the difference between obese people who seek treatment and those who do not. When investigating depression, one must differentiate moderators from mediators. *Moderators* include the severity of depression, the severity of obesity, gender, ethnicity, age, socioeconomic status, gene-environment interactions, and experiences in childhood. Moderators "specify for whom and under what conditions" an effect occurs (Stunkard et al. 2003). *Mediators*, on the other hand, include eating (and even disturbed eating), physical activity, and stress. These mediators "identify why and how" the moderators exert these effects. A moderator according to one researcher may be a mediator according to another. The treatment of obesity can often result in an improvement in depression (e.g., mood improvement after bariatric surgery); the treatment of depression, though, may have a negative impact on obesity.

Vogelzangs et al. (2008) investigated longitudinally over 5 years whether "clinically relevant" depressive symptoms can predict an increase specifically in abdominal obesity, as diagnosed by computed tomography scan. Over 2,000 older people ages 70–79 in the Pittsburgh area were studied. Nearly 53% of subjects in the study were women; over 63% were white and over 46% were college educated, and use of antidepressant medications was controlled for. It should be noted that depression was measured by the 20-item Center for Epidemiologic Studies Depression Scale, a scale that has been shown to be a valid measurement of depression in the elderly but does not specifically reflect a "psychiatric definition of depression." Depression was present in 4% of the subjects initially, which is lower than the 10%–15% normally seen in elderly people. Neuroendocrine disturbances (i.e., dysregulation of the HPA axis), such as high levels of cortisol and lower levels of the sex steroid hormones, have been reported in some depressed people as well as in those with abdominal obesity (Vogelzangs et al. 2008). And of course the excess visceral fat of abdominal obesity, as we have earlier noted, is associated with type 2 diabetes, cardiovascular disease, the metabolic syndrome, and even increased mortality (see Chapter 2, "Obesity in the United States").

Baseline depression was associated with an increase in abdominal obesity specifically over the 5 years of the study. This was the first longitudinal (rather than cross-sectional) study to examine the relationship between depressive symptoms and the development of abdominal obesity. Waist circumference, unlike actual computed tomography scanning, did not accurately predict the presence of abdominal fat because this measurement includes abdominal *subcutaneous* fat as well as visceral fat. Even though depression has often been associated with weight loss, even in an elderly population where there was often a decrease in fat (the researchers did not mention the loss of muscle that is typical as well in this population), there was more visceral fat specifically in those with depressive symptoms—that is, depressive symptoms correlated with visceral fat accumulation specifically. And even in those who lost weight during the study, those who had depression retained their visceral fat accumulation. Depressed people "frequently" have an increased risk of diabetes and cardiovascular disease. Visceral fat is particularly sensitive to cortisol because of the increased number of glucocorticoid receptors in visceral fat. The mechanism by which cortisol promotes visceral fat accumulation is activation of lipoprotein lipase and inhibiting of lipid metabolism, and this is more apt to happen when sex steroid levels are lower. A "certain amount of distress" is required before visceral fat will accumulate, but in this study there did not need to be recurrent episodes of depression or even persistent depression for visceral fat to accumulate (Vogelzangs et al. 2008).

Vaccarino et al. (2008) also looked at the connection between depression and the metabolic syndrome. The mechanisms underlying the observation that depression is associated with cardiovascular disease or mortality are unknown and could be related to unhealthy lifestyles among depressed individuals as well as dysregulation of the HPA axis that leads to insulin resistance and accumulation of visceral fat. This study, with almost 6 years of follow-up, aimed to clarify whether the metabolic syndrome and depression were associated in women who were suspected of having had myocardial ischemia (they had "chest discomfort"), as well as whether the metabolic syndrome "explains the effect of depression" on the incidence of cardiovascular disease events over the years of the study. The metabolic syndrome was defined by the criteria of the American Heart Association and the National Heart, Lung, and Blood Institute. Over 600 women were available for follow-up. Depression was assessed by the Beck Depression Inventory (21-item scale).

Depression severity was associated with the number of metabolic syndrome risk factors. Women with both an elevated Beck Depression Inventory score and a history of depression (including current level and treatment history) had twice the risk for cardiovascular disease of women without depression. Both depression and the metabolic syndrome remained significant but independent predictors of cardiovascular disease in the women in this study. The use of medications, such as beta-blockers (which can lead to weight gain and depression as well) and antidepressants, did not change the results significantly: even when these medications were considered, those women with depression still had a 60% higher chance of having the metabolic syndrome than nondepressed women did. In women with suspected coronary artery disease, there was a "strong association" between depression and the prevalence of the metabolic syndrome, independent of lifestyle and demographic factors, and there was a dose-response pattern, suggesting a causal relationship (Vaccarino et al. 2008). But it could not be determined whether depression was causal or rather a consequence of, or even simply a marker of, the metabolic syndrome. Notably, no interviews were conducted to diagnose depression, nor was there information on the length of any depressive episode or information on the type or course of antidepressant medication used. The researchers concluded that the metabolic syndrome "only explains a small portion of the association between depression and incident cardiovascular disease," suggesting that each increases the risk for cardiovascular disease independently of the other (Vaccarino et al. 2008).

Vagus nerve stimulation (VNS) is a treatment technique devised originally for intractable epilepsy. More recently it has been used for treatment-resistant depression as well as for pain syndromes. According to Bodenlos et al. (2007), VNS, which has just received U.S. Food and Drug Administration approval for use in treating intractable depression, involves the implanting of a small generator in a patient's chest just under the skin. An electrode connects the generator to the left cervical vagus nerve, one of our 10 cranial nerves that send impulses to and from the brain to organs, including the heart and gastrointestinal system. The vagus nerve has been implicated in short-term control of food regulation. Research in both animals and humans (with epilepsy) found that VNS led to weight loss (with greater stimulation leading to greater weight loss), though it was not clear whether this was related to changes in hunger and satiety signals, food cravings, or other changes in metabolism (Bodenlos et al. 2007). In earlier research with depressed patients, VNS did not lead to consistent weight loss. Bodenlos et al. (2007) studied a total of 33 patients in one of three groups to assess the effect of VNS on food cravings: VNS with depression; depressed patients without VNS; and healthy control subjects. They found that half of their VNS subjects had increased cravings for sweets and half had decreased cravings. They speculate that it is possible that initially cravings are increased but that over time, there may be a downregulation of cravings. Obviously more research is needed, but VNS may eventually offer a treatment modality for a subgroup of those patients with intense cravings that lead to overweight or obesity.

In another small study, Pardo et al. (2007) also made the "serendipitous observation" that those given VNS for treatment-resistant depression lost a "significant" amount of weight over 2 years of the study, even without dieting or exercise. The higher the initial BMI value, the greater the weight loss. Patients reported they felt "satiated" with less food, though actual food cravings were not discussed. Interestingly, the patients' weight loss did not correlate with changes in their depression. Pardo et al. (2007) suggest that VNS be studied as a potential treatment for "severe obesity."

Hypochondriasis

The following case example illustrates hypochondriasis in a patient with anxiety and binge eating disorder.

Hypochondriasis With Anxiety and Binge Eating Disorder

Dan, a 50-year-old married, successful, somewhat overweight businessman, recently felt faint on a tennis court. He had not eaten breakfast before his tennis game, as his physician had suggested he always do, and this was the logical initial explanation for his feeling faint in the midst of strenuous exercise; however, Dan's immediate thought was that he was having a heart attack. His father had had his first myocardial infarction in his early 60s (and died in his late 60s). Dan just assumed his turn would come soon enough. He became concerned enough to see his physician, an internist, that day, who took some blood samples and reassured him that his heart was fine. This was Dan's third visit to his physician in the past 2 weeks—and his fifth in the past 6 months. His physician kept referring to Dan as his "hypo" patient each time his secretary told him Dan had made another appointment. It seemed each time the stock market lost another hundred points, Dan became more symptomatic.

Dan was clearly preoccupied with all aspects of his body, including his weight, not just his heart, and he was not reassured by any medical workup, no matter how thorough it had been over the past 6 months. For example, on one visit the internist did not think an electrocardiogram (ECG) was indicated. Dan, as soon as he got home from the appointment, kept ruminating about this. He went back the following day to demand an ECG, "just to be on the safe side." The internist, who actually specialized in cardiology, was so frustrated that he found himself ordering another stress test and echocardiogram, both of which were unnecessary because Dan had had normal results on both in the past 6 months.

It was at this point that his internist recommended Dan consider speaking to a psychiatrist. The internist suggested a psychiatrist, rather than another type of mental health professional, because he assumed, rightly, that Dan should be on medication for the considerable anxiety related to his hypochondria and an apparent eating disorder. Dan had been loath to accept any medication the internist had suggested.

Dan finally accepted the suggestion to see a psychiatrist because even he began to realize that his anxiety kept mounting and nothing was reassuring him. He would have been dead many times over had he actually had all the diseases he had imagined in the past 6 months.

When he saw the therapist, he began by saying, "How can this be happening to me? I am as reasonably fit a person as one can be at my age. Okay, I could lose 10 pounds, but I play tennis and racquetball all the time. I have regular indoor court time throughout the year. I play with pros, mind you, pros! You know what kind of a game those characters can give you? Believe me, I give as good as I take.

WHAT IS HYPOCHONDRIASIS?

- *Essential feature*: preoccupation with fears of having a serious medical illness based on misperceptions of one or more bodily signs or symptoms

- Fears persist despite thorough medical evaluation to the contrary; in other words, reassurance is not helpful

- The fears, although quite intense, do not reach a delusional level; the person can acknowledge the *possibility* that there might not be a medical disease

- The fears cause considerable distress and/or impairment in a person's functioning

- Often the symptoms are vague, e.g., pain, headache, fatigue, which may be part of many diseases

- The fears can involve one body system or many different ones, or switch from one disease to another

- People with hypochondriasis may go from one doctor to another, subjecting themselves to many unnecessary tests and examinations ("doctor shopping")

- There may be a chronic course, with periods of waxing and waning, due to stress

- Often associated with a cluster of symptoms including suggestibility, unrealistic fear of infection, fascination with medical information, fear of prescribed medication, rumination about illness, and preoccupation with their bodies

- May develop a compulsive desire to seek medical information on the Internet

Source: DSM-IV-TR, p. 507; Fink et al. 2004

If I lost the weight, I could readily kick some serious ass. Yet I am a psychiatric mess! I am constantly thinking that I'm having a heart attack or I have some deadly form of cancer. I am always thinking the worst. And the Internet just makes everything even more horrible. It is really a terrible liability for someone like me. Whenever I have any symptom, I look it up on one of those medical searches and know it must be lymphoma or leukemia or something even more esoteric. My doctor told me the old joke they used to tell when he was in medical school: 'If you hear hoofbeats, think horses, not zebras.' Well, I'm not even thinking zebras, I'm thinking unicorns!

"Then I gorge myself! Lately, like everyone else, I am really worried about the economy. I have always been successful, but you never know. If General Motors needs a government bailout and Lehman Brothers can go bankrupt, anything is possible. I realize my bingeing is getting more frequent—probably several times a week now—and I can pack in at least a thousand calories at a sitting—mostly crap when I am alone—and I am usually not even really hungry. I'm not really very discriminating when I get in one of those states—anything sugary and fatty will do—even Twinkies, would you believe? And this is from someone who loves to eat at the Four Seasons! Mind you, I never vomit—that would actually be disgusting—but sometimes I wish I could because I realize if this bingeing continues, I really will be a lot more than 10 pounds overweight. I feel so out of control while I am eating and so disgusted with myself and embarrassed and even depressed afterward.

"I'm sorry. I know I've talked too much about this. My wife says I am a hypochondriac and am always talking about my health, my food, my weight, my tennis games and that all this stress may, in fact, really cause a heart attack. I really may end up being the boy who cried wolf. Remember that Aesop's fable? When the wolf finally came, the townsfolk wouldn't even believe him that that time there really was a wolf.

"But, by the way, another bizarre thing happened the other day. In the court, playing an easy double, I tripped over my own foot, fell, and almost broke my wrist. Maybe I am getting multiple sclerosis or Lou Gehrig's disease—isn't that the one with muscle weakness and incoordination? Maybe I am just getting old? But the other three people, all were older than I am. My knees hurt, my right hip bothers me. Damn! I feel I am just not as coordinated as I used to be. What is so confusing is that I have been an athlete all my life. Despite my father's death in his late 60s, I expected to be in good shape until my late 80s."

Of course, Dan needed to talk. His wife and even his internist were getting impatient with his physical complaints and preoccupations with his body. Now only a therapist would listen to him. Dan immediately assumed he had a serious physical disease after experiencing only transient and usually nondescript, vague symptoms, and each week the symptoms changed. Here a psychiatrist could help correct some of Dan's misperceptions about these illnesses and their implications, confront him about some of his cognitive beliefs, and provide him with corrective medical information. Reassurance, though, with patients like Dan does not work for more than a few minutes. Patients like Dan are so prone to assume the worst that they often ignore inconsistencies and distortions in making their case for serious illness. And they often believe that they know more than most physicians—that, in fact, physicians are just incompetently failing to find what is ailing them. For these patients, every cough is lung cancer; every headache is an inoperable brain tumor.

Luckily, Dan was so troubled by his symptoms at this point that he was eager to accept psychiatric help. Many people with hypochondriacal symptoms would rather believe they have a serious medical problem than a problem that is primarily psychological. They are usually completely reluctant to take psychiatric medication for anxiety or depression—or sometimes any prescribed medication—and it often takes considerable coaxing on the part of the psychiatrist. In Dan's case, after eight sessions of cognitive therapy he was finally amenable to the use of a selective serotonin reuptake inhibitor (SSRI) like fluoxetine (Prozac) to alleviate some of his excessive anxiety as well as his binge eating. The psychiatrist taught Dan to use the phrase "wasted worry" each time he decided he had some deadly disease and suggested Dan could use this phrase hundreds of times a day if he needed to.

Dan, who had never been in therapy previously, was also motivated for psychoanalytically oriented therapy because he became intellectually curious about the relationship of his hypochondriacal symptoms to issues involving his father. After the initial sessions of cognitive therapy and several weeks of medication, Dan decided he wanted to explore some of the more dynamic connections, including issues related to his being overweight. He realized he tended to eat when he felt anxious and stressed, and that, of course, only made him feel worse and reminded him of his father, who also had anxiety and used to overeat when he was stressed.

Dan ate when he felt anxious or stressed; he ate when he thought he had some physical illness; he ate when he was tired; he ate when he was happy or unhappy. He ate when he thought he might be hungry. Furthermore, Dan never skipped the standard three-meals-a-day regimen.

Dan's major defenses to ward off anxiety included *rationalization*, such as when he would check the Internet saying he would "just read a little" about some medical disease even though this approach only made his anxiety worse and, of course, he really could not stop his reading. Likewise, with eating, he would say he would "just eat a little" cake and find himself finishing an entire cake. He actually described needing a sense of closure, and couldn't let himself eat only some. He had the same experience eating cookies—he would have to eat at least an entire row of cookies within a package. For him, the 100-calorie packaging became ideal, unless he found himself, almost automatically, eating several packages in one sitting. With considerable embarrassment he once told the psychiatrist that he had had his wife pay a lot extra for these individually wrapped quantities in order to prevent himself from eating an entire larger package, only to sabotage himself by eating six individual packages, which was even more than the quantity in the larger package.

He also used *intellectualization* in his Internet searches, attempting to master a subject by trying to learning all there was to know about it. However, the information he found on the Internet was often not helpful (and sometimes misleading or downright incorrect), all of which made him more anxious. And he used *identification*, wherein he behaved just as his father had, without even knowing it. The problem was that all these defenses were not working. They were having the opposite effect: instead of easing his anxiety, as defenses are supposed to do, they made him extraordinarily more stressed. Luckily, he had not used the defense of denial primarily, for that would have prevented him from finally accepting his internist's suggestion to seek psychiatric help.

Issues concerning weight may appear, for example, when a patient loses a pound or two and automatically thinks he or she must have cancer. Likewise, a small gain in weight may also send patients into a panic, thinking that they are developing some other illness or condition that leads to weight gain. Further, their anxiety, as in Dan's case, may lead them to eating disorders such as overeating or actual bingeing.

COMORBIDITY OF EATING DISORDERS WITH PSYCHIATRIC SYMPTOMS

Please note that our book is not about eating disorders, though a book about weight by psychiatrists must include them. Our discussion here provides the bare essentials, and we refer the reader to the excellent book by Yager and Powers (2007), *Clinical Manual of Eating Disorders*, and the American Psychiatric Association's (2006) treatment guidelines for eating disorders, both of which provided much of the material below.

There are essentially three major eating disorders, all of which affect weight— binge eating disorder, anorexia nervosa, and bulimia nervosa—although binge eating disorder, the most common clinically, is not yet classified separately in our latest DSM nomenclature beyond "eating disorder not otherwise specified" (American Psychiatric Association 2000; see individual sections on each of these disorders below). The night eating syndrome, although described many years ago in the 1950s by Stunkard, is also not yet officially recognized in DSM (see Stunkard et al. 1955, 2008) but is discussed in Chapter 9 of this volume ("Circadian Rhythms, Sleep, and Weight").

Tanofsky-Kraff and Yanovski (2004) differentiate actual eating disorders from "disordered, or non-normative eating." Disordered eating, for example, does not necessarily cause distress and hence should not be considered an eating disorder. It may include "objective" overeating without loss of control, eating without being hungry, eating without a regular pattern, or continual grazing, all of which may eventually contribute to weight gain and even the development of obesity.

But specific eating disorders are important because they frequently present with other comorbid psychiatric symptoms and are frequently undertreated (Hudson et al. 2007). Physicians, in general, as well as psychiatrists, often fail to inquire about the possibility of eating disorders when confronted with patients who have personality disorders or symptoms of anxiety or depression. In a sample of obese men and women who had binge eating disorder, Yanovski et al. (1993) found significantly higher rates of affective disorder, panic disorder, and personality disorders such as borderline and avoidant personality disorders in the subjects themselves, as well as substance use disorders in family members of almost half of the subjects. In fact, in their study, 60% of these obese subjects with binge eating disorder had an Axis I diagnosis. Kaye et al. (2004) noted the presence of anxiety disorders, often originating in childhood before the onset of the eating disorder, in a large nonclinical sample of more than 650 individuals (predominantly women) with anorexia and/or bulimia. Many described symptoms of anxiety "as long as they can remember." Two-thirds of the subjects had one or more anxiety disorders, most commonly obsessive-compulsive disorder (in 41%, with symptoms including the need for symmetry, exactness, and order) and social phobia (in 20%). Even those without a diagnosed disorder tended to be anxious and harm avoidant.

Godart et al. (2006) studied a population of young French women who sought treatment for eating disorders. There were 271 subjects, of whom 111 had restrictive anorexia nervosa, 55 had symptoms of anorexia and bulimia, 86 had bulimia nervosa, and 19 had binge eating disorder without purging. Godart and his group found an "extremely high frequency" of both depressive and anxiety disorders among the subjects. Furthermore, when a subject had at least one anxiety disorder (generalized anxiety was the most common) she had a significantly greater chance (2.4–4.2 times greater) of developing depression. The other two common anxiety disorders were obsessive-compulsive disorder, which increased the risk of depression by 350%, and social phobia, which increased depressive risk by 300%. When considering the decision to hospitalize a patient with an eating disorder, a physician should therefore consider not only the patient's weight but her depressive status as well, something not commonly done in the United States or in France (Godart et al. 2006).

Grilo et al. (2007) noted significant comorbidity of Axis II disorders with bulimia nervosa and the general category of eating disorders not otherwise specified. They studied 92 female subjects for 5 years as part of a personality disorder study to ascertain the natural course of personality disorders in real-world clinical settings. Of all subjects with an eating disorder, 15 had no personality disorder and 77 had at least one of the four personality disorders studied (borderline, avoidant, schizotypal, and obsessive). The two categories of eating disorders showed similar patterns of remissions and relapses, and the presence of a personality disorder "counterintuitively" seemed not to have a significant impact on prognosis of the eating disorder. Almost 75% of those with bulimia had a remission, but 47% of them relapsed during the course of the study; 83% of those with nonspecified eating disorder had a remission, and of those, about 42% relapsed within the 5-year period. The study did not explore or focus on what treatments were given.

And in a sample of almost 3,000 respondents in a nationally representative survey, the first national survey to study eating disorders specifically, comorbidity was high: more than half of those with anorexia nervosa, over 94% with bulimia nervosa, almost 80% with binge eating disorder, and almost 65% with subthreshold binge eating disorder met criteria for at least one other DSM-IV diagnosis, such as mood disorder, anxiety disorder, impulse control disorder, or substance use disorder (Hudson et al. 2007). Surprisingly, there were more men than in previous assessments of eating disorders (one-fourth of the individuals with anorexia nervosa and one-fourth of those with bulimia nervosa). As would be predicted, a lifetime prevalence of anorexia led to a persistently low BMI value (<18.5), even after resolution of the disorder, and in those with binge eating disorder there was a strong association with severe obesity (BMI value >40. Further, fewer than half of those with bulimia or binge eating disorders had ever sought treatment specifically for their eating disorder, though the majority of those with all three (including anorexia) had sought help for other emotional disturbances. Binge eating disorder seems to be a chronic condition that occurs more commonly than either anorexia or bulimia and represents a "public health problem at least equal to that of the other two better established [disorders]" (Hudson et al. 2007).

Food is neither an antidepressant nor an antianxiety agent, though temporarily it may seem so. Many persons, particularly those with a tendency to binge, characteristically reach for the so-called comfort foods when they are in psychological distress. Most never choose a salad when under stress, just as the subjects in Baumeister and Härter's (2008) experiments never impulsively bought light bulbs or toilet paper when they were stressed. When we shift to psychological survival mode, we go for the fats and the sweets—

> No one eats salad under stress; we go for the comfort food, especially the sweets. This psychological survival mode alters the intricate biochemical feedback system, setting the stage for obesity.

and not the sweets of fruits. We indulge in the super sweets—cakes, cookies, pies—because we confuse the *psychological* survival mode with *biological* survival.

Some researchers, like Dallman and colleagues (2003), theorize that we eat "comfort food" (highly caloric foods high in fat and carbohydrates) to reduce our levels of anxiety that result from excessive activity of the chronic stress system (the HPA axis). Dallman et al. (2003) suggest that we tend to eat comfort foods in the context of chronic stress because glucocorticoids produced during stress increase the "salience" of both pleasurable activities (e.g., eating sugar and fatty foods) and compulsive activities (e.g., taking drugs). These researchers note that although chronic stress tends to increase glucocorticoid production in rats, it usually leads to a decrease in their weight. In humans, by contrast, chronic stress can lead either to increased intake of comfort foods and subsequent weight gain, or to decreased intake of food and subsequent weight loss. Those who gravitate toward comfort foods, according to the researchers, may be attempting to self-medicate by changing this intricate biochemical feedback system. Eating comfort foods is often seen in the extreme in those with binge eating disorder.

So far, this section has discussed comorbidity of psychiatric symptoms with eating disorders in general. Below, each of the three major eating disorders is considered specifically.

Binge Eating Disorder

Stunkard introduced the term *binge eating* in the late 1950s (Stunkard 1959). He spoke of patients he had seen who had an "irresistible compulsion to overeat" and noted the eating had an "orgiastic quality to it." It is ironic that though this syndrome was first described 50 years ago, it has yet to make it into our psychiatric nomenclature as an official diagnosis. In other words, DSM-IV-TR does not include binge eating as an eating disorder. As mentioned earlier, at this point it is classified as an "eating disorder not otherwise specified" (American Psychiatric Association 2000). Although some still question the validity of the diagnosis, others see it as a stable

Binge eating disorder is a chronic condition; although it occurs more commonly than anorexia and bulimia it receives less attention, and it is closely associated with obesity.

syndrome, presenting a single continuous episode across a person's lifetime rather than multiple episodes. It seems to be the most common of the eating disorders, with reports that about 2.8% of adults are affected (Pope et al. 2006).

Aspects of the definition are, though, at best quite arbitrary and inexact. Bingeing requires eating a quantity of food greater than normal in a restricted (2-hour) time period. Bingeing may occur many times a week and, if serious enough, many times in one day. Several thousands of calories can be eaten at one sitting. Though researchers such as Pope et al. (2006) describe the course as stable and chronic, others have noted it can be episodic and made worse by stresses in a person's life. If the condition is troubling enough, a person may have comorbid depression and even consider suicide. Recently, *New York Times* health columnist Jane Brody (2007) admitted she had been a binge eater years ago (eating 3,000 calories at one sitting) and had thought of suicide. Though Brody sought psychotherapeutic help from a psychologist, she said she had to stop the binges on her own.

Yanovski (1995) found that those with binge eating disorder have an "all-or-none" attitude in their food intake: when they have "lapses in adherence," as she called them, these lapses are considerable. The primary mechanism underlying binge eating in those who are obese is *disinhibition*, that is, a loss of control due to cognitive or emotional factors.

We do not really know what leads a person to develop binge eating disorder, but there are probably both psychological and biological factors involved. For example, there seems to be some genetic component because eating disorders and mood disorders often run in families of binge eaters. There may be a disorder of the neurotransmitter serotonin; cerebrospinal fluid levels of a metabolite of serotonin have been found to be abnormal in binge eaters, and positron emission tomography scans have shown abnormalities. Branson et al. (2003) report that some patients with binge eating disorder have phenotype abnormalities in their melanocortin 4 receptor gene (*MC4R*), though others have disputed the connection (Gotoda 2003). There have not been consistent findings, but there are reports of abnormalities in the secretion of certain hormones such as cortisol, which has a diurnal rhythm in all of us. There has also been speculation that vagal dysfunction may play a role in bingeing (Yanovski 1995). The urge to binge can seem completely out of control for a person when he or she is alone, and yet if another person enters the room, the binge is likely to stop.

Binge eating is considered one of those intermittent excessive behaviors that are continued despite the possibility of negative consequences. It has been associated with gambling, drug abuse, alcoholism, aberrant sexual behavior, and other harmful behaviors. Excessive eating has been induced in rats when the animals were given limited access (e.g., 2 hours, three times a week) to a more palatable food than their typical food. The pattern, interestingly enough, took 4 weeks to develop in the rats, but it was "easily maintained" once it was established, and the researchers believe this limited-access protocol has specific relevance to binge eating in humans (Corwin 2006). These researchers also found in rat experiments that certain neuropeptides that regulate fat intake, such as galanin and enterostatin, behave differently under conditions of limited access—that is, the actual neurobiology of fat intake is different during binge eating. For example, enterostatin, believed to be involved in fat-mediated satiety, did not have the same effect when the availability of fat was limited. Eventually this difference may lead to novel therapeutic approaches.

Successful treatment currently often involves both medication—usually a trial of a medication that increases the neurotransmitter serotonin, an SSRI such as fluoxetine or sertraline or citalopram—and psychotherapy. Even the opioid antagonists, such as naltrexone (100 mg), have been used, in combination with an SSRI, to reduce bingeing (Neumeister et al. 1999). Reas and Grilo (2008) evaluated randomized, placebo-controlled studies of pharmacological treatments for binge eating disorder. They evaluated 14 studies that included over 1,200 patients. Their tentative conclusion was that medications (SSRIs, tricyclics, and others), at least in the short term, are more effective than placebo for binge eating disorder; combination treatment with medication and cognitive or behavioral therapy (tested in only eight studies), however, did not improve the bingeing disorder beyond medication itself. They also found that although medication treatment may have increased the likelihood of eliminating or reducing bingeing, it did not necessarily lead to weight loss. Significantly, to date none of the studies reported follow-up data after the initial medication was discontinued. Only the addition of specific weight loss medications, such as orlistat or topiramate, led to weight loss in these studies. It should be noted that 12 of these 14 studies were funded by drug manufacturers, and therefore one should interpret these conclusions cautiously (Reas and Grilo 2008).

Another aspect of treating those with binge eating disorder is the importance of establishing "normal" patterns of eating. Allison et al. (2005) note that binge eaters are particularly prone to chaotic eating patterns, characterized by irregular patterns of meals, grazing, and skipping meals entirely, as well as actual binges.

Anorexia Nervosa

Some researchers, such as Halmi and Attia, believe anorexia nervosa has been around at least since the time of the fourteenth-century Saint Catherine of Siena (who supposedly could live on air). The disease was identified independently by Sir William Gull and Charles Lasègue around the 1870s when they each saw cases of "self-starvation" in young girls (Andersen and Yager 2009, p. 2130). Though people often shorten its name, the full name of the disorder is *anorexia nervosa*. The name implies a lack of appetite with an origin involving the nerves and is actually a misnomer, because anorexia is not necessarily a disease of appetite loss or diminishment.

Many diseases can present with reduced appetite without body image distortion. A differential diagnostic workup is obviously essential to rule out tumors, endocrine disorders, and other physical conditions.

Anorexia nervosa is a potentially fatal disease and in fact has the highest mortality rate among all psychiatric disorders (Yager and Powers 2007, p. 10–11). In one follow-up study of more than 10 years, there was a mortality rate of almost 7.5%, and almost one-quarter of these deaths were by suicide (Keel et al. 2003). It is an eating disorder that typically begins in adolescence (though it can begin as early as prepuberty and in adulthood), characterized by severe distortions in body image and an intense fear of gaining weight, despite maintaining a weight 85% of normal. In those who have reached puberty, it is also characterized by a loss of regular menstrual periods (amenorrhea). It is overwhelmingly more common in females, with up to 95% of those diagnosed being females. Andersen and Yager (2009, p. 2129) describe three major components to the diagnosis: 1) the behavioral component of self-starvation; 2) a psychopathological component of a "relentless drive for thinness" combined with a "morbid fear" of becoming fat; and 3) a physiological component of medical signs and symptoms, such as amenorrhea. The distortions in body image can be psychotic in that the person literally cannot distinguish perception from reality and, no matter how often confronted with reality, maintains that she or he is fat even when actually emaciated. There are two major subtypes of anorexia nervosa: the *restricting type* and the *binge eating/purging type*. Those who have the restricting type restrict their calories, often to starvation rations, without vomiting, bingeing, or engaging in any other compensatory behaviors such as laxative or diuretic use, excessive exercise, or use of enemas. Those who have the binge eating/purging type (the majority of those with anorexia nervosa) have symptoms of bulimia, including inducing vomiting and/or the use of laxatives, diuretics, enemas, or excessive exercise as compensatory behaviors. Although both forms are potentially deadly, the binge eating/purging type is more commonly associated with suicide and other impulse control disorders such as substance abuse. There can also be those with anorexia nervosa who have a mixture of both types in that they sometimes restrict and sometimes purge. This is called *diagnostic migration* (Yager and Powers 2007, p. 10).

Anorexia nervosa can affect every system in the body, mostly because of the effects of starvation, and in fact, it is sometimes difficult to tease out those effects from the actual effects of anorexia. There can be cardiac arrhythmias, endocrine abnormalities (including amenorrhea, infertility, and thyroid dysfunction), osteoporosis, abnormal electrolyte levels (including elevated blood urea nitrogen levels, indicative of failing kidney function), anemia, and even abnormalities in the brain's gray matter, among others. One of the most serious long-term complications is osteoporosis, and apparently the longer someone has the disease, the more intractable is the osteoporosis. In other words, though many other symptoms resolve with refeeding, the osteoporosis does not in those who have had the disease longer than a year (Attia and Walsh 2007).

Years ago, those who studied anorexia nervosa, such as Hilde Bruch in the 1950s, thought that strong dynamic factors were involved in the etiology. More recently, researchers have focused on risk factors such as early feeding difficulties, symptoms of anxiety, and the need for perfection in the context of demanding parents (Attia and Walsh 2007). Initially there was the belief that cultural issues were involved, but the disorder is no longer considered specific to a type of culture. There is a strong genetic component, with estimates of up to 84% for heritability (Attia and Walsh 2007). There also is a strong indication of abnormalities in neurotransmitters, particularly serotonin, though it is not clear whether this is the cause or the result of the disorder. Some with anorexia nervosa have significantly lower levels of serotonin metabolites in their cerebrospinal fluid while the disease is active, but after recovery these levels increase. Other serotonin receptor activity shows persistent abnormalities even after recovery, and there is speculation that differences in certain receptors may be involved in the different subtypes of anorexia (restrictive vs. bingeing/purging). Further, those with anorexia nervosa may have symptoms of anxiety and obsessional symptoms (that predate the anorexia and begin in childhood) because of a dysregulation of their serotonin system. There is even the suggestion that medications like the SSRIs work better after recovery (i.e., after "nutritional restoration") because of the particular serotonin system of the anorexic individual. Further, it is not clear why the disorder seems to be so much more common in women than men (with a ratio of 10 to 1) (Kaye et al. 2005).

More recent research has focused on brain imaging studies in patients with anorexia nervosa to assess the effect of the disease on the brain. Mühlau et al. (2007) looked at brain scans of women who had recovered from anorexia (having attained BMI values > 17 and regular menstrual periods for 6 months). There was generalized loss of gray matter (but not white matter) across the entire brain, but particularly in the region of the anterior cingulate cortex, the area of the brain involved in emotion, reward seeking, attention, language, motor behavior, and learning, among other functions. It was not clear, though, whether this specific decrease in gray matter was a cause of the anorexia (and hence involved in its pathophysiology) or an effect of the anorexia, or even whether this decrease in gray matter in the anterior cingulate cortex stemmed from environmental or genetic factors. The specific changes in this region did correlate with the severity of the anorexia the patients had experienced. Follow-up of 6 months may not have been long enough to ascertain whether the brain changes were permanent (Mühlau et al. 2007).

Other recent research has focused on ways to predict outcomes and the potential for relapse in patients with anorexia nervosa. In a study of 32 women who had been hospitalized, patients with a lower percentage of body fat at the time of discharge (after weight restoration) did significantly worse. Among all the variables studied, including serum cortisol levels, serum leptin levels, BMI values, and waist-to-hip ratios, only percentage of body fat predicted outcomes. Even the distribution of body fat (as noted in the waist-to-hip measurement) was not predictive of outcome. The percentage of body fat may be particularly important because that may involve restoration of reproductive function (related to leptin, though not a factor here). It is possible that body composition testing may eventually be seen as a worthwhile predictive assessment (Mayer et al. 2007).

Steinhausen et al. (2009) more recently also emphasized the importance of monitoring a patient's weight, as measured by BMI. In their study of 212 adolescents (ages 10–18, with almost 95% female), they conclude, "Recovery from anorexia nervosa in the short and the long-term run cannot be achieved without the interventions aiming at restoration of normal weight," since being so substantially underweight (BMI <17.5 kg/m^2) has "far-reaching consequences for health and wellbeing."

Earlier, Steinhausen (2002) had conducted a meta-analysis (with > 5,500 patients and almost 30 years of follow-up) and found only half of the patients were able to have a full recovery, and of these, one-third had relapses. Another one-third reported some improvement but were still plagued with symptoms (Yager and Powers 2007, p. 10). Furthermore, 20% remained "chronically ill." Steinhausen (2002) concluded that "anorexia remains a mental illness with a serious course and outcome." In general, he found that patients with anorexia nervosa had other psychiatric illnesses as well, such that one-fourth had anxiety disorders, one-fourth had affective disorders, and "substance use disorders, OCD, and obsessive-compulsive personality disorder were very common diagnoses at outcome." Steinhausen (2002) found "almost unanimous evidence" that the symptoms of vomiting, bulimia and purging, chronicity, and "features" of obsessive-compulsive personality disorder were poor prognostic signs; patients with a histrionic personality disorder, though, apparently are more apt to have a positive prognosis. He reports that early age of onset, short duration of symptoms prior to coming for treatment, a "good parent-child relationship" and high socioeconomic status did not have any consistent significance across studies in terms of prognostic value. Steinhausen (2002) further emphasized that patients, in general, do better prognostically with "extended" follow-up (i.e., more than 4 years and even 10 years or more).

In an editorial in the *American Journal of Psychiatry*, Halmi (2008) noted that when she reviewed the research conducted with randomized, placebo-controlled treatment trials for anorexia nervosa, she found "a dismal state of affairs." One of the major problems in conducting research, besides the fact that the disease is rare (Bissada et al. 2008), is the significantly high rate of refusals by adults to participate in a treatment study. Another is the dropout rate (~40% in most treatment trials with adults). Bissada et al. (2008) illustrated this dramatically with a flowchart in their study of the efficacy of olanzapine for weight gain and relief of psychiatric symptoms, such as depression, anxiety, and obsessions and compulsions: of 147 patients referred for treatment, between those who were excluded, those who would not participate in a day hospital treatment trial, and those who failed to complete the 13-week trial, only 14 patients receiving the medication (and 14 control subjects who did not) remained. Incidentally, results from this study indicated that olanzapine was effective in producing greater and more rapid weight gain in the anorexic patients who did complete the study, and there were also improvements in the patients' symptoms of depression, anxiety, and obsessive and compulsive symptoms. However, there is the concern, with use of atypical psychotics, that type 2 diabetes may develop, as well as cardiac disease. A 13-week trial may be too short to elicit these potentially dangerous symptoms.

Family studies, with younger patients, have a lower dropout rate (10%–20%), probably only because parents have the "authority legally to compel underage patients to participate" (Halmi 2008). Halmi does not believe there will be effective treatments for anorexia "until we decipher the reinforcing neurobiological mechanisms sustaining the disorder."

Despite the difficulties in conducting research, there are specific aims in treatment for anorexia nervosa (American Psychiatric Association 2006). Most important, obviously, given that this is potentially a life-or-death situation, is to restore patients to a healthy weight (*nutritional rehabilitation*) in order to restore normal endocrine system functioning, as well as to treat all the physical complications. Many times this requires an inpatient treatment setting with a team of specialists. Only then can physicians turn their attention to treating psychological issues. Cognitive therapy, medication management (particularly using the SSRIs, with fluoxetine doses of up to 60 mg), and family therapy all have a place in the treatment of anorexia nervosa. Because of the likelihood of recurrence, a treatment team must have a long-term plan.

Bulimia Nervosa

The word *bulimia*, not used until the 1980s, literally means "ox-hunger," and like *anorexia nervosa*, the full name implies an origin in the nervous system. Also like anorexia nervosa, it is a disorder that often begins in adolescence, but bulimia nervosa is characterized by recurrent, discrete, uncontrollable episodes of eating huge quantities of food (binges), sometimes as much as thousands of calories at one time. An average binge may have been reported to consist of 1,500 to 2,000 calories when self-reports were obtained, but up to 4,500 calories in one episode (and up to 9,000 calories within 24 hours) when inpatient records were kept (Kaye et al. 1993). What differentiates bulimia from binge eating disorder is the use of inappropriate compensatory mechanisms to avoid weight gain, such as vomiting. Vomiting is a fairly effective means of ridding the body of all the extra calories eaten. Those with bulimia may retain a similar number of calories irrespective of the number of calories actually eaten: one study showed that no matter how many calories were eaten, only

> Researchers in one study found that no matter how many calories people with bulimia nervosa ate, they retained only about 1,200 of these calories after vomiting.
>
> **Source: Kaye et al. 1993**

about 1,200 of these calories were retained after vomiting, for reasons that were not clear to the examiners (Kaye et al. 1993).

Bulimia nervosa, just like anorexia nervosa, is overwhelmingly more common in females. Up to 95% of those with the disorder are females, and the disorder occurs in up to 4% of some populations (Yager and Powers 2007, p. 17). No one knows the etiology of bulimia nervosa, but there is definitely a genetic component and there is some evidence of hormonal abnormalities, such as elevated levels of neuropeptide Y (the intestinal hormone that increases appetite) and lower levels of cholecystokinin, as well as abnormalities on functional magnetic resonance imaging (MRI) scans (see Bailer and Kaye 2003; Kaye 2008). Marsh et al. (2009) investigated functional MRI scans of 20 women with bulimia nervosa and 20 healthy control subjects while they were performing a task involving self-regulation. The investigators are cautious in interpreting their results (and recommend future studies of larger samples) because they were studying only adult women who had had bulimia chronically and were in different stages of treatment (some who were inpatients, some not receiving treatment but still having symptoms, and others). Further, the researchers did not have a control group of women who had impulse disorders but normal weight. Nevertheless, those women who had bulimia nervosa had diminished activity in certain areas of the brain such as the prefrontal cortex (i.e., frontostriatal areas) that are related to impulse control—that is, self-regulatory mechanisms. Furthermore, those who were more symptomatic (had more bulimic episodes) had even less activity in these areas, so there seems to be a "dose-dependence" relationship. Those with bulimia may have abnormal transmission of serotonin, and possibly abnormal dopaminergic transmission as well, which may be responsible for the impaired self-control regarding their bingeing.

About 80%–90% of bulimic individuals induce vomiting; this is called the *purging type*. They may also abuse laxatives, enemas, and/or diuretics. The *nonpurging* bulimic individuals compensate by overdoing exercise or fasting, but not by vomiting. During a binge, the food is eaten rapidly, often voraciously, as if nothing could satisfy. Arbitrarily, the DSM-IV-TR diagnosis specifies that the enormous (also completely arbitrary) quantity of food is eaten in a discrete period of time (within 2 hours; American Psychiatric Association 2000, p. 589). Typically the binges consist of fats and carbohydrates, particularly cakes, cookies, ice cream, and bread, but sometimes just any food available. Bingeing is overwhelmingly more common in women than men. The binges are often done in secret, and they are often followed by feelings of anxiety and remorse at the uncontrollable behavior. Because of the compensatory behavior and their preoccupation with their body shape and weight, those with bulimia nervosa often stay within a normal weight range, although their weight may fluctuate over time. This population has higher comorbidity with other disorders of impulse control, including stealing and even cutting behavior, as well as anxiety disorders such as obsessive-compulsive disorder. In some studies, the lifetime prevalence rate for obsessive-compulsive disorder in bulimic individuals has been greater than 40% (Kaye et al. 2004).

Bulimia nervosa, although significantly less deadly than anorexia nervosa, is nevertheless a serious disorder. Only half of patients achieve a full recovery, and of those who recover, about one-third have a relapse (Yager and Powers 2007, p. 20). There are many potential medical complications, including electrolyte imbalances, electrocardiographic abnormalities, muscle weakness, erosion of tooth enamel and possibly gum recession, abdominal symptoms (e.g., esophagitis, irritable bowel, or even esophageal rupture), and infertility problems (Yager and Powers 2007, p. 14).

Treatment usually does not require hospitalization, but a multimodal treatment team approach may be crucial. A team may consist of a nutritionist (for nutritional rehabilitation), a psychiatrist (to prescribe medication such as an SSRI), a psychologist (e.g., for cognitive therapy), and a social worker (e.g., for family therapy). Because of the potential for recurrence, a long-term treatment plan is essential.

Comorbidity of Eating Disorders With Alcohol and Drug Abuse

Comorbidity with abuse of alcohol and other drugs is fairly common in eating disorders. Abuse and dependence prevalence rates can be as high as 38% in individuals who have the binge eating/purging type of anorexia nervosa, compared with prevalence rates of only about 17% in those who have the restricting type of the disorder (Yager and Powers 2007, p. 82). The prevalence of alcohol abuse and dependence can be considerably higher in those with bulimia nervosa, with rates as high as 46% reported (Yager and Powers 2007, p. 83). Other substance abuse is also fairly commonly seen in patients with eating disorders, particularly in those with bulimia and anorexia nervosa; the lifetime prevalence is 22%–26% (Yager and Powers 2007, pp. 82–83). Substance abuse in binge eating disorder is less common, because the same reward systems in the brain may be involved in these two types of behavior and they show an inverse relationship.

The following case illustration describing a young female with bulimia nervosa, a substance abuse disorder, and borderline personality disorder brings to mind Leon Kass's observation "The hungry soul wants more than food" (Kass 1994, p. 52).

Bulimia Nervosa and Substance Abuse in Borderline Personality Disorder

Carolyn, a 17-year-old college student, had had bulimia since she was 14. In her preadolescent years, she was short and chubby but she didn't really care because she considered herself a tomboy. Her weight and strength, in fact, helped her wrestle with her brothers, play soccer and baseball, and be accepted by other boys—especially by friends of her older brother. The only unhappy people in the picture were Carolyn's parents. They cajoled her to lose weight, they pleaded with her, threatened her, embarrassed her, deprived her, you name it—nothing helped. Carolyn either remained relatively indifferent to their anxiety and totally oblivious to her own weight situation, or she became oppositional and defiant and ate even more. When she turned 15 years old, all of a sudden her weight became her own problem and it hit her like a ton of bricks.

Her brother's friends began avoiding her. They neither wanted to play nor to socialize with her. They were now clustering around more attractive and thinner girls and fiercely competing for their attention. She tried to join those girls, in whom she had had no interest in the past; they didn't want anything to do with her and even openly mocked her. Carolyn felt rejected and isolated.

Her parents, both fairly narcissistic and preoccupied with their own appearance, were rejecting also, with a "we told you so" attitude. Nonetheless, they took her to a pediatrician and to a number of dietitians who tried to restrict her calorie intake, but to no avail. She couldn't give up her old habit of gorging herself no matter what kind of food was in front of her.

Gradually the girl who had been sweet, affectionate, and good-natured turned into an angry and hostile adolescent. She cursed her mother for giving her such hefty thighs and blamed her father for marrying a woman of Polish genes.

She would hit her thighs and her buttocks to the point of making them black and blue. She hated everyone, especially herself. She relentlessly demanded breast reduction surgery and liposuction, and this became another source of conflict with her parents, who refused to consider allowing them. She stole her younger brother's Ritalin to suppress her appetite. Of course, this was quickly discovered and she was reprimanded.

It is not clear how or from whom she learned, but one day she figured out that by putting her fingers deep into her throat, she could vomit most of the food she had eaten. Eventually, that became her daily routine after practically every meal. She would eat everything in sight and then go to the bathroom and vomit whatever she could. Even in restaurants, as soon as she finished one course, she would excuse herself to leave the table. Her parents detected the faint odor of vomit, but initially did not confront her because they actually were pleased to see she was losing some weight. Carolyn also began abusing laxatives to get rid of any food left in her gastrointestinal tract.

Now that she had found "the solution," she would binge on the worst possible food, the unhealthiest stuff, sometimes several times a day, for she declared her body "enemy territory." To the question "Why are you torturing your stomach?" she tersely replied that it was only "a fair reciprocation."

Her weight now hovered around normal because of all her bingeing, but she looked terrible and she was very malnourished. Her health was deteriorating—the enamel of her teeth was even beginning to erode from the acidic bile of her vomit, and her breasts and buttocks were sagging. She would not exercise, because exercise builds muscles and she had heard that muscle weighs more than fat; she was anemic and looked tired and depressed. Her parents finally grew concerned and took her to an internist, who prescribed an SSRI, but she never took it because she had heard that these medications cause you to put on weight (sometimes they do, particularly over time). Meanwhile, as thin as she became, boys were still avoiding her. The internist grew particularly concerned when Carolyn's routine blood tests showed evidence of low potassium levels (hypokalemia). An ECG actually showed an arrhythmia and a chest X ray showed an enlarged heart (cardiomegaly). It was at that point that the internist called in both Carolyn and her parents and told them that she and the family needed to seek psychiatric consultation.

Carolyn was not an easy patient. Her major defense was that of *regression;* that is, she often resorted to an earlier level of functioning by having temper tantrums and even refusing to come to the initial consultation. Her parents, finally desperate to help, ultimately persuaded her to come with them. The psychiatrist recommended family therapy with a social worker to deal with the dynamics in the family, including the fact that Carolyn's mother had serious eating issues herself (she tended to restrict her calories and had actually bordered on anorexia nervosa much of her own life). The psychiatrist also recommended that Carolyn take an SSRI because her eating disorder had reached life-threatening proportions. When her parents threatened to hospitalize her if she did not comply, Carolyn finally agreed.

When the biological balance of the body is severely disrupted, no psychological approach alone can be effective. Even if the patient's eating problem originated, in part, from psychological conflicts, it can no longer be undone exclusively by psychological means. The biophysiological system of the person has to be stabilized first by some medical interventions. Only afterward can psychotherapy combined with pharmacotherapy become useful and effective. A psychiatrist must work with a treatment team (including a nutritionist, a cognitive therapist, and a social worker) in concert to address the potentially destructive behavior.

Carolyn's treatment was further complicated by her *borderline personality disorder:* she had strong fears of abandonment and a chronic sense of emptiness, as well as a history of very unstable relationships with her peers. She tended to idealize some of her friends, only to devalue them later, and she was quite impulsive and self-destructive, not only in her eating pattern, but also in a tendency to abuse alcohol and even diet pills when she could obtain them. Getting her to understand her mind was difficult and time-consuming because Carolyn was quite reluctant to do so. But eventually she had a significant insight: she was still throwing up not just "the bad food" but also her "bad old self-image." She needed to go back psychologically to her preadolescent years to recapture her love of herself. After that the result was remarkable. Now all she needed was to feed "her loved body" with good stuff. Providing that information was the easiest task.

ALCOHOL AND WEIGHT

Alcohol is a carbohydrate without any nutritional value. In effect, it is liquid sugar but with a higher calorie count than most other carbohydrates (7 cal/g compared with 4 cal/g). It is true that a substance in red wine, resveratrol, has properties that promote good health, and some researchers suggest a glass of red wine daily can be part of a healthy diet, particularly for the heart, but in general alcohol has more negative than positive effects in weight control.

Any alcohol excess, though, besides putting weight on the belly, will fatten the liver and damage the dendrites (communication wires) of the brain cells. By interfering with the absorption of vitamin B, it also causes peripheral neurological damage and central neurological atrophies, resulting in unsteadiness, weakness, inattentiveness, and loss of memory.

Furthermore, excessive, chronic use of alcohol can lead to weight gain because of its own caloric impact, as well as the fact that people often do not realize how much they are actually eating when they drink simultaneously. And alcohol can cause sleep disturbances, which (as we discuss in Chapter 9 of this volume) can have their own impact on weight gain.

As we have noted earlier, those with a predisposition to sugar abuse *may* be more likely to be predisposed to alcohol abuse, because the reward circuits in the brain are similar. (See "Reward, Cravings, and Addiction" section in Chapter 4, "The Psychology of the Eater.") Kalarchian et al. (2007) suggest that prospective studies involving "diverse, community-based cohorts" are needed. Warren and Gold (2007), using chart reviews, report that those with a weight problem were *less* prone to substance abuse difficulties. They believe that obesity (and even being overweight) may actually be protective against drug addiction, as well as alcohol and even marijuana use. Because both alcohol and marijuana may act as stimulants to appetite acutely, they acknowledge that the relationship of substance abuse, weight, and the reward circuitry of the brain is a complex one. Wadden and Phelan (2002, p. 198) also reported that their obese women patients were less likely to abuse alcohol, with fewer than 10%

ALCOHOL AND WEIGHT

- Alcohol is a carbohydrate with a high calorie count (7 cal/g) and without any nutritional value.

- At 7 calories per gram, alcohol provides more calories than proteins or carbohydrates (each about 4 calories per gram).

- The body has no capacity to store alcohol, but while waiting for oxidation, it circulates in the blood and can reach toxic levels.

- If protein, fat, or carbohydrates are consumed simultaneously with alcohol, their oxidation will be suppressed because alcohol is preferentially oxidized, leading to fat accumulation in the body.

- Alcohol stimulates appetite, prolongs meal duration, and leads to continued eating even after one is full.

Source: Melanson and Dwyer 2002, p. 278

having a history of substance abuse or dependence. Though their obese male patients abused alcohol somewhat more than their female patients, Wadden and Phelan note that substance abuse was also "uncommon" in their male patients. Patients with concomitant substance abuse had a poorer prognosis. These authors recommend that substance abuse be treated prior to attempts at weight reduction. Lundgren et al. (2006), in contrast to the studies by Warren and Gold (2007) or Wadden and Phelan (2002, p. 198), in a study of the night eating syndrome, found substance abuse, particularly

- Nonalcoholic beer has the same number of calories as alcoholic beer (~150 per pint).

- Dry wine and champagne (100 calories) have fewer calories than a sweet dessert wine.

- The number of calories in hard liquor depends on the proof.

- Large mixed drinks, such as margaritas, can have about 400 calories each, a piña colada has about 260 calories, and a Bloody Mary has about 115 calories.

Source: Grieger 2009

ALCOHOL AND HEALTH

- Severe complications of alcohol withdrawal can include visual, tactile, or auditory hallucinations (commonly called "the DTs," or delirium tremens), seizures, and even death.

- Because of the short half-life of alcohol, symptoms of alcohol withdrawal peak in intensity during the second day of abstinence and likely improve by the fourth or fifth day.

- Blackouts—period of amnesia for events that occur during alcohol intoxication when there is a high blood alcohol level—can be seen in heavy drinkers.

- Alcohol affects every organ in the body, including the brain, liver, gastrointestinal system, and skin: you are virtually pickling your body the more you drink; if you have a concentration of 100 milligrams of alcohol per deciliter of blood and do not show signs of intoxication, you are drinking too much and have probably developed some degree of tolerance.

- Alcohol during pregnancy can lead, in the child, to a specific syndrome of varying severity called *fetal alcohol syndrome* (distinctive, specific facial abnormalities; small head and deformities of the brain; learning disabilities and possibly mental retardation; hyperactivity; cardiac abnormalities).

- Women tend to develop higher blood alcohol levels than men with the same amount of consumption because of their higher percentage of body fat and their tendency to metabolize alcohol more slowly; they may therefore be at greater risk of developing alcohol-related health problems.

Source: DSM-IV-TR, pp. 214–222

alcohol abuse, among their population, and lifetime substance abuse was "more likely to occur" among patients with night eating syndrome (the majority of whom were overweight or obese) than in those patients without it (see Chapter 9, "Circadian Rhythms, Sleep, and Weight"). The connection between substance abuse and obesity is obviously a complex one, and there may be overlap among subsets of patients.

REFERENCES

Allison KC, Grilo CM, Masheb RM, et al: Binge eating disorder and night eating syndrome: a comparative study of disordered eating. J Consult Clin Psychol 73:1107–1115, 2005

American Psychiatric Association: Diagnostic and Statistical Manual of Mental Disorders, 4th Edition, Text Revision. Washington, DC, American Psychiatric Association, 2000

American Psychiatric Association: Treatment of patients with eating disorders, third edition. American Psychiatric Association. Am J Psychiatry 163 (7 suppl):4–54, 2006

Andersen AE, Yager J: Eating disorders, in Kaplan & Sadock's Comprehensive Textbook of Psychiatry, 9th Edition, Vol I. Edited by Sadock B, Sadock V, Ruiz P. Philadelphia, PA, Lippincott Williams & Wilkins, 2009, pp 2128–2149

Atlantis E, Baker M: Obesity effects on depression: systematic review of epidemiological studies. Int J Obes (Lond) 32:881–891, 2008

Atlantis E, Ball K: Association between weight perception and psychological distress. Int J Obes (Lond) 32:715–721, 2008

Attia E, Walsh BT: Anorexia nervosa: treatment in psychiatry. Am J Psychiatry 164:1805–1810, 2007

Bailer UF, Kaye WH: A review of neuropeptide and neuroendocrine dysregulation in anorexia and bulimia. Curr Drug Targets CNS Neurol Disord 2:53–59, 2003

Baumeister H, Härter M: Overweight and obesity are associated with psychiatric disorders: are they? (letter) Psychosom Med 70:1060; author reply 1060–1061, 2008

Bissada H, Tasca GA, Barber AM, et al: Olanzapine in the treatment of low body weight and obsessive thinking in women with anorexia nervosa: a randomized, double-blind, placebo-controlled trial. Am J Psychiatry 165:1281–1288, 2008

Bodenlos JS, Kose S, Borckardt JJ, et al: Vagus nerve stimulation acutely alters food craving in adults with depression. Appetite 48:145–153, 2007

Branson R, Potoczna N, Kral JG, et al: Binge eating as a major phenotype of melanocortin 4 receptor gene mutations. N Engl J Med 348:1096–1103, 2003

Brody JE: Out of control: a true story of binge eating. The New York Times, Personal Health section, February 20, 2007

Bruch H: Psychological aspects of reducing. Psychosom Med 14:337–346, 1952

Buescher LS, Buescher KL: Body dysmorphic disorder. Dermatol Clin 24:251–257, 2006

Corwin RL: Bingeing rats: a model of intermittent excessive behavior? Appetite 46:11–15, 2006

Crisp AH, McGuiness B: Jolly fat: relation between obesity and psychoneurosis in general population. Br Med J 1:7–9, 1976

Dallman MF, Pecoraro N, Aakana SF, et al: Chronic stress and obesity: a new view of "comfort food." Proc Natl Acad Sci U S A 100:11696–11701, 2003

Fink P, Ørnbol E, Toft T, et al: A new, empirically established hypochondriasis diagnosis. Am J Psychiatry 161:1680–1691, 2004

Foster GD, Kendall PC, Wadden TA, et al: Psychological effects of weight loss and regain: a prospective evaluation. J Consult Clin Psychol 64:752–757, 1996

Friedman MA, Brownell KD: Psychological correlates of obesity: moving to the next research generation. Psychol Bull 117:3–20, 1995

Godart NT, Perdereau F, Curt F, et al: Is major depressive episode related to anxiety disorders in anorexics and bulimics? Compr Psychiatry 47:91–98, 2006

Gold PW, Chrousos GP: Organization of the stress system and its dysregulation in melancholic and atypical depression: high vs low CRH/NE states. Mol Psychiatry 7:254–275, 2002

Gotoda T: Binge eating as a phenotype of melanocortin 4 receptor gene mutations. N Engl J Med 349:606–609, 2003

Grieger L: Is beer or wine making you fat? iVillage.co.uk Diet and Fitness. Available at: http://www.ivillage.co.uk/dietandfitness/nutrition/fooddiet/articles/0,9544,238_160400,00.html. Accessed November 13, 2009

Grilo CM, Pagano ME, Skodol AE, et al: Natural course of bulimia nervosa and of eating disorder not otherwise specified: 5-year prospective study of remissions, relapses, and the effects of personality disorder psychopathology. J Clin Psychiatry 68:738–746, 2007

Halmi KA: The perplexities of conducting randomized, double-blind, placebo-controlled treatment trials in anorexia nervosa patients (editorial). Am J Psychiatry 165:1227–1228, 2008

Hasler G, Pine DS, Gamma A, et al: The associations between psychopathology and being overweight: a 20-year prospective study. Psychol Med 34:1047–1057, 2004

Herman CP, Mack D: Restrained and unrestrained eating. J Pers 43:647–660, 1975

Hewig J, Cooper S, Trippe RH, et al: Drive for thinness and attention toward specific body parts in a nonclinical sample. Psychosom Med 70:729–736, 2008

Hudson JI, Hiripi E, Pope HG Jr, et al: The prevalence and correlates of eating disorders in the National Comorbidity Survey Replication. Biol Psychiatry 61:348–358, 2007

Kalarchian MA, Marcus MD, Levine MD, et al: Psychiatric disorders among bariatric surgery candidates: relationship to obesity and functional health status. Am J Psychiatry 164:328–334, 2007

Kass L: The Hungry Soul: Eating and the Perfecting of Our Nature. Chicago, IL, University of Chicago Press, 1994

Kaye W: Neurobiology of anorexia and bulimia nervosa. Physiol Behav 94:121–135, 2008

Kaye WH, Weltzin TE, Hsu G, et al: Amount of calories retained after binge eating and vomiting. Am J Psychiatry 1:969–971, 1993

Kaye WH, Bulik CM, Thornton L, et al; Price Foundation Collaborative Group: Comorbidity of anxiety disorders with anorexia and bulimia nervosa. Am J Psychiatry 161:2215–2221, 2004

Kaye WH, Frank GK, Bailer UF, et al: Neurobiology of anorexia nervosa: clinical implications of alterations of the function of serotonin and other neuronal systems. Int J Eat Disord 37 (suppl 1):S15–S19, 2005

Keel PK, Dorer DJ, Eddy KT, et al: Predictors of mortality in eating disorders. Arch Gen Psychiatry 60:179–183, 2003

Keys A, Fidanza F, Karvonen MJ, et al: Indices of relative weight and obesity. J Chron Dis 25:329–343, 1972

Lowe MR, Levine AS: Eating motives and the controversy over dieting: eating less than needed versus less than wanted. Obes Res 13:797–806, 2005

Lu XY: The leptin hypothesis of depression: a potential link between mood disorders and obesity? Curr Opin Pharmacol 7:648–652, 2007

Lundgren JD, Allison KC, Crow S, et al: Prevalence of the night eating syndrome in a psychiatric population. Am J Psychiatry 163:156–158, 2006

Marsh R, Steinglass JE, Gerber AJ, et al: Deficient activity in the neural systems that mediate self-regulatory control in bulimia nervosa. Arch Gen Psychiatry 66:51–63, 2009

Mather AA, Cox BJ, Enns MW, et al: Associations between body weight and personality disorders in a nationally representative sample. Psychosom Med 70:1012–1019, 2008

Mayer LE, Roberto CA, Glasofer DR, et al: Does percent body fat predict outcome in anorexia nervosa? Am J Psychiatry 164:970–972, 2007

McElroy SL, Kotwal R, Malhotra S, et al: Are mood disorders and obesity related? A review for the mental health professional. J Clin Psychiatry 65:634–651, 2004

McKinley NM: Resisting body dissatisfaction: fat women who endorse fat acceptance. Body Image 1:213–219, 2004

McLaren L, Beck CA, Patten SB, et al: The relationship between body mass index and mental health: a population-based study of the effects of the definition of mental health. Soc Psychiatry Psychiatr Epidemiol 43:63–71, 2008

Melanson K, Dwyer J: Popular diets for treatment of overweight and obesity, in Handbook of Obesity Treatment (Chapter 12, Appendix 1). Edited by Wadden TA, Stunkard, AJ. New York, Guilford, 2002, pp 249–282

Moore ME, Stunkard A, Srole L: Obesity, social class, and mental illness. JAMA 181:962–966, 1962

Mühlau M, Gaser C, Ilg R, et al: Gray matter decrease of the anterior cingulate cortex in anorexia nervosa. Am J Psychiatry 164:1850–1857, 2007

Neumeister A, Winkler A, Wöber-Bingöl C: Addition of naltrexone to fluoxetine in the treatment of binge eating disorder (letter). Am J Psychiatry 156:797, 1999

Occhiogrosso M: "Gourmandizing," gluttony and oral fixations: perspectives on overeating in the American Journal of Psychiatry, 1844 to the present, in Food for Thought: Essays on Eating and Culture. Edited by Rubin LC. Jefferson, NC, McFarland, 2008, pp 265–276

Pardo JV, Sheikh SA, Kuskowski MA, et al: Weight loss during chronic, cervical vagus nerve stimulation in depressed patients with obesity: an observation. Int J Obes 31:1756–1759, 2007

Petry NM, Barry D, Pietrzak RH, et al: Overweight and obesity are associated with psychiatric disorders: results from the National Epidemiologic Survey on Alcohol and Related Conditions. Psychosom Med 70:288–297, 2008

Phillips KA: Body dysmorphic disorder: the distress of imagined ugliness. Am J Psychiatry 148:1138–1149, 1991

Phillips KA, Pinto A, Menard W, et al: Obsessive-compulsive disorder versus body dysmorphic disorder: a comparison study of two possibly related disorders. Depress Anxiety 24:399–409, 2007

Phillips KA, Didie ER, Feusner J, et al: Body dysmorphic disorder: treating an underrecognized disorder. Am J Psychiatry 165:1111–1118, 2008

Pickering RP, Grant BF, Chou SP, et al: Are overweight, obesity, and extreme obesity associated with psychopathology? Results from the National Epidemiologic Survey on Alcohol and Related Conditions. J Clin Psychiatry 68:998–1009, 2007

Pope HG Jr, Lalonde JK, Pindyck LJ, et al: Binge eating disorder: a stable syndrome. Am J Psychiatry 163:2181–2183, 2006

Reas DL, Grilo CM: Review and meta-analysis of pharmacotherapy for binge-eating disorder. Obesity (Silver Spring) 16:2024–2038, 2008

Roberts RE, Deleger S, Strawbridge JW, et al: Prospective association between obesity and depression: evidence from the County Study. Int J Obes (Lond) 27:514–521, 2003

Saguy AC, Riley KW: Weighing both sides: morality, mortality, and framing contests over obesity. J Health Polit Policy Law 30:869–921, 2005

Sarwer DB, Thompson JK: Obesity and body image disturbance, in Handbook of Obesity Treatment. Edited by Wadden TA, Stunkard AJ. New York, Guilford, 2002, pp 447–464

Simon GE, Von Korff M, Saunders K, et al: Association between obesity and psychiatric disorders in the US adult population. Arch Gen Psychiatry 63:824–830, 2006

Smoller JW, Wadden TA, Stunkard AJ: Dieting and depression: a critical review. J Psychosom Res 31:429–440, 1987

Stefan N, Kantartzis K, Machann J, et al: Identification and characterization of metabolically benign obesity in humans. Arch Intern Med 168:1609–1616, 2008

Steinhausen H-C: The outcome of anorexia nervosa in the 20th century. Am J Psychiatry 159:1284–1293, 2002

Steinhausen H-C, Grigoroiu-Serbanescu M, Boyadjiva S, et al: The relevance of body weight in the medium term to long-term course of adolescent anorexia nervosa: findings from a multisite study. J Eat Disord 42:19–25, 2009

Straus R: Public attitudes regarding problem drinking and problem eating. Ann N Y Acad Sci 133:792–802, 1966

Stunkard AJ: The dieting depression: incidence and clinical characteristics of untoward responses to weight reduction regimens. Am J Med 23:77–86, 1957

Stunkard AJ: Eating patterns and obesity. Psychiatr Q 33:284–295, 1959

Stunkard A, Mendelson M: Obesity and the body image, I: characteristics of disturbances in the body image of some obese persons. Am J Psychiatry 123:1296–1300, 1967

Stunkard AJ, Messick S: The three-factor eating questionnaire to measure dietary restraint, disinhibition, and hunger. J Psychosom Res 29:71–83, 1985

Stunkard AJ, Rush J: Dieting and depression reexamined. Ann Intern Med 81:526–533, 1974

Stunkard AJ, Grace WJ, Wolff HG: The night-eating syndrome: a pattern of food intake among certain obese patients. Am J Med 19:78–86, 1955

Stunkard AJ, LaFleur WR, Wadden TA: Stigmatization of obesity in medieval times: Asia and Europe. Int J Obes (Lond) 22:1141–1144, 1998

Stunkard AJ, Faith MS, Allison KC: Depression and obesity. Biol Psychiatry 54:330–337, 2003

Stunkard AJ, Allison KC, Lundgren J: Issues for DSM-V: the night eating syndrome (editorial). Am J Psychiatry 165:424, 2008

Sullivan S, Cloninger CR, Przybeck TR, et al: Personality characteristics in obesity and relationship with successful weight loss. Int J Obes (Lond) 31:669–674, 2007

Tanofsky-Kraff M, Yanovski SZ: Eating disorder or disordered eating? Non-normative eating patterns in obese individuals. Obes Res 12:1361–1366, 2004

Vaccarino V, McClure C, Johnson D, et al: Depression, the metabolic syndrome and cardiovascular risk. Psychosom Med 70:40–48, 2008

van den Bree MB, Przybeck TR, Cloninger CR: Diet and personality: associations in a population-based sample. Appetite 46:177–188, 2006

Vogelzangs N, Kritchevsky SB, Beekman AT, et al: Depressive symptoms and change in abdominal obesity in older persons. Arch Gen Psychiatry 65:1386–1393, 2008

Wadden TA, Phelan S: Behavioral assessment of the obese patient, in Handbook of Obesity Treatment. Edited by Wadden TA, Stunkard AJ. New York, Guilford, 2002, pp 186–226

Wadden TA, Stunkard AJ: Social and psychological consequence of obesity. Ann Intern Med 103:1062–1067, 1985

Wadden TA, Stunkard AJ, Smoller JW: Dieting and depression: a methodological study. J Consult Clin Psychol 54:869–871, 1986

Wadden TA, Womble LG, Stunkard AJ, et al: Psychosocial consequences of obesity and weight loss, in Handbook of Obesity Treatment. Edited by Wadden TA, Stunkard AJ. New York, Guilford, 2002, pp 144–163

Warren MW, Gold MS: The relationship between obesity and drug use (letter). Am J Psychiatry 164:1268; author reply 1268–1269, 2007

Weinberg N, Mendelson M, Stunkard A: A failure to find distinctive personality features in a group of obese men. Am J Psychiatry 117:1035–1037, 1961

Willemen MJ, Mantel-Teeuwisse AK, Straus SM, et al: Psychiatric and cardiovascular comorbidities in patients with diabetes mellitus starting antiobesity drugs. Obesity (Silver Spring) 16:2331–2335, 2008

Yager J, Powers PS (eds): Clinical Manual of Eating Disorders. Washington, DC, American Psychiatric Publishing, 2007

Yanovski SZ: Biological correlates of binge eating. Addict Behav 20:705–712, 1995

Yanovski SZ, Nelson JE, Dubbert BK, et al: Association of binge eating disorder and psychiatric comorbidity in obese subjects. Am J Psychiatry 150:1472–1479, 1993

7

MEDICAL CONDITIONS AND WEIGHT

*Every reasonable being, understanding that health is the greatest blessing of all,
must know how to help himself in disease.*

Hippocrates, *On Hygiene*, #9 (Precope 1952, p. 191)

SOME PHYSICAL CAUSES OF WEIGHT GAIN

When a health care professional encounters a person who is overweight or obese, that professional must consider the importance of a diagnostic workup, not only to assess the consequences of the excess fat, but also to eliminate potentially reversible and treatable conditions. For the most part, serious medical conditions, and particularly chronic ones such as AIDS, cancer, and chronic lung or kidney disease, lead to a cachectic, wasting state. There are a few medical conditions, though, that actually lead to weight gain. A careful history, beginning from birth and including family history for a genetic contribution, is obviously the place to start when presented with a patient with overweight or obesity (Atkinson 2002; Wadden and Phelan 2002).

Obesity has been considered (and is still considered by some) to be a metabolic disturbance. There are several endocrine disorders that may lead to significant changes in weight, among myriad other symptoms, including psychiatric symptoms such as depression and anxiety. For example, thyroid disease may lead to weight loss if thyroid hormone levels are high or weight gain if thyroid hormone levels are low. Less commonly (Williams and Dluhy 2008, p. 2255), Cushing syndrome such as caused by adrenal hyperplasia or a tumor, in which there is excessive abnormal secretion of the adrenocortical hormones (e.g., cortisol), also produces weight gain in

94% of those afflicted, whereas a deficiency of cortisol secretion, as in Addison disease, produces considerable weight loss in 97% of patients (Williams and Dluhy 2008, p. 2263). Other uncommon endocrine disorders associated with weight changes include hypogonadism and polycystic ovary syndrome. Polycystic ovary syndrome is a rare genetic syndrome characterized by infertility, amenorrhea or irregular periods, hirsutism, and obesity in 40% of women with this syndrome; and even in those not obese, most have insulin resistance (Flier and Maratos-Flier 2008, p. 467). A leptin deficiency, which is an even more exceedingly rare genetic disorder, also produces massive obesity, beginning in early childhood and often with accompanying abnormalities of the reproductive system. The hormone leptin, produced by adipose tissue, can be given exogenously for replacement therapy, with substantial reversal of the massive obesity. (Leptin is discussed also in Chapter 5, "The Metabolic Complexities of Weight Control.")

ENDOCRINE DISORDERS THAT CAUSE WEIGHT GAIN

- Hypothyroidism
- Cushing syndrome
- Hypogonadism
- Polycystic ovary syndrome

An unusual, but interesting, cause of weight gain occurs as a postoperative side effect of subthalamic deep brain stimulation surgery in patients with Parkinson disease. This surgical procedure is a radical alternative treatment when the L-dopa treatment for parkinsonism, itself, produces disabling dyskinesias and drastically affects a patient's quality of life. The most common postsurgical side effects are speech disturbances such as dysarthria and hypophonia, postural instability, apathy, and weight gain (Guehl et al. 2006). In the 6 months following surgery in one small study, patients gained a mean of 10 pounds and almost one-fourth gained more than 20 pounds. In patients followed for a full year, weight gain continued (Tuite et al. 2005). Here it is speculated that weight gain seems associated with the decreased chronic tremor (and hence decreased resting energy expenditure) that is seen postoperatively (Macia et al. 2004).

SEXUAL AND REPRODUCTIVE FUNCTIONING AND OBESITY

> *When unnaturally fat women cannot conceive, it is because the fat presses the mouth of the womb, and conception is impossible until they grow thinner.*
>
> Hippocrates, *Aphorisms* V, xlvi

Obesity can have a major impact on the reproductive functioning of both men and women. Some studies indicate that prostate cancer is more common in obese men than in nonobese men, and particularly that death from prostate cancer is more likely (Calle 2008, pp. 202, 204). Obese women are more prone to gynecological cancers such as endometrial cancer and postmenopausal breast cancer than nonobese women are (Calle 2008, pp. 198–199). Furthermore, obese women are less likely to schedule proper gynecological screenings, including routine mammograms (Calle 2008, p. 203).

Though we might not agree with Hippocrates' mechanical theory underlying why "unnaturally fat women" have difficulty conceiving (that fat literally presses on the womb), we can support his conclusion. Today we would theorize that metabolic abnormalities, such as insulin resistance and imbalances in sex hormone levels, as are commonly seen in obesity, are a more likely etiology for infertility. Studies have shown that obese women, particularly when their obesity started in adolescence, are more likely to have irregular menstrual periods, chronic cycles without ovulation, and eventually even infertility (Pasquali and Gambineri 2006; Pasquali et al. 2007; Zain and Norman 2008). And if they do become pregnant, obese women with a body mass index (BMI) value greater than 30 kg/m^2 are more likely to have miscarriages and even poorer outcomes with artificial insemination or other assisted reproduction techniques. Further, those obese women who are able to sustain a pregnancy are more likely to have complications during pregnancy (e.g., diabetes, hypertension), as well as complications in the perinatal period (Zain and Norman 2008) (see "Pregnancy" section below).

Esposito and Giugliano (2005) suggest that obesity is a risk factor for sexual dysfunction in both men and women. Esposito et al. (2008) report that obesity, and specifically the amount of fat rather than its distribution, affected arousal, lubrication, satisfaction, and orgasm in at least one study they conducted. They also found, in a preliminary study, that women with the metabolic syndrome (e.g., hypertension, dyslipidemia, insulin resistance, and abdominal obesity) had significantly more sexual dysfunction than a group of matched female control subjects, though the researchers acknowledged they did not yet fully understand the reason. And Esposito et al. (2008) report on an older study of 171 postmenopausal women in whom the higher a woman's BMI level, the less sexual interest she had. It is certainly plausible, in a culture that values impossible levels of thinness, that from a psychological perspective, obese women might have more conflictual feelings about their bodies and be less willing to expose them to others and hence have less interest in sex. It is also possible that obese women derive much of their gratification from food, so that sexual gratification becomes less important to them. Esposito et al. (2008) recommend more prospective studies to determine the relationship between sexual functioning and obesity in women.

Obesity may also affect reproductive functioning in men. For example, obese men may have lower testosterone levels and, if very obese, even decreased sperm production (Pasquali et al. 2007). Dallal et al. (2008) suggest that morbidly obese men, for example, "commonly suffer from profound but reversible sexual dysfunction." They found that sexual drive, erectile functioning, ejaculation, and even sexual satisfaction were significantly improved after gastric bypass surgery in a study involving almost 100 men and 19 months of follow-up. The men had a mean preoperative BMI value of 51 kg/m^2 and lost 67% of their excess weight after surgery.

More commonly, obesity is associated with erectile dysfunction, which is the most frequent sexual disorder in men ages 50–80 years. Esposito and Giugliano (2005) report that up to about 80% of men who complain of erectile dysfunction are either overweight or obese. About 43% of men with erectile dysfunction meet criteria for the metabolic syndrome (Esposito et al. 2008). Furthermore, it is estimated that 29% of men who present with different symptoms of sexual dysfunction, such as decreased libido, premature ejaculation, or delayed ejaculation, as well as erectile dysfunction, have evidence of the metabolic syndrome (Esposito et al. 2008). Hannan et al. (2009) found, though, that erectile dysfunction could be significantly improved with lifestyle intervention (physical exercise and diet). And Esposito et al. (2008) found that "very intensive" intervention, including diet, exercise, and regular meetings with a trainer and nutritionist, significantly improved weight, metabolic abnormalities, and erectile function in their own study of 110 obese men at 2-year follow-up.

Pregnancy

The most common and most natural condition that leads to weight gain, of course, is pregnancy. In a sense, pregnancy is an example of weight cycling—gaining and losing weight in this case, though, as a normal biological function. It is not uncommon for women to have issues regarding the change in size and shape of their bodies, during and after pregnancy, and up to 5% of pregnant women actually have "significant eating disorders" that may lead to potentially serious medical conditions for both the fetus and the mother, as well as a significantly increased risk of postpartum depression in the mother (Berg and Andersen 2007, pp. 340–342). Many women never regain their shape or prepregnancy weight, especially after having more than one child. In fact, fewer than 40% of pregnant women gain only the recommended amount of weight during their pregnancy, and studies have shown that obese women can retain over 20 pounds after each pregnancy (Olson 2008).

> Obese women can retain over 20 pounds after each pregnancy.

Proximity to fast food restaurants may be a factor in pregnancy weight gain. Recent research by Currie et al. (2009) found that pregnant women are more likely to gain over about 45 pounds during pregnancy if they live within a tenth of a mile of a fast food restaurant. There was a 4.4% increase in the probability of this substantial weight gain in women living in this proximity. Their study included over 3.5 million pregnancies and was conducted over a period of about 13 years in Michigan, New Jersey, and Texas. Currie et al. (2009) do acknowledge that those pregnant women who live closer to fast food restaurants are more likely to be younger, less educated, and unmarried. The researchers believe their results demonstrate a link between proximity to a fast food restaurant and an increased risk of obesity, both in their sample of pregnant women and in a sample of schoolchildren.

Over the years, physicians have reconsidered weight gain recommendations for women during pregnancy. Gaining too much or too little obviously can be potentially detrimental to the developing fetus. Most studies of weight gain during pregnancy conducted in recent years, however, have still used the guidelines recommended by the U.S. Institute of Medicine (IOM) in 1990. The recommendations are as follows (for a single birth, not multiple births), based on BMI levels: If a woman has a low BMI value (<19.8 kg/m^2), the IOM recommends a pregnancy gain of 28–40 pounds. For those with a normal BMI value (19.8–26 kg/m^2), a weight gain of 25–35 pounds is recommended; for those who are overweight (BMI value, 26–29 kg/m^2), a gain of 15–25 pounds is recommended; and for those who are obese, with a BMI value of greater than 29 kg/m^2, a gain of no more than 15 pounds is recommended (Olson 2008). Please note that the ranges of BMI levels reported in this study are slightly different from the standard definition. (See Chapter 2, "Obesity in the United States," on BMI norms.)

Research has demonstrated that those women who gain weight within these guidelines are less likely to have a baby that is either small or large for the gestational age. Further, when pregnant women gain more, they are at greater risk for preeclampsia, failed induction, cesarean delivery, seizures, and hypoglycemia (and increased risk of diabetes), as well as meconium aspiration, low Apgar scores, and a greater possibility of overweight or obese children. In other words, increased weight gain is "significantly associated with a range of unfavorable pregnancy, labor, and delivery outcomes" and is even associated with breast-feeding for shorter periods postnatally (Olson 2008). Even though weight does tend to increase with age, pregnancy can have a significant impact on women's "weight gain trajectory" (Amorim et al. 2007). Power and Schulkin (2009, p. 302) note that the uterine environment is particularly sensitive to a mother's nutrition, including, of course, glucose regulation, but also weight gain. It is "a form of 'inheritance of acquired characteristics'" (p. 302) when a woman's weight or glucose regulation during pregnancy has an impact on her growing fetus not only in utero but for years later.

Rössner and his colleagues (Amorim et al. 2007; Linné et al. 2004) conducted 15-year follow-up studies in Sweden (the Stockholm Pregnancy and Women's Nutrition studies) to evaluate whether a woman's BMI level prior to pregnancy, as well as weight gain during pregnancy, would correlate with her weight 1 year after pregnancy and then 15 years later. What they found is that women who were overweight prior to pregnancy did not necessarily have a greater risk of retaining excessive weight postpartum than normal-weight women. But they did find that those who gained excessively (per IOM recommendations), as well as those who had not lost their pregnancy weight by 1 year, were more likely to have a higher BMI level at 15 years. Of the initial 2,342 women, 38% dropped out after 1 year but ultimately 483 women were available for follow-up at 15 years. The women in the study had, on average, two to three children over the course of the study. One-half of the women who gained the most during their pregnancy had the greatest weight retention at follow-up 1 year after delivery, and the 1-year weight was the best predictor of overweight 15 years later. In other words, if women had not lost their pregnancy weight by 1 year, they were more likely to keep that weight throughout their lives. One significant limitation of this study, though, is that there was not a control group of women who had not had any children over the course of the 15 years, to assess weight gain without pregnancy (Linné et al. 2004).

More recently, Chu et al. (2009) assessed gestational weight gain among more than 52,000 women (with a single-birth as opposed to a multiple birth-pregnancy) in a population-based sample in 29 states during 2004–2005. Over 40% of the women who were of normal weight and over 60% of those who were overweight initially, as measured by self-reported BMI levels, gained excessive weight during pregnancy (according to the IOM guidelines). Though obese women tended to gain less weight than others during pregnancy, still, one-quarter of them gained 35 pounds or more (rather than the ≤15 pounds recommended). A woman's prepregnancy BMI level became the strongest predictor of the amount of gestational weight gained. Chu et al. predict that this bodes badly for the future in regard to overweight and obesity in this country. For statistics reported for 2004–2005, significantly, one in five women who gave birth in the United States was obese, such that obesity in a woman has become a "common obstetrical condition" (American College of Obstetricians 2005). Many normal-weight women eventually become overweight and many of those who start out as overweight become obese as a result of pregnancy by not losing excessive gestational weight. Returning to a prepregnancy weight obviously becomes "particularly challenging" for those women who gain excessively (Chu et al. 2009).

The psychological impact of postpregnancy weight gain can be significant, as illustrated in the case below.

Pregnancy With Weight Gain Postpregnancy and Mild Depression and Anxiety

Elisa, a 40-year-old married woman, left her successfully evolving money management career to take care of her two children, now ages 1 year and 4 years.

Until her first pregnancy, she had maintained a healthy weight easily, with a BMI level of 21. She used to go regularly to the gym near her workplace and enjoyed working up a sweat on the treadmill, as well as the camaraderie with other young married women. During her first pregnancy, she managed to continue to go to the gym and was proud that she had gained only 25 pounds—"a perfect weight gain," she called it—as recommended by her obstetrician. By 6 months after delivery, she had lost all of it.

After the birth of her baby girl, she continued to work at her money management career, though now only part-time, and balanced work with spending time with her husband and daughter, so it was much more difficult to get to the gym regularly to see her friends.

Over the following 3 years, she began to gain weight, "inexplicably," as she put it. She had always been proud of her looks and maintained them without much effort. She had never really had weight problems, except during her freshman year at college when the new environment exposed her to eating many more calories than she had ever been used to eating. By sophomore year, she was able to gain control of her eating again and lost the weight she had gained.

She had never even owned a scale, but did monitor her weight regularly at the gym. One day, though, with the change of seasons, she realized that her clothes were considerably tighter than they had been the previous year. And when she went for her yearly physical shortly after noticing how her clothes were fitting, she found, on her internist's scale, that she was now 8 pounds heavier than her prepregnancy weight. She finally realized that often, without much thought, she would finish the leftover food on her young daughter's plate. And now that she was working only part-time, she was more apt to make dinner and found herself noshing when she prepared food for the family.

In the last 2 months, now that her daughter was in a half day of school and liked to be picked up by her mother, Elisa had not gotten to the gym at all. She actually felt somewhat panicked and began to watch her diet much more strictly and to be sure to get to the gym for jogging at least three times a week (though less than she had done prior to her first pregnancy). She managed to lose some of her postpregnancy weight but was still about 5 pounds heavier than her prepregnancy weight.

Then she got pregnant with her second child. She had had some trouble conceiving this time, now that she was in her late 30s, and her obstetrician suggested that she give up jogging, at least temporarily. She put on 35 pounds during this second pregnancy, for a total weight gain of 40 pounds, and about 6 months after the delivery of her son she had lost only lost 14 pounds of it. She had also decided she would stop working so as to be able to spend more time with her children. She would put the same drive and determination into motherhood that she had put into her business career earlier.

But Elisa now felt "out of control." What had worked for her before was just not working now. She thought the second pregnancy had somehow changed her metabolism. She kept gaining weight. Even breast-feeding, which enables a woman to eat about 500 additional calories a day, did not help control her weight. She had dependent and avoidant personality traits that were making the situation worse. She became clingy with her husband, somewhat helpless, and even unable to make decisions. She began to feel hypersensitive to criticism and socially inhibited whenever she did go out. She now detested getting dressed up to go to her husband's law firm functions (her dressy clothes no longer fit her), something she would have eagerly looked forward to earlier in their marriage. She felt people would not even recognize her now, with her new shape after the two pregnancies, and she felt she had nothing intelligent to say to her husband's colleagues. A year after the birth of her second child, she was 15 pounds heavier than her prepregnancy weight.

In fact, Elisa's weight gain was quite explicable. When she described her eating habits, an obvious pattern emerged. A number of issues were making her unhappy and anxious: although she believed that a woman with two young children should be a full-time mother, Elisa missed the excitement of the office, the successes and failures, the broad engagement with others, and adult conversations. She had bought into the idea that motherhood involves what Judith Warner has described as "perfect madness," in which mothers create a kind of "parenting pressure cooker" for themselves (Warner 2005, p. 23). In fact, Warner describes how "massive professional ambition and massively ambitious parenting" are mutually exclusive. Elisa, to the exclusion of almost any of her own interests, felt she needed to provide constant enrichment for her children. She became extremely oversolicitous and overprotective of her children as she hid her tremendous resentment toward them. Defensively, she was employing the psychological defense of *reaction formation* (being overly solicitous), as well as *displacement,* as she also took her anger and resentment out on her husband, who was confused by her change of personality.

> Massive professional ambition and massively ambitious motherhood are "perfect madness."
>
> **Source: Warner 2005, p. 262**

During the past 4 years, she had seen her vocabulary shrink and her topics of interest narrow down to that of her children. Her husband felt she had not much interest in him (and he was about to start an affair with an office mate). Even her pillow talk with him was devoid of adult content: she and her husband had hardly any sexual life. She claimed she was just too exhausted for sex after a day of being with the children. Whenever she was not completely enraged, she just wanted to cuddle.

Elisa was at times a mother and at times a child, and always distressed. She had *regressed* to a much earlier level of functioning than when she was working. She found some momentary solace in eating, often highly caloric food she kept in the house for the children. She didn't really binge, but was grazing constantly and had given up on keeping the figure of which she had been so proud. She was just taking in many more calories than she required. She seemed a needy child herself and was mildly depressed and anxious for feeling she was reduced to being a full-time nanny. "I don't even have time to get my hair cut anymore," she said.

Elisa needed to have more social contact with adults—by giving and going to dinner parties, joining a book club, and taking short vacations with her husband without the children. Her life had become totally child focused, to the exclusion of her own identity. She also had to learn that her anxiety, depression, and loneliness needed to be faced squarely and dealt with, rather than her continuing to use her maladaptive defenses (avoidance, reaction formation, displacement) that reinforced her dependent and avoidant personality traits.

Her internist, a woman who had known Elisa for years and was quite sensitive to her issues, suggested she might want to return to work, at least part-time, and insisted Elisa make time for herself by going to the gym. This gave Elisa the permission she seemed to need. Her internist also recommended that she speak to a psychotherapist about her conflicts regarding motherhood. Elisa, who had been in therapy years ago prior to her marriage and had had a positive therapeutic experience, willingly accepted the idea. Within the year, Elisa was able to lose most of the weight she had gained and was back to feeling more like herself.

SMOKING AND WEIGHT

Another common cause of weight gain is cessation of smoking. In fact, many people smoke in order to keep their weight down, and the possibility of weight gain after stopping actually discourages some from quitting (Lerman et al. 2004). Even rats given nicotine ate less initially and lost weight. Over the time of nicotine exposure, the rats eventually returned to eating normally but their weight still remained 8%–12% below normal. Once nicotine exposure was removed, these rats became hyperphagic until their body weight normalized (Schwid et al. 1992). Nicotine exposure also inhibits neuropeptide Y, which, as we have discussed, is a potent stimulator of appetite (Nicklas et al. 1999) (see Chapter 5 in this volume).

Nicklas et al. (1999) demonstrated that male smokers have significantly higher leptin levels (60% higher for a given BMI level) than nonsmokers, and leptin levels decrease after smoking cessation. The speculation is that cigarette smoking elevates leptin levels and this elevated level

> Individuals exposed to nicotine had less pleasure in eating sweets and rapidly achieved sensory satiety, that is, *negative alliesthesia*.
>
> **Source: Cabanac and Frankham 2002**

may be one physiological factor contributing to lower body weight in those who smoke. Not all studies, though, have found lower leptin levels in smokers and not all researchers believe leptin levels are involved (Al Mutairi et al. 2008; Cabanac and Frankham 2002). Cabanac and Frankham (2002), in a small study, found that although smoking did not decrease pleasure in eating sweets, it significantly accelerated self-reported displeasure (called *negative alliesthesia*) on repeated exposure to the sweets. In other words, individuals exposed to nicotine had less pleasure in eating sweets sooner and experienced a kind of sensory satiety more rapidly.

Smoking does increase a person's resting metabolic rate, and smoking cessation does result in some lowering of this rate, but the primary mechanism for weight gain in those who have stopped smoking is similar to that in rats: increased eating (Lerman et al. 2004). Sackey and Rennard (2009) reported that people typically gain 2–5 pounds within the first 2 weeks of quitting and an additional 4–7 pounds over the next 5 months; the average long-term weight gain after quitting is between 8 and 10 pounds. Williamson et al. (1991) found that men typically gain 6 pounds and women typically gain over 8 pounds, though a major weight gain (>25 pounds) can occur in almost 10% of men and over 13% of women. These results came from a survey of 748 men and 1,137 women in the National Health and Nutrition Examination Survey (NHANES I), conducted by Williamson et al. (1991). And Lerman et al. (2004) found in their study of 71 adults that one in four smokers who had quit smoking had gained 15 pounds.

> Food and nicotine stimulate the same dopamine reward system and can substitute for each other.

Like all addictive drugs, though, nicotine elicits the release of dopamine, the neurotransmitter most associated with reward circuits in the brain (Kauer 2005) (see Chapter 4, "The Psychology of the Eater," in this volume), and some believe that weight gain after smoking cessation is really related to genetically determined changes in this reward system. Food, after all, stimulates the identical dopamine reward path that nicotine does. And we are all particularly good at substitution: increasing the behavioral cost (Epstein and Leddy 2006) (e.g., the dangers of cigarette smoking) to obtain something reduces our response to it (e.g., cigarettes) and can lead to increasing the response to something different (a substitute such as food).

Reinholz et al. (2008) believe some overeating, in general, may be related to dopaminergic hypofunctioning, either genetically based or possibly a compensatory mechanism (an "adaptive downregulation") after dopamine hyperstimulation, such as from certain medications or cigarettes. For example, Pålhagen et al. (2005) believe that the medication L-dopa, itself, and not the disease or the typical excessive motor activity, is responsible for weight loss in patients with parkinsonism, a disease characterized by symptoms such as tremor, rigidity, and impaired balance. When L-dopa (which obviously induces a hyperdopaminergic state and even weight loss) is discontinued in Parkinson disease patients, rebound weight gain may result from the newly created hypodopaminergic state. Lerman et al. (2004) noted that abstinent former smokers who did gain weight had an abnormal genotype associated with fewer and weaker dopamine type 2 (D_2) receptors: individuals with this genetic allele have demonstrated significant increases in the reward response to food when they were no longer smoking, although not when smoking. In other words, "as a result of decreased activation of reward circuitry" following their smoking cessation, these people "may compensate" with food instead of cigarettes in order "to stimulate the dopamine reward pathway" (Lerman et al. 2004). Epstein and Leddy (2006) also found that ex-smokers with this allele were more likely to substitute food as their reinforcer and hence more likely to gain weight when they stopped smoking. Genotyping might be used as a screening tool to identify those particularly vulnerable to gaining weight after smoking cessation. Furthermore, the antidepressant bupropion, which increases dopamine release and blocks the reinforcing value of food that occurs in some who have quit smoking, may be particularly useful in preventing weight gain in those genetically predisposed (Epstein and Leddy 2006; Lerman et al. 2004).

INFECTIOUS AGENTS AND WEIGHT GAIN

There are over one billion people worldwide who are now overweight (Fulurija et al. 2008). No one really knows what causes weight gain to occur in some people and not in others. Though it is far more complicated, most researchers in the field acknowledge there are three major components to weight gain. First, there is a genetic component, as evidenced from adoptive studies of twins (see "Genetics and Obesity" section in Chapter 2 of this volume). Second, we have a toxic environment with an extraordinary array of highly caloric foods rich in fat and sugar. And third, the conveniences of the modern world have led most people to get considerably less exercise than our ancestors. The standard belief is that weight gain results from an increased intake of calories relative to the number of calories expended (primarily through resting metabolic rate, the thermogenic effect of digestion, and physical activity) (Turnbaugh et al. 2006). Haskell (1996) suggests, for example, that even the use of e-mail, rather than getting up and walking around to a colleague's office as we might have done just a few years ago, can lead to an 11-pound weight gain over the course of 10 years!

Keith et al. (2006) suggest that we have been concentrating far too much on our toxic environment (which exposes us to enormous portions and foods loaded with high-fructose corn syrup) and the decreased energy expenditure common in modern society. They question whether increases in the number of vending machines and fast food restaurants and the amount of television viewing—though all contributory—are really causative of the extraordinary increase in the prevalence of obesity seen in the past 30 years. Perhaps, instead, one could speculate that several other factors are contributing to the increase in obesity, including changes in our sleep patterns (e.g., many more people are sleep deprived and have a *sleep debt;* see Chapter 9, "Circadian Rhythms, Sleep, and Weight," in this volume), a tremendous increase in the use of prescription medications that lead to weight gain, changes in the prevalence of smoking, and even more time spent in "thermoneutral zones" such as air-conditioned spaces, where less energy is expended (Keith et al. 2006).

What we do know is that the prevalence of obesity has increased worldwide: between 1980 and 1990 the prevalence of obesity increased by 30%, and between 1990 and 2000 it increased by 61% (Greenway 2006). Could there be other mechanisms involved?

One controversial theory that has received some attention, even in the lay press (*The New York Times Magazine;* Henig 2006). is that the obesity epidemic is exactly that—an epidemic caused by an infectious agent. In other words, the rapid spread of obesity worldwide, particularly since 1980, is "compatible with an infectious origin" (Atkinson 2007). There are at least eight different viruses that appear to increase adipose tissue experimentally in animals (Atkinson 2008). One virus, though, the human adenovirus 36, first isolated in the late 1970s, is not only responsible for increased obesity in chickens, mice, and nonhuman primates, it is the only one to date to induce obesity in humans (Atkinson et al. 2005). Because humans cannot be directly inoculated with the virus due to ethical considerations, researchers have to infer the relationship from adenovirus 36 antibodies. Atkinson (2007) has found human subjects with antibodies to this virus actually had lower serum cholesterol and triglyceride levels than subjects without the antibodies, but more importantly, obese individuals had an almost threefold higher level of adenovirus 36 antibodies than nonobese individuals. Antibodies to adenovirus 36 were found in 30% of obese people and in only 11% of lean people in one study involving three U.S. cities (Atkinson 2007). Furthermore, in twin studies, twins who had adenovirus 36 antibodies had significantly higher BMI levels and body fat percentages than the discordant twins (i.e., those without the antibodies; Atkinson et al. 2005). The mechanism by which adenovirus 36 may induce increased adipose tissue is not known, but adenovirus 36 apparently accelerates the process by which preadipocytes become adipocytes. If this adenovirus 36 is in fact responsible for at least some cases of obesity, a vaccination against it may ultimately become a viable treatment for obesity. Whigham et al. (including Atkinson; 2006), in experiments with chickens, evaluated whether three other human adenoviruses could increase adiposity, as well as affect serum triglyceride and cholesterol levels. They found that adenovirus 37 could increase fat in these chickens (and decrease triglyceride levels), and their recommendation was that other human adenoviruses should be studied. Atkinson, though, seems to be the main proponent of (and major researcher of) a viral theory for obesity, and only further studies will determine the validity of his theory. It is an intriguing etiology. After all, when the infectious agent *Helicobacter pylori* was first proposed as a cause of stomach ulcers, that theory was met with disbelief and skepticism by most in the field.

Another approach has been to examine variations in gut flora in obese as compared with lean individuals. Bacteroidetes spp. and Firmicutes spp. are both beneficial bacteria present in the human gut, but Bacteroidetes levels have been found to be lower in obese persons than in lean ones, and Firmicutes levels have been found to be higher in obese individuals (Bajzer and Seeley 2006).

> Obese people's gut flora may increase their capacity to absorb energy from their diet.

In a small study, when obese people had lost a certain percentage of body weight (with percentages varying with the type of diet: on a fat-restricted diet, at least 6% was lost; on a carbohydrate-restricted diet, at least 2% was lost), their levels of Bacteroidetes spp. increased and their levels of Firmacutes spp. approached the levels seen in nonobese people. The "potentially revolutionary" speculation (Bajzer and Seeley 2006) is that obesity may have a microbial component in some people and that the levels of certain bacteria may possibly affect how many calories can be extracted from dietary intake (Ley et al. 2006). In other words, obese people may have an "increased capacity to absorb energy from their diet" and this may be genetically determined (Turnbaugh et al. 2006). Experiments in mice have also indicated that gut flora may lead to differences in how efficiently calories are extracted from food and hence to differences in body weights (Bajzer and Seeley 2006). Potentially, treatments for obesity might involve manipulations of the gut flora.

Still another area of research for obesity involves a potential vaccine against gastric inhibitory polypeptide (GIP), also called *glucose-dependent insulinotropic polypeptide*, an amino acid polypeptide released in the duodenum and jejunum parts of the gastrointestinal tract after ingestion of food (Fulurija et al. 2008). GIP specifically facilitates the digestion of glucose and fat and stimulates the release of insulin from beta cells in the pancreas, such that there is prompt glucose uptake by the tissues. GIP also fosters both fat deposition and triglyceride accumulation in adipose tissue. Experiments in mice demonstrated that a vaccine incorporating GIP and viruslike particles was able to prevent the accumulation of excessive body weight in mice given a high-fat diet (35% fat) and even led to weight loss in obese mice without negatively affecting glucose homeostasis. These mice, though, did not eat less, nor did they have a greater activity level. Presumably, this anti-GIP vaccine increases energy expended by increasing the resting metabolic rate. It is noteworthy, though, that vaccinating normal-weight mice that were fed a regular diet did not affect their weight. Because it takes about 10–12 weeks on a high-fat diet (i.e., prolonged high-fat feeding) for mice to start to deviate from normal and begin to gain weight (and eventually become obese), there is speculation that GIP itself acts to increase fat tissue, particularly in an environment of a prolonged high-fat diet such as those typical in many countries worldwide. Potentially, this vaccine as well could eventually have a role in obesity treatment.

MEDICATIONS THAT CAUSE WEIGHT GAIN

Weight gain secondary to medication use is not uncommon in either medical or psychiatric practices. Medications are more likely to cause weight gain than weight loss. Table 7–1 lists medications that typically lead to weight gain and those that are more typically weight neutral, or even known to produce some weight loss, and can be substituted for them. Powers and Cloak (2007, p. 256) speculate that weight gain might be more common, from an evolutionary perspective, because energy storage would provide a survival advantage. Sansone et al. (2004)

> Medications are more likely to cause weight gain than weight loss.

conducted a study to assess patients' stated tolerance to medication-induced weight gain. In a sample of over 200 people (79% women) in a predominantly white, suburban, Midwestern primary care practice, the average number of pounds that patients said they were willing to gain to treat a non-life-threatening medical condition was 5½ pounds, and about 5⅓ pounds for a non-life-threatening psychiatric condition. For life-threatening psychiatric conditions, they were willing to gain slightly less than 13 pounds, and for life-threatening medical conditions, they were willing

Table 7–1. Weight gain–inducing drugs and alternatives

Drug class	Drugs that may induce weight gain	Drugs that are weight-neutral or promote weight loss
Diabetes drugs	Insulin, glipizide, glyburide, glimepiride, pioglitazone, rosiglitazone, nateglinide, repaglinide	Metformin,[b] acarbose, miglitol, pramlintide, exenatide, sitagliptin phosphate
Antidepressants	SSRIs (initial weight loss, then weight gain), monoamine oxidase inhibitors, tricyclic antidepressants, mirtazapine, trazodone	Bupropion, venlafaxine, nefazodone
Mood stabilizers	Lithium, valproic acid *Less weight gain:* quetiapine	Lamotrigine, tiagabine, ziprasidone, aripiprazole
Antipsychotic drugs	Clozapine, olanzapine, thioridazine/mesoridazine, sertindole, chlorpromazine, risperidone, haloperidol, fluphenazine *Less weight gain:* quetiapine	Molindone, ziprasidone
Anticonvulsants	Valproic acid, gabapentin, carbamazepine, oxcarbazepine	Topiramate, lamotrigine
Migraine prevention drugs	Anticonvulsants and antidepressants (as above), beta-blockers	Topiramate, verapamil
Contraceptives and hormone replacement therapy	Hormonal contraceptives (progestin-containing)	Barrier methods, copper IUD
	Hormone replacement therapy (progestin-containing)	No alternative
Anti-inflammatory drugs	Corticosteroids (oral)	NSAIDs, inhaled corticosteroids
Antihypertensive agents	Alpha- and beta-blockers	Thiazide diuretics, ACE inhibitors, angiotensin receptor blockers
Antiretroviral therapy	All agents	No alternatives

Drug class	Drugs that may induce weight gain	Drugs that are weight-neutral or promote weight loss
Allergy drugs	Diphenhydramine	Inhaled corticosteroids
Thyroid drugs	PTU, methimazole	No alternatives

Table 7–1. Weight gain–inducing drugs and alternatives (*continued*)

Note. ACE = angiotensin converting enzyme; IUD = intrauterine device; NSAID = nonsteroidal anti-inflammatory drug; PTU = propylthiouracil; SSRI = selective serotonin reuptake inhibitor.

[a]Off-label uses of drugs are not listed in the table.
[b]Metformin is the first-line pharmacological treatment for type 2 diabetes unless contraindicated.

Source. Reprinted from the New York City Department of Health and Mental Hygiene: "Preventing and Managing Overweight and Obesity in Adults." *City Health Information* 26:23–30, 2007, p. 28. Available at: http://www.nyc.gov/html/doh/downloads/pdf/chi/chi26-4.pdf. Used with permission.

to gain slightly more than 13 pounds. In this particular study, the responses were no different in men than in women. In this sample, more than 5% were not willing to gain any weight under any of the theoretical circumstances. It was suggested that health care providers emphasize the seriousness of a condition in order to increase compliance among their patients.

Unfortunately, many of the medications that do cause considerable weight gain are those used for psychiatric disorders (and therefore these medications are the main focus of this section). Schwartz et al. (2004), for example, report that they found "solid evidence" that psychiatric medications like mood stabilizers, antidepressants, and antipsychotics lead to weight gain. This is quite unfortunate because there is substantial prejudice and social stigma against both mental illness and obesity.

Antipsychotics

Reportedly, up to half of those on antipsychotic medications gain weight (Khazaal et al. 2008). The Clinical Antipsychotic Trials of Intervention Effectiveness (CATIE) schizophrenia studies (with over 1,400 patients receiving medications for up to 18 months) found that in Phase I of the study, the mean BMI level was 30 kg/m^2— that is, in the obese range—and 46% had abdominal obesity, with an abnormal waist circumference (Citrome 2007). Those who were distressed by their weight gain were less likely to be compliant with medication and more likely to miss doses. In the CATIE Phase I study, 74% of patients actually discontinued medication given in the study before the 18-month period ended (Henderson 2007).

Though the first generation of antipsychotic medications, such as chlorpromazine and thioridazine, is associated with weight gain, the second-generation medications, such as clozapine, olanzapine, and risperidone, have produced substantially worse metabolic side effects, including potentially significant weight gain. For example, Citrome (2007) reports on a meta-analysis's results regarding mean weight gain after only 10 weeks of treatment using standard doses: clozapine produced almost a 10-pound weight gain; olanzapine produced about a 9-pound gain; and risperidone produced about a 4½-pound gain. Though medication doses are not necessarily related to weight gain, one predictor for substantial weight gain is rapidity: those who gained more than 7% of their initial weight (usually > 10 pounds) within 6 weeks were more likely to continue gaining significantly. Patients taking quetiapine or ziprasidone fared somewhat better, but all antipsychotic medications have the potential to produce weight gain in at least some patients and it is not always predictable which patients will be affected (Zimmermann et al. 2003). There is some suggestion that weight gain is associated with response to the medication (Henderson 2007). Weight gain with psychotropic drugs has also been reported in some studies to be more common in those who already have a weight problem and possibly more common in women (Zimmermann et al. 2003).

The mechanism for weight gain with the atypical antipsychotic medications is not known. It is likely that genetic variability is involved. There are apparently more than 300 genes possibly involved in the weight gain associated with the use of antipsychotic medications (Chagnon 2006). What we do know is that, predominantly, patients increase their food intake. In a small study, Khazaal et al. (2008) found that those who gained weight while taking the atypical antipsychotics had delayed negative alliesthesia for sweet substances, not unlike those who gained weight after cigarette cessation. Negative alliesthesia functions as a physiological satiety mechanism; if that mechanism is delayed, a person will continue to eat sugary foods and hence ingest more calories, with potential subsequent weight gain.

In experiments with mice, Kim et al. (2007) have found that atypical antipsychotic medications "potently stimulate" the enzyme adenosine monophosphate–activated protein kinase (AMP kinase) specifically in the hypothalamus. This enzyme has a role in regulating food intake as well as in regulating (and inactivating) other enzymes involved in fatty acid and cholesterol synthesis. Minokoshi et al. (2004) calls AMP kinase the "fuel gauge" that specifically monitors the body's cellular energy status, and found that AMP kinase suppression in the medial part of the hypothalamus is a necessary condition for leptin to have its anorectic and even weight loss effects. When there is no suppression of AMP kinase, for example, there is leptin resistance. Significantly, leptin levels have been reported to be elevated with treatment with some of the atypical antipsychotics, such as clozapine and olanzapine. For example, in several studies, leptin levels increased within a few weeks of treatment with these medications, as patients' weights increased about 5 pounds with clozapine and over 7 pounds with olanzapine. In the same studies, haloperidol did not lead to either increased leptin levels or increased weight (Zimmermann et al. 2003).

With the atypical antipsychotics, histamine type 1 (H_1) receptors are involved. Increased appetite, then, results from an activation of AMP kinase that is linked to H_1 receptor blockade. When mice no longer have H_1 receptors (because the receptors were experimentally deleted), the atypical antipsychotic medications no longer stimulate AMP kinase and no longer create increased appetite. Antihistamines in humans (and rats) can increase appetite, but they tend to be used sporadically and at considerably lower doses, so their appetite-enhancing effects are of less significance than the effects of the atypical antipsychotics (Kim et al. 2007). An atypical antipsychotic such as clozapine, which causes the greatest weight gain, is also able to reverse the reduced levels of AMP kinase that anorectic hormones such as leptin produce. It is possible, therefore, that by manipulating H_1 receptors and AMP kinase, researchers could develop alternative medications that would retain their antipsychotic potential without the complications of serious weight gain. Incidentally, medications like the biguanides (e.g., metformin) and thiazolidinediones, both used to treat type 2 diabetes, work through the AMP kinase system (Hardie et al. 2006).

But weight gain with the atypical antipsychotics is not the only problem: abnormal glucose metabolism and overt insulin resistance and type 2 diabetes, seen particularly with clozapine and olanzapine, have become major concerns (Henderson 2007). Further, in a retrospective large study published in the *New England Journal of Medicine*, with over 44,000 subjects in each cohort, investigators found a significant dose-related increase in the risk of sudden cardiac death (most likely by ventricular arrhythmias) in those who used either the older antipsychotics or the newer atypical antipsychotics, compared with matched nonusers of these drugs (Ray et al. 2009).

Gentile (2009) reviewed studies from 1966 through January 2009, with 39 peer-reviewed studies specifically focusing on the effects of the second-generation antipsychotics on weight. Gentile concluded that being overweight or obese was more likely due to the effects of medication and not to any underlying psychiatric illness or even necessarily an unhealthy lifestyle. Gentile noted that weight changes due to these antipsychotics were related to "complex overlapping of different factors," including patient-specific variables such as age, sex, initial BMI, concomitant use of other medications, and drug-specific variables such as timing of changes in weight, dose, and differences in receptor affinities. Furthermore, Gentile said that many studies suffered from methodological difficulties, such as lack of controls and small samples. Gentile concluded that the "true impact" of the relationship between weight gain and specific second-generation antipsychotics is far from being definitely established (Gentile 2009).

Mood Stabilizers

Many other medications used to treat psychiatric disorders also cause weight gain. The mood stabilizers, such as lithium and valproate, can cause substantial weight gain. Valproic acid, a medication also used for seizure disorders, reportedly causes weight gain in over 70% of those taking it, and an average weight gain is over 12 pounds (Powers and Cloak 2007, p. 259). The mechanism here seems to involve activation of γ-aminobutyric acid type A ($GABA_A$) receptors (Harvey and Bouwer 2000). Lithium was associated with weight gains of more than 20 pounds over a 10-year period, and 20% of patients gain even more over longer periods of time

(Powers and Cloak 2007, p. 259). Lithium may also lead to hypothyroidism, which may contribute to weight gain. The serious weight gain seen with lithium seems to be dose dependent and can affect compliance with drug treatment (Torrent et al. 2008). In some research it has been seen more commonly in those who are genetically predisposed to obesity and those who have preexisting obesity. For example, Bowden et al. (2006) compared lithium to the mood stabilizer and antiseizure medication lamotrigine during a year of follow-up in 155 obese patients and 399 nonobese patients with bipolar disorder. They found that lithium produced a significant increase in weight among the obese (as much as 6 kilograms, or ~14 pounds) but not among those not obese; lamotrigine, though, actually produced moderate weight loss in the obese (as much as 4.2 kilograms, or ~10 pounds).

Antidepressants

Antidepressant medications, particularly the older tricyclic medications like amitriptyline and imipramine, and the newer ones like mirtazapine, are also associated with weight gain. For example, it has been reported that approximately 10% of patients taking mirtazapine gained more than 7% of their baseline weight (Powers and Cloak 2007, p. 263). Food cravings and increased appetite have both been reported with mirtazapine, and there are also some reports of a decreased resting metabolic rate with some antidepressants (Zimmermann et al. 2003). Though trazodone is not typically associated with weight gain, Schwartz et al. (2004) report that even this medication can lead to a 1- to 2-pound gain over time. These researchers suggest that the antidepressants "may collectively carry the most weight gain burden" because they are so much more commonly prescribed than medications like the antipsychotics. The mechanism for weight gain with the antidepressants, however, is not known. There is speculation that histamine receptor blockade, with decreased satiety, may be involved, as well as activation of the tumor necrosis factor α (TNF-α) system. For example, Hinze-Selch et al. (2000) found (though the study was neither randomized nor blinded) that TNF-α is activated even before there is weight gain with the tricyclics amitriptyline and nortriptyline, and this may serve as a marker for subsequent weight gain. Zimmermann et al. (2003), who reviewed other studies, believe that activation of the TNF-α system is specifically associated with those psychotropic drugs that do cause weight gain.

Harvey and Bouwer (2000) have emphasized the complications involved in assessing the relationship among antidepressants, weight gain, and appetite regulation, particularly because symptoms of the depression itself can lead to weight gain and increased appetite, such as with atypical depression, or loss of appetite and weight loss. In other words, separating the pathology of the disease from any treatment effects, especially when weight changes are involved, can be difficult.

The selective serotonin reuptake inhibitor (SSRI) antidepressants generally tend to lead to weight loss initially (in the first 12 or so weeks of treatment) and subsequent weight gain over time for reasons that are not completely understood. Furthermore, "subtle yet significant pharmacological differences" exist between one SSRI and another vis-à-vis weight (Harvey and Bouwer 2000). For example, citalopram, with its particularly high affinity for H_1 receptors, has been associated with carbohydrate cravings and subsequent weight gain; nefazodone, on the other hand, has affinity for serotonin 5-hydroxytryptamine type 2 ($5-HT_2$) receptors but not H_1 receptors and hence tends not to cause the same weight gain. And fluoxetine, unlike other SSRIs, has particular affinity for $5-HT_{2C}$ receptors; this affinity, as well as the altered sensitivity that develops over prolonged exposure to fluoxetine, may contribute to its potential for causing weight gain over time (Harvey and Bouwer 2000). Zimmermann et al. (2003) report that in one placebo-controlled, double-blind study of fluoxetine, patients on average lost about a pound during the first weeks but gained over 6 pounds within the first year of treatment. Surprisingly, the placebo group also gained the same amount of weight. Powers and Cloak (2007, pp. 262–263) reviewed studies on the SSRIs and found that paroxetine seems more likely than others to cause weight gain, particularly in women, though there is considerable variation in weight change for individual patients with all of the SSRIs. For example, sertraline, unlike most of the other SSRIs, blocks the reuptake of dopamine and as a result tends to lead to appetite suppression (Malone 2005). Significantly, weight gain associated with antidepressant medications has not been found to be related to treatment outcome, sex, age, weight prior to treatment, or severity of depression (Zimmermann et al. 2003). Also significant is that, unlike what happens with some of the atypical antipsychotics, leptin levels tend not to change with antidepressant medications, despite weight gain in patients; this seems to represent a "differential drug effect on leptin regulation" (Zimmermann et al. 2003).

> ### SSRIs AND WEIGHT
>
> - The selective serotonin reuptake inhibitors, such as fluoxetine, sertraline, and paroxetine, allow the neurotransmitter serotonin to build up at nerve endings.
>
> - Initially these medications cause weight loss of several pounds, but over time they do tend to add weight in those prone to gaining weight.

The antidepressant serotonin-norepinephrine reuptake inhibitors (SNRIs), such as duloxetine and venlafaxine, are less likely to cause weight gain than α_1 agonists and β_3 receptor agonists, because of the specific receptors involved. They tend to suppress appetite and even have thermogenic properties (Harvey and Bouwer 2000). Sibutramine, a medication used for weight loss, has the same mechanism of action.

Other Medications

Other medications known to be associated with weight gain include the corticosteroids, the beta-blockers, the oral contraceptives, and insulin and some of the other medications used to treat type 2 diabetes, such as the sulfonylureas (e.g., glyburide).

The beta-blocker propranolol, for example, causes a weight gain of about 5 pounds over the course of a year. The mechanisms suspected include decreased sympathetic nervous system activity, as well as decreased physical activity possibly related to propranolol's side effects of fatigue and shortness of breath (Malone 2005). The sulfonylureas stimulate insulin secretion and have been known to cause a weight gain of almost 10 pounds over the course of 6 months. The thiazolidinediones, also used to treat type 2 diabetes, can produce edema and fluid retention in about 5% of patients, and these medications can also promote increases in insulin-sensitive adipocytes (Malone 2005). Injections of insulin were associated with significant weight gain in almost three-quarters of patients receiving three or more injections a day over the course of 10 years (Malone 2005).

> Among psychotropic medications, bupropion and the SNRIs (reuptake inhibitors of norepinephrine and serotonin; e.g., duloxetine, venlafaxine) are the least likely to cause weight gain.

CELLULITE (GYNOID LIPODYSTROPHY)

Rossi and Vergnanini (2000) describe cellulite as an "alteration of the topography of the skin" that occurs primarily in the thighs, abdomen, and buttocks of women. They note the term was first used in the 1920s to describe an aesthetic condition that was not thought to be inflammatory (but rather a disturbance of water balance) that resulted in a "padded and orange peel appearance of the skin." Some women describe cellulite as giving a "cottage cheese-like," uneven, or dimpling look to their skin. According to Rossi and Vergnanini (2000), cellulite involves structural changes in the dermis as well as in the blood microcirculation of the tissues and adipose tissue. As such, it seems to be a "localized metabolic disorder of the subcutaneous tissue" that results in visible external changes to the skin, as well as to a "granular (i.e. nodular) texture" when the skin is touched. And it is not synonymous with obesity or merely excessive fat tissue where fat cells increase in number (i.e., hyperplasia) and/or size (i.e., hypertrophy) without the accompanying other effects (Altabas et al. 2009). In fact, cellulite is not seen only in overweight or obese women (Altabas et al. 2009)With cellulite, small blood vessels are compressed, and when that happens, there occurs inflammation, increased collagen synthesis, and tissue hypoxia. Rawlings (2006) calls cellulite a "condition of altered connective tissue." Excess subcutaneous fat does not help the process and it "bulges" into the dermis layer of the skin (Rawlings 2006).

The condition is a common one, thought to be found in up to 85% of women after puberty, although it is more commonly seen in Caucasian than in Asian or black women. It evolves over years, with an initial alteration in fat cells (adipocytes) and a proliferation of fibrocytes, with poor lymph drainage of the tissue, to an actual "sclerosis" involving the fibrous bands of the subcutaneous tissue and deeper skin layers.

Many factors predispose women to develop cellulite, including genetic factors, hormonal factors (including increased estrogen levels), and lifestyle factors (e.g., lack of exercise, obesity, constipation, excessive salt intake) (Rossi and Vergnanini 2000). To date, no treatment is completely effective, though many systemic and local therapies have been utilized. Van der Lugt et al. (2009) report that a variable radiofrequency is one new approach. It works by a combination of electrical and heat stimulation (that can be somewhat painful) reaching different depths of tissue of the affected areas. These researchers claim their patients were "satisfied" with the results that could also be seen in before-and-after photographs. Maintenance treatments, though, are required. Ultrasound therapy, as well as vigorous massage to the affected areas, has also been temporarily successful in some patients.

Topical creams with combinations of aminophylline, caffeine, or herbal substances such as lemon, fennel, and barley (combinations often advertised in health food stores and magazines) have had limited or no success (Rawlings 2006). Peroxisome proliferator-activated receptors (PPARs), which can increase collagen and improve the texture and the appearance of the epidermis as well as decrease inflammation, are also being considered. It is likely that oral and topical products could be used together synergistically (Rawlings 2006). One of the newest theoretical approaches involves use of the phosphodiesterase inhibitors. The most common one, of course, is sildenafil (Viagra). Altabas et al. (2009) hypothesize that sildenafil, through its vasodilation effects, may have a beneficial effect on cellulite. The authors suggest that a topical formulation might eventually be developed to minimize deleterious systemic side effects like hypotension.

Although cellulite is not seen only in overweight or obese women, there are many diseases of the skin that are "aggravated by obesity" (Yosipovitch et al. 2007). These researchers describe that obesity can result in changes in sebaceous and sweat glands, lymphatics, collagen structure, wound healing, both micro- and macrocirculation, and subcutaneous fat, among other changes. For example, they note there can be alterations in the epidermis leading to increased water loss and drier skin in the obese. But the obese can also sweat more profusely because of increased activity of their sweat glands, and acne can be exacerbated in those who are obese. Wound healing impairment (e.g., slower wound healing due to collagen alterations) may make plastic surgery (including liposuction or abdominoplasty) more difficult in obese patients (Joseph Rabson, personal communication, August 2009). (For more on surgical treatments in the obese, see Chapter 12 in this volume.)

Some diseases of the skin are actually associated with obesity, such as acanthosis nigricans, described by Yosipovitch et al. (2007) as "symmetric, velvety, hyperpigmented plaques" that can occur anywhere but most commonly appear in the groin, neck, or axilla. These abnormalities can be associated with increased blood insulin levels and insulin resistance. Furthermore, there is a "significantly higher prevalence of obesity" among patients who have psoriasis, and obesity is also associated with gout.

REFERENCES

Al Mutairi SS, Mojiminiyi OA, Shihab-Eldeen AA, et al: Effect of smoking habit on circulating adipokines in diabetic and non-diabetic subjects. Ann Nutr Metab 52:329–334, 2008

Altabas K, Altabas V, Berković MC, et al: From cellulite to smooth skin: is Viagra the new dream cream? Med Hypotheses 73:118–125, 2009

American College of Obstetricians and Gynecologists (ACOG) Committee on Obstetric Practice: Obesity in pregnancy (paper # 315). Obstet Gynecol 106:671–675, 2005

Amorim AR, Rössner S, Neovius M, et al: Does excess pregnancy weight gain constitute a major risk for increasing long-term BMI? Obesity (Silver Spring) 15:1278–1286, 2007

Atkinson RL: Medical evaluation of the obese patient, in Handbook of Obesity Treatment. Edited by Wadden TA, Stunkard AJ. New York, Guilford, 2002, pp 173–185

Atkinson RL: Viruses as an etiology of obesity. Mayo Clin Proc 82:1192–1198, 2007

Atkinson RL: Could viruses contribute to the worldwide epidemic of obesity? Int J Pediatr Obes 3:37–43, 2008

Atkinson RL, Dhurandhar NV, Allison DB, et al: Human adenovirus-36 is associated with increased body weight and paradoxical reduction of serum lipids. Int J Obes (Lond) 29:281–286, 2005

Bajzer M, Seeley RJ: Physiology: obesity and gut flora. Nature 444:1009–1010, 2006

Berg SL, Andersen AE: Eating disorders in special populations: medical comorbidities and complicating or unusual conditions, in Clinical Manual of Eating Disorders. Edited by Yager J, Powers PS. Washington, DC, American Psychiatric Publishing, 2007, pp 335–356

Bowden CL, Calabrese JR, Ketter TA, et al: Impact of lamotrigine and lithium on weight in obese and nonobese patients with bipolar I disorder. Am J Psychiatry 163:1199–1201, 2006

Cabanac M, Frankham P: Evidence that transient nicotine lowers the body weight set point. Physiol Behav 26:539–542, 2002

Calle E: Obesity and cancer, in Obesity Epidemiology. Edited by Hu FB. New York, Oxford University Press, 2008, pp 196–215

Chagnon YC: Susceptibility genes for the side effect of antipsychotics on body weight and obesity. Curr Drug Targets 7:1681–1695, 2006

Chu SY, Callaghan WM, Bish CL, et al: Gestational weight gain by body mass index among US women delivering live births, 2004–2005: fueling future obesity. Am J Obstet Gynecol 200(3):271.e1–271.e7, 2009

Citrome L: The effectiveness criterion: balancing efficacy against the risks of weight gain. J Clin Psychiatry 68:12–17, 2007

Currie J, DellaVigna S, Moretti E, et al: The effect of fast food restaurants on obesity. NBER Working Paper No 14721. February 2009. Cambridge, MA, National Bureau of Economic Research, 2009

Dallal RM, Chernoff A, O'Leary MP, et al: Sexual dysfunction is common in the morbidly obese male and improves after gastric bypass surgery. J Am Coll Surg 207:859–864, 2008

Epstein LH, Leddy JJ: Food reinforcement. Appetite 46:22–25, 2006

Esposito K, Giugliano D: Obesity, the metabolic syndrome, and sexual dysfunction. Int J Impot Res 17:391–398, 2005

Esposito K, Giugliano F, Ciotola M, et al: Obesity and sexual dysfunction, male and female. Int J Impot Res 20:358–365, 2008

Flier JS, Maratos-Flier E: Biology of obesity, in Harrison's Principles of Internal Medicine, 17th Edition. Edited by Fauci A, Kasper DL, Longo DL, et al. New York, McGraw-Hill, 2008, pp 462–468

Fulurija A, Lutz TA, Sladko K, et al: Vaccination against GIP for the treatment of obesity. PLoS One 3:e3163, 2008

Gentile S: Contributing factors to weight gain during long-term treatment with second-generation antipsychotics: a systematic appraisal and clinical implications. Obes Rev 10:527–542, 2009

Greenway F: Virus-induced obesity. Am J Physiol Regul Integr Comp Physiol 290:R188–R189, 2006

Guehl D, Cuny E, Benazzouz A, et al: Side-effects of subthalamic stimulation in Parkinson's disease: clinical evolution and predictive factors. Eur J Neurol 13:963–971, 2006

Hannan JL, Maio MT, Komolova M, et al: Beneficial impact of exercise and obesity interventions on erectile function and its risk factors. J Sex Med 6:254–261, 2009

Hardie DG, Hawley SA, Scott JW: AMP-activated protein kinase—development of the energy sensor concept. J Physiol 574:7–15, 2006

Harvey BH, Bouwer CD: Neuropharmacology of paradoxic weight gain with selective serotonin reuptake inhibitors. Clin Neuropharmacol 23:90–97, 2000

Haskel WL: Physical activity, sport, and health: toward the next century. Res Q Exerc Sport 67:S37–S47, 1996

Henderson DC: Weight gain with atypical antipsychotics: evidence and insights. J Clin Psychiatry 68:18–26, 2007

Henig MR: Fat factors. The New York Times Magazine, August 13, 2006

Hinze-Selch D, Schuld A, Kraus T, et al: Effects of antidepressants on weight and on the plasma levels of leptin, TNF-alpha and soluble TNF receptors: a longitudinal study in patients treated with amitriptyline or paroxetine. Neuropsychopharmacology 23:13–19, 2000

Hippocrates: Aphorisms V, xlvi, in Works, Vol IV (The Loeb Classical Library). Translated by Jones WHS. Cambridge, MA, Harvard University Press, 1967, p 171

Kauer JA: A home for the nicotine habit. Nature 436:31–32, 2005

Keith SW, Redden DT, Katzmarzyk PT, et al: Putative contributors to the secular increase in obesity: exploring the roads less traveled. Int J Obes (Lond) 30:1585–1594, 2006

Khazaal Y, Chatton A, Claeys F, et al: Antipsychotic drug and body weight set-point. Physiol Behav 95:157–160, 2008

Kim SF, Huang AS, Snowman AM, et al: Antipsychotic drug-induced weight gain mediated by histamine H1 receptor-linked activation of hypothalamic AMP-kinase. Proc Natl Acad Sci U S A 104:3456–3459, 2007

Lerman C, Berrettini W, Pinto A, et al: Changes in food reward following smoking cessation: a pharmacogenetic investigation. Psychopharmacology (Berl) 174:571–577, 2004

Ley RE, Turnbaugh PJ, Klein S, et al: Human gut microbes associated with obesity: microbial ecology. Nature 444:1022–1023, 2006

Linné Y, Dye L, Barkeling B, et al: Long-term weight development in women: a 15-year follow-up of the effects of pregnancy. Obes Res 12:1166–1178, 2004

Macia F, Perlemoine C, Coman I, et al: Parkinson's disease patients with bilateral subthalamic deep brain stimulation gain weight. Mov Disord 19:206–212, 2004

Malone M: Medications associated with weight gain. Ann Pharmacother 39:2046–2054, 2005

Minokoshi Y, Alquier T, Furukawa N, et al: AMP-kinase regulates food intake by responding to hormonal and nutrient signals in the hypothalamus. Nature 428:569–574, 2004

Nicklas BJ, Tomoyasu N, Muir J, et al: Effects of cigarette smoking and its cessation on body weight and plasma leptin levels. Metabolism 48:804–808, 1999

Olson CM: Achieving a healthy weight gain during pregnancy. Annu Rev Nutr 28:411–423, 2008

Pålhagen S, Lorefält B, Carlsson M, et al: Does L-dopa treatment contribute to reduction in body weight in elderly patients with Parkinson's disease? Acta Neurol Scand 111:12–20, 2005

Pasquali R, Gambineri A: Metabolic effects of obesity on reproduction. Reprod Biomed Online 12:542–551, 2006

Pasquali R, Patton L, Gambineri A: Obesity and infertility. Curr Opin Endocrinol Diabetes Obes 14:482–487, 2007

Power ML, Schulkin J: The Evolution of Obesity. Baltimore, MD, Johns Hopkins University Press, 2009

Powers PS, Cloak NL: Medication-related weight changes: impact on treatment of eating disorders, in Clinical Manual of Eating Disorders. Edited by Yager J, Powers PS. Washington, DC, American Psychiatric Publishing, 2007, pp 255–285

Precope J: Hippocrates on Diet and Hygiene. London, Zeno, 1952, p 191

Rawlings AV: Cellulite and its treatment. Int J Cosmet Sci 28:175–190, 2006

Ray WA, Chung CP, Murray KT, et al: Atypical antipsychotic drugs and the risk of sudden cardiac death. N Engl J Med 360:225–235, 2009

Reinholz J, Skopp O, Breitenstein C, et al: Compensatory weight gain due to dopaminergic hypofunction: new evidence and own incidental observations. Nutr Metab (London) 5:35–38, 2008

Rossi ABR, Vergnanini AL: Cellulite: a review. J Eur Acad Dermatol Venereol 14:251–262, 2000

Sackey JA, Rennard SI: Patient information: smoking cessation. UpToDate, Edition 17.2. Available (by subscription) at: http://www.uptodate.com. Accessed October 29, 2009.

Sansone RA, Sansone LA, Gaither GA, et al: Patient attitudes toward weight gain with medications. Gen Hosp Psychiatry 26:487–489, 2004

Schwartz TL, Nihalani N, Jindal S, et al: Psychiatric medication-induced obesity: a review. Obes Rev 5:115–121, 2004

Schwid SR, Hirvonen MD, Keesey RE: Nicotine effects on body weight: a regulatory perspective. Am J Clin Nutr 55:878–884, 1992

Torrent C, Amann B, Sánchez-Moreno J, et al: Weight gain in bipolar disorder: pharmacological treatment as a contributing factor. Acta Psychiatr Scand 118:4–18, 2008

Tuite PJ, Maxwell RE, Ikramuddin S, et al: Weight and body mass index in Parkinson's disease patients after deep brain stimulation surgery. Parkinsonism Relat Disord 11:247–252, 2005

Turnbaugh PJ, Ley RE, Mahowald MA, et al: An obesity-associated gut microbiome with increased capacity for energy harvest. Nature 444:1027–1031, 2006

Van Der Lugt C, Romero C, Ancona D, et al: A multicenter study of cellulite treatment with a variable emisión radio frequency system. Dermatol Ther 22:74–84, 2009

Wadden TA, Phelan S: Behavioral assessment of the obese patient, in Handbook of Obesity Treatment. Edited by Wadden TA, Stunkard AJ. New York, Guilford, 2002, pp 186–226

Warner J: Perfect Madness: Motherhood in the Age of Anxiety. New York, Riverhead, 2005

Whigham LD, Israel BA, Atkinson RL: Adipogenic potencial of multiple humna adenoviruses in vivo and in vitro in animals. Am J Physiol Regul Integr Comp Physiol 290:R190–194, 2006

Williams GH, Dluhy RG: Diseases of the adrenal cortex, in Harrison's Principles of Internal Medicine, 17th Edition. Edited by Fauci AS, Kasper DL, Longo DL, et al. New York, McGraw-Hill, 2008, pp 2247–2266

Williamson DF, Madans J, Anda RF, et al: Smoking cessation and severity of weight gain in a national cohort. N Engl J Med 324:739–745, 1991

Yosipovitch G, DeVore A, Dawn A: Obesity and the skin: skin physiology and skin manifestations of obesity. J Am Acad Dermatol 56:901–916, 2007

Zain MM, Norman RJ: Impact of obesity on female fertility and fertility treatment. Womens Health (Lond Engl) 4:183–194, 2008

Zimmermann U, Kraus T, Himmerich H, et al: Epidemiology, implications, and mechanisms underlying drug-induced weight gain in psychiatric patients. J Psychiatr Res 37:193–220, 2003

8

EXERCISE

Walking also is a natural exercise.... Walking after food prevents abdominal fat. Morning walks help in the same way, they clear the head....Running long distances, gradually increased, helps to burn excess of food in the body and is suitable for people who eat much.

Hippocrates, *Regimen,* Book II (Precope 1952, pp. 66–67)

EXERCISE AND NONEXERCISE ACTIVITY THERMOGENESIS

As we saw in Chapter 3 on the basic principles of calories, there are three major components involved in how the body expends energy: 1) the resting metabolic rate, which accounts for about 60% of our daily expenditure; 2) the thermogenic effect of food, including its digestion, absorption, and storage, which accounts for about 10%–15% of our daily expenditure; and 3) all physical activity, the most variable component, which accounts for the remainder (see "Factors Involved in Daily Energy Requirements" in Chapter 3). For very active individuals, this third component can account for about 50% of the daily expenditure, whereas for sedentary people it can be about 15% (Levine 2004). In other words, people who are naturally highly active can expend three times as many calories daily as those who are fairly sedentary. This can translate into variations in daily energy expenditure of 2,000 calories a day (Levine 2007b). Unfortunately, though, we have overall become a fairly physically inactive population.

Eaton and Eaton (2003) make the comparison between the modern world and that of our Paleolithic ancestors some 50,000 to 20,000 years ago. Before agriculture developed around 10,000 years ago, the Stone Age people were mostly nomadic. From the work of physical anthropologists, who examined skeletal remains, researchers believe their regular activities of daily living might have included considerable physical activity, such as walking from one hunting location to another, walking while gathering food, building shelters, butchering animals and cleaning carcasses for food, digging for roots, carrying firewood as well as children, and dancing for play or religious ceremonies. Eaton and Eaton (2003) believe that their physical activity patterns resembled those of people today who cross-train, incorporating different forms of exercise that make them quite muscular, and that Stone Age people's physiques were close to "those of contemporary elite athletes." Furthermore, it is estimated that people in the Stone Age used about 1,300 calories per day in the physical activity of living; in comparison, sedentary people in our society use only about 550 calories each day in this way (Eaton and Eaton 2003). Clearly, our Paleolithic ancestors got all their physical activity naturally. Today, however, we can divide human activity into *exercise* and *nonexercise* activity.

> "In terms of physical energy expenditure, the experiences of Stone Agers were probably more uniform than are those of contemporary Americans, whose propensities range from exercise fanaticism to near total sedentism."
>
> **Source: Eaton and Eaton 2003**

Exercise

Exercise is a specific form of physical activity that is "purposeful," repetitive, structured, and planned exertion for the specific function of maintaining or improving physical fitness or health (Dishman et al. 2006; Hill et al. 2004, p. 632). According to Diehl and Choi (2008), although this figure varies by age, fewer than 50% of individuals in the American population exercise on a regular basis. In fact, Levine (2007b) makes the point that many people worldwide do not engage in any exercise at all and many more expend only about 100 calories a day in exercise.

Dishman et al. (2006) note that the type of exercise and the extent to which it is voluntary may determine its effect on the body's homeostasis. For example, when considering research on the effects of exercise, we must distinguish the exertional stress of the actual physical exercise from the emotional or psychological stress that may be part of some coercive process (e.g., forced swimming in animal experiments). Identifying what mechanisms are actually involved in determining the effects of exercise on humans is challenging, according to Woods et al. (2006). For example, we have to consider individual differences, including genetics, as well as the many different kinds of exercise, their relationship to other forms of physical activity, and the subjective nature of the intensity of exercise, among other variables.

Exercise can be further divided into 1) aerobic exercise; 2) anaerobic exercise, usually referred to as resistance or strengthening exercise; and 3) flexibility exercise, or stretching. Effects of aerobic and anaerobic exercise are outlined in Table 8–1.

Aerobic exercise is endurance exercise, and it is exercise in which the muscles use oxygen (hence "aerobic"). According to Rouzier and Mancini (2009a) aerobic exercise is any exercise done for longer than 3 minutes at a time. It increases blood flow to the lungs, increases cardiac output so that the heart pumps more efficiently, increases heart-healthy cholesterol (high-density lipoprotein), and ultimately de-creases our resting heart rate, respiratory rate, and blood pressure. It also helps maintain bone density and increases sensitivity to insulin (e.g., decreases in insulin response to glucose and decreases in baseline levels of insulin are seen) and can decrease the percentage of body fat. Examples of aerobic exercise include jogging, walking, swimming, biking, and playing basketball.

Resistance exercise, or *strengthening exercise*, on the other hand, is exercise done in less than 3 minutes, in which the muscles do not use oxygen (anaerobic exercise, "without oxygen"). It consists of bursts of exercise, as seen in weight lifting with either free weights or machines (exercise in which specific muscles are moved re-peatedly against a resisting force), or throwing a medicine ball, or pulling on elas-tic cords (Howley and Franks 2007, p. 518), but it can also be done with so-called *interval training*, in which any activity can be done in short spurts. Examples include purposely running to catch a bus, shoveling snow, and running up a flight of stairs. Resistance exercise involves contractions of specific muscle groups. Contractions can be *isometric*, such as pushing against a wall, in which the length of the muscle does not change; *concentric*, which shortens the muscle, such as by lifting a weight up; or *eccentric*, which lengthens the muscle, such as by lowering a weight against the force of gravity (Simon 2008). Resistance exercise tends to increase muscle strength considerably, increase lean body mass (and decrease fat), and maintain bone density. In fact, even in older people, who tend to lose muscle, resistance ex-ercise is able to increase muscle mass and strength (M. A. Williams et al. 2007). Just like aerobic exercise, though, it also increases the body's sensitivity to insulin such that it reduces the insulin response to glucose and also decreases baseline insulin levels. Resistance exercise can also improve balance and coordination, even in older people (M. A. Williams et al. 2007).

M. A. Williams et al. (2007) note, "The extent to which an activity is predomi-nantly aerobic or anaerobic depends primarily on its intensity relative to the person's capacity for that type of exercise." Most exercises involve both aerobic and anaerobic mechanisms, but they can be classified to a certain extent by which mechanism is predominant. For example, an exercise is more anaerobic when resistance train-ing involves lifting heavier weights with longer periods of rest after, but it is more aerobic when a person lifts lighter weights with less rest after (M. A. Williams et al. 2007). Or it can be a few minutes of intense exercise (anaerobic) followed by a less intense period (aerobic) in interval training.

Flexibility exercises involve stretching the muscles to improve the range of mo-tion of muscles and joints. These exercises may be particularly helpful for persons with back problems. Root (1991) has prescribed a series of exercises that take about 15 minutes daily that have helped many patients avoid back surgery. Yoga and tai chi are examples of more regimented stretching exercises. Some believe that stretching before any exercise helps prevent injuries and stiffness (Simon 2008). Herbert and Gabriel (2002), however, surveyed five studies and concluded that stretching before

AEROBIC (ENDURANCE) VS. ANAEROBIC (STRENGTH OR RESISTANCE) EXERCISE

- *Aerobic exercise,* also called *endurance exercise,* is an exercise that makes the muscles use oxygen; it should be the main kind of exercise done; an exercise that lasts more than 3 minutes is considered aerobic.
  - Makes the heart stronger because it has to work harder to get more oxygen to the muscles; increases blood flow to the lungs (allowing more oxygen into the blood with every breath); decreases blood pressure, maintaining a sense of well-being (an excellent antidepressant); and burns calories
  - Examples (note that "low to moderate impact" and "high impact" are terms relative to a person's fitness level, but in general):

    Low to moderate impact exercises: walking, rowing, swimming, cross-country skiing, step classes

    High-impact exercises: running, squash, raquetball, dance exercising

  - Some studies suggest that walking briskly for ≥3 hours/week reduces the risk of coronary heart disease by 65%

- *Anaerobic exercise* (strength training) is any exercise that lasts less than 3 minutes, in which time the muscles do not use oxygen.
  - Does not build endurance as aerobic exercise does, but does strengthen muscles, burn fat, maintain bone density, and improve digestion
  - Examples: interval training, such as running or weight lifting in short bursts of exercise (run for 30 seconds, then walk for 2 minutes, then repeat pattern)
  - Other examples of anaerobic exercise: walking a flight of stairs, running to catch a bus, shoveling snow—all for purpose of maintaining or improving fitness

- Anaerobic exercise boosts metabolic rate considerably longer afterward than does aerobic exercise.

Source: Holloszy and Kohrt 1996; Rouzier and Mancini 2009a, 2009b; Simon 2008

or after exercising did not significantly prevent injury or muscle soreness that occurred later.

When we measure exercise, we can measure its frequency (how often it is done), its duration (how long it lasts), and its intensity (how hard the heart is pumping, usually measured by a person's pulse). Maximum heart rate is usually calculated by the formula of 220 minus a person's age. So if you are 60 years old, your maximum heart rate is $220 - 60 = 160$ beats per minute. The target heart rate is usually between 60% and 85% of one's maximum heart rate, and it is recommended that people exercise aerobically at a pace such that they are able to talk while they exercise—in other words, you should not be gasping for breath.

Another measurement of exercise intensity is maximal oxygen uptake, or Vo_2max, which is the maximum rate at which oxygen is delivered to exercising

Table 8–1.	Effect on the body of aerobic (endurance) exercise compared with anaerobic (resistance, strengthening) exercise	
Health parameter	**Aerobic exercise**	**Anaerobic exercise**
Lean body mass	Unchanged	Moderate increase
Percent body fat	Moderate decrease	Small decrease
Muscle strength	Unchanged to slight effect	Large increase
Bone density	Moderate increase	Moderate increase
Insulin sensitivity	Moderate increase	Moderate increase
Baseline insulin levels	Small decrease	Small decrease
Insulin response to glucose	Moderate decrease	Moderate decrease
Resting heart rate	Moderate decrease	Unchanged
Vo_2max (maximum rate oxygen delivered to muscles)	Large increase	Unchanged to small increase

Source: Adapted from M.A. Williams et al. 2007.

muscles and is related to the greatest capacity of the heart to pump blood to the muscles. It is influenced by age, heredity, altitude, pollution, and level of fitness, and it decreases about 1% per year as we age. It is also about 15% lower in women than men, mostly because of differences in fat percentages and hemoglobin levels. People with cardiovascular and pulmonary diseases have lower Vo_2max levels than people without these diseases, but levels can be improved with aerobic endurance exercise. Endurance training typically can increase Vo_2max by 5%–25%, depending on a person's initial level of fitness. Some people are genetically predisposed to be world-class athletes (e.g., long-distance runners), but for most of us there is a certain point at which our Vo_2max will not increase any further no matter how much we train (Howley and Franks 2007, pp. 456–457). Vo_2max determines how we categorize exercise—as high intensity, moderate intensity, or low intensity—and of course an exercise that is very difficult (high intensity) for an elderly untrained person can be considered fairly easy (low intensity) for a well-trained athlete.

Nonexercise Physical Activity

Nonexercise physical activity is also called *spontaneous* physical activity or *NEAT* (for nonexercise activity thermogenesis) and is any bodily movement that increases energy expenditure over the basal level. Levine (2007b) notes that how many calories someone burns in this type of activity is genetically based.

Levine (2007b) distinguishes *NEAT activators*, who are constantly expending energy and tend to be lean (i.e., "the signals that stimulate NEAT are plentiful and potent even in the presence of caloric excess"), from *NEAT conservers*, who tend to expend minimal energy and hence tend toward obesity ("obesity as a state of central NEAT resistance"). As Levine sees it, some people tend to be lean walkers and some do practically everything from their chairs, though he acknowledges most people are somewhere between these two extremes. He recommends environmental re-engineering (e.g., wearing sneakers to work; he even suggests using vertical desks attached to treadmills) to get people to be more physically active.

Of course, environmental factors, such as where someone lives or what occupation she or he has, as well as biological factors, such as someone's weight, body composition, and even sex, may all have an impact on a person's spontaneous activity. For example, Hill (2006) reports on studies that have shown that men from the Amish culture walk 18,000 steps daily and women from that culture walk about 14,000 steps, whereas by comparison, those who live in Colorado walk only about 6,300 to 6,700 steps daily—and Colorado has one of the thinnest populations. These differences translate into substantial differences in the number of calories burned (400–600 cal/day).

Furthermore, it requires more energy to move a heavier or larger person, so when a person gains weight that person's NEAT increases, and when a person loses weight that person's NEAT decreases, though it is not yet clear how NEAT is actually regulated (Levine 2007b). Nonexercise activity includes maintaining posture, fidgeting, talking, walking, shopping, performing one's job, sitting, standing, playing a musical instrument, and other activities not undertaken with the goal of physical fitness. Of course, all these activities burn calories (i.e., expend energy), but they do not necessarily provide the cardiovascular and other health benefits that sustained exercise of a certain intensity provides (Brooks et al. 2004). Even chewing sugarless gum (i.e., nonnutritional chewing) burns calories. Levine and colleagues found that gum chewing increased energy expenditure by 11 (±3) calories, more than standing (Florman 2000; Levine et al. 1999).

> "If a person chewed gum during waking hours and changed no other components of energy balance, a yearly loss of more than 5 kg of body fat might be anticipated."
>
> **Levine et al. 1999**

There have been attempts to codify and systematize the amount of energy expended in daily activities. The "Compendium of Physical Activities" (Ainsworth et al. 2000) is a list of thousands of activities, divided into categories like sports, occupation, home repair, music playing, and self-care, that a person in our society might engage in during the day. The unit of measurement is the MET, for metabolic equivalent, and it is the ratio of the energy involved in performing an activity to the energy involved when a person is at rest sitting quietly; the latter is given a standard MET of 1. Values in this compendium range from 0.9 METs for sleeping to 18 METs for running. The values are based on the actual movement, that is, the energy expenditure, involved in the activity. This measure was originally derived more scientifically from laboratory studies involving doubly labeled water (Di Pietro et al. 2004).

Outside of the laboratory, estimates of energy expenditure are fairly rough estimates. Vacuuming gets a value of 3.5 METs and carrying groceries upstairs gets a MET value of 7.5, whereas a person sitting and playing the flute gets a MET value of 2.0. But do two people really vacuum exactly the same way or, for that matter, even sleep the same way? There is obviously considerable individual variability, and the cost of energy expenditure in an activity is higher among heavy people than thin people. This compendium of values would underestimate the energy expended for a heavier person and overestimate the activity value for a thinner person (Ainsworth et al. 2000). Furthermore, there is also considerable variation dependent on one's age, fitness level, amount of adipose tissue, and even environmental conditions. The physical activity level (PAL) is the standard method of assessing total energy expenditure for a period of time. It is the ratio of the average daily

EXAMPLES OF PHYSICAL ACTIVITY AND ENERGY COSTS

- Moderate-effort bicycling (12–14 miles/hour): 8.0 METs

- Dancing (ballet, modern, tap): 4.8 METs

- Watering plants: 2.5 METs

- Making a bed: 2.0 METs

- Reclining (while talking on the telephone): 1.0 MET

- Shoveling snow: 6.0 METs

- Playing violin: 2.5 METs

- Grooming (brushing teeth, shaving, urinating): 2.0 METs

- Golfing (including walking and carrying clubs): 4.5 METs

- Playing tennis (doubles): 5.0 METs

- Kayaking: 5.0 METs

Source: Howley and Franks 2007, pp. 483–496

energy expended to the resting metabolic rate. Any kind of physical activity that expends calories over the basal resting level—whether recreational or occupational, intentional or spontaneous—is part of the daily PAL total. In other words, the PAL "reflects a summation of all accumulated physical activity in a 24-hour day" (Brooks et al. 2004).

As you can see, it is exceptionally difficult to quantify daily physical activities, given the infinite possibilities in the ways the human body can move and the infinite number of different variables. Lanningham-Foster et al. (2003) tried to quantify some of the tasks involved in household chores in recent years in contrast with the same tasks without modern conveniences such as a dishwasher or clothes washing machine. These labor-saving devices led, on average, to 111 fewer calories burned per day. Though this may not seem like much, this difference could lead to a 10-pound weight increase over the course of a year if no other variables were changed (Lanningham-Foster et al. 2003). Along those lines, Matthews et al. (2008) sought to quantify the actual amount of sedentary behavior in a large ($N > 6,000$) representative U.S. population. Sedentary behavior, defined as involving no more than 1.5 times the resting metabolic rate, included sitting, reclining, or lying down during waking hours (and might include time watching television or using the computer). It was measured by means of an Actigraph, a small instrument that records acceleration information as an activity count, providing an objective measurement of the intensity of the body's movement. In general, people in this survey spent almost 55% of their nonsleeping time (>7 hours/day) in sedentary activities. Adults who were between age 70 and 85 years, were, not surprisingly, the most sedentary, with almost 68% of men's time (9½ hours/day) and over 66% of women's time (just over 9 hours/day) spent in such low-level energy expenditure (Matthews et al. 2008). These studies point to the fact that our environment not only provides a toxic array of high-sugar and high-fat foods, but also is conducive to spending extensive periods every day expending very few calories. This is a perfect setup for small but significant weight gain over time, no matter what one's genetic influences. Other examples of the energy cost of various activities include making the bed, 2.0 METs; ironing, 2.3 METs; watering plants, 2.5 METs; and bathing a dog, 3.5 METs (Howley and Franks 2007, p. 485).

DETERMINANTS OF EXERCISE

Many factors are involved in whether a person decides to exercise regularly. For example, environmental, demographic, and social factors—such as access to exercise facilities, socioeconomic status, gender and cultural norms, support of family or peers, or attitudes regarding health and leisure time—may all be contributing elements. Psychological factors, such as preoccupation with body image or even feelings someone had about gym class as a child, may contribute to conflicts regarding exercise. Many people use lack of time as an excuse for not engaging in exercise, but this can be "a true barrier, a perceived barrier, a lack of time management skills, or merely an excuse" (Lee et al. 2004).

Lewis and Lynch (1993), in a short-term study of 2 months, found that primary care physicians who advised their patients to exercise had a positive impact in getting them to exercise for a longer duration, though not necessarily more frequently. Genetics may also play a role. De Moor et al. (2007), in studying a large sample of twins and siblings in the Netherlands, found that different genes may be responsible for genetic effects in males as opposed to females. They hypothesized that genes may be involved in three specific ways in a person's willingness to exercise: 1) genes may influence actual ability (i.e., whether someone is good at exercise or not), and then indirectly influence exercise behavior; 2) genes may influence personality traits (e.g., conscientiousness, self-discipline, or motivation) or even mood (i.e., whether a person is depressed), both of which may affect exercise behavior; and 3) genes may predispose a person to experience more of a rewarding feeling from exercise (e.g., a sense of well-being). It is speculated that many genes may be involved but that each gene may have small effects. Likewise, Stubbe et al. (2006) studied exercise behavior in over 37,000 pairs of monozygotic and dizygotic twins, ages 19–40, in seven countries. They found a median high heritability of 62% across the seven countries: Australia, Denmark, Finland, the Netherlands, Norway, Sweden, and the United Kingdom. They speculated that genes that favor an interest in fitness (to be strong) may be more important in whether males exercise, whereas genes that favor an interest in weight loss (to "stay in shape") may be more significant with females. Shared environmental factors in the home or school seemed to be less significant. Of note, Stubbe et al. (2006) found that only about 44% of males and 35% of females in the study actually exercised regularly.

For some people, environmental factors can have a significant impact on the motivation to exercise. Perri and Corsica (2002, pp. 368–369) report on several studies that indicate people with exercise equipment in the home are more apt to exercise (and continue doing so over time), particularly if they are encouraged to do short bouts of exercise. And personal trainers and monetary incentives work for some people. More recently, though, D. M. Williams et al. (2008) studied psychosocial factors involved in predicting who would begin an exercise program and who would continue to maintain it over time in a group of previously sedentary subjects, predominantly—about 84%—women. They found that access to exercise equipment in the home may be helpful in *beginning* an exercise program, but that it became less important as a motivating factor over the course of time (in their case, 12 months of follow-up). Those who were more likely to *maintain* a program over time had a sense of self-efficacy, that is, the sense of confidence in being able to exercise, even in the face of obstacles, such as bad weather, vacations, fatigue, time constraints, or mood. Those who maintained their exercise were also more likely to have a sense of perceived satisfaction with exercising. Of the sample of just over 200 subjects, though, only about half (98) were regularly exercising at 6 months and only 64 maintained their exercise at 12 months. Among the 107 non-exercisers at 6 months, 24 had become active by 12 months but 83 remained inactive (D. M. Williams et al. 2008).

> "There is no diet that will allow us to maintain the low level of energy intake required to achieve energy balance at a healthy body weight, given the current [sedentary] level of physical activity."
>
> **Source: Hill and Wyatt 2005**

METABOLIC CONSEQUENCES OF EXERCISE

What we eat is one of many factors (such as genetics) that determine our stamina and endurance when we exercise. The primary fuels our bodies use are carbohydrates and fat. Protein utilization, for example, accounts for only 5% of the fuel used during exercise (Howley and Franks 2007, p. 452). Carbohydrates come from blood glucose as well as from the breakdown of muscle glycogen stores. When there is inadequate muscle glycogen during high-intensity, prolonged exercise (~2 hours), we become fatigued and hypoglycemic. If we exercise for 3 or more hours, blood

glucose is the source of fuel for the muscles, and many athletes engaged in prolonged exercise utilize carbohydrate drinks (energy drinks) as a supply of blood
glucose. Athletes employ *carbohydrate loading*—a diet with 65%–70% of calories
from carbohydrates—before prolonged exercise (>60 minutes) to maximize their
energy sources (i.e., increase muscle glycogen stores). If there are no carbohydrates
available to be used as fuel, the body breaks down glycogen in the liver and produces
more glucose in the liver (gluconeogenesis) (Holloszy and Kohrt 1996). When exercise is prolonged and strenuous, there occurs a "progressive decrease in muscle glycogen stores until, at the point of exhaustion, they are almost completed depleted"
(Holloszy and Kohrt 1996).

When someone fasts or eats a low-carbohydrate diet, that person has a reduced
ability to engage in "vigorous prolonged exercise" because, say Holloszy and Kohrt
(1996), hypoglycemia develops quickly due to initially low glycogen and due to the
fact that gluconeogenesis "cannot keep pace" with the amount of glucose utilized.

What else causes skeletal muscle fatigue? Cairns (2006) notes that the accumulation of lactic acid in muscles has long been implicated as a cause of muscle fatigue.
He defines *fatigue* as "a decline in muscle force or power output leading to impaired
exercise performance." But, he adds, many of the cited experiments were done on
amphibian muscle, which generates more lactic acid accumulation than in humans.
In fact, says Cairns, accumulation of lactic acid may even have some beneficial effects for us in protecting against increased potassium levels. His conclusion is that
lactic acid accumulation in skeletal muscles "should not be taken as fact that lactic
acid is the deviant that impairs exercise performance" (Cairns 2006).

Fat is used as a fuel during exercise, particularly at a certain intensity. Many
regular users of exercise equipment such as an elliptical machine or a treadmill will
see a *fat-burning* zone demarcated. Fat oxidation, from the breakdown of muscle
triglycerides and the release of free fatty
acids from adipose tissue, provides
about half of a person's energy when he
or she is exercising at a moderate intensity of about 50%–70% of Vo_2max, with
blood glucose providing about 15%–
35% of one's energy in this range. When
exercising at a high intensity, such as
from 75% to 85% of Vo_2max, we are oxidizing fat less than at the moderate intensity
level. Endurance training enables an athlete to have "carbohydrate sparing" during
prolonged exercise and increase the oxidation of fat as a fuel, but carbohydrates are
still the main fuel during very strenuous exercise (Holloszy and Kohrt 1996).

> Exercise at a moderate intensity
> (50%–70% of Vo_2max) burns more fat
> than carbohydrates. Exercise at a high
> intensity (75%–80% of Vo_2max) burns
> more carbohydrates than fat.
>
> **Source: Holloszy and Kohrt 1996**

In a discussion of the severity and extent of the obesity epidemic, not only in
the United States but also worldwide, Hill et al. (2003) speak of the *energy gap*,
the amount of greater activity (energy expenditure) relative to calorie intake that a
person requires in order to not continue to gain weight every year. It is estimated,

for example, that people from ages 20–40 gain an average of about 2 pounds a year (1.8–2.0 pounds) (Colditz et al. 1990; Yanovski et al. 2000). In a large, population-based study of over 1,800 middle-aged women over the course of 5 years, Brown et al. (2005) found that women tended to gain about half a kilogram or just over a pound each year, so that by 5 years they had gained, on average, 2½ kilograms or about 5½ pounds. This amounted to an energy imbalance of about 10 calories a day. Those who quit smoking had an almost 3-fold increase in their odds of gaining more than 11 pounds compared with women who had never smoked, and those who sat for more than 4½ hours a day were also likely to gain more than 11 pounds over the 5 years. Even for those women who gained more than 11 pounds, their weight gain reflected an imbalance of only 20–40 calories per day over the 5 years (Brown et al. 2005).

Hill et al. (2003) suggest that by some combination of decreasing calories and increasing energy expenditure by 100 calories a day, we could severely curtail the typical weight gain seen year after year. This is the same principle that Wansink (2006, pp. 30–31) has noted in his book *Mindless Eating*. This amounts to walking an extra mile a day or leaving a few bites of a hamburger uneaten (Hill et al. 2003). It sounds fairly simple, but obviously it is not.

First, the human body is extraordinarily able to store excess energy in body fat: even a lean person has enough energy stored to support the person's basic needs for 2–3 months, and an obese person has a year's worth of energy stored (Levine 2004). And women tend to be more efficient at preserving their level of fat, so it is more difficult for them to lose weight than it is for men (Westerterp 1998). Many researchers have been interested in the effects of exercise on body composition.

- Our bodies are very efficient.

- Even a lean person has 2–3 months' worth of energy storage; an obese person, a year's worth.

After all, weight loss from exercise, unlike weight loss from diet alone, has the potential additional benefit of improving cardiovascular fitness (Irwin et al. 2003). One study by Irwin et al. (2003) examined the effect of exercise (45-minute sessions of moderate exercise, such as walking or biking, for 5 days/week) on body fat in about 175 overweight women, ages 50–75 years, after menopause. In a randomized, controlled study over the course of a year, women who exercised for about 200 minutes per week at moderate intensity had dose-dependent, significant improvements in their amount of intra-abdominal fat specifically and lost over 4% of their total body fat (vs. 0.4% in control subjects who did not exercise). Although these women improved their body composition significantly, their actual weight loss was described as modest.

After exercise, the body does continue to burn calories. This is called the *excess postworkout oxygen consumption*, or EPOC, and depends on both the intensity and duration of the exercise as well as the type: aerobic exercise tends to burn more calories during the actual exercise whereas anaerobic exercise (resistance exercise) continues to burn more after the exercise is completed. There is controversy, however, about the importance of this calorie expenditure in terms of the body's overall expenditure, and researchers disagree about how long this effect actually lasts—whether it continues for extended periods of time or just minutes (Hill et al. 2004, p. 637). Exercise over the course of years, even those exercises that have a low EPOC, can have a cumulative effect (LaForge 2006). In general, the EPOC effect is greater with the duration and intensity of the exercising. EPOC tends to return to baseline within 2–15 minutes, but may last up to 90 minutes (Herring et al. 1992). Ralph LaForge (2006, and personal communication, January 4, 2010) emphasizes, though, that even though anaerobic exercise may boost the metabolic rate for a longer period of time than does aerobic exercise, it is not the calories expended "during recovery" but the calories burned during the actual exercise that "represent the most important factor in total exercise energy expenditure."

> Aerobic exercise tends to burn more calories during the actual exercising, whereas anaerobic (i.e., strength or resistance) exercise continues to burn calories after the exercise is completed.

Geliebter et al. (1997) compared aerobic exercise (cycling) with strength training (weight resistance exercise) to assess differences over 8 weeks in body composition, resting metabolic rate, and oxygen consumption in moderately obese dieting men and women. Neither aerobic exercise nor strength training was able to prevent the decline in resting metabolic rate that occurred with weight loss in the subjects. Strength training, however, tended to preserve lean body tissue more than aerobic exercise, whereas aerobic exercise tended to enhance peak oxygen consumption, a marker of cardiovascular fitness.

Exercise for Initial Weight Loss Versus Minimizing Weight Regain

Many studies have shown that those who fail to get regular physical exercise are much more likely to gain weight over the long term (sometimes three times as likely) than those who do even low-level to moderate amounts of exercise (Hill and Wyatt 2005). For example, Donnelly et al. (2003) studied 74 previously sedentary and overweight or obese young men and women (ages 17–35) over the course of 16 months to evaluate the effects of exercise alone, without any dietary recommendations. The types of exercise that this randomized, controlled study evaluated were primarily exercise on a treadmill, stationary bike, or elliptical machine. By month 6, the exercise group was expending about 2,000 calories per week in 45-minute sessions 5 days of the week. Significantly, the men in the exercise group lost weight (~11 or more pounds); by the end of the study, though, they were expending about 3,300 calories per week. The women who exercised maintained a fairly stable weight (but without weight loss), though they were expending about 2,200 calories per week.

The control subjects in the study gained over 6 pounds on average. This study shows how very difficult it is for women to lose weight, even with extensive exercise. Say Donnelly et al. (2003), "The suggestion that women might need to obtain an even greater amount of exercise to promote weight loss is not likely to be well received or executed and may in fact be a barrier, discouraging women from contemplating an exercise program." Significantly, this study had a large attrition rate, as have many others involving either diet or exercise: of the original 131 people screened, only 44% completed the 16-month study.

Di Pietro et al. (2004) studied over 2,500 men, ages 25–55, over the course of about 5 years, to assess just how active these people had to be on a daily basis to maintain their weight and prevent weight gain over time. Di Pietro et al. (2004) found that their subjects had to improve their fitness level over time in order to avoid weight gain—"simply maintaining the same level of fitness (even among the most fit subjects) was not sufficient." In other words, "at least some" of their middle-aged subjects had to maintain a daily activity level ≥60% above the resting metabolic rate to avoid weight gain. This could translate into 45–60 minutes a day of brisk walking or even working in the garden—hardly much, but only barely what most people do every day.

Levine (2007a) makes the point that our bodies were designed for walking all day. Think about the fact, for example, that the earth was populated by people walking across it. In general, though, exercise is not a particularly effective means of weight loss. Our bodies are just too efficient and the availability of highly caloric food is too plentiful for exercise to make a substantial difference. Miller et al. (1997) performed a meta-analysis of the previous 25 years of research (1969–1994) comparing diet alone, exercise alone, or combined diet-exercise interventions in almost 500 study groups. Most of those studies evaluated only moderately obese, middle-aged populations for less than 6 months. Not surprisingly, though, the diet alone

---

REGULAR PHYSICAL EXERCISE

- Researchers do not agree on how much exercise is beneficial, but most recommend ≥30 minutes of moderate physical exercise 5 or 6 days a week.

- During aerobic exercise, you should keep your heart rate up but be able to talk or sing at the same time; your maximum heart rate is 220 minus your age; you can take your own pulse by pressing your fingers (not thumb) on the thumb side of your wrist and counting the number of beats within 60 seconds.

- An exercise routine should consist of aerobic exercise, anaerobic exercise (strength training with contraction of muscles in intense, short bursts) and flexibility training (prevents stiffness, cramping, injuries; allows greater range of motion; relieves stress—e.g., yoga).

Source: Rouzier and Mancini 2009a; Simon 2008

and the combined diet-exercise intervention programs yielded considerably better results. For example, exercise alone tended to produce a weight loss of about 1–2 kilograms (< 5 pounds) whereas there was a 9- to 12-kilogram weight loss with diet or diet combined with exercise. Notably, for the studies providing 1 year of follow-up, subjects in the diet-exercise combination group maintained 77% of their initial weight loss, whereas those in the diet alone group maintained only 56% and those in the exercise alone group maintained only 53% of their initial weight loss. In other words, there is something important about exercise for preventing weight regain. A more recent meta-analysis by Anderson et al. (2001), addressing long-term weight loss maintenance in U.S. studies from the years 1970–1999, with six studies addressing the role of exercise, found that those who exercised more were able to maintain a weight loss of over 30 pounds during 2–3 years of follow-up. And Christiansen et al. (2007) confirmed these earlier findings of the importance of exercise in preventing weight regain in a study with over 4 years of follow-up: those who maintained a 10% or greater weight loss (considered successful) engaged in significantly more daily physical activity than those who did not. Significantly, though, in this study of very obese subjects with average initial body mass index (BMI) values of over 47 kg/m^2 and initial weights of over 300 pounds, 4 years after subjects experienced an intensive lifestyle intervention at a weight loss camp, only between 20% and 29% were able to maintain a weight loss of 10% of their initial weights.

The importance of exercise is also seen in follow-up data on those in the National Weight Control Registry. Since it began in 1993, the Registry has accumulated over 6,000 members who have all lost at least 30 pounds and kept that weight off for at least a year (and most for substantially longer periods of time). In other words, these members not only were successful at weight loss but have been successful at preventing weight regain over time. Those who continue to be most successful at preventing weight regain, by self-reports, do substantial physical exercise daily (Catenacci et al. 2008). In this subgroup of almost 900 men and over 2,700 women, subjects report walking, including power walking, more than a mile per day as the most common exercise; more than half of the subjects report engaging in this type of exercise. On average, these people expend more than 2,600 calories per week in exercise, with a range of 25% expending less than 1,000 calories to almost 35% expending more than 3,000 calories per week. This is equivalent to about 60–75 minutes of moderate-intensity daily activity. About 29% of the members of this subgroup report doing resistance training (and over 90% do this in addition to other activities). Resistance exercise seems to be more helpful in avoiding weight regain than in accomplishing initial weight loss. Catenacci et al. (2008) note that the majority do not engage in resistance training, and this type of exercise does not seem to be required to prevent weight regain.

Hill and Wyatt (2005) also found that most people may need to expend from 2,500 to 2,800 calories per week, spending 60–90 minutes per day in moderate-intensity exercise, in order to avoid weight regain after substantial weight loss. And the greater the weight loss initially, the more physical activity may be required for weight maintenance at the lower weight. According to Johannsen et al. (2007), when we lose 10% or more of our body mass, we reduce our energy expenditure even more than what we would expect. So, for example, when we lose 10% of our weight, we decrease our energy expenditure (in skeletal muscle primarily) by 20%–30%. It is the body's mechanism for preserving weight. No one really knows why the resting metabolic rate, and hence total amount of energy expended, decreases when we lose weight. It takes more energy to move a larger body than a smaller one. So to maintain weight loss over time, we have to either increase our physical activity or decrease how much we eat. Physical activity has another advantage, however: it potentially changes body composition and gives us more fat-free mass, which is more metabolically active than fat (Hill and Wyatt 2005).

Studies on the effects of exercise and metabolic rate, though, do not show consistent results. Many factors may be involved, including differences in levels of weight or other differences in the populations studied. For example, Byrne and Wilmore (2001) suggest that researchers may get contradictory results regarding the effect of exercise on resting metabolic rate because some studies do not take into account the level of training of their subjects: when the premenopausal women in their particular study were grouped by training level, only those who were "highly trained" had an increased resting metabolic rate, regardless of whether aerobic or resistance exercise was used.

Geissler et al. (1987) found that a group of obese women who had lost weight and maintained that loss for ≥6 months had a 15% decrease in metabolic rate compared with lean women who had never been obese, and they ate significantly less than those who had never been obese. The researchers figured that this 15% decrease in subjects' metabolic rates would lead to a weight gain of approximately 14 kilograms (~30 pounds) in just 1 year if calorie intake did not decrease. Furthermore, in this study, aerobic exercise did not have any lasting stimulating effects on metabolic rate in either group after exercise. Other studies, however, have shown different results. For example, Bielinski et al. (1985) demonstrated that after a period of intense exercise (in this case, 3 hours on a treadmill at 50% of Vo_2max—i.e., within the fat-burning range), the resting metabolic rates of young, healthy male volunteers were elevated 9 hours after the exercise period ended. Furthermore, the subjects had been given a mixed meal of 18% protein, 27% fat, and 55% carbohydrates. After the exercise period, there was an increase in fat oxidation (for 18 hours postexercise)—that is, a shift toward fat oxidation—and a decreased insulin response. There was a significant increase in protein catabolism in the postexercise period as well.

Another study, by Hunter et al. (2001), examined the effects of exercise (resistance training or aerobic exercise versus no exercise) on resting metabolic rate in a group of previously overweight premenopausal women (with initial BMI values of 27–30) who had each lost about 12 kilograms (~25 pounds) through significant calorie restriction, an 800-calorie diet. All testing was done during the follicular stage of menses (within 10 days of the women's periods), as it usually is when women are tested, because the phase of the menstrual cycle can affect metabolic measurements. This study, unlike most others, in which populations are often predominantly white, had equal numbers of African American and European American women. After weight loss, the African American women lost less fat-free mass (i.e., muscle) than European American women. Resistance training, regardless of race, enabled women to preserve substantially more muscle and strength after weight loss than aerobic exercise did, and it did not result in a decrease in resting metabolic rate. However, both aerobic exercise (walking or jogging on a treadmill for 40 minutes at 80% of Vo_2max, which did preserve cardiovascular fitness) and no exercise resulted in a loss of muscle mass after weight loss, as well as a decrease in resting metabolic rate, as is generally typical after weight loss (Hunter et al. 2008).

LaForge (2006) emphasizes the difficulty in calculating just how many calories are actually expended by exercise and hence how much a person might lose by exercise alone. Both the amount of time taken for a particular exercise and the intensity must factor in the calculations. He distinguishes the *net energy cost* of an exercise from the *gross energy cost*. The net energy cost is how many calories are expended, taking into account the number of calories that might have been expended had the person not been doing any exercise (e.g., sitting, standing—"doing what you would have been doing anyway"). The longer it takes to do an exercise, the more the net energy cost and the gross energy cost will differ. In other words, walking slowly for an hour is not the same as running for half an hour because during that 1 hour of slow walking, you are not doing all those other things that "you would have been doing anyway" for a much longer period of time. Says LaForge (2006), "Think of the net cost as being the actual *added* calorie expenditure of an exercise program to your daily living routine." He gives examples: the net energy cost (calories expended) per mile for moderate-paced walking (≤3.5 miles/hour) is 0.77 cal/kg per mile, whereas the gross energy cost might be 0.9–1.0 cal/kg per mile. For fast walking (3.5–5 miles/hour), the net energy cost is 1.38 cal/kg per mile. And the net energy cost of running 1 mile is almost twice that for walking 1 mile at a moderate pace. Furthermore, the calorie counter on a treadmill usually displays the gross number of calories expended. The actual number of calories burned is usually 10%–15% lower than what the treadmill indicates.

It takes about 10,000 steps per day to maintain general cardiovascular health and 12,000–15,000 steps to lose weight (LaForge 2006). There are roughly 2,000 steps per mile as measured by a device like a pedometer, and Bravata et al. (2007) suggest that use of this kind of device significantly increases the amount of physical activity done in a day. In fact, Bravata et al. (2007) note that using a pedometer motivates people to take approximately 2,100–2,500 additional steps per day.

Other aspects that affect how many calories are actually expended during exercise include the muscle fibers and muscle groups used. Exercises such as cross-country skiing or long-distance running and even some dance exercises that involve many muscle groups in weight-bearing exercises (i.e., involving gravity) expend more energy. Exercises like swimming or stationary bike cycling that are non–weight bearing (and involve gravity less) expend less energy. Even how well someone performs an exercise can affect the number of calories expended. For example, someone who is not as skilled may tend to expend more calories by making more unnecessary movements, but this may lead to metabolic fatigue (higher oxygen costs and faster heart rate), all of which may reduce the actual time the person exercises. In other words, someone who is more coordinated tends to exercise longer and more efficiently (LaForge 2006).

EXERCISE AND APPETITE

The relationship between exercise and appetite (and hence subsequent food intake) is a complex one. Exercise or any increased physical activity can affect meal size, meal frequency, and even specific choice of food. And many factors—such as the mode, duration, and intensity of exercise as well as the age, sex, and fat percentage of a person, and even what foods are available—may affect whether exercise increases or decreases appetite and to what extent and for what period of time (King et al. 1997). Blundell et al. (2003) note that physical activity can affect appetite by making a person more sensitive to the body's satiety signals, changing food preferences, or even changing a person's "hedonic response" (i.e., whether the food seems more pleasant). For example, Marcus et al. (1999) reported that exercise can be used effectively both as an adjunct to a cognitive-behavioral program to stop smoking and to help prevent the weight gain typically seen after cessation of smoking. And more recently, Taylor and Oliver (2009) reported that exercise can also be used to suppress chocolate cravings.

DOES EXERCISE AFFECT HOW MUCH YOU EAT?

- Following intense exercise, most people experience an immediate suppression of hunger, but this effect does not last long and does not affect how much a person will eat in a day.

- In one study, nonobese subjects ate significantly less immediately after strenuous exercise compared with nonobese subjects who did only moderate exercise. Obese subjects, however, showed no decrease in what they ate after strenuous exercise. The researchers believed psychological factors (e.g., rewarding oneself for difficult exercise) might have been involved in overriding the short-term exercise-induced suppression of food consumption in the obese subjects.

- How much a person, even when exercising, eats in the course of a day may be more a function of available fattening food and psychological factors than any lasting physiological effect from exercising.

Source: King et al. 1997

Both anecdotal and experimental data have shown that exercise, and particularly strenuous exercise, can suppress feelings of hunger, but exercise-induced suppression of hunger does not seem to last very long and does not necessarily lead to decreased food intake. Blundell et al. (2003) summarize the data by noting that in the very short term, "very intense bouts of exercise" can suppress hunger but that exercise essentially has a "marked lack of effect" on appetite and energy balance. When study results differed in whether exercise increased, decreased, or had no effect on hunger, the differences may have been related to differences in methodologies, protocols, or subjects. Over the longer term (e.g., >2 weeks), though, some people are more sensitive to changes in energy balance than others; those who are more sensitive are called *compensators* and are more likely to increase their food intake, whereas the less sensitive *noncompensators* are less likely to change their food intake, even over time. In general, humans are much more tolerant of too much food ("energy surfeits") than too little ("energy deficits") (Blundell et al. 2003).

King et al. (1997) found that obese women, as opposed to nonobese women, did not reduce their food intake after strenuous exercise. The speculation was that psychological factors were involved: the obese women "rewarded" themselves by eating more because of their "perception of the strenuous exercise as very difficult."

More recently, Hagobian et al. (2009) reported differences between men and women in the effects of exercise on appetite: the women in their study tended to increase their food intake, whereas appetite was inhibited in men. These differences are apparently related to differences in hormone secretions. For example, in another study, women showed higher levels of the acylated form of the hormone ghrelin in response to exercise than men and also differences in insulin secretion. (Acylated ghrelin is able to cross the blood-brain barrier, and its measurement provides a more sensitive indicator of the body's response to exercise than does total ghrelin level [Broom et al. 2009].) The speculation is that exercise alters these energy-regulating hormones such that appetite is stimulated in women regardless of whether they are in "energy balance," and that "mechanisms to maintain body fat are more effective in women" than in men (Hagobian et al. 2009).

Broom et al. (2009) investigated the immediate effects of both aerobic exercise and resistance (strength) exercise on hunger and the hormones acylated ghrelin and peptide tyrosine-tyrosine (PYY) in non-overweight young men ages 19–23. They found that both aerobic exercise and resistance exercise suppressed hunger in their subjects transiently, though strenuous aerobic exercise (e.g., running on a treadmill) did so to a greater extent. The transient decrease in appetite might be explained by the fact that both aerobic exercise and resistance exercise suppressed acylated ghrelin levels. PYY levels were significantly increased with aerobic exercise but not with anaerobic exercise (weight lifting). Broom et al. (2009) acknowledge, though, that they measured total PYY, which may not have been quite as sensitive as fractionated forms. Clearly, more research is needed.

GENERAL HEALTH EFFECTS OF EXERCISE

Exercise, Depression, and Anxiety

In some ways, it may seem counterintuitive to think of exercise as a treatment for psychiatric symptoms, particularly depression. After all, people with serious depression may be immobilized by their pessimism and anhedonia. They tend to withdraw socially and become helpless and hopeless. They may not want to get up out of bed in the morning. At best, they are physically much less active than nondepressed individuals. Because of their feelings of low self-confidence and worth, they are not motivated to do much. They are less likely to initiate any activity and may have an "all-or-none" mentality (Seime and Vickers 2006). And exercise is hard enough to initiate and maintain over the long run even in most healthy people.

But for years now, reports have appeared that exercise can, in fact, be an effective treatment for psychiatric disorders, particularly depression and anxiety. Early studies, though, suffered from methodological problems. For example, sometimes the exact nature of the exercise prescribed was not noted or the intensity was not specified or the dropout rate was not provided (Stathopoulou et al. 2006). Sometimes these early studies were observational and not randomized, controlled studies that had adequate follow-up (Daley 2008). Furthermore, it was often difficult to compare studies when frequency and duration of exercise varied from study to study. More recently, though, there have been meta-analyses evaluating the more methodologically sound studies (Daley 2008). One result that seems to be emerging is a dose-response effect: for example, high-intensity aerobic exercise (e.g., expending 17.5 cal/kg) for 5 days per week was more effective for major depressive disorder than lower-intensity exercise (7 cal/kg) for only 3 days per week (Dunn et al. 2005). And high-intensity anaerobic exercise (resistance training, with an 80% maximum load) was more effective than lower-intensity anaerobic exercise (with a 20% load). Howley and Franks (2007, pp. 191–192) define the overload principle as follows: "to enhance muscular performance, the body must exercise at a level beyond that at which it is normally stressed...overload is typically manipulated by changing the exercise intensity, duration, or frequency over the course of a training program. This process is often referred to as "*progressive overload* and is the basis for maximizing long-term training adaptations" (Stathopoulou and Powers 2006). When anaerobic and aerobic exercise were compared directly, they were equally effective in improving fitness and decreasing symptoms of depression (Stathopoulou et al. 2006).

Other studies have used exercise as an adjunct to other therapies, such as antidepressant medication or cognitive-behavioral approaches. Though some studies have shown that exercise alone can work more effectively than the combination of exercise and pharmacotherapy, these results may have been due to medication discontinuation. In general, combined treatment has "strong beneficial results," though the addition of exercise to cognitive-behavioral therapy "often has little advantage" over either modality used separately (Stathopoulou et al. 2006). Daley (2008) makes the point that exercise, which is "relatively side-effect free" and "comparatively cheap," can have an important place in treating patients with depression, particularly when patients are averse to taking medication and when medication is not as useful as exercise in improving symptoms of cognitive functioning or fatigue. And Dunn et al. (2005) believe exercise can sometimes be a more viable treatment because it does not have the "negative social stigma" that other treatments may have. Furthermore, there are reports that exercise continues to exert its antidepressant effect even months after an exercise program has stopped (Ernst et al. 2006).

Exercise has also been used as an adjunctive treatment for eating disorders and even alcohol abuse. For example, alcoholics who had been in a program of rehabilitation combined with an exercise program had better abstinence rates on followup and reported few cravings. And patients with eating disorders such as bulimia nervosa or anorexia nervosa who had tended to "abuse" exercise were able to have more sensible attitudes toward exercise when an exercise component was part of their treatment. Exercise has also been used effectively as an adjunctive therapy with cognitive-behavioral treatment for binge eating disorder (Stathopoulou et al. 2006).

Stathopoulou et al. (2006) report that in studies of anxiety disorders, antidepressant medications may have improved symptoms of anxiety sooner than exercise did, but at least in one 10-week study (see Broocks et al. 1998) comparing exercise and clomipramine treatment, by the end of the study, exercise was as effective in relieving symptoms. Furthermore, exercise can be helpful in allowing patients with anxiety to deal with the typical body responses associated with both exercise and anxiety, like tachycardia and rapid breathing, because they occur "in the absence of anticipated negative consequences."

De Moor et al. (2006, 2008), with a genetic model in mind, evaluated the relationship of symptoms of anxiety and depression to exercise in a large population-based sample in the Netherlands from 1991 to 2002. They questioned the causal effect of exercise on symptoms of anxiety and depression, calling it "folk wisdom." As noted, they believe that there is a heritable component to symptoms of anxiety and depression (40%–50% heritability) as well as exercise behavior (50%–60% heritability). Using longitudinal data from their large twin and family member study (almost 6,000 twins, > 1,300 additional siblings, and > 1,200 parents), they did note that there were "modest, but significant" associations, both cross-sectionally and prospectively, between exercising and having fewer anxiety and depressive symptoms. But their impression was that this association was genetic rather than causal; they stated that "there is a common genetic vulnerability to lack of regular exercise and risk for anxiety and depression in the population" (De Moor 2008). They found that in identical twins, for example, the twin who exercised more was not less anxious or depressed than the twin who exercised less. They realized that their study was "at odds" with some other studies, including randomized, controlled studies. They make a distinction, though, between voluntary leisure-time exercise in a large population sample, which has a genetic component, and exercise prescribed and monitored as part of a program ("environment driven"). In other words, exercise may have antidepressant or antianxiety effects only when the exercise is part of a monitored treatment.

There are many theoretical explanations for the positive effect exercise has on mood and other psychiatric symptoms. For example, exercise can improve sleep and this may make patients less anxious or depressed. Or exercise may make patients feel they can cope and have greater self-efficacy by making them take action. Or exercise may create a distraction from the typical ruminating thoughts seen in many psychiatric disorders (Stathopoulou et al. 2006). Over the past 20 years, researchers have appreciated the physiological effects that exercise has not only on the body but on the brain. In the 1980s, for example, researchers focused on the effects of the β-endorphins, opiate peptides formed from the protein pro-opiomelanocortin, found in the pituitary, which gives rise to the melanocortins and the opiates. They saw that some people became "addicted" to running (Ernst et al. 2006).

More recently, though, several other substances, including serotonin, vascular endothelial growth factor (VEGF), and brain-derived neurotrophic factor (BDNF), have received attention. All of these substances seem to be involved in *neurogenesis*, the synthesis of new neurons, in certain areas of the brain such as the hippocampus. Originally, researchers did not believe that any new neurons could be synthesized after an initial early developmental period, but adult neurogenesis is now thought to be characteristic of the brains of all mammals, including humans. Adult neurogenesis occurs, at least in animal models, under certain conditions, such as when animals can exercise *voluntarily* (and not when they are forced to swim, for example) (Ernst et al. 2006). The hypothesis is that major depression, and stress in general for that matter, is associated with decreased adult neurogenesis (Duman 2005) and that both antidepressant medications and exercise are able to reverse this decrease (Duman 2005). In other words, perhaps one mechanism involved in the effectiveness of both exercise and certain antidepressants is that they increase substances like VEGF, BDNF, and serotonin, which, in turn, support and facilitate adult neurogenesis. BDNF, for example, is involved in the survival and regeneration of nerve cells (and their "synaptic plasticity" [Vaynman et al. 2006]) and is typically low in animal models of depression but increases with exercise. The speculation, given that this has been done only with animal models to date, is that β-endorphins and serotonin enhance the creation of new nerve cells whereas VEGF and BDNF act as mediators, and that they all enhance the survival of the nerve cells. It remains to be seen how this theory of the relationship of adult neurogenesis to exercise and depression is relevant to depression in humans (Ernst et al. 2006). Researchers such as Hunsberger et al. (2007) are optimistic that substances like VEGF and BDNF, new "potential therapeutic targets," may eventually lead to successful treatments for major depressive disorder.

Exercise and Cognitive Functioning

Along the same lines, researchers are now beginning to appreciate the role of exercise in preserving cognitive functioning, or at least in "reducing the risk of cognitive decline" in older adults (Lautenschlager et al. 2008). Ferris et al. (2007) measured serum levels of BDNF and cognitive functioning in humans after different intensities of exercise. They found that BDNF did increase in humans after exercise and that this was "dose-dependent"; that is, the higher the intensity of the exercise, the greater the magnitude of BDNF increase. Furthermore, cognitive functioning increased after exercise of all intensities, but this was not related to changes in BDNF blood levels. Ferris et al. (2007) speculate that the potential impact of exercise on the brain has considerable implications. For example, if exercise-induced increases in BDNF levels can lead to improved functioning of neurons, then exercise can become a "potent weapon" in treating diseases of cognition, mood, or even neuromuscular disorders. BDNF does cross the blood-brain barrier but these levels have been measured so far only in animals, so we do not yet know what effect exercise actually has on levels of BDNF in the human brain. Brain levels, though, can be inferred from cerebrovascular blood volume, which can be measured by magnetic resonance imaging (MRI). MRI scans can detect areas of increased density of new blood vessels (*angiogenesis*) and the process of angiogenesis has been correlated with neurogenesis. Pereira et al. (2007) found that aerobic exercise (on a treadmill, stair-climbing machine, or elliptical trainer for 40 minutes four times per week, with extra time for warm-up and cool-down periods) did selectively increase blood volume in a particular area of the brain (the dentate gyrus of the hippocampus) in humans who were initially below average in aerobic fitness level. Furthermore, their cognitive functioning also improved after exercise. The researchers caution that we still do not have direct confirmation that the increased cerebral blood volume seen in the hippocampus in humans definitely reflects neurogenesis, as it does in mice (Pereira et al. 2007). After all, only autopsy findings confirm the process in mice.

Traustadóttir et al. (2004) found that increased aerobic fitness can lead to a blunted reaction to psychological and physical stresses (i.e., less hypothalamic-pituitary-adrenal axis reactivity) in previously physically unfit older women, who usually have a stronger reaction to stress. In this case, researchers produced stress by mental arithmetic tests, color-word interference tasks (the Stroop test, in which a word for a certain color is printed in an ink of a different color; e.g., the word *red* may be written in blue ink), and even exposure of the subject's hand to cold water. In general, older people have an increased cortisol response to psychological stresses (e.g., a longer duration of response), but this increased stress response was attenuated or even prevented with increased levels of aerobic fitness (Traustadóttir et al. 2004).

Research on the relationship between exercise and improved cognitive functioning (and specifically, preventing or delaying the development of dementia), though, is mixed. Some studies have found a connection (e.g., Chan et al. 2005; Larson et

al. 2006; Lautenschlager et al. 2008). One large population-based prospective longitudinal study (Larson et al. 2006), sought to determine whether regular exercise
could reduce a person's risk for developing dementia, including Alzheimer disease.
This study population was a fairly homogeneous sample of mostly white and well-
educated subjects (>1,700 individuals) who were older than age 65 and without
cognitive impairment initially. Over the course of the 6-year study, 158 developed
a type of dementia (mostly Alzheimer disease but also vascular dementia and other
types). They found that those who exercised three or more times per week had a
32% lower risk of developing dementia than those who did not (exercise was self-
reported). Unfortunately, the researchers did not measure intensity of exercise or
duration, but merely frequency. They were cautious, as well, to observe that "modest
levels" of regular exercise do not necessarily prevent the development of dementia,
but may delay its onset.

Lautenschlager et al. (2008) conducted an 18-month randomized, controlled
study to determine whether individuals age 50 or older who already had subjective
complaints of memory impairment, as well as subjects for whom there had already
been objective findings of mild cognitive decline, could benefit from 6 months of
participation in an exercise program. The 138 people in this study showed a "modest" improvement in cognitive functioning with an extra 150 minutes of moderate-
intensity aerobic exercise per week (home-based exercise, most commonly walking).
In another study of older people (140 people, mostly women, age 56 or older), Chan
et al. (2005) compared cardiovascular exercises such as jogging or swimming to
mind-body exercises such as tai chi—where each movement is consciously performed, slowly and with a relaxed mind—or both. The combination of these types
of exercises, even when practiced as little as once a month each, was more helpful
in improving learning and memory than either type practiced alone.

The results suggestive of a connection between exercise and improved cognitive
functioning are encouraging but far from definitive, and more research is warranted.
Many of these studies are based on self-reports and do not include standardization
of intensity of exercise or other factors. It certainly makes sense that exercise can
improve blood flow to the brain, with improved oxygenation, and can possibly induce new nerve growth in areas particularly vulnerable to aging such as the areas
of the hippocampus involved in memory and learning.

Exercise and Medical Consequences

Osteoporosis

Osteoporosis is a serious condition that can affect any age and either sex but is much
more common in women than men and especially in postmenopausal women. It is
defined by a specific decrease in bone mineral density, a measure of bone mass that
predisposes a person to bone fragility and a significant increase in the risk of fracture.

Both kinds of bone, cortical and trabecular (cancellous), lose mass in osteoporosis. About 10 million adults in the United States have osteoporosis, and another 34,000 reportedly have *osteopenia*, lower bone mass that is not yet at the level diagnosed as osteoporosis. About 80% of people with osteoporosis are women (Simon 2009). In the elderly, fractures may result not only from decreased bone mass but also from difficulties with balance and eyesight as well as loss of muscle (*sarcopenia*) or loss of muscle strength. Osteoporosis is a leading cause of disability and even mortality in both elderly men and elderly women. For example, there are about 300,000 hip fractures in the United States annually (Jackson et al. 2006). Though people with osteoporosis are typically elderly and can have concomitant illness, more than 1% of all deaths after the age of 50 are related to hip fractures specifically, and most deaths occur between 1 and 6 months after the fracture (Kanis et al. 2003). Men have an even higher rate of mortality (74% greater) after hip fracture than women. And 20% of both men and women are not able to return to their own homes after the fracture, but require nursing home care (Trombetti et al. 2002). Osteoporosis is often a silent disease in which the first sign of the disease is a bone fracture.

There are several ways to measure bone mineral density, but the method of choice is dual-energy X-ray absorptiometry (DXA), which is also one of the most accurate measures of percentage of fat in the body. Measurements are taken most commonly of the spine, hip, and wrist bones. Bones have to be light enough for movement and yet strong enough to resist fractures. Their design is a "compromise between strength and mass," particularly with their marrow cavity (Borer 2005). Obviously, someone does not have to have osteoporosis to sustain a fracture, as evidenced by injuries in young athletes. Bones can also weaken (i.e., become fragile) and osteoporosis can develop secondarily with organ transplantation, chronic liver or kidney disease, rheumatoid arthritis, epilepsy, leukemia, lymphoma, and diabetes. Even certain medications, such as corticosteroids, antiepileptic medications, and heparin, can predispose a person to bone loss. Both excessive alcohol consumption and cigarette smoking have been associated with increased rates of bone loss as well (Kanis et al. 2003; Trombetti et al. 2002). Furthermore, men who have decreased levels of testosterone (hypogonadism) secondary to illness such as a pituitary tumor may also be at risk for developing osteoporosis (Simon 2009).

Even though osteoporosis typically occurs in the elderly, it can also occur as a result of nutritional deprivation as seen in patients with anorexia nervosa. The hormone leptin, a signal for puberty initiation, as well as a marker of the amount of fat in the body, is also hypothesized to be involved in the proliferation and differentiation of bone cells, as well as in stimulating longitudinal bone growth. But if there is insufficient calorie intake, bone growth can be permanently stunted, as seen in individuals with short stature due to malnutrition. Leptin levels are low in patients with anorexia nervosa, and these low levels are correlated with low bone mass in young female athletes who no longer have their menstrual periods (Borer 2005). Even women who are not anorexic but are on the lean side tend to have lower bone mass and be more susceptible to fractures than those of normal weight and even those who are overweight. Furthermore, dieting results not only in the loss of adipose tissue but also in the loss of lean tissue; up to 25% of weight lost during dieting may be lean tissue, including bone mass (Borer 2005).

In general, women tend to lose bone mass in the perimenopausal time, after age 40. In fact, some researchers believe that sufficient calcium—from 1,000 to 2,000 mg a day (the usual dosage is 1,200 mg/day in divided doses)—and concomitant vitamin D_3 (cholecalciferol) intake (up to 1,000 IU/day [Bordelon et al. 2009]), necessary for calcium absorption, are even more important in this earlier period than after menopause, which typically occurs between ages 45 and 55 (Borer 2005). But once menopause comes, with the fall of estrogen and progesterone levels, there is marked bone loss, with increased calcium levels in the blood and increased excretion of calcium in the urine. Even in the late postmenopausal phase, bone mass density still decreases at a rate of about 1% a year (Borer 2005).

Calcium is most plentiful in dairy products like milk and cheese, including non-fat or low-fat varieties, whereas vitamin D_3 (cholecalciferol) can be obtained when skin is exposed to sunlight, by eating liver, or when milk is fortified with the vitamin. Bordelon et al. (2009) note, though, that a vitamin D deficiency can occur at any age and is manifested by "symmetric low back pain, proximal muscle weakness, muscle aches, and throbbing bone pain" when pressure is exerted on either the sternum or the tibia. Although a vitamin D deficiency can affect all ages, Bordelon

OSTEOPOROSIS

- Bones become brittle and fracture easily in both men and women as we age, partly related to a decrease in both testosterone and estrogen; osteoporosis occurs 5–10 years earlier in women, especially after menopause.

- It is often a silent disease that appears only with the onset of a serious fracture.

- Both excess alcohol use and cigarette smoking are associated with increased rates of bone loss.

- Between 25% and 36% of women who experience a hip fracture die within a year, and the percentage is even higher in men.

- Moderate, weight-bearing exercise (2–3 times a week) and muscle-strengthening exercise reduce the risk of osteoporosis in men and women.

- Calcium supplements of 1,200 mg/day, in divided doses, are recommended for those over age 50: calcium citrate (Citracal) is better absorbed but is only 24% calcium, whereas calcium carbonate (Os-Cal) is 40% calcium; vitamin D_3 400 IU/day is needed for calcium absorption; recommendations for vitamin D are now up to 800–1,000 IU/day.

Source: Bordelon et al. 2009; Simon 2009

et al. (2009) emphasize that it is more common in those older than 65 years, people with dark skin, those with insufficient exposure to sunlight, those on medications that change vitamin D metabolism (e.g., anticonvulsants or glucocorticoids), and those with obesity (e.g. with a body mass index value greater than 30 kg/m².) The authors recommend obtaining vitamin D levels, with a deficiency defined as a serum level of less than 20 ng/mL of 25 hydroxyvitamin D (the major circulating form of vitamin D). Even when there is no deficiency, Bordelon et al (2009) recommend at least 700–800 IU/day of vitamin D_3 (cholecalciferol) for adults and even up to 1,000 IU/day "from dietary or supplemental sources." Calcium is also in oily fish (e.g., sardines, salmon, fresh tuna, and mackerel), almonds, and molasses. Calcium absorption can be lowered by antacids. Too much calcium can lead to kidney stones. Dr. Andrew Weil, on his health Web site (2009) notes that many people take Tums as a calcium supplement because it is less expensive. He recommends against using Tums (which provides calcium in the form of calcium carbonate) for calcium supplementation because it is not as easily absorbed as calcium citrate.

Some believe that calcium found in food is superior to supplemental calcium. If calcium is taken as a supplement, it should be taken in divided doses, with food. There are two preparations: calcium citrate (Citracal), which is better absorbed but is only 24% calcium, and calcium carbonate (Os-Cal), which is 40% calcium. Patients after bariatric surgery require calcium supplementation, and calcium citrate is the recommended form because calcium carbonate requires stomach acid, which is lower after surgery, for absorption (Shah et al. 2006).

Borer (2005) reports on many studies that have shown that calcium supplementation can substantially reduce bone mineral loss in postmenopausal women in their 50s, 60s, and beyond. Other studies have questioned whether calcium supplementation actually leads to a decrease in the number of fractures. In a 5-year, double-blind study of women older than 70 years, Prince et al. (2006) found that calcium carbonate (600 mg twice daily) supplementation did not necessarily reduce the risk of fractures in a large population (>1,400 women), but primarily because there was poor long-term compliance with taking the calcium supplements; 43% of women in this study were noncompliant. In those who took at least 80% of the pills prescribed each year, there was almost a 57% reduced rate of fracture, and Prince et al. (2006) do recommend supplementation for those willing to continue taking calcium supplements long term. Another long-term population study by Jackson et al. (2006), with an average of 7 years of follow-up at multiple centers in the United States, found that supplementation with calcium carbonate (~1,000 mg/day) and vitamin D_3 (only 400 IU/day), both taken in divided doses, diminished hip bone loss but not significantly, and it did not have a significant effect on vertebral fractures or fractures of other bones. But again, noncompliance was an issue. Only 59% of the treated population was still taking the prescribed doses by the end of the study. Jackson et al. (2006) noted that this trial of over 36,000 healthy, postmenopausal women ages 50–79 was not able to differentiate the effects of calcium from the effects of vitamin D_3 supplementation, and also suggested that the vitamin D_3 supplementation may not have been high enough. Furthermore, supplementation increased the risk of kidney stones. Bordelon et al. (2009) also note that too much vitamin D can lead to toxicity, with headache, a metallic taste, nausea, vomiting, and even pancreatitis, as well as kidney stones.

Though calcium and vitamin D_3 supplementation seems to be helpful in strengthening bone and preventing some fractures to some degree, at least when the supplements are taken regularly, most researchers do believe that moderate physical exercise is extremely important as we age and become prone to osteoporosis. Low-impact, non-weight-bearing exercises such as swimming and biking improve cardiovascular fitness but do not increase bone density. And high-impact exercise, such as step aerobics, can increase the risk of fractures (Simon 2008). Borer (2005) reviewed studies that indicate that the mechanical stress that exercise provides, particularly in postmenopausal women at later ages, actually enables more uptake of calcium by bones and complements the increased calcium absorption and bone mineralization that supplemental calcium provides. For example, Borer (2005) reported that subjects who engaged in high-intensity walking (>90% of maximum heart rate), three times per week for 30 minutes each time over a period of months, increased their bone density, unlike subjects who walked at a lower intensity, who even lost some density. Jogging and stair-climbing 3 days a week for about an hour were also effective. Once people stopped exercising, though, the increased bone density did not remain. Borer (2005) recommends short but intense exercise for maximum effect in strengthening bone, with at least 6–8 hours of recovery time between exercise periods. Exercise is most effective when it subjects the bone to unusual patterns of exercise, that is, greater magnitude and a different orientation from what the bone is used to. For example, using greater stress (greater intensity) is more effective than conventional patterns of flexion and extension of an arm in building bone mass. Resistance exercises (strength exercises) and flexibility exercises are also important in maintaining the health of bones and joints and in improving balance. As noted above, M. A. Williams et al. (2007) reported that resistance training moderately increased bone density. Borer (2005), though, clarified that "higher exercise intensities (e.g., 3 weekly sessions of 15–20 minutes) and unusual loading patterns" (e.g., loading the forearm with tensing, compressing, and bending stresses) produced an increased bone density of 3.8% in the distal part of the radius, whereas lower intensities did not.

Overall Benefits for Physical Health

Brown et al. (2007) did a 10-year overview update of evidence linking the importance of physical activity in preventing certain diseases in women. Their conclusion, in a review from 1997 through early 2006, was that there was "strong evidence for the role of physical activity in the primary prevention of cardiovascular disease, diabetes, and some cancers in women," though they found no evidence for "additional health benefits" for more vigorous exercise than walking at moderate intensity. For example, they found reductions ranging from 28% to 58% in cardiovascular disease in 12 of 17 studies they examined, risk reductions from 14% to 46% in 7 of 8 studies of diabetes, and risk reduction of 11% to 67% in 7 of 10 studies involving breast cancer. "As little as 60 minutes of moderate-intensity physical activity per week" had "protective benefit" for cardiovascular disease and diabetes (Brown et al. 2007). But in reviewing these many studies, Brown et al. (2007) emphasized how difficult it is to compare and summarize data from different studies. For example, questions about physical activity varied from study to study (including even what constituted physical activity), and different researchers might elicit information through one general question or multiple questions (e.g., "How active are you?" versus "How many blocks do you walk?"). The researchers also mention that earlier studies used measurements in kilocalories or kilojoules, whereas more recent studies used METs (i.e., activity compared to resting.) And different studies recorded data at various times, with different lengths for follow-ups, and different frequency of assessments. In fact, because of the "wide variations in measurement and reporting of physical activity," Brown et al. (2007) could not conduct a meta-analysis of the studies, but could do only a "narrative review."

Many studies have concluded that exercise, as well as all strenuous physical activity, has substantial benefits for physical health. For example, even moderate-intensity exercise such as walking regularly—as little as 1 hour per week, but 30 minutes per day on most days—can have a major impact, with a 31% reduction in cardiovascular disease, the main cause of death in the United States (Bauman 2004; Brown et al. 2007; Diehl and Choi 2008). In a large study of over 15,000 people in 52 countries (the INTERHEART study), people who engaged in exercise of moderate intensity (e.g., walking, bicycling, or swimming) 4 or more hours per week "significantly decreased" their risk for developing cardiovascular disease, regardless of sex, age, or country (Diehl and Choi 2008). And exercise can reduce both systolic and diastolic blood pressure. Nemoto et al. (2007) reported that high-intensity walking (at 70% of subjects' peak aerobic capacity; i.e., 70% Vo_2max) for intervals of several minutes, combined with low-intensity walking (at 40% of peak capacity),

> The best exercise is the one you will do regularly.

taking 8,000 steps per day at least 4 days per week, improved blood pressure and also increased thigh muscle strength and peak aerobic capacity in a group of men and women in their 60s. In addition, Diehl and Choi (2008) reported that women who engage in regular exercise (>3 hours/week) have fewer menopausal symptoms of hot flashes (i.e., decreased "vasomotor symptom frequency and severity").

A large study of over 3,200 people, the Diabetes Prevention Program, concluded that regular, moderate exercise can also improve insulin sensitivity, blood glucose levels, and levels of hemoglobin A_{1c}, a marker for diabetes (Diehl and Choi 2008).

Those who exercised at moderate intensity for 150 minutes per week and also modified their diets were significantly more successful (58% vs. 31%) in reducing the incidence of or preventing the onset of diabetes than subjects who were taking the antidiabetic medication metformin—so much so that researchers stopped the study early. Moderate exercise (30–60 minutes/day) can substantially cut a woman's risk for postmenopausal breast cancer and decrease the risk for colon cancer in both sexes (Diehl and Choi 2008).

Woods et al. (2006) have reviewed the many studies suggesting that increased physical activity, and particularly exercise, works by decreasing low-grade systemic inflammatory responses in the body. For example, levels of C-reactive protein, a nonspecific marker of inflammation, have decreased significantly with exercise in some studies. Obesity, as well as the metabolic syndrome, has been considered a disease of inflammation; in fact, macrophages, the cells in the body associated with inflammation, are produced by adipose tissue, as are the inflammatory cytokines tumor necrosis factor α and

> Obesity may be considered a disease of inflammation, and regular exercise decreases systemic inflammation.

interleukin-6. Leptin, among its many functions in the body, is also associated with inflammation, and leptin levels fall with exercise. But Woods et al. (2006) distinguish chronic exercise, which leads to a decrease in systemic inflammation, from acute exercise, which may lead to mild inflammatory responses due to muscle and tissue damage in individuals not accustomed to exercise. Damaged tissue requires time for repair, and rest periods are essential when someone is beginning an exercise program, or else one can develop a chronic inflammatory situation that has been called the *overtraining syndrome*, with symptoms of fatigue, muscle and joint pain, and even loss of appetite and depression.

Many studies have shown that regular vigorous exercise is associated with longevity. Lee et al. (1995), in a famous prospective study of over 13,000 male Harvard University alumni who matriculated between 1916 and 1950, found an inverse relationship between vigorous exercise—but not nonvigorous exercise—and mortality. This study has continued through the years (Lee and Paffenbarger 2000); those engaging in light activities (defined as activities involving < 4 METs, such as housework, bowling, boating) did not have lower mortality rates; moderate activities (4–<6 METs, such as golfing, dancing, gardening) provided some bene-

> Regular exercise may promote longevity even in overweight people.

fit; and vigorous activity (≥6 METs, such as jogging, swimming laps, shoveling snow) "clearly predicted" lower mortality rates. The largest decrement in mortality occurred with calorie expenditures of greater than 1,000 calories in vigorous exercise per week. Lee et al. (2004) looked at the same population and wondered whether the "weekend warriors," so called because they exercised only 1 or 2 days on the weekends, were obtaining any benefit from this sporadic pattern of exercise in regard to mortality. Most commonly, weekend warriors engaged in golf (13%), ten-nis (38%), and gardening (9%). Even this pattern, if it generated an expenditure of 1,000 calories or more per week, was helpful in postponing mortality as long as the men were not considered at high risk. Those at "high risk" had one or more risk factors: smoking, being overweight or obese (BMI ≥ 25 kg/m^2), hypertension, or having high cholesterol levels. Those who were more "regularly active" (expending $>1,000$ cal/week) had a 36% lower mortality rate than those who were completely sedentary. Lee et al. (2004) found, though, that those men who were high risk "may not benefit from sporadic physical activity, such as the weekend warrior pattern." They found, for example, that the effects of the physical activity were short-lived: there were decreases in systolic blood pressure immediately after the exercise, but these decreases were not maintained even as soon as 3 hours after exercise.

Hu et al. (2004) looked at mortality in a group of over 115,000 middle-aged women over a period of 24 years of follow-up. In their study, any activity that ex-pended more than 3.5 METs per hour (e.g., brisk walking for 3.5 to >7 hours/week) was considered vigorous activity. Those who were lean (defined as a BMI value of 22–23.4 kg/m^2) and physically active (at least 3.5 hours per week exercising) had the lowest level of mortality. Significantly, weight gain during adulthood, even "modest" weight gain, was a risk factor for earlier mortality regardless of activity level. "Our data do not support the hypothesis that a higher level of physical activity eliminates the excess mortality associated with increased body fat," said Hu et al. (2004). Both BMI value and physical activity level were "strong and independent predictors of death." Hu also added, "Some unusually muscular persons with a body mass index over 30 who are active and fit may have a relatively low risk of death, but such per-sons must be rare: only 2 percent of women in our study were both physically active and obese, and the overall risk of death in this group was twice that among lean and active women." In a letter to the *New England Journal of Medicine*, Jacobs and Pereira (2004), though, took issue with Hu et al.'s (2004) conclusions, namely that someone had to be both physically fit and of normal weight (i.e., that a high body mass index does, indeed, necessarily convey extra risk even in most fit people) rather than just fit. Jacobs and Pereira (2004) noted that "imprecision in the measurement of physi-cal activity may have caused some misinterpretation of the data." For example, they noted that physically fit women (but with a high body mass index) would be "harder to identify" when researchers used self-reported data rather than actual tests of fitness on a treadmill test. And Hu et al. did not include measurement of physical activity that was "light-to-moderate intensity—which constitutes the bulk of energy expenditure in most people's lives" (and which varies, as we have also said, consider-ably from one person to another.) Furthermore, Jacobs and Pereira (2004) also noted that self-reported data of weights (as we have also discussed—see Chapter 2) can be notoriously inaccurate. The discussion by Jacobs and Pereira of Hu et al.'s (2004) research just highlights the extraordinary complexities involved in obesity research: the number of variables may seem infinite. As Cairns (2006) very poignantly stated (in his discussion of experiments measuring lactic acid in exercise), "Scientists usually endeavor to do experiments by systematically changing one factor and keeping all aspects constant, but this is not the situation during whole-body exercise."

Leitzmann et al. (2007) came to different conclusions in their large prospective study of men and women ages 50–71. With over 250,000 subjects, they found a 27% lower risk of mortality when a person engaged in at least moderate-intensity exercise (3 METs/hour) at least 3 days per week. For those who engaged in vigorous exercise for 20 minutes three or more times per week, there was a 32% lower mortality risk. The researchers defined *vigorous* exercise as exercise that increased heart rate or breathing or caused a sweat. Unlike the Hu et al. study (2004), this study found that BMI status did not seem to affect the reduction in mortality risk with exercise, such that the results supported the "value of regular exercise in promoting longevity not just for normal-weight individuals but also for those who are overweight or obese" (Leitzmann et al. 2007).

Most of the studies regarding mortality and physical activity have used self-reported data, which can be inaccurate measures of actual activity level. Manini et al. (2006) sought to rectify this by studying just over 300 high-functioning men and women, ages 70–82, over a period of 8 years (but follow-up actually averaged just over 6 years). The researchers measured their subjects' levels of activity by means of the gold standard measurement of doubly labeled water, in which analysis of body fluids measures the differences in disappearance rates of the isotopes (as a measure of total body expenditure) and "captures *any form* [our emphasis] of physical activity ranging from purposeful exercise to simple fidgeting" (Manini et al. 2006). Physical activity questionnaires, on the other hand, record only "basic volitional activities," such as exercise (e.g., running, walking) or household chores. Body fat was also measured accurately, by DXA. Manini et al. (2006) found that "any activity energy expenditure" in this older population was associated with lower mortality rates. Specifically, for every 287 calories per day expended in "free-living activity" (not even necessarily exercise), the mortality risk was 30% lower.

RECOMMENDATIONS: HOW MUCH, HOW OFTEN, WHAT KIND?

Recommendations for an exercise program depend primarily on a person's physical and psychological health and what the person wants to achieve. Goals may include building and/or maintaining strength (and maintaining fat-free mass; i.e., muscle); increasing flexibility and/or improving balance; improving health and/or preventing disease (e.g., cardiovascular disease, type 2 diabetes, or osteoporosis); building and/or maintaining aerobic fitness; preventing natural weight gain as we age; maintaining psychological well-being; training for endurance or sports performance; and increasing weight loss and/or preventing weight regain. Recommendations also depend on age, sex, level of fitness, previous training, psychological factors like motivation, and even practical limitations such as availability of exercise facilities (including in the home) and time. According to Church et al. (2007), lack of time is the major excuse people give for not exercising, despite their appreciating the considerable health benefits of exercise. Ultimately, the best exercise for someone is an exercise the person will continue to do. Recommendations can go only so far if people find them too burdensome and stop adhering to them over time.

Trainers often recommend a warm-up and cool-down period before extensive exercise. For aerobic exercise, this is a period of several minutes of low-intensity aerobic exercise, such as walking on a treadmill or slow cycling, before and after the period of greater intensity. For strength training, it may include several minutes of lifting lighter weights than those to be used in the full exercise, and for flexibility, it might include various movements like skipping or jumping. The idea of a warm-up or cool-down period is that these lower-intensity movements increase blood flow and increase body and muscle temperature, as well as potentially increasing flexibility and reducing the possibility of injury (Howley and Franks 2007, p. 200). It may also put a person in the proper mindset psychologically. For some, when time is crucial, the idea of 5 or so minutes tagged onto either end of a workout seems daunting. As noted earlier, whether stretching prior to exercise really prevents injury is still open to question; at least one review did not find stretching particularly useful (Herbert and Gabriel 2002).

Researchers have also questioned the importance of the intensity of exercise. Tremblay et al. (1994), for example, studied the intensity of exercise. In comparing vigorous exercise to moderate exercise in a small population of healthy young men and women, they found that after 15–20 weeks, vigorous exercise led to a greater loss of subcutaneous fat. The speculation was that vigorous exercise leads to more postexercise utilization of fat than does moderate-intensity exercise.

Church et al. (2007) evaluated changes in aerobic fitness in a group of over 450 previously overweight, postmenopausal women who participated in different levels of aerobic exercise over the course of 6 months (with ~92% of subjects in follow-up at 6 months). This was not a weight loss study, and no lifestyle changes, including diet, were recommended. Not surprisingly, all groups increased their cardiovascular fitness levels, including women who engaged in only 72 minutes of moderate-intensity exercise per week, and the more they exercised, the greater the increase in cardiovascular fitness.

Jakicic et al. (2007) studied aerobic exercise intensity and duration and a calorie-restricted diet (1,200–1,500 calories) in almost 200 premenopausal, sedentary, overweight women over the course of a year. Exercise ranged from less than 150 minutes to more than 200 minutes per week and from moderate to high intensity. Women in all groups lost weight, but there were no significant differences in weight loss with different durations and intensities of exercise. Cardiovascular fitness levels improved in all groups. Slentz et al. (2004), in STRRIDE (Studies of Targeted Risk

Reduction Interventions through Defined Exercise), also assessed exercise intensity and duration in subjects who were previously sedentary. In this study of an 8-month exercise program in more than 100 overweight men and women, the subjects were told not to change their eating habits and to maintain their initial weight. There was a dose-response effect such that those who exercised a greater amount—walking or jogging 17 versus 11 miles per week (averages based on adherence)—lost more weight and fat, but the effect of intensity (walking vs. jogging) was not as clear. Even without dieting, 85% of subjects who exercised a greater amount lost

> Overweight people who lose weight only by high-dose exercise (17 miles of walking or jogging per week), without dieting, may have to walk or jog 6–7 miles/week afterward to prevent regaining their weight.
>
> **Source: Slentz et al. 2004**

weight. There was, though, a tendency (though not significant) for a greater increase in fat-free mass (lean muscle) in those who exercised at a higher intensity. Slentz et al. (2004) suggest that walking or jogging 6–7 miles per week may be required just to prevent weight gain. And almost three-quarters of the control subjects, who did not exercise, gained weight (~2 pounds) over the course of the 8 months. Slentz et al. (2004) noted, as well, that although exercise did not decrease the amount of abdominal (i.e., central, visceral) fat over peripheral fat accumulation, the controls who did not exercise "appeared" to increase their fat "preferentially" in "central body skinfolds more than peripheral body skinfolds" but the effect was "small" and the "difference was not significant."

Tate et al. (2007) compared different activity levels, as measured by expenditure of calories, in a group of about 200 overweight (≤70 pounds overweight initially), middle-aged men and (58%) women followed over the course of 30 months. Those who expended more than 2,500 calories in exercise per week (e.g., walking 75 minutes per week), as opposed to 1,000 calories per week, and continued this level of exercise for at least 18 months—*high-adherence subjects*—lost an average of 15 pounds from their initial weight. Those who expended fewer calories had an average weight loss of about 2 pounds over the same period. But even the subjects in the 2,500-calorie per week group regained an average of about 5 pounds. And of the original sample of about 200, only 13 (out of the 75 subjects in the high-adherence group) maintained the high level of exercise throughout the follow-up period, and only 4 were able to maintain their entire weight loss. For a year, the amount of weight regained correlated with the amount of fat in the diet and calorie intake. (For more on the differences between initial weight loss and minimizing weight regain, see Chapter 2, "Obesity in the United States.")

This study points to one of the problems with exercise, namely compliance. It is very difficult to get most people to continue an exercise program indefinitely when they are not being directly supervised in a clinical study or given some incentive (including financial incentive) to continue a program. For example, Jakicic et al.

(2007) provided treadmills to all their participants, and Church et al. (2007) gave a monetary incentive of $150 to those who completed the study. Tate et al. (2007) suggest a "chronic care model," in which supervision extends for considerably longer periods of time (and we would add, perhaps indefinitely), "may be necessary to sustain the behaviors necessary for long-term weight regulation."

Blair et al. (2004) reviewed many of the difficulties involved in "specifying with confidence" exactly how much, what type, and what intensity of exercise should be prescribed to achieve health benefits, especially when many studies have employed self-reports, which can be notoriously inaccurate. What does seem to emerge from the research is that there is a dose-response relationship—that is, there is a minimal amount of exercise required for any benefit, but also "relatively small changes" in activity, particularly in individuals who are almost completely sedentary, "might produce large reductions in disease risk at the population level" (Blair et al. 2004). Blair et al. (2004) take issue with some of the recommendations proposed in 2002 by the Institute of Medicine (Trumbo et al. 2002), particularly that people need to get 60 minutes of exercise a day to prevent weight gain. There is obviously a major genetic component involved, in that some people are able to control their weight without much exercise whereas others can be active and still gain weight. And of course some people, even in our obesogenic environment, can regulate their weight, whereas others seem unable to prevent weight gain no matter what they do. The point is, we have to take into account individual differences. Blair et al. (2004) and Blair and Leermakers (2002, p. 288) recommend 30 minutes of moderate-intensity exercise every day, but acknowledge that this will not be enough for some and "perhaps many," at which point individuals have to either reduce their calorie intake or increase their exercise to prevent weight gain. For additional health benefits, the recommendation is to increase the amount of time spent exercising to 60 minutes per day, and to do resistance training and flexibility exercises at least twice a week to build and maintain muscle, strength, and endurance, as well as to slow bone loss in middle age. Duncan et al. (2005) reached similar conclusions, namely that "various combinations of intensity and frequency" may lead to increased cardiovascular fitness, but in their 2-year study they, like so many other researchers, observed diminished adherence to exercise over the course of follow-up.

Haskell et al. (2007), a panel representing the American College of Sports Medicine and the American Heart Association, have updated their organizations' recommendations, which were originally published in 1995. These recommendations, summarized below, are for adults ages 18–65. Obviously, individuals with special circumstances, such as pregnant or breast-feeding women, must discuss these guidelines with their physicians and adjust them accordingly.

First, Haskell et al. (2007) acknowledge that U.S. adults are still a fairly sedentary group. Though proportions vary with age, ethnic background, and education level (e.g., those with college degrees are more likely to be more active), overall, fewer than half of Americans are getting the amount of physical activity recommended (and women are even somewhat less likely to do so than men). The panel recommends, "to promote and maintain health," moderate-intensity aerobic exercise (e.g., brisk walking with increased heart rate) for a minimum of 30 minutes, 5 days per week, or vigorous exercise (e.g., jogging with rapid breathing and increased heart rate) for a minimum of 20 minutes on 3 days of the week. Aerobic exercise that is done intermittently in segments, as long as each period is at least 10 minutes in length, "can be as effective as single, longer bouts" in its beneficial effects on health and risk factors (e.g., blood pressure, blood lipid profile, insulin levels, and weight control). The panel also allows daily, routine activities that are of moderate or even high intensity (e.g., carpentry, walking to work), as long as they are longer than 10 minutes in duration, to count as part of the daily total amount. Those of light intensity (e.g., taking out the trash), although contributing to the daily activity level, cannot be counted as part of the recommended amount of aerobic exercise. The panel also recommends 8–10 exercises (e.g., resistance weight training, calisthenics, or stair-climbing), on two or more nonconsecutive days for increasing muscle strength and endurance and to promote health and physical independence.

> To control weight and reduce risk factors (e.g., an abnormal blood lipid profile or elevated insulin levels), an average person needs 30 minutes of moderate-intensity exercise (e.g., brisk walking) 5 days a week or 20 minutes of vigorous (high-intensity) exercising (e.g., jogging) 3 days a week.

Haskell et al. (2007) also use the system of tabulating energy expenditure (and accumulating credit for various physical activities done over the course of a week) by using METs, or metabolic equivalents (the system that compares any activity to sitting quietly, which has a MET value of 1). The minimum goal for moderate activities (values of 3–6 MET) or vigorous activities (>6 MET), is 450–750 MET.min per week (MET.min is calculated by multiplying the intensity of the exercise times the number of minutes the exercise is done). These recommendations are, of course, the minimal amount, and adults are encouraged to engage in more.

In regard to preventing weight gain over time, the panel acknowledges tremendous individual variation, with some suggestion that up to 60 minutes "on most days" may be required, but "the specific types and amounts of activity required to prevent weight gain in the majority of people have not been well established" by prospective studies (Haskell et al. 2007). For those who want to prevent weight regain, particularly after substantial weight loss (30–50 pounds), the panel believes that 60–90 minutes of moderate-intensity exercise daily may be warranted.

Strenuous physical activity, though, is not without risk. As the intensity and duration of exercise increase, so does the likelihood of injury and even the possible risk of cardiac arrest. This risk is estimated to be 56 times higher among those who exercise vigorously but infrequently than among those who exercise regularly (Haskell et al. 2007).

REFERENCES

Ainsworth BE, Haskell WL, Whitt MC, et al: Compendium of physical activities: an update of activity codes and MET intensities. Med Sci Sports Exerc 32 (9 suppl):S498–S504, 2000

Anderson JW, Konz EC, Frederich RC, et al: Long-term weight-loss maintenance: a meta-analysis of US studies. Am J Clin Nutr 74:579–584, 2001

Bauman AE: Updating the evidence that physical activity is good for health: an epidemiological review, 2000-2003. J Sci Med Sport 7 (1 suppl):6–19, 2004

Bielinski R, Schutz Y, Jéquier E: Energy metabolism during the postexercise recovery in man. Am J Clin Nutr 42:69–82, 1985

Blair SN, Leermakers EA: Exercise and weight management, in Handbook of Obesity Treatment. Edited by Wadden TA, Stunkard AJ. New York, Guilford, 2002, pp 283–300

Blair SN, LaMonte MJ, Nichaman MZ: The evolution of physical activity recommendations: how much is enough? Am J Clin Nutr 79:913S–920S, 2004

Blundell JE, Stubbs RJ, Hughes DA, et al: Cross talk between physical activity and appetite control: does physical activity stimulate appetite? Proc Nutr Soc 62:651–661, 2003

Borer KT: Physical activity in the prevention and amelioration of osteoporosis in women: interaction of mechanical, hormonal and dietary factors. Sports Med 35:779–830, 2005

Bordelon P, Ghetu MV, Langan RC: Recognition and management of vitamin D deficiency. Am Fam Physician 80:841–846, 2009

Bravata D, Smith-Spangler C, Sundaram V, et al: Using pedometers to increase physical activity and improve health: a systematic review. JAMA 298:2296–2304, 2007

Broocks A, Bandelow B, Pekrun G, et al: Comparison of aerobic exercise, clomipramine, and placebo in the treatment of panic disorder. Am J Psychiatry 155:603–609, 1998

Brooks GA, Butte NF, Rand WM, et al: Chronicle of the Institute of Medicine physical activity recommendation: how a physical activity recommendation came to be among dietary recommendations. Am J Clin Nutr 79:921S–930S, 2004

Broom DR, Batterham RL, King JA, et al: Influence of resistance and aerobic exercise on hunger, circulating levels of acylated ghrelin, and peptide YY in healthy males. Am J Physiol Regul Integr Comp Physiol 296:R29–R35, 2009

Brown WJ, Williams L, Ford JH, et al: Identifying the energy gap: magnitude and determinants of 5-year weight gain in midage women. Obes Res 13:1431–1441, 2005

Brown WJ, Burton NW, Rowan PJ: Updating the evidence on physical activity and health in women. Am J Prev Med 33:404–411, 2007

Byrne HK, Wilmore JH: The relationship of mode and intensity of training on resting metabolic rate in women. Int J Sport Nutr Exerc Metab 11:1–14, 2001

Cairns SP: Lactic acid and exercise performance: culprit or friend? Sports Med 36:279–291, 2006

Catenacci VA, Ogden LG, Stuht J, et al: Physical activity patterns in the National Weight Control Registry. Obesity (Silver Spring) 16:153–161, 2008

Chan AS, Ho YH, Cheung MC, et al: Association between mind-body and cardiovascular exercises and memory in older adults. J Am Geriatr Soc 53:1754–1760, 2005

Christiansen T, Bruun JM, Madsen EL, et al: Weight loss maintenance in severely obese adults after an intensive lifestyle intervention: 2- to 4-year follow-up. Obesity (Silver Spring) 15:413–420, 2007

Church TS, Earnest CP, Skinner JS, et al: Effects of different doses of physical activity on cardiorespiratory fitness among sedentary, overweight or obese postmenopausal women with elevated blood pressure. JAMA 297:2081–2091, 2007

Colditz GC, Willett WC, Stampfer MJ, et al: Patterns of weight change and their relation to diet in a cohort of healthy women. Am J Clin Nutr 51:1100–1105, 1990

Daley A: Exercise and depression: a review of reviews. J Clin Psychol Med Settings 5:140–147, 2008

De Moor MH, Beem AL, Stubbe JH, et al: Regular exercise, anxiety, depression and personality: a population-based study. Prev Med 42:273–279, 2006

De Moor MH, Posthuma D, Hottenga JJ, et al: Genome-wide linkage scan for exercise participation in Dutch sibling pairs. Eur J Hum Genet 15:1252–1259, 2007

De Moor MH, Boomsma DI, Stubbe JH, et al: Testing causality in the association between regular exercise and symptoms of anxiety and depression. Arch Gen Psychiatry 65:897–905, 2008

Diehl JJ, Choi H: Exercise: the data on its role in health, mental health, disease prevention, and productivity. Prim Care 35:803–816, 2008

Di Pietro L, Dziura J, Blair SN: Estimated change in physical activity level (PAL) and prediction of 5-year weight change in men: the Aerobics Center Longitudinal Study. Int J Obes Relat Metab Disord 28:1541–1547, 2004

Dishman RK, Berthoud HR, Booth FW, et al: Neurobiology of exercise. Obesity (Silver Spring) 14:345–356, 2006

Donnelly JE, Hill JO, Jacobsen DJ, et al: Effects of a 16-month randomized controlled exercise trial on body weight and composition in young, overweight men and women. Arch Intern Med 163:1343–1350, 2003

Duman RS: Neurotrophic factors and regulation of mood: role of exercise, diet and metabolism. Neurobiol Aging 26 (suppl 1)S:S88–S93, 2005

Duncan GE, Anton SE, Sydeman SJ, et al: Prescribing exercise at varied levels of intensity and frequency: a randomized trial. Arch Intern Med 165:2362–2369, 2005

Dunn AL, Trivedi MH, Kampert JB, et al: Exercise treatment for depression: efficacy and dose response. Am J Prev Med 28:1–8, 2005

Eaton SB, Eaton SB: An evolutionary perspective on human physical activity: implications for health. Comp Biochem Physiol A Mol Integr Physiol 136:153–159, 2003

Ernst C, Olson AK, Pinel JP, et al: Antidepressant effects of exercise: evidence for an adult-neurogenesis hypothesis? J Psychiatry Neurosci 31:84–92, 2006

Ferris LT, Williams JS, Shen CL: The effect of acute exercise on serum brain-derived neurotrophic factor levels and cognitive function: psychobiology and behavioral strategies. Med Sci Sports Exerc 39:728–734, 2007

Florman DA: More on chewing gum (comment on Levine et al. 1999). N Engl J Med 342:1531–1532, 2000

Geissler CA, Miller DS, Shah M: The daily metabolic rate of the post-obese and the lean. Am J Clin Nutr 45:914–920, 1987

Geliebter A, Maher MM, Gerace L, et al: Effects of strength or aerobic training on body composition, resting metabolic rate, and peak oxygen consumption in obese dieting subjects. Am J Clin Nutr 66:557–563, 1997

Hagobian TA, Sharoff CG, Stephens BR, et al: Effects of exercise on energy-regulating hormones and appetite in men and women. Am J Physiol Regul Integr Comp Physiol 296:R233–R242, 2009

Haskell WL, Lee IM, Pate RR, et al; American College of Sports Medicine; American Heart Association: Physical activity and public health: updated recommendation for adults from the American College of Sports Medicine and the American Heart Association. Circulation 116:1081–1093, 2007

Herbert RD, Gabriel M: Effects of stretching before and after exercising on muscle soreness and risk of injury: systematic review. BMJ 325:468–470, 2002

Herring JL, Molé PA, Meredith CN, et al: Effect of suspending exercise training on resting metabolic rate in women. Med Sci Sports Exerc 24:59–65, 1992

Hill J: Understanding and addressing the epidemic of obesity: an energy balance perspective. Endocr Rev 27:750–761, 2006

Hill J, Wyatt HR: Role of physical activity in preventing and treating obesity. J Appl Physiol 99:765–770, 2005

Hill JO, Wyatt HR, Reed GW, et al: Obesity and the environment: where do we go from here? Science 299:853–855, 2003

Hill J, Saris WH, Levine JA: Energy expenditure in physical activity, in Handbook of Obesity: Etiology and Pathophysiology, 2nd Edition. Edited by Bray GA, Bouchard C. New York, Marcel Dekker, 2004, pp 631–653

Holloszy JO, Kohrt WM: Regulation of carbohydrate and fat metabolism during and after exercise. Annu Rev Nutr 16:121–138, 1996

Howley ET, Franks BD: Fitness Professional's Handbook, 5th Edition. Champaign, IL, Human Kinetics Publishers, 2007

Hu FB, Willett WC, Li T, et al: Adiposity as compared with physical activity in predicting mortality among women. N Engl J Med 351:2694–2703, 2004

Hunsberger JG, Newton SS, Bennett AH, et al: Antidepressant actions of the exercise-regulated gene VGF. Nat Med 13:1476–1482, 2007

Hunter GR, Weinsier RL, McCarthy JP, et al: Hemoglobin, muscle oxidative capacity, and VO2max in African-American and Caucasian women. Med Sci Sports Exerc 33:1739–1743, 2001

Hunter GR, Byrne NM, Sirikul B, et al: Resistance training conserves fat-free mass and resting energy expenditure following weight loss. Obesity (Silver Spring) 16:1045–1051, 2008

Irwin ML, Yasui Y, Ulrich CM, et al: Effect of exercise on total and intra-abdominal body fat in postmenopausal women: a randomized controlled trial. JAMA 289:323–330, 2003

Jackson RD, LaCroix AZ, Gass M, et al: Calcium plus vitamin D supplementation and the risk of fractures. N Engl J Med 354:669–683, 2006

Jakicic JM, Marcus BH, Gallagher KI, et al: Effect of exercise duration and intensity on weight loss in overweight, sedentary women: a randomized trial. JAMA 290:1323–1330, 2007

Jacobs DR, Pereira MA: Physical activity, relative body weight, and risk of death among women. N Engl J Med 351:2753–2755, 2004

Johannsen DL, Redman LM, Ravussin E: The role of physical activity in maintaining a reduced weight. Curr Atheroscler Rep 9:463–471, 2007

Kanis JA, Oden A, Johnell O, et al: The components of excess mortality after hip fracture. Bone 32:468–473, 2003

King NA, Tremblay A, Blundell JE: Effects of exercise on appetite control: implications for energy balance. Med Sci Sports Exerc 29:1076–1089, 1997

LaForge R: Key considerations for metabolic syndrome and diabetes prevention programs: exercise determinants of weight loss. Online clinical articles of the National Lipid Association. 2006. Available at: http://www.lipid.org/clinical/tlc/1000002.php. Accessed February 10, 2009.

Lanningham-Foster L, Nysse LJ, Levine JA: Labor saved, calories lost: the energetic impact of domestic labor-saving devices. Obes Res 11:1178–1181, 2003

Larson EB, Wang L, Bowen JD, et al: Exercise is associated with reduced risk for incident dementia among persons 65 years of age and older. Ann Intern Med 144:73–81, 2006

Lautenschlager NT, Cox KL, Flicker L, et al: Effect of physical activity on cognitive function in older adults at risk for Alzheimer disease: a randomized trial. JAMA 300:1027–1037, 2008

Lee IM, Paffenbarger RS Jr: Associations of light, moderate, and vigorous intensity physical activity with longevity: the Harvard Alumni Health Study. Am J Epidemiol 151:293–299, 2000

Lee IM, Hsieh CC, Paffenbarger RS Jr: Exercise intensity and longevity in men: the Harvard Alumni Health Study. JAMA 273:1179–1184, 1995

Lee IM, Sesso HD, Oguma Y, et al: The weekend warrior and risk of mortality. Am J Epidemiol 160:636–641, 2004

Leitzmann MF, Park Y, Blair A, et al: Physical activity recommendations and decreased risk of mortality. Arch Intern Med 167:2453–2460, 2007

Levine JA: Nonexercise activity thermogenesis (NEAT): environment and biology. Am J Physiol Endocrinol Metab 286:E675–E685, 2004

Levine JA: Exercise: a walk in the park? Mayo Clin Proc 82:797–798, 2007a

Levine JA: Nonexercise activity thermogenesis—liberating the life-force. J Intern Med 262:273–287, 2007b

Levine J, Baukol P, Pavlidis I: The energy expended in chewing gum (letter). N Engl J Med 341:2100, 1999 [Comment: Florman 2000]

Lewis BS, Lynch WD: The effect of physician advice on exercise behavior. Prev Med 22:110–121, 1993

Manini TM, Everhart JE, Patel KV, et al: Daily activity energy expenditure and mortality among older adults. JAMA 296:171–179, 2006

Marcus BH, Albrecht AE, King TK, et al: The efficacy of exercise as an aid for smoking cessation in women: a randomized controlled trial. Arch Intern Med 159:1229–1234, 1999

Matthews CE, Chen KY, Freedson PS, et al: Amount of time spent in sedentary behaviors in the United States, 2003–2004. Am J Epidemiol 167:875–881, 2008

Miller WC, Koceja DM, Hamilton EJ: A meta-analysis of the past 25 years of weight loss research using diet, exercise or diet plus exercise intervention. Int J Obes Relat Metab Disord 21:941–947, 1997

Nemoto KI, Gen-No H, Masukis S, et al: Effects of high-intensity interval walking training on physical fitness and blood pressure in middle-age and older people. Mayo Clin Proc 82:803–811, 2007

Pereira AC, Huddleston DE, Brickman AM, et al: An in vivo correlate of exercise-induced neurogenesis in the adult dentate gyrus. Proc Natl Acad Sci U S A 104:5638–5643, 2007

Perri MG, Corsica JA: Improving the maintenance of weight lost in behavioral treatment of obesity, in Handbook of Obesity Treatment. Edited by Wadden TA, Stunkard AJ. New York, Guilford, 2002, pp 357–379

Precope J: Hippocrates on Diet and Hygiene. London, Zeno, 1952

Prince RL, Devine A, Dhaliwal SS, et al: Effects of calcium supplementation on clinical fracture and bone structure: results of a 5-year, double-blind, placebo-controlled trial in elderly women. Arch Intern Med 166:869–875, 2006

Root L: No More Aching Back: Dr. Root's New Fifteen-Minute-a-Day Program for a Healthy Back. New York, Signet, 1991

Rouzier P, Mancini L: Starting an exercise program. MDConsult. Available (by subscription) at: http://www.mdconsult.com/das/patient/body/119813694-5/802797486/10068/18186.html. Accessed February 10, 2009a.

Rouzier P, Mancini L: Strength training basics. MDConsult. Available (by subscription) at: http://www.mdconsult.com/das/patient/body/135136932–11/836712431/10068/18199.html. Accessed October 29, 2009b.

Seime RJ, Vickers KS: The challenges of treating depression with exercise: from evidence to practice. Clinical Psychology Science and Practice 13:194–197, 2006

Shah M, Simha V, Garg A: Review: long-term impact of bariatric surgery on body weight, cormorbidities, and nutritional status. J Clin Endocrinol Metab 91:4223–4231, 2006

Simon H: Exercise. MDConsult, Patient Education. 2008. Available (by subscription) at: http://www.mdconsult.com/das/patient/body/135136932–12/836713261/10041/9446.html. Accessed February 8, 2009.

Simon H: Review: Osteoporosis. MDConsult, Patient Education. Available (by subscription) at: http://www.mdconsult.com/das/patient/view/0/10041/9435.html/top. Accessed February 16, 2009.

Slentz CA, Duscha BD, Johnson JL, et al: Effects of the amount of exercise on body weight, body composition, and measures of central obesity: STRRIDE—a randomized controlled study. Arch Intern Med 164:31–39, 2004

Stathopoulou G, Powers MB, Berry AC, et al: Exercise interventions for mental health: a quantitative and qualitative review. Clinical Psychology: Science and Practice 13:179–193, 2006

Stubbe JH, Boomsma DI, Vink JM, et al: Genetic influences on exercise participation in 37,051 twin pairs from seven countries. PLoS One 1:e22, 2006. Available at: http://www.plosone.org.

Tate DF, Jeffery RW, Sherwood NE, et al: Long-term weight losses associated with prescription of higher physical activity goals: are higher levels of physical activity protective against weight regain? Am J Clin Nutr 85:954–959, 2007

Taylor AH, Oliver AJ: Acute effects of brisk walking on urges to eat chocolate, affect, and responses to a stressor and chocolate cue: an experimental study. Appetite 52:155–160, 2009

Traustadóttir T, Bosch PR, Cantu T, et al: Hypothalamic-pituitary-adrenal axis response and recovery from high-intensity exercise in women: effects of aging and fitness. J Clin Endocrinol Metab 89:3248–3254, 2004

Tremblay A, Simoneau JA, Bouchard C: Impact of exercise intensity on body fatness and skeletal muscle metabolism. Metabolism 43:814–818, 1994

Trombetti A, Herrmann F, Hoffmeyer P, et al: Survival and potential years of life lost after hip fracture in men and age-matched women. Osteoporos Int 13:731–737, 2002

Trumbo P, Schlicker S, Yates AA, et al: Dietary reference intakes for energy, carbohydrate, fiber, fat, fatty acids, cholesterol, protein, and amino acids. J Am Diet Assoc 102:1621–1630, 2002

Vaynman SS, Ying Z, Yin D, et al: Exercise differentially regulates synaptic proteins associated to the function of BDNF. Brain Res 1070:124–130, 2006

Wansink B: Mindless Eating: Why We Eat More Than We Think. New York, Bantam Books, 2006

Weil A: Tums for calcium? Available at: http://www/drwweil.com/drw/u/id/QAA400065. Accessed October 31, 2009

Westerterp KR: Alterations in energy balance with exercise. Am J Clin Nutr 68:970S–974S, 1998

Williams DM, Lewis BA, Dunsiger S, et al: Comparing psychosocial predictors of physical activity adoption and maintenance. Ann Behav Med 36:186–194, 2008

Williams MA, Haskell WL, Ades PA, et al: Resistance exercise in individuals with and without cardiovascular disease: 2007 update: a scientific statement from the American Heart Association Council on Clinical Cardiology and Council on Nutrition, Physical Activity, and Metabolism. Circulation 116:572–584, 2007

Woods JA, Vieira VJ, Keylock KT: Exercise, inflammation, and innate immunity. Neurol Clin 24:585–599, 2006

Yanovski, JA, Yanovski SZ, Sovik KN, et al: A prospective study of holiday weight gain. N Engl J Med 342:861–867, 2000

9

CIRCADIAN RHYTHMS, SLEEP, AND WEIGHT

The idea of having an internal biological clock might sound weird, but if we consider the number of times that we wake up automatically before the alarm clock rings, or we experience the feeling of hunger, even without seeing food, at a precise time…

Jorge Mendoza, "Circadian Clocks" (2007)

BIOLOGICAL CLOCKS

What Are Circadian Rhythms?

One of the most interesting associations (and one that we found rarely discussed in detail in any other book on weight control) is the relationship of weight regulation to the natural rhythms of our body. Whether we are talking about food intake or cravings that occur at certain times of day, or the effects of sleep deprivation on weight, or want to identify the most efficacious time to administer a medication to maximize its benefit and minimize deleterious effects (i.e., the relatively new science of "chronopharmacology"), we have to be cognizant of the multitude of ways our bodies interact with our natural environment.

What is remarkable about humans as well as animals is that we have elaborate internal systems that regulate the daily metabolic rhythms of our bodies. Even the lowly fruit fly (*Drosophila* spp.) has evidence of this kind of biological regulation and rhythm (Allada 2008), and photosynthesis in plants has a biological regularity as well. In other words, virtually all light-sensitive organisms, from certain kinds of bacteria to humans, have their own built-in biological rhythms (Levi and Schibler 2007). Hastings et al. (2007) call these systems our "self-sustaining endogenous biological timekeepers." Strubbe and Woods (2004) suggest that this pattern evolved as an adaptation to "idiosyncratic environmental constraints and opportunities" found

WHAT ARE CIRCADIAN RHYTHMS?

- Our body has a natural, built-in biological clock—a kind of pacemaker, in the hypothalamus—that is regulated by internal and external factors and that regulates many of our body's processes. This biological clock is particularly sensitive to the day-night/light-darkness 24-hour (diurnal) cycle of our rotation around the sun. Many external factors, such as the timing of eating, can affect our circadian rhythms, as can our body temperature.

- This normal diurnal pattern begins in infants, in the first year of life.

- We know, however, from those who are blind and others deprived of light, that this biological clock actually has a slightly longer periodicity of 24½–25 hours. *Circadian*, in fact, means "about a day."

- Many of our hormones—particularly ACTH, cortisol, and melatonin—are secreted on a specific daily cycle, with peaks and valleys, set by this clock. Even secretion of leptin, the major hormone that is involved in feeling full, is on a diurnal schedule. Researchers have found that night shift workers are much more likely to develop the metabolic syndrome than daytime workers.

- Jet lag is a syndrome, most commonly brought on by airplane travel involving time zone changes, in which circadian rhythms are disrupted, resulting in considerable fatigue and malaise. The syndrome can also be seen in night-shift workers and others whose sleep is disrupted. Depending on the nature of the sleep disruption, it may take days for a person to feel normal again.

Source: National Institute of Neurological Disorders and Stroke 2007

in nature (e.g., predators, food availability, harsh conditions) and it is partly based on genetics and partly based on learning. Levi and Schibler (2007) speculate that one of the major functions of these biological rhythms is the timing of metabolism, including energy utilization and detoxification, to ensure an organism's survival. Because of the body's extraordinarily complex signals involving eating, for example, there can be considerable flexibility in the number of meals we eat and the timing of individual meals, as well as the size of one meal versus another. Most of us have a fairly consistent meal pattern, though our own pattern may differ considerably from that of other people.

Even in the animal world, there are advantages to confining "food-seeking behavior" to specific times in order to avoid wasting energy on "fruitless hunting" (Moore-Ede 1986). Moore-Ede believes, as well, that our human ability, unlike many other species', to consolidate our sleep-wake cycle into a "sustained period of alert wakefulness" throughout our day, "may have been one of the most significant evolutionary adaptations which permitted the development of human intellect."

The major influence involved in setting the timing of our biological rhythms, including eating, is light, namely our planet's natural 24-hour light-dark cycle—the rotation of the earth around the sun. This is the concept of a circadian rhythm (*circadian*, from the Latin words *circa* and *dies* for "about a day," because it is not exactly a 24-hour rhythm). Because the system is not set exactly on a 24-hour day, the cycle is reset, as it were, to the light-dark cycle each day as light hits the retina in our eyes (Froy 2007). In other words, there is a daily rhythm in animals, including humans, that is genetically entrained or synchronized with our environment's light cycle, a "temporal anchor," if you will (Strubbe and Woods 2004). Of course, not all animals are active during the day like humans; rodents, for example, are nocturnal animals whose main activity, including eating, occurs at night. When light is experimentally manipulated, feeding patterns can change and a "free-running rhythm" that may be somewhat longer or shorter than our 24-hour pattern results. But even when we (or animals) do not have the sun or our customary social routine as an anchor, our daily rhythms (i.e., our biological clock) of hormone secretion, sleeping, eating, and so on do not become completely disorganized (Hastings et al. 2007). In other words, we are all affected by, or balance, the extraordinarily complex interactions among the sun, our social clocks of daily routines, and our biological clocks (Roenneberg et al. 2003). And what about those who are totally blind, without any light perception at all? Even when they have social cues and time cues (and a regular sleep-wake cycle), they have a "free-running system," with an average circadian period ranging from 23.9 to 25.1 hours, that is similar to that of people kept experimentally in total isolation (Sack 2009).

> The disruption of our environmental light cycle (e.g., jet lag)—the temporal anchor—changes our eating patterns.

The Master Clock: The Suprachiasmatic Nucleus

For years researchers believed the only "clock" in the body was the one that is located in the anterior part of the hypothalamus, near the optic chiasm, called the *suprachiasmatic nucleus* (SCN)—the "circadian pacemaker" (Strubbe and Woods 2004) or "master clock" (Zvonic et al. 2007). When there is extensive damage to the SCN, such as by experimental disruption, animals may lose many of their biological rhythms and their eating pattern may become immediately and permanently arrhythmic. The SCN consists of about 20,000 cells in mammals and has a core component and an outer shell. These cells have a set of what are referred to as *clock genes*—with names like *Clock, BMAL1, Cry1, Cry2, Per1, Per2,* and *Per3*—that researchers began to isolate in the mid 1990s, with the likelihood that others will be found (Ramsey et al. 2007).

Experimental animals can be rendered what is called *clock mutant* to study the effects of circadian rhythm disruptions (Prasai et al. 2008). Clock-mutant mice, for example, will eat almost as much during their typically inactive period as during the time of their usual food intake, for reasons we don't fully understand. As a result, they will eat more and gain weight. Those made mutant in the *mPer2* gene lose their normal feeding rhythm (and hence develop hyperphagia when it is light) as well as their usual corticosterone rhythm, though when under stress they can produce corticosterone (Yang et al. 2009). Furthermore, because ovulation and reproduction are also under circadian control, rats made clock mutant have been shown to have hormonal abnormalities (e.g., decreased progesterone levels, no luteinizing hormone surge, and abnormal prolactin secretion), with irregular estrous cycles and a higher rate of difficulties maintaining their pregnancies. These abnormalities were all related to circadian rhythm disorders and not to any abnormalities in the pituitary of the rats (Miller et al. 2004).

As long as 15%–25% of the SCN is not destroyed, the rhythms remain (Antle and Silver 2005). This area has many neuronal connections to other parts of the hypothalamus that have been shown to be involved in food intake, such as the lateral hypothalamus (where a lesion causes experimental animals to stop eating and lose weight) or the ventromedial nuclei of the hypothalamus (where a very large lesion causes increased eating, obesity, and disruption of the regular pattern of food intake). Interestingly, rodents that have been made genetically obese (Zucker rats), but do not have damage to or disruption of their circadian rhythms, increase their food intake at meals (i.e., become hyperphagic) but do not have any disruption in their feeding pattern regularity (Strubbe and Woods 2004).

Other Clocks (Central and Peripheral)

We now know that there are actually other biological clocks, with their own so-called clock genes, throughout the body and other parts of the brain besides the anterior part of the hypothalamus where the SCN is located. For example, it is believed that this ventromedial area of the hypothalamus has a separate clock that functions independently of the one in the SCN and is entrained not to light but to food, and perhaps even more to carbohydrates than to fats. The speculation is that this area of the brain enables the body to make meal-anticipatory responses (also called *food-anticipatory activity*) (e.g., changes in glucose and insulin levels, salivation, and secretion of digestive enzymes, even prior to eating) that allow for our eating meals of different sizes (Strubbe and Woods 2004). In fact, research has found that when animals are given food only at certain times of day, they come to anticipate the food 2–4 hours before by increased motor activity, body temperature, digestive enzymes, and corticosterone secretion (Froy 2007).

> Food-anticipatory activity changes glucose and insulin levels, salivation, and secretion of digestive enzymes, prompting eating of different-sized meals.

Researchers now believe that there are circadian clocks (*peripheral tissue oscillators*) in many cells throughout the body. It is as if each tissue can "sense time," as Kohsaka and Bass (2007) poetically describe. In fact, there is evidence for circadian clocks in most of our organ systems, including our liver, heart, lungs, and skeletal muscle

(Hastings et al. 2007). Ramsey et al. (2007) report, for example, that about 20% of proteins in the liver are under circadian control. In addition, Hastings et al. (2008) note that major areas of the brain other than just the hypothalamus, including the cerebral cortex, cerebellum, and hippocampus, all contain evidence of circadian clocks. It is significant that circadian rhythms, particularly with disruptions in the normal sleep-wake cycle, are dysfunctional in many disease states involving degeneration of the brain, such as Alzheimer and Huntington disease (Hastings et al. 2008). There is even the suggestion that patients with bipolar disorder, in whom sleep abnormalities and diurnal variations in mood are common, have "abnormally shifted or arrhythmic circadian" rhythms (Harvey 2008). In fact, Plante and Winkelman (2008) note that sleep disturbances are the most commonly reported prodromal symptom for a manic episode and an inadequate amount of sleep can actually trigger a manic episode in individuals predisposed to them. Furthermore, even after patients become euthymic, the overwhelming majority still have sleep disturbances (Plante and Winkelman 2008). Abe et al. (2000) have shown in mice that lithium, one of the major treatments for mania in bipolar disorder, actually works directly on some (but not all) of the cells of the SCN and lengthens circadian rhythms. The speculation is that lithium's ability to stabilize mood may be partly related to its effect on the circadian rhythm.

> There are circadian clocks in most of our organs, including in our brain, liver, heart, lungs, and skeletal muscles as well as our digestive system—the last one keeping an "eye" on meal times.
>
> **Strubb and Woods 2004**

Plante and Winkelman (2008) report that those with depression may have a genetic "chronobiological vulnerability" to becoming depressed. A study by Parry et al. (2008) found that levels of melatonin, "the best measure of circadian rhythmicity," were lower in pregnant women who were depressed than in pregnant women who were not depressed, whereas melatonin levels were elevated in women who were depressed postpartum compared with postpartum levels in women who were not depressed. The differences in blood levels of melatonin during pregnancy and postpartum may be related to changes in sex hormones. Furthermore, depression has been alleviated, at least temporarily, by sleep deprivation, and seasonal affective illness has been treated by artificial light therapy, but Wirz-Justice (2007) suggests that light therapy might have much broader potential in conditions involving sleep disruptions.

As the master clock, the SCN generally synchronizes the circadian rhythms in the body's peripheral clocks by means of synaptic networks and hormones (Fuller et al. 2008). For example, there is evidence that adipose tissue has a circadian component, because tumor necrosis factor α (TNF-α), interleukin-6 (IL-6), adiponectin, and leptin—all mediators produced by adipose tissue—have distinct circadian rhythms (Zvonic et al. 2007). Insulin, glucagon, cortisol, adrenocorticotropic hormone (ACTH), melatonin, and ghrelin all have circadian rhythms as well (Froy

2007). Our blood pressure has a circadian rhythm, such that it typically is lower at night (Prasai et al. 2008). Even cell division, including division of tumor cells, can have a circadian rhythm. Froy (2007) goes as far as to say that circadian rhythms regulate "nearly all aspects of physiology and behavior"—including sleep-wake cycles, endocrine functioning, body temperature, cardiovascular activity, and gastrointestinal functioning—in all mammals. Significantly, the most common time for sudden death from myocardial infarction or heart failure is the early morning, when blood levels of plasminogen activator inhibitor type 1 are highest (Zvonic et al. 2006). Further, increased sympathetic nervous system activity (e.g., increased blood pressure and heart rate) and decreased parasympathetic (vagal) nervous system activity, which may lead to rupturing of atherosclerotic plaques and an acute myocardial infarction, have been reported in the early morning. This pattern, though, is not seen in patients who have had type 1 or type 2 diabetes for more than 5 years; in these individuals, sudden death is as likely to occur at any time throughout the day. The speculation is that these patients already have autonomic dysfunction and disturbed circadian rhythm patterns secondary to the chronic disease (Rana et al. 2003).

> Diabetic patients whose circadian rhythm is disturbed may be vulnerable to sudden death from heart-related conditions throughout the day, not just in the early mornings as is common in those with a regular circadian rhythm.

Zeitgebers

Though our biological rhythms are primarily synchronized (entrained) to the natural light of the sun, many other environmental signals can affect these rhythms and phase-shift them one way or the other. These environmental signals are called *zeitgebers*, from the German word meaning "time givers" (Kohsaka and Bass 2007). Think how different our world has become from the primitive world of the Paleolithic Age and even since the incandescent electric light bulb was invented at the end of the nineteenth century. We are now a 24/7 world with computers, the Internet, and jet travel. Our artificial lights can phase-shift our rhythms significantly. For example, if we are exposed to bright light earlier than our usual awakening time, we can advance our circadian rhythms; inversely, we can cause a phase delay if we expose ourselves to bright lights early in the night.

The physical activity of exercise can act as a zeitgeber (Zee and Manthena 2007). There is even the suggestion that caloric restriction (restricting calories to 25%–60% below what is normally eaten, while maintaining proper nutrition), which has been found to prolong life in rodents, can affect the SCN master clock. Glucose and alcohol have both been shown to affect circadian rhythms (Froy 2007). And apparently, so can the reward and arousal properties of chocolate: Mendoza et al. (2005) demonstrated that rats, kept in total darkness and given chocolate at a certain time every day for weeks, adjusted (i.e., synchronized) their motor activity to the chocolate treat, though how long the changes took to occur varied with individual rats (5–21 days). Stephan and Davidson (1998) showed that rats with lesions of the SCN that were given glucose, but not vegetable oil, at a particular time of day came to anticipate it by increased motor activity such as increased wheel running and approaches to where the glucose would appear. Glucose, then, has zeitgeber qualities, the ability to synchronize or entrain or phase-shift a biological rhythm—in this case, a feeding pattern. Interestingly, in these experiments saccharin (a nonnutritive sweetener) did not phase-shift eating patterns. Fuller et al. (2008) also demonstrated that when animals were subjected to conditions of restricted food availability, the clock in the dorsomedial hypothalamus (which entrains to food rather than to light) takes over as the master clock. This adaptive measure protects the organism from starvation by enabling the animal to change its patterns of behavior.

> Calorie restriction, physical activity, glucose, and alcohol and other addictive substances have the ability to phase-shift eating patterns.

Bray and Young (2006) suggest that the timing of feeding is one of the most powerful zeitgebers. And Kretschmer et al. (2005) have demonstrated, at least in rats, that the timing of food has a strong impact on how much they eat and how much weight they gain. When rats were given a high-fat/carbohydrate diet at a time they were not usually fed (when lights were on, their typically inactive period), they gained more weight very quickly than when fed at their usual time. It took rats 3 weeks of the high-fat/high-carbohydrate diet to gain weight when fed at their usual time whereas it took only 2 hours for them to gain weight when fed at their typically inactive time.

Along those lines, Sleipness et al. (2007) demonstrated that *drug-seeking for cocaine* in rats—acquisition, extinction, and reinstatement of drug-seeking—is also affected by circadian rhythms. They concluded that cocaine craving varies with the time of day (there is a "window of high reward potential") and cravings may last longer when attempts at extinction are carried out at certain times rather than at others. The speculation is that the SCN works in concert with dopamine secretion. Anecdotally, there is no question that those who crave certain foods, drugs, or alcohol are more apt to do so at certain times of day and that being in a different time zone can change the timing of these cravings. For example, rarely does someone want to eat an entire chocolate cake when first awakening in the morning, whereas this may seem inviting considerably later in the day. And rarely does someone reach for alcohol immediately on awakening unless the addiction is so far gone that there is the possibility (and fear) that delirium tremens might occur.

Chronotypes

Some individuals are more "night people" and some are more "morning people." In other words, humans have different chronotypes (though there are degrees) that more commonly are called the owls, or nightowls, and the larks. In the extreme, owls can stay up all night, go to sleep in the wee hours of the morning, and sleep all day, whereas people of the lark chronotype spontaneously arise at an early hour and fade out by early night (Wittmann et al. 2006). Roenneberg et al. (2003) devised the Munich Chronotype Questionnaire to assess these categories more accurately; they emphasize that *chronotype* refers to sleep phase and not sleep duration, though people can obviously differ in both. Because most work schedules are based on starting work early in the morning, night owls may find themselves out of sync with a society that demands an early wake-up time. Not surprisingly, these people may begin to accumulate what is called a *sleep debt*, with feelings of daytime sleepiness and the inability to fall asleep at a so-called normal time. They may need to sleep many extra hours on the weekends to try to compensate for their chronic sleep deprivation (Wittmann et al. 2006). Adolescence is a time when many teenagers find their circadian rhythms shift toward the owl pattern. Despite reports in the literature that indicate this shift toward going to sleep later and getting up later is related to pubertal development and hormonal changes in adolescence, Gau and Soong (2003) did not find that pubertal status was as significant as environmental factors, such as grade level (the change occurs most commonly around the seventh grade), decreased attention of parents to their adolescents' bedtime, part-time jobs, and increased homework. Of course, many people find themselves phase-shifted on Monday mornings so that it is particularly difficult to awaken to go to work when they have slept even a little later on weekend mornings.

> Night shift workers and "owls" tend to develop the metabolic syndrome (e.g., abdominal obesity, diabetes, abnormal lipid profile).

Working out of synchrony with our society can prove to be quite stressful. Significantly, those who work at night are more prone to develop metabolic abnormalities, like the metabolic syndrome (e.g., abdominal obesity, hypertension, diabetes, abnormal lipid profile), than those who work during the day as is customary (Zvonic et al. 2007). A higher incidence of drug and alcohol abuse has been reported in people who work at night and may have circadian dysfunction (Sleipness et al. 2007). There have also been reports of increased risk of breast and colon cancer in those who do night-shift work (Boivin et al. 2007; Haus and Smolensky 2006), though not all researchers agree that the evidence is strong enough to make those claims (Kolstad 2008).

When there is a chronic mismatch or discrepancy between a person's biological clock and his or her societal clock, we can speak of *social jet lag* (Wittmann et al. 2006), analogous to the common jet lag we experience when we change time zones.

Jet Lag

Circadian rhythm disruptions, such as those seen in what is commonly called "jet lag," can also have an impact on the timing of our meals. Though most people in our culture eat three meals a day, there is considerable variability in how we define meals, what foods seem appropriate for which meals, and even what temporal pattern we follow. Obviously, many variables influence the timing of our food intake, including physiological, genetic, and even social, cultural, and psychological factors (de Castro 2004). Conditioning may also play a role: we are just used to eating certain foods at certain times. Boston et al. (2008) make the point that breakfast, for example, has many meanings and can be defined as the first meal of the day after we awaken, a meal eaten at a certain time, and even a certain kind of food eaten. Illustrating the latter point, years ago there was the orange juice advertising campaign, "Orange juice: it's not just for breakfast anymore."

The timing of meals can have a significant impact on us. A patient once spoke of a memorable experience years earlier when she was an adolescent and she returned from her first trip to Europe. She remembers that her plane from Italy landed in New York at 8 A.M., and the first thing she and her family did when they left the airport was to go to straight to a Burger King and eat hamburgers with Coca-Cola. Is that so strange? Well, normally the idea of eating a hamburger or even drinking a cola at 8:00 in the morning seems almost disgusting, she said. After all, breakfast usually consists of cereal or maybe eggs. But this family was still on Italian time (7 hours ahead) and for them, it was no longer breakfast time; they were behaving as if it were late in the afternoon and they had missed lunch. Their circadian clocks had been shifted.

Though our circadian clocks can be shifted, most people feel the effects of shifts quite strongly when they exceed 3 hours' delay or 2 hours' advance. That is because the SCN has limited phase-shifting capacity (Levi and Schibler 2007). Of course, the most common condition in humans that affects circadian rhythms and causes discomfort with these time shifts is *jet lag*. Jet lag is considered "circadian misalignment" (Sack 2007, 2009). It is a syndrome that is recognized by the American Academy of Sleep Medicine (2008; see also Sack et al. 2007) as well as DSM-IV-TR (American Psychiatric Association 2000) as one of the subtypes of circadian rhythm disorders (the "shift work" type is another). It is manifested by a pattern of sleep disruption, including insomnia and excessive sleepiness, that is due to a mismatch between the person's current environment and his or her usual circadian sleep-wake pattern. A person experiencing jet lag usually also experiences general malaise, somatic symptoms such as gastrointestinal disturbances, and impaired daytime functioning (Sack 2009).

When the term *jet lag* is used concretely, it refers to a syndrome brought on by jet travel across different time zones (i.e., crossing time zones too quickly for our circadian systems to acclimate) though as we have seen above, it can be used metaphorically for any mismatch between a person's environment and his or her circadian rhythms. Eventually, our systems adjust as they resynchronize to the new environment. Jet lag is usually a transient and self-limiting condition. How long the syndrome lasts depends on several factors, including individual sensitivity, how many time zones are crossed (one day is needed to adjust per time zone crossed), the direction of the travel, how much and how well a person can sleep during the jet travel, and even the availability and intensity of time cues when the person arrives in the new time zone (Sack 2009). Most of us have had the experience of seeing how the airplane staff prepares us for our destination by either turning off all the lights and shutting the curtains or else turning all of them on and opening up the plane's curtains. Traveling east (advancing sleep-wake hours), for example, is usually more problematic for most people than traveling west (delaying sleep-wake hours).

As noted, light exposure is the most powerful environmental cue to phase-shift our circadian rhythms. The effectiveness of light exposure depends primarily on its timing and intensity but also varies with factors such as its wavelength (light in the blue-green wavelength is most effective), duration, and pattern (e.g., continuous or intermittent) (Sack 2009). As modern life is spent more and more indoors in artificial light, we are exposed to light that is far less intense than midday sunlight (<400 lux with indoor lighting vs. up to tens of thousands of lux with sunlight) (Roenneberg et al. 2003). A *lux* is an international unit of illumination that is equal to the light exposure we get by looking at a candle from a distance of 1 meter; *watts* are international units of power that measure intensity. Usually lights of more than 1,000 lux are required to phase-shift our circadian rhythms, but there is considerable variation, and some people have a greater sensitivity to phase shifting (i.e., lower *phase tolerance*) than others (Sack et al. 2007).

Most people know when their circadian rhythms are disrupted, but there are scientific means of measuring circadian rhythms. Originally, a person's core body temperature was used as a circadian marker, but our core body temperature can be affected by sleep, eating, and activity levels. (Incidentally, the lowest core body temperature occurs between 3 A.M. and 5 A.M. and continues to rise throughout the day until evening, when it starts to fall; Reite et al. 2009, p. 98.) The measure most commonly used now is melatonin levels in the blood or saliva (Sack 2009). Melatonin is a hormone secreted by the pineal gland for 10–12 hours in humans each night in the dark. The beginning of melatonin secretion, the *melatonin onset*, measured in dim light, is a marker for the circadian phase. Interestingly, because of the path of neurons from the SCN to the pineal gland (involving noradrenergic neurons), melatonin secretion is inhibited by beta-blockers (e.g., propranolol) and other antihypertensives as well as medications used to decrease pulse and respiratory rate. Caffeine intake and nonsteroidal anti-inflammatory medications may also affect melatonin levels.

Melatonin has also been used to aid in phase-shifting circadian rhythms affected by jet lag or shift work; melatonin and light work synergistically. The use of dark glasses and hypnotic medications can be helpful, as can avoiding eating on a plane. Reite et al. (2009, pp. 118–119) describe research in which mice subjected to starvation adjusted more quickly to phase-shifts. Castillo et al. (2004), through their experiments with mice, suggest that strictly regimented meal times may be useful in treating circadian rhythm disorders seen in patients with jet lag or on shift work, and even the blind. They caution that because food is not as powerful a zeitgeber as light, this kind of entrainment may take time: some of the mice in their experiments took 12 weeks to adapt. (Also, some mice had "sloppy circadian organization" and there was considerable variation among them.) They speculate that many mechanisms, including hormonal signals or neuronal connections, but even nonspecific signals like cleaning the cages or handling the food of the mice, may have been involved in entrainment to scheduled feeding.

Chronopharmacology

One of the most interesting new developments in the study of circadian rhythms is the recognition that a medication may have different effects, from beneficial to toxic, depending on the time of day the drug is administered. In other words, there may be a time schedule that leads to optimal therapeutic effect and minimal toxicity. This is the field of *chronopharmacology*. Experiments in both rodents and humans have shown that a drug's efficacy may be affected by the organism's circadian rhythms that affect such things as gastric pH, liver metabolism, and kidney functioning. These rhythms, in turn, affect the timing of the drug's uptake and metabolism, and even the sensitivity of particular tissues. All aspects of drug intake—absorption, distribution, metabolism, and elimination—may be involved, and chronopharmacokinetics can be more important in determining a drug's exposure in the body than even *how* it is administered (e.g., orally vs. intravenously) or how quickly it is eliminated from the body (Levi and Schibler 2007).

For example, Levi and Schibler (2007) report that because of specific renal rhythms, the antibiotic gentamicin is tolerated best when given in the afternoon, and the effects of the anticoagulant heparin have been shown to be twice as effective when it is given between early morning and 4 P.M. Levi and Schibler (2007) speculate that the cyclooxygenase-2 inhibitor celecoxib (Celebrex), withdrawn from the market because of toxic reactions, might have been less toxic if administered in the evening. Furthermore, chemotherapeutic medications for treatment of cancers are more toxic when cells are undergoing cell division, and sometimes even at specific phases of this process, all of which are controlled by circadian rhythms. Devastating side effects from anticancer therapy, such as peripheral neuropathy, can be minimized by attention to circadian schedules (Levi and Schibler 2007). That drug administration effects would be under circadian control makes sense, say Levi and Schibler (2007) inasmuch as a "xenophobic detoxification…defense system" may have evolved to eliminate and inactivate any "noxious food components" from our environment. The science, though, is exceptionally complicated and still fairly inexact because there is considerable variation in circadian rhythms from one person to another (see "Chronotypes" section above) and even between men and women, because of the influence of the sex hormones. "Personalizing chronotherapy" (Levi and Schibler 2007) is still in its infancy.

Along those lines, back in the early 1980s Halberg presented research in which subjects ate one meal a day and the timing of the meal was found to determine whether a subject lost weight (Halberg 1983). Participants in this small study acted as their own control subjects. Those who ate their one meal in the morning lost weight, whereas some of those who ate their meal in the evening—four of the six subjects who did so—gained weight. There is also some suggestion that fats are utilized before other food groups in the evening, such that "a calorie appears to be utilized differently" depending on the time of day (Halberg 1983). It is likely that some people are more genetically sensitive to timing of meals than others. (For a discussion of the metabolic complexities of eating all our daily food in one meal as opposed to multiple meals, see Chapter 10, "Diet and Weight.")

HORMONES, SLEEP, AND WEIGHT

Orexins

As we have seen from the previous discussion "Hormones of Food Intake" in Chapter 5, the orexins, also referred to as hypocretins, come in two forms: orexin A and orexin B. Discovered in 1998, the orexins, from the Greek *orexis* for appetite, are so named because they increase appetite. They are a novel peptide family found predominantly in the lateral hypothalamus, one of the areas of the brain involved in food intake. The orexins are found in many mammalian species besides humans, including rodents, dogs, sheep, cows, and pigs. The A and B forms originate from a common polypeptide precursor; it is speculated that levels of glucose as well as of the hormone leptin, and particularly low levels of glucose and leptin as seen during fasting, may regulate the conversion into the active A and B forms (Ohno and Sakurai 2008). It is now fairly clear that the orexins are involved in regulating sleep and states of wakefulness, as well as in energy homeostasis, through pathways that involve reward and even emotional arousal (Harris and Aston-Jones 2006). This connection makes sense when you think that an animal in the fasting state requires vigilance and motivation (reward-seeking behavior) to search for food sources that will ensure its survival. Ohno and Sakurai (2008), though, speculate that this reinforced pattern of alertness and motivation to seek food when fasting may counteract the dieter's attempt at weight control by fasting. After all, when in a state of food deprivation, as one dieter said, "Everything makes me think of food."

> The dieter's attempt to control weight by fasting is counteracted by appetite-increasing hormones—orexins—which reinforce food-seeking patterns.

Fadel et al. (2002) have suggested that orexin neurons are heterogeneous and that a subset of them in the lateral hypothalamus may be involved in weight gain with the atypical antipsychotics as well as with some of the older antipsychotics. The antipsychotics that are most likely to cause substantial weight gain, such as clozapine, olanzapine, risperidone, and chlorpromazine, are also most likely to activate orexin neurons, whereas those that do not lead to increased weight (e.g., ziprasidone, fluphenazine) do not activate orexin

> Antipsychotics such as clozapine, olanzapine, risperidone, and chlorpromazine cause weight gain either by directly or indirectly (by H_1 receptor blockade) activating orexins.

neurons. Fadel et al. (2002) also note that histamine type 1 (H_1) receptors are involved.

Interestingly, orexin levels (mostly orexin A levels) are low in the cerebrospinal fluid in those patients with *narcolepsy*. Narcolepsy, a disorder found in 1 of 2,000 people in the United States, is characterized by excessive daytime sleepiness with sudden attacks of sleep, cataplexy (sudden loss of muscle tone) without a loss of consciousness, and fragmented, disrupted sleep (profound dysregulation of rapid eye movement [REM] sleep). It has even been suggested that measuring levels of orexin A in the cerebrospinal fluid may be a test for narcolepsy. Further, individuals with narcolepsy also have a higher body mass index (BMI) value than individuals without this disorder, with an accumulation of abdominal fat (and a greater waist measurement) and an increased risk of type 2 diabetes. Ironically, though, those with narcolepsy have been found to eat *fewer* calories. The reason for their increased risk of obesity is not clear, and researchers have speculated that there may be abnormalities in their metabolism or they may be getting less physical activity (i.e., expending less energy). But not all patients with narcolepsy have obesity, so there is the suggestion that genetic and environmental factors are involved as well (Sakurai 2006).

Orexin neurons increase appetite but also increase metabolic rate. Mice that were rendered orexin deficient had decreased energy expenditure and decreased food intake but increased body weight (Ohno and Sakurai 2008). The orexins are involved in increasing food-seeking behavior ("appetitive" behaviors such as exploration, foraging, and even "willingness to work for food" in animal experiments) and may be involved in the emotional, rewarding aspects of eating. The orexins increase appetite, length of a meal, and meal frequency (i.e., "consummatory" behaviors) (Baird et al. 2009). Continuous infusions of orexin A over several days produced disrupted feeding patterns in mice such that they ate more in the daytime and less in the evening, the reverse of what they usually do. Significantly, though, they did not gain weight. The suggestion, then, is that orexin A is involved in regulating short-term feeding patterns rather than long-term homeostasis (Sakurai 2006). There is also the suggestion that the orexins, in combination with dopamine, may be involved in addiction, that is, drug-seeking or reward-seeking behaviors. Interestingly, those with narcolepsy are treated with amphetamine-like medications and it is significant that they typically do not become addicted to these medications (Harris and Aston-Jones 2006).

Researchers speculate that orexin neurons increase appetite by interfering with the signals for satiety in the gastrointestinal tract. Though orexin neurons are found near the neurons of melanin-concentrating hormone (MCH), which is also involved in increasing appetite, they work differently. MCH apparently increases appetite by altering taste rather than by interfering with satiation (Baird et al. 2009).

Ghrelin

Leidy and Williams (2006) found that levels of the hunger hormone ghrelin have their own diurnal rhythm. In their study of nonobese, premenopausal women, ghrelin levels varied with the quantity of food eaten at a particular meal, and the levels tended to increase later in the day, reflecting our tendency to eat more food as the day progresses. It is possible that these higher ghrelin levels later in the day may be a compensatory response for insufficient food intake throughout the day. Ghrelin levels after eating fell much further after higher-calorie meals. The researchers speculate that ghrelin acts as an acute sensor of energy balance. Leidy and Williams (2006) also found that ghrelin levels were highest at night, and they may be involved in promoting sleep, particularly slow-wave sleep, rather than just food intake. When ghrelin is given experimentally, levels of both cortisol and growth hormone (but not leptin) rise (Weikel et al. 2003). Yannielli et al. (2007), who studied the effects of administering ghrelin in mice, speculate that circadian rhythms may respond to "food-related cues" like ghrelin only when other cues, such as light or plentiful food, are not available. There is also the suggestion that ghrelin, produced primarily in the stomach, may act directly on the SCN master clock and act as an "intermediary" with the stomach such that it affects circadian rhythms when there is limited or even no food (Yannielli et al. 2007).

Rising ghrelin levels (usually in the evenings) may trigger increased eating and drinking.

Further, when ghrelin was administered experimentally to rats, it stimulated vigilance and wakefulness, possibly related to its ability to stimulate cortisol, and ghrelin caused a significant decrease in both REM and non-REM sleep for several hours. There is the speculation that rising ghrelin levels trigger an entire behavior pattern, at least in rodents, characterized by increased eating and drinking, as well as increased activities such as exploring and grooming (Szentirmai et al. 2006).

Serotonin

An experiment done years ago also demonstrates the relationship among hormone secretion, circadian rhythms, and feeding. Leibowitz et al. (1989) injected serotonin directly into rats' paraventricular nucleus, an area of the brain involved in the control of satiety, at different times during a 24-hour period. They found that serotonin suppressed food intake very specifically, depending on the type of food, dose, and the time administered. Their speculation was that serotonin has a circadian pattern: when it was given at the *start* of the animals' feeding time (in the case of rats, the night cycle), it inhibited intake of carbohydrates selectively but promoted later protein and fat intake. Significantly, rats and humans seem to have a strong natural preference for carbohydrate intake at the first meal (e.g., our breakfast cereal or pancakes) after a period of not eating—a finding also noted by de Castro in 1987, who felt that there was a circadian rhythm to satiety, such that we tend to eat more as the day progresses toward evening. Years later, in a study of almost 600 subjects, de Castro (2004) found that those who ate more in the morning hours, particularly of foods of lower density, tended to feel more satiated and eat less overall for the day than those who ate more in the late evening. In general, though, most people tend to increase their meal size as the day goes on and decrease the time interval between meals. This is the opposite of the recommendation to eat like a king at breakfast, a prince at lunch, and a pauper at dinner. De Castro (2004) cautions that his results do not provide a causative link between eating more foods with a lower density in the morning (and feeling more satiated) and eating less food later in the day, but merely a correlation.

Histamine

Histamine is a substance synthesized from one of the amino acids. It is found in mast cells, where it is involved in our body's immune responses (thus antihistamines are used to treat allergic reactions), and it is also found in a posterior part of the hypothalamus, where it is a neurotransmitter (Jørgensen et al. 2007). It has direct projections to the SCN, or master clock, as well as throughout other areas of the brain, and has been implicated in the regulation of sleep-wake cycles, feeding cycles, and even body temperature (Yoshimatsu 2008). There are three major types of histamine receptors: H_1, H_2, and H_3 receptors. H_1 and H_3 receptors are the ones that seem to be involved in regulating eating. An infusion of histamine experimentally, for example, led to a suppression of appetite in rodents, and prevented the development of obesity in rats that were genetically bred to become diabetic and obese or that were given an obesity-inducing diet (Jørgensen et al. 2007). In fact, as we noted in the "Orexins" section above, it has been suggested that H_1 receptor blockade is responsible for the fact that the atypical antipsychotics (e.g., clozapine, olanzapine) cause weight gain by stimulating appetite (Fadel et al. 2002). There is speculation that histamine and its receptors mediate both orexin A neurons (for arousal) and the hormone leptin (for its satiety effects) (Yoshimatsu 2008).

Yoshimatsu (2008) demonstrated that mice rendered deficient in H_1 receptors developed abnormal circadian rhythms for activity, as well as for feeding, and they became obese. Interestingly, they tended to lose their circadian rhythms even before they developed obesity. When researchers placed these mice on scheduled feeding, rather than allowing them to eat whenever they chose, the mice were able to lose weight, but this was probably because of increased activity (Yoshimatsu 2008). Masaki and Yoshimatsu (2006) believe that by controlling diurnal rhythms of eating, histamine and H_1 receptors are "crucial for the regulation of obesity" and they speculate that histamine and its receptors may eventually provide a pharmaceutical control for human obesity.

Hibernating Animals and a Model for Human Obesity

One of the most intriguing theories about obesity in humans is Neel's theory that insulin resistance and obesity actually evolved genetically as a survival mechanism to ensure energy stores in times of food shortage. As Neel (1962) explains it, overproduction of insulin was, "at an earlier stage in man's evolution, an asset in that it was an important energy-conserving mechanism, when food intake was irregular and obesity rare." Neel analogizes to the initial benefits that sickle cell disease conferred benefits against malaria, but because we are now able to treat malaria for the most part, we are left with only the deleterious effects of sickle cell disease. Neel's "thrifty gene" theory remains controversial, and some have suggested that around the Paleolithic Age food may not even have been in short supply.

Nevertheless, Scott and Grant (2006) have revisited Neel's theory and adapted it analogously to hibernating mammals (e.g., ground squirrels, marmots, and woodchucks) with which we share some genes that are "homologous to hibernating genes." Martin (2008) suggests that man probably evolved from a hibernating ancestor and sees hibernation as a natural model of reversible obesity in humans. Scott and Grant (2006) differentiate a cycle of adaptive, physiologically beneficial, short-term (seasonal) weight gain—that is, *fat loading*, as seen in hibernating mammals—from long-term, physiologically maladaptive weight gain as seen in human obesity. Some hibernating mammals, such as marmots, actually seasonally develop insulin resistance, an increase in secretion of the fat hormone leptin, and a decrease in secretion of the fat hormone adiponectin. This pattern works to suppress hunger and appetite during winter's hibernation, and the energy sources switch from carbohydrates to fat. Eventually, though, there is increased melatonin secretion and increased insulin sensitivity such that these mammals are leaner and more insulin sensitive in the spring after hibernation. Martin (2008) believes the seasonal changes ("circannual cycles") in metabolism and hormone secretion, including secretion of thyroid and reproductive hormones, "orchestrate a sliding setpoint."

> We are nonhibernating; nevertheless, we are *fat-loading* mammals.

SLEEP DISRUPTION AND WEIGHT

Normal Sleep Architecture

Normally, we tend to sleep in 90-minute cycles that are repeated several times throughout the night. These cycles are divided into REM and non-REM sleep, and non-REM sleep is divided further into Stages 1–4; this is referred to as *sleep architecture*. Stages 3 and 4 are considered *slow-wave sleep* (characterized by delta waves seen on electroencephalograms), thought to be the most restorative (Tasali et al. 2008). It is primarily during slow-wave sleep that hormone secretion patterns, as well as decreased sympathetic activity and increased parasympathetic tone (e.g., vagal tone), occur. As we age past 60 years, the percentages of REM and non-REM sleep change, and we can actually be awake as much as 30% of the time during the night (Van Cauter et al. 2007). For a more thorough discussion of sleep architecture, we recommend the Reite et al. (2009) *Clinical Manual for Evaluation and Treatment of Sleep Disorders*.

WHAT ARE THE STAGES OF SLEEP?

- STAGE 1: 5% of sleep; light sleep from which one can be easily awakened; some eye movements and muscle contractions may occur

- STAGE 2: 20%–25% of sleep spent in stages 2 and 3) eye movements stop and our brain waves become slower, although there may still be some bursts of rapid waves

- STAGE 3: Extremely slow waves, called delta waves, beginning; this is the first stage of deep sleep

- STAGE 4: Also a stage of deep sleep from which it is difficult to be awakened; delta waves predominate and no eye movements or muscle movements; if awakened, we feel groggy and somewhat disoriented; this is also the stage when night terrors, sleepwalking, or bedwetting can occur, as well as secretion of growth hormone in children and adolescents

- REM (rapid eye movement) sleep: 20%–25% of sleep; called "paradoxical sleep" because the EEG during REM is similar to the waking state; this is the stage of dreaming, jerky eye movements, and rapid breathing, as well as increased heart rate, increased blood pressure, and temporary paralysis; men can have erections during this phase; alcohol, caffeine, nicotine, and many drugs can interfere with REM sleep; cardiac arrhythmias are more common
  As night progresses, our REM stages lengthen; we still do not know exactly why we dream; Freud thought dreams represented the "royal road to the unconscious" and each dream always contained a wish fulfillment

- The entire cycle of sleep takes about 90–110 minutes and is repeated throughout the night

Source: Benca et al. 2009, p.361; DSM-IV-TR, pp. 597–604

Fragmented Sleep, Excessive Daytime Sleepiness, and Obstructive Sleep Apnea

> *Some of the people who overeat present the following signs: at first they fre-*
> *quently fall into a prolonged and pleasant sleep at night, and at short intervals*
> *during the day. As the condition get worse, their sleep becomes less agreeable,*
> *more disturbed, and in their dreams they struggle.*

Hippocrates, *Regimen*, Book III (Precope 1952, p. 75)

Most adults require 7–9 hours of sleep a night, but the amount of sleep required varies considerably among individuals: some require less than 6 hours to feel rested and some require more than 9 hours (Benca et al. 2004, p. 282). Sleep requirements change throughout the life span; for example, infants require considerably more sleep, as do pregnant women, than the elderly do. Although we do not really know all the functions of sleep, we do know that sleep is useful for consolidation of memories as well as maintaining synaptic connections in the brain, and total sleep deprivation can lead to death within weeks (Reite et al. 2009, p. 38).

We can speak of inadequate duration of sleep and/or poor sleep quality (disturbed or fragmented sleep) when we speak of sleep deprivation. Sleep deprivation can be a serious condition and lead to life-threatening consequences. For example, those who are sleep deprived perform as badly on eye-hand coordination tests as someone who is intoxicated with alcohol, and driving while sleep deprived accounts for about 100,000 motor vehicle accidents each year, as well as 71,000 injuries and 1,550 fatalities, according to the National Highway Transportation Safety Administration (Knipling and Wang 1995). Furthermore, sleep deprivation affects cognitive functioning dramatically. It affects logical thinking, speed of response, attention, ability to think flexibly, memory, and speech, among other things (Benca et al. 2009, pp. 370–371).

When we get an inadequate amount of sleep or have poor sleep quality, we can have excessive daytime sleepiness. Excessive daytime sleepiness can, of course, be caused by narcolepsy, but one of the most common causes of fragmented sleep quality and hence daytime sleepiness is obstructive sleep apnea, a syndrome characterized by loud snoring, episodic airway obstruction (or collapse) that is either partial or complete, and sleep fragmentation (Subramanian and Strohl 2004, p. 939). Sometimes loud snoring and fatigue are the only symptoms (Strollo and Rogers 1996).

Back in the mid 1950s, Burwell et al. (1956) described a syndrome manifested by marked obesity, periodic respiration, and somnolence, among other signs and symptoms, that they designated the *Pickwickian syndrome*, after a character in a Charles Dickens novel. What was striking about this syndrome, said Burwell et al., was that many of the symptoms were reversible when the patient lost a "sufficient" amount of weight. Their conclusion was that in some vulnerable people "there is a critical degree of obesity at which ventilatory insufficiency appears."

Subramanian and Strohl (2004, p. 939) noted that the link between obesity and obstructive sleep apnea is such a strong one that it was thought sleep apnea did not occur without obesity. It can, in fact, occur without obesity (and at any age and in both genders) but is obviously much more commonly linked to obesity as originally described. Up to 15% of individuals who are obese (with a BMI value of >35 kg/m^2) have the Pickwickian syndrome, with carbon dioxide retention (i.e., a hypoventilation condition) when they are awake (Subramanian and Strohl 2004, p. 940). Furthermore, those with obesity can have excessive daytime sleepiness without actually having sleep apnea.

Reite et al. (2009, p. 228) define apnea as a stopping of airflow for at least 10 seconds, and when this occurs oxygen saturation falls. Those with severe sleep apnea can have about 30 of these episodes an hour (Pack and Gislason 2009), leading to restless, nonrefreshing, fragmented sleep. There is an increase in sympathetic nervous system activity with elevated catecholamine levels—this can also happen throughout the day—and when this happens during sleep the person awakens (Pack and Gislason 2009). Spiegel et al. (2005) reported that about 24% of men and 9% of women in middle age have this disorder. It is not at all common in women prior to menopause except in those who have polycystic ovary syndrome; in one study, these women were found to have obstructive sleep apnea 30 times more frequently than control subjects (insulin resistance also occurred in half of women with polycystic ovary disorder) (Vgontzas 2008). In general, though, this syndrome is seen more commonly in those who are overweight or obese. Reite et al. (2009, p. 226) report that about 70% of people diagnosed with sleep apnea are at least 20% overweight. In fact, the greater the degree of abdominal (visceral) obesity, the greater the prevalence of obstructive sleep apnea. Obstructive sleep apnea is associated with the metabolic syndrome, and sleep apnea has been described as part of a syndrome called *syndrome Z* when added to the diagnosis of abdominal obesity, insulin resistance, hypertension, and abnormal

> *Syndrome Z*: sleep apnea, abdominal obesity, insulin resistance, and abnormal lipid and blood glucose profile

lipid and blood glucose profiles (Hu 2008, p. 149). Reite et al. (2009, pp. 226–227) note there are reports that about half of adults with obstructive sleep apnea have hypertension, and they suggest that those who have high blood pressure without an apparent cause should be evaluated for obstructive sleep apnea.

Vgontzas (2008) makes the point that obstructive sleep apnea has often been considered a "local abnormality" of the respiratory tract rather than a systemic disease, as he considers it to be. Even though there may be local abnormalities—for example, a larger than average neck circumference is sometimes seen in these patients—there are also systemic markers of inflammation such as higher levels of IL-6, TNF-α, and C-reactive protein. In fact, Vgontzas (2008) notes that a large neck may be reflective of an increased BMI value and obesity. He believes that the abnormalities in respiration seen in patients with sleep apnea are caused by central neural mechanisms such as decreased functioning of the hypothalamic-pituitary-adrenal (HPA) axis. Furthermore, Vgontzas speculates that sleep apnea may be a heterogeneous disorder. And Pack and Gislason (2009) speculate that increased sympathetic activity may be one of the physiological mechanisms responsible for the increase in cardiovascular disease, including an increased risk of myocardial infarction and stroke, seen in those with obstructive sleep apnea. When the condition was treated by nasal continuous positive airway pressure (CPAP), catecholamine levels decreased, and Pack and Gislason (2009), in reviewing several studies, found that nasal CPAP only sometimes improves insulin sensitivity, but the "interventional data are less compelling." Pack and Gislason (2009) explained the discrepancy among studies by noting that better results with CPAP were found in patients who were less obese, namely with a BMI of less than 31 kg/m^2, and they added, "In most obese subjects there was no change in insulin sensitivity. In such cases the effects of obesity may be so overwhelming that treatment of OSA has no effect." Basta et al. (2008) emphasized the importance of screening for depression in those with obstructive sleep apnea because both depression and obstructive sleep apnea can contribute to excessive daytime sleepiness. They recommended regular exercise as part of the treatment approach. They pointed out that the prevalence of depression (as measured by the General Health Questionnaire) in their study of over 1,100 men and women with sleep apnea was high: over 18% in men and over 37% in women. Furthermore, undiagnosed depressive symptoms may interfere with compliance with a treatment such as CPAP (Basta et al. 2008).

Strollo and Rogers (1996) recommend that a sleep study using polysomnography be conducted to verify the diagnosis for those who snore, report daytime sleepiness, or have been observed to have episodes of apnea. Both alcohol and benzodiazepines can make obstructive sleep apnea worse.

> The word *fatigue* should be used for depressed obese patients who complain of tiredness and disturbed sleep; *sleepiness* should be used for obese patients who complain of tiredness but are not depressed and do not have disturbed sleep.

Excessive daytime sleepiness is sometimes not related to *objectively* measured sleep duration, but rather to *perceived* short sleep duration, particularly in those who are depressed. Vgontzas (2008) noted that obese people who report short sleep duration are more apt to be chronically emotionally stressed. In other words, an individual's perception of how long he or she sleeps may be determined by emotional factors (Vgontzas et al. 2008). Vgontzas (2008) differentiates fatigue from objectively measured sleepiness, and recommends we use the word *fatigue* for those with emotional distress—for depressed obese patients who complain of tiredness and disturbed sleep—and *sleepiness* for those without emotional stress, that is, for obese patients who complain of tiredness but are not depressed and do not have disturbed sleep. He believes that on this basis we can differentiate two categories of obese patients, as he did in a review of studies of patients with sleep disorders: one group of obese patients (47%) who complained of poor sleep and emotional stress and had depression and fatigue (with "low sleep efficiency" and a hyperactive HPA axis), such as seen in patients with chronic insomnia, and another group of obese patients (53%) who slept well and were not depressed or otherwise emotionally stressed (and had "high sleep efficiency" and a hypoactive HPA axis) but did have objective sleepiness, such as seen in disorders like sleep apnea, narcolepsy, and sleep deprivation (Vgontzas et al. 2008).

Inadequate Sleep and Hormone Secretion

Disrupted, poor-quality sleep, such as occurs in obstructive sleep apnea, can be associated with changes in metabolic functioning. Inadequate amounts of sleep ("chronic partial sleep loss") can cause dysregulation of our metabolic processes (Van Cauter et al. 2007), and even the lay press has run stories suggesting that sleep deprivation can make us fat (ScienceDaily 2006). Some have suggested that chronic inadequate sleep, which is seen increasingly in our hectic, 24/7 environment, may be seriously contributing to the obesity epidemic, at least in the United States. For a discussion of the rising rates of obesity (and with these rates, of type 2 diabetes) over the past decade, not only in the United States but worldwide, please see discussions in Chapters 1 and 2 of this volume. The World Health Organization (2006) reported that there are "approximately 1.6 billion adults over the age of 15 who are overweight and at least 400 million who are obese" (by BMI data), and it predicts that by 2015, 2.3 billion will be overweight and more than 700 million will be obese. Most recently, Aronne et al. (2009), in discussing these statistics, call obesity "increasingly prevalent and now considered a 'pandemic.'" They add, "This situation is more than a mere crisis of aesthetics, since obesity is causally associated with several chronic diseases, most notably type 2 diabetes and cardiovascular disease."

For example, Spiegel et al. (2005) call it intriguing that the dramatic increase in obesity and diabetes has occurred in the time period when many have been reporting sleeping considerably fewer hours. They point to the fact that human sleep—unlike that of most other mammals, which sleep in bouts—usually occurs in a consolidated 7- to 9-hour block. During that time, an extended fasting period, our blood glucose levels must remain stable. During early sleep, especially slow-wave sleep, our brains need considerably less glucose, but as morning approaches and we have more periods of REM sleep, we begin to use more glucose. How, when, and how much glucose the body utilizes is even more significant in those who experience the metabolic consequences of abdominal obesity, particularly people who have developed type 2 diabetes or even those with abnormalities of insulin (includ-

HORMONES AND CIRCADIAN RHYTHMS

- The lowest levels of leptin occur before noon and highest levels occur in the middle of the night.

- Ghrelin, growth hormone, and prolactin levels all increase substantially during sleep.

- Melatonin levels are highest during the first half of the night.

- Cortisol and thyrotropin (thyroid-stimulating hormone) decrease during sleep.

- Cortisol levels peak in the morning; prolactin levels fall upon awakening.

- Adiponectin levels, like those of cortisol, also peak in the morning but about 2 hours later than cortisol.

Source: Allison et al. 2005a; Gavrila et al. 2003; Van Cauter et al. 2007

ing high but ineffective levels—the state of insulin resistance) and abnormally high blood glucose levels (see Chapter 5, "Metabolic Consequences of Obesity").

Van Cauter et al. (2007) point out that secretion of growth hormone, prolactin, and ghrelin increases substantially during sleep, whereas secretion of cortisol and thyrotropin (thyroid-stimulating hormone, or TSH) decreases. Leptin (a satiety hormone) also has a "striking" diurnal pattern (Bray and Young 2006). When the quality of sleep is disrupted, changes occur in these secretions. In other words, hormone secretion when we are asleep is actually dependent on our sleep quality. For example, leptin levels are reportedly about 18% lower and levels of ghrelin (the appetite-stimulating hormone) are as much as 28% higher when we get several hours less sleep (Spiegel et al. 2005). Bray and Young (2006) suggest that leptin resistance seen in obesity may be a function of a "blunted" pattern in diurnal variation. They note that up to 5% of obese individuals have a mutation of the melanocortin 4 receptor gene (*MC4R*)—the same percentage that have the BRAt genetic variation for breast cancer. In general, leptin levels, as we have said (see Chapter 5, "The Metabolic Complexities of Weight Control"), are higher in women than in men and are higher in obese women than in nonobese women. Interestingly, Perfetto et al. (2004) have found that leptin circadian rhythms show a 3-hour difference in women with the android pattern of abdominal obesity (in the midsection) compared with women with the more common gynoid (lower body) pattern of obesity. In other words, body fat distribution is a factor in leptin rhythms, and Perfetto et al. (2004) suggest further studies in this area. Leptin level circadian patterns also seem to be related to meal timing rather than to light, as well as to insulin secretion. (Cortisol levels, on the other hand, which are highest in the morning, are related to the light-dark cycle and not to meals.) Furthermore, Perfetto et al. (2004) report on studies that demonstrate that leptin levels that rise at night can be shifted forward by jet lag and a day-night reversal, but cortisol levels do not shift, at least not over a short period of time. And orexin levels, at least in animals, increase with sleep deprivation. Knutson and Van Cauter (2008) suggest that because orexin is involved in our reward and motivation systems, it is possible that increased sleep deprivation encourages us to eat irregularly and to eat foods with poor nutritional value (e.g., eating snack foods rather than fruits or vegetables, and not in response to "actual caloric need"). They report on studies that indicate individuals who are sleep challenged do tend to have dysregulation, or "nonhomeostatic control," of eating, and there is some evidence that they also tend to overeat. Paradoxically, when animals are sleep deprived, they are hyperphagic but they lose weight (due to increased physical activity and stress) whereas sleep-deprived humans tend to be hyperphagic but to gain weight, often due to being fatigued and getting less physical activity.

Mice that are genetically altered so that they become obese, diabetic, and leptin resistant (a model for leptin resistance in humans) have been shown to have dramatic changes in their sleep patterns. Laposky et al. (2008) found these mice slept longer but had considerably more fragmented and less restful sleep, and they were less able to compensate for sleep deprivation when they were allowed to sleep (as is usually the case). Furthermore, they had abnormal diurnal patterns of their sleep architecture, with changes in both REM and non-REM sleep.

Gavrila et al. (2003) have found that adiponectin levels, as we have mentioned (see Chapter 5, on metabolic complexities), also have a "clear" diurnal rhythm, with significantly lower levels at night and reaching their lowest levels (nadir) in the early morning (i.e., around 3 A.M.). Adiponectin levels, after peaking in the late morning, decrease slightly for most of the day and plateau until late evening when they begin to fall more significantly. These levels are apparently not in phase with the diurnal rhythm of leptin. According to Gavrila et al. (2003), adiponectin and cortisol have "similar but not overlapping diurnal variations" with each other, such that cortisol levels progressively also increase during morning hours and peak in the late morning. Cortisol levels, though, have more of a continuous decline during the day with their nadir in the early night (around 1 A.M.), whereas adiponectin levels are lowest about two hours after cortisol's (Gavrila et al. 2003).

High-Fat Feeding and Disrupted Rhythms

The effects of high-fat diets on circadian rhythms has been studied in mice. Jenkins et al. (2006) found that high-fat feeding disrupted the sleep pattern of mice during a 6-week experimental period. Not only did the mice increase their weight compared with control animals, they also had significant increases in non-REM sleep and had difficulty remaining awake during the time when they were usually active, a pattern seen in some obese humans. Furthermore, Kohsaka et al. (2007) found that feeding mice a high-fat diet disrupted the usual circadian pattern of feeding. The mice were more likely to eat during the period when they usually did not eat (during the day) and ate less during their usual eating period (at night). Their motor activity also changed, but not as significantly as their eating pattern. The researchers speculate that when animals receive increased calories and there is a disruption of circadian rhythms, they may be less able to regulate their weight effectively.

Can Inadequate Sleep Lead to Obesity?

Both sleep and sleeplessness, when beyond due measure, constitute disease.

Hippocrates, *Aphorisms* VII, lxxii

Significantly, though, researchers are finding that incurring a sleep debt by a pattern of recurrent inadequate sleep, as is commonly seen today, seems to result in a marked decrease in insulin sensitivity and eventually in overt insulin resistance if the pattern continues. Men in particular seem sensitive to developing type 2 diabetes (Van Cauter et al. 2007). In an analysis of data from a large study of almost 9,000 men and women between the ages of 32 and 86, with 8–10 years of follow-up—the First National Health and Nutrition Examination Survey (NHANES I)—Gangwisch et al. (2007) found that men and women whose sleep duration was either too short (<5 hours) or too long (>9 hours) were significantly more likely to develop type 2 diabetes over time. The researchers, though, are willing to entertain the possibility that reverse causation may be involved, namely that either too much sleep or too little sleep is perhaps a "prodromal symptom" of diabetes, rather than causative itself.

Spiegel et al. (2005) reviewed the literature on large studies involving thousands of people over many years in different countries, including Germany, and found that a chronic pattern of inadequate sleep does seem to increase the risk of developing obesity and/or type 2 diabetes. Patel et al. (2006) looked at data on almost 70,000 middle-aged women over the course of 16 years (beginning in 1986) in the Nurses' Health Study. In general, just over 4% of women reported sleeping 5 or fewer hours, 25.5% slept 6 hours, 42% slept 7 hours, 23.5% slept 8 hours, and 4.5% slept 9 hours or more per night. Women who reported sleeping less than 5 hours a night had a 32% greater chance of gaining more than 30 pounds over the 16 years of follow-up. Those who reported sleeping 7 to 8 hours a night had the lowest risk of gaining weight over time. In general, those who slept 5 or fewer hours a night tended to gain over 2 pounds more than those who reported sleeping 7 to 8 hours.

> Individuals who sleep either too little or too long may develop type 2 diabetes.

More recently, Patel et al. (2008) studied about 6,000 older men and women (ranging in age from their mid 60s through their 90s) cross-sectionally to assess the relationship of shortened sleep and obesity. The researchers objectively monitored sleep by having their subjects wear an actigraph, a device that measures movement and correlates with more accurate measures of sleep such as a polysomnograph. What is also interesting about this study is that sleep duration was similar on weekdays and weekends in this older and, presumably, mostly retired population (unlike the pattern in most working people, who typically sleep longer on weekends). Patel et al. (2008) found that these older men and women who slept 5 or fewer hours a night were significantly more likely to be obese (men, 3.7 times more likely; women, 2.3 times more likely) as measured by BMI value, with increased waist circumferences and more abdominal fat. Their conclusion was that the effects of sleep deprivation on weight seemed to be independent of the etiology of the sleeping difficulty (e.g., psychiatric disorder or obstructive breathing), but because their study was cross-sectional they could not establish a causal connection between decreased sleep and weight.

Cappuccio et al. (2008) performed a meta-analysis of studies from 1996 to 2007 involving sleep duration and obesity. Of almost 700 studies, they found 18 adult studies (with >600,000 people from different countries) that could provide data to meet the criteria for their meta-analysis. They found that a person is indeed more likely to be a so-called short sleeper if he or she is obese, and that there is a dose-response effect—the greater a person's BMI value, the less sleep the person gets. It has been speculated that increased appetite, decreased physical activity, and/or deleterious effects on glucose control may be involved in the connection between chronic sleep loss and weight (Knutson et al. 2007).

Chaput et al. (2008) studied 276 men and women over the course of 6 years to investigate the connection between sleep length and a person's weight. They, too, found that those who had too much sleep (defined as 9–10 hours a night) were 25% more likely, and those with too little sleep (defined as 5–6 hours a night) were 35% more likely, to have a weight gain of 5 kilograms (11 pounds) over the course of the study.

In an earlier paper, Knutson et al. (2006) had introduced the concept of "perceived sleep debt," which incorporates a person's habitual sleep time as compared to his or her subjective sleep need. In their study of a group of almost 300 men and women (mostly African Americans) who already had type 2 diabetes, these researchers found that decreased sleep duration was related to poorer glucose control and higher levels of hemoglobin A_{1c}, a marker of diabetes control. They could not infer causality, though, because poor glycemic control can lead to increased awakenings, due to the need to urinate (nocturia) or to pain from diabetic neuropathy, and hence decreased sleep duration or quality. Nevertheless, they suggest that sleep should be considered a potential factor that may influence glucose control in patients with diabetes. Trento et al. (2008), in a controlled study, looked at a population of just under 50 men and women with type 2 diabetes. They excluded those with peripheral neuropathies. Nevertheless, they found that type 2 diabetes is significantly associated with more disrupted and poorer-quality sleep compared with sleep in individuals without diabetes.

Patel and Hu (2008a) reviewed the connection between weight gain and sleep duration in a literature search that covered 1966 through early 2007. They found clearer connections between short sleep duration and obesity in children, with more mixed results in adults. However, they noted inconsistencies in their review. For example, some studies have shown a gender effect (in some, men were more likely to have the connection between short sleep duration and obesity, and in others, women were more likely to have the connection); other studies have not shown an effect of gender. Furthermore, ethnic differences may affect results such that African Americans may be more susceptible to weight gain with short sleep duration and Japanese populations less so. Patel and Hu (2008a) also note that there may be considerable variability in sleep from night to night, and studies often do not consider afternoon naps (more common among some populations than others) when they consider sleep.

Marshall et al. (2008) also reviewed the connection between obesity and sleep duration. Their conclusion was that it is premature to consider sleep duration a "modifiable risk factor" when we consider obesity (though there may be a somewhat clearer connection in children). For example, studies have not yet demonstrated that alterations in sleep duration lead to changes in a person's weight, nor is it even clear just how much sleep should be recommended.

Tasali et al. (2008) looked specifically at slow-wave sleep (stages 3 and 4, the most restorative stages of sleep). The amount of slow-wave sleep a person gets is variable and "highly heritable." In their very small study of nine healthy, lean men and women, they found that a "selective and profound" reduction in slow-wave sleep produced decreased glucose tolerance and decreased insulin sensitivity, and that these decreases were related to a person's baseline level of slow-wave sleep. They speculated that both sleep duration and sleep quality can have such impacts and that some people may have a genetic predisposition to develop diabetes in the context of decreased slow-wave sleep. In fact, Tasali et al. (2008) add, "Furthermore, our data suggest that reduced sleep quality with low levels of slow wave sleep, as occurs in aging and in many obese individuals, may contribute to increase the risk of type 2 diabetes."

There are many methodological problems, though, when we study sleep. For one thing, studies define sleep deprivation inconsistently. In some studies, less than 5 hours a night is considered a short amount of sleep, whereas others draw the line at 6 hours and still others define inadequate sleep duration as anything less than 7 hours. Furthermore, when studies are cross-sectional they do not account for changes in sleep over time, and individual studies often do not control consistently for various confounders such as psychiatric comorbidity (e.g., depression) or other chronic illnesses, use of medications, and so on. Another problem is that most large sleep studies use self-reports of sleep duration and these, of course, are notoriously subjective and can be inaccurate (Knutson and Van Cauter 2008).

So we are left with the suggestion that both too much sleep and too little sleep may be contributing to obesity and metabolic abnormalities, but the evidence, particularly for adults, is far from definite. It is still difficult, for example, to determine whether obesity causes short sleep duration or whether short sleep duration causes obesity, particularly because there are so many conditions associated with obesity that could contribute to disrupted sleep (e.g., cardiac disease, osteoarthritis, gastroesophageal reflux, chronic pain syndromes, depression) (Patel and Hu 2008a; Patel and Hu 2008b, pp. 320–341).

THE NIGHT EATING SYNDROME (DISORDER OF CIRCADIAN RHYTHMS)

Over 50 years ago, Stunkard and his colleagues (Stunkard et al. 1955) identified what they called a "distinctive syndrome," characterized by nocturnal hyperphagia, insomnia, and morning anorexia, in a small group of obese patients (in 20 of 25 patients) they had been seeing in their New York clinic. They noticed that these patients did not sleep until midnight, took in at least one-quarter of their total daily calories after their evening meal, and had nothing more than coffee and maybe some orange juice for breakfast. They further noted that these patients had particularly intractable weight problems, with failure to control their weight by "dietary regimens." At the time, Stunkard and his colleagues noted the connection to life stresses in many of their patients. Presciently, they appreciated that their patients had apparent alterations in their diurnal rhythms, such as are sometimes seen in cases of depression or after encephalitis, and they even suggested that a person's normal circadian eating pattern "may be important in the maintenance of caloric balance" (Stunkard et al. 1955).

> Night eating syndrome may be a pathway to obesity.

The two most important features, though, seem to be that 1) 25% of total daily calories are eaten after the evening meal, and 2) individuals experience multiple awakenings from their sleep and they eat during at least half of these episodes (Allison et al. 2005b). The syndrome seems to begin in early adulthood and often predates the development of obesity (in more than half of patients) and may be a "pathway" to obesity (Stunkard et al. 2005). In fact, These researchers (Stunkard et al. 2005) compared night eaters of normal weight with obese individuals and found that the normal-weight night eaters were a full 10 years or more younger and had had the disorder a shorter period of time.

By convention, researchers differentiate night eating syndrome from what is referred to as *nocturnal sleep-related eating disorder*, particularly by the fact that those with night eating syndrome are conscious and aware when they awaken and eat (Tanofsky-Kraff and Yanovski 2004). Those with a nocturnal sleep-related eating disorder, on the other hand, are only partly conscious, and their eating is considered involuntary and not in their control. Those afflicted are not easily aroused and have been known to eat inedible or even dangerous substances (e.g., raw bacon) and can be amnestic for the experience the next morning (Howell et al. 2009). Recently, this disorder came into the news when reports surfaced that the medication zolpidem (Ambien), used to treat insomnia, was associated with episodes of "sleep eating." The night eating syndrome is also to be distinguished from binge eating disorder, which is also not yet an official DSM diagnosis but is included in DSM-IV-TR as a criteria set for further study (American Psychiatric Association 2000, pp. 785–787). These conditions can be seen concomitantly (Tanofsky-Kraff and Yanovski 2004), and patients who have both have considerably higher levels of anxiety than those diagnosed with night eating syndrome alone (Napolitano et al. 2001).

Allison et al. (2005b), including Stunkard, compared almost 300 people who were binge eaters or nighttime eaters versus a control group of overweight people to assess their patterns of disordered eating as well as their level of psychological distress. The researchers' conclusion was that there is "strong evidence" that the two syndromes are quite distinct. (See below for controversies regarding these diagnoses.) For example, even though both groups experienced subjective feelings of loss of control over their eating, subjects with night eating syndrome ate considerably less food at one time than those with binge eating disorder. Furthermore, many of those with night eating syndrome seemed to have control over their eating during the day, unlike those with binge eating disorder, who had "greater disinhibition" and reported more hunger, as well as more concerns over their weight and shape. Both groups, with reports of mild to moderate depression, may be at risk for mood disorders (Allison et al. 2005b).

In an editorial in the *American Journal of Psychiatry*, Stunkard et al. (2008) argued for inclusion of the night eating syndrome in DSM-V, particularly because it affects about 1.5% of people in the general population; up to 16% of people in weight reduction programs; and, in some studies, as many as 42% of obese people who present for bariatric surgery (though the statistics vary considerably). Rand et al. (1997), for example, found that night eating was present in about 30 of 111 individuals (27%) in a sample of patients having bariatric surgery for their weight. Allison et al. (2006) make the point that an evaluation of disordered eating is particularly relevant in patients considering surgery for extreme obesity because eating patterns may ultimately affect how much weight a person will lose after bariatric surgery. Reports of having either night eating syndrome or binge eating disorder were lower than in other previously reported studies in a population of over 200 candidates presenting for bariatric surgery when the researchers (Allison et al. 2005b) used particularly strict definitions for each condition. They speculated that the prospective surgical candidates tended to minimize their symptoms of disordered eating lest they be refused surgery, or possibly that the patients had had these patterns so long they no longer considered them distressing (Allison et al. 2006). Colles et al. (2007), in a study in Australia, also looked at patients presenting for bariatric surgery ($n = 180$) and compared these patients to a group of control subjects from the community ($n = 158$) and people seeking nonsurgical intervention for excess weight (e.g., a weight loss support group; $n = 93$). These researchers found that over 4% of the total group had binge eating disorder concomitant with night eating syndrome. Of the subgroup with the night eating syndrome, 40% reported binge eating. They also distinguished a special subgroup of more severely impaired night eating patients who snacked frequently in the middle of the night and were more likely to be depressed.

The night eating syndrome is also seen among psychiatric outpatients. Lundgren et al. (2006) found that among almost 400 patients (from two states, Pennsylvania and Minnesota), more than 12% met the researchers' criteria for the night eating syndrome, "greatly exceeding the prevalence of such well-known eating disorders as anorexia nervosa (0.3%) and bulimia nervosa (1.0%)." Those with the night eating syndrome were more likely to have a substance use disorder, particularly alcohol abuse. Lundgren et al. (2006) found that a lifetime substance use disorder "was more likely to occur among patients with night eating syndrome (30.6%) than among those without the syndrome (8.3%.)" Alcohol abuse was found in 46.7% of those with the night eating syndrome and in 66.7% of those without the night eating syndrome. In this study by Lundgren et al. (2006), obesity (with a body mass index value of 30 kg/m² or greater) was found in 57% of night eaters, and an additional 29% of the night eaters were found to be overweight.

NIGHT EATING SYNDROME

- Originally described in the 1950s by Albert Stunkard

- Most striking aspect of syndrome: unusual food intake pattern; in Tanofsky-Kraff and Yanovski (2004) study, by 6:00 P.M. night eaters had consumed only 30% of their daily calories, whereas control subjects had consumed 74%

- Food intake of non–night eaters in that study slowed after evening meal, whereas food intake of night eaters continued after midnight: from 10 P.M. until 6 A.M., night eaters consumed 56% of their daily calories, compared with 15% for control subjects

- Night eaters awaken several times during the night and more than half of the awakenings are associated with eating food, whereas non–night eaters do not eat if they awaken

- Does not appear to be a disorder of sleep but rather a disorder of the circadian rhythm of eating: night eaters sleep same length of time as non–night eaters and have same time of onset of sleep

- Night eaters are more likely to become obese or already be obese than non–night eaters

- Night eaters usually have no interest in eating in the morning

- Syndrome has been responsive to treatment with SSRIs and melatonin in some patients

Source: Tanofsky-Kraff and Yanovski 2004

The study by Lundgren et al. (2006) that highlights the co-occurrence of substance abuse disorder (and particularly alcohol abuse) in a population of those with night eating disorder (over 85% of their population being either overweight or obese) is at variance with data such as those by Warren and Gold (2007), who reported that those with a weight problem were less prone to substance abuse difficulties. Warren and Gold (2007) even suggested that obesity may be protective against substance abuse. Likewise, Wadden and Phelan (2002, p. 198) also thought that substance abuse was "uncommon" in their patient populations though it predicted a poorer outcome. But neither research group was studying the night eating syndrome patients. The point is that there may be subsets of those with a weight problem who may be more vulnerable to substance abuse (see Chapter 6, "Psychiatric Disorders and Weight").

Stunkard et al. (2005) suggest that the night eating syndrome is a circadian rhythm disorder involving eating but not sleep. O'Reardon et al. (2004) measured sleep in these patients and "unexpectedly" found they did not differ from control subjects in total sleep time, in the time of sleep onset, or even by much in the time of morning awakening, even though they may have had many awakenings throughout the night (during which they may have eaten). They were much more likely to eat during the first awakening (almost 90% of the time) than during the fourth awakening (~40% of the time). These patients had a food intake pattern that was "out of phase" with their sleep pattern (O'Reardon et al. 2004). In other words, there was a *dissociation* of the circadian sleep-awake rhythm from the biological rhythm for eating (Stunkard et al. 2005).

Allison et al. (2005a) measured hormonal levels in a group of 15 obese women with the night eating syndrome and a group of obese control subjects. Both groups had BMI values greater than 36 kg/m². Those with night eating syndrome consumed about half of their total daily calories after their evening meal and awoke to eat during the night three or more times per week. Control subjects had no nocturnal awakenings to eat and ate less than one-quarter of their total daily calories after their evening meal. The researchers found that the two groups ate about the same number of calories, so the night eaters did not take in a greater number of calories but rather had a "shift" in when they ate them. Furthermore, morning ghrelin levels were lower in those with night eating syndrome, presumably a consequence of their nocturnal eating. In this study, insulin levels were significantly higher and glucose levels "marginally" higher when measured at night (compared with control subjects) in those with night eating syndrome. This study *did not* find differences in melatonin, cortisol, prolactin, or leptin levels between night eaters and the control subjects, although levels of TSH (thyrotropin) tended to be higher in night eaters. The researchers' conclusion was that any differences in terms of hormone levels between those with night eating and the control subjects were most likely the result, rather than the cause, of the differences in timing of food intake. Allison et al. (2005b) did not know why previous studies had found blunted levels of melatonin and leptin in those with nighttime eating, and obviously further research is warranted.

A more recent study by Goel et al. (2009) of 15 female overweight or obese patients with the night eating syndrome (and 14 female matched control subjects) found that both melatonin and leptin rhythms were significantly phase-delayed (each by an hour or more), though not different in amplitude, compared with those in control subjects. Ghrelin levels, on the other hand, not only were significantly phase-shifted (advanced by > 5 hours), but had half the amplitude of the control group levels; insulin

> Dysfunction of peripheral clocks such as in the stomach (e.g., ghrelin rhythms) and the one in adipose tissue (e.g., leptin rhythms) as well as within the central nervous system (i.e., melatonin rhythms) may be responsible for circadian rhythm abnormalities in patients with night eating syndrome.

levels were phase-delayed by almost 3 hours, also with half the amplitude of the control subjects'. And leptin and ghrelin rhythms were "markedly" out of synchrony (by ~ 6 hours) with each other, which could be a physiological marker specifically for the night eating syndrome. Goel et al. concluded that patients with the night eating syndrome had "significant abnormalities" in circadian rhythms, in terms of both phase and amplitude. They speculate that these abnormalities represent a dysregulation among the so-called peripheral oscillators (i.e., clocks) such as the one in the stomach (e.g., for ghrelin) and the one in adipose tissue (e.g., for leptin), as well within the central SCN master clock (e.g., for melatonin). Furthermore, they noted that glucose and insulin levels were also markedly out of phase with each other ("mismatched") in this study, which could represent metabolic difficulties related to switching from day to evening eating, particularly regarding metabolism of carbohydrates (Goel et al. 2009).

Stunkard et al. (2006) speculate that the night eating syndrome stems from a genetic vulnerability that leads to decreased levels of serotonin, and they note that studies have demonstrated that the selective serotonin reuptake inhibitors (e.g., paroxetine, fluvoxamine, and sertraline) can be effective treatments. They report on a "new paradigm" in which night eating syndrome was treated effectively with sertraline (mean dose, ~125 mg/day). Patients from different geographical locations were assessed by telephone and prescribed medication by their local physicians in consultation with the Penn group (Stunkard et al. 2006). Other researchers have had success treating this syndrome with the antiseizure medication topiramate, though it is not a medication that is easily tolerated (e.g., paresthesias and even kidney stones are known side effects) (Howell et al. 2009).

Experiments with mice might yield other therapies. For example, Yang et al. (2009) noted that mice made mutant for one of the genes involved in circadian rhythms, *mPer2-l*, developed a feeding abnormality whereby they ate excessively, particularly when mice do not usually eat, that is, during the day. The researchers found that administering α–melanocyte-stimulating hormone (α-MSH) could reverse this pattern of hyperphagia. They speculate that α-MSH might be given to people who have the night eating syndrome. And Goel et al. (2009) suggest that night eating syndrome, though clearly primarily a circadian rhythm eating disorder, may have features in common with seasonal affective illness (e.g., mood and sleep symptoms). These researchers further speculate that morning bright light therapy, which is used to phase-shift circadian rhythms, might have a place in treatment of this syndrome, and they recommend further studies.

Despite over 50 years of clinical observations, the night eating syndrome still has not made it into the official DSM nomenclature—neither as an eating disorder nor as a disorder of circadian rhythms. Allison et al. (2009) note there are many major reasons for recognizing disorders officially, including providing a framework to aid in the diagnosis of a particular syndrome, enabling clinical research trials, creating evidence-based guidelines for treatment, and even improving reimbursement for treatment. With these reasons in mind, investigators (Allison et al. 2009) have reached a consensus on "a set of provisional diagnostic criteria" for the night eating syndrome. These researchers even believe there may be subtypes of this disorder.

PROPOSED RESEARCH DIAGNOSTIC CRITERIA FOR NIGHT EATING SYNDROME

A. Daily pattern of significantly increased food intake in evening and/or nighttime as manifested by at least 25% of food intake consumed after evening meal and/or two episodes of nocturnal eating per week

B. Awareness and recall of evening and nocturnal eating episodes

At least three of following:

1. Lack of desire to eat in morning and/or skipping breakfast four or more mornings/week

2. Strong urge to eat between dinner and sleep onset and/or during night

3. Sleep onset and/or sleep maintenance insomnia four or more nights/week

4. Belief that one must eat in order to initiate or return to sleep

5. Mood frequently depressed and/or worse in evening

C. Associated with significant distress and/or impaired functioning

D. Pattern present for at least 3 months

E. Disorder not secondary to any other psychiatric or medical disorder or medication or other substances

Source: Adapted from Allison et al. 2009

REFERENCES

Abe M, Herzog ED, Block GD: Lithium lengthens the circadian period of individual suprachiasmatic nucleus neurons. Neuroreport 11:3261–3264, 2000

Allada R: How flies time when they're having brunch. Cell Metab 8:279–280, 2008

Allison KC, Ahima RS, O'Reardon JP, et al: Neuroendocrine profiles associated with energy intake, sleep, and stress in the night eating syndrome. J Clin Endocrinol Metab 90:6214–6217, 2005a

Allison KC, Grilo CM, Masheb RM, et al: Binge eating disorder and night eating syndrome: a comparative study of disordered eating. J Consult Clin Psychol 73:1107–1115, 2005b

Allison KC, Wadden TA, Sarwer DB, et al: Night eating syndrome and binge eating disorder among persons seeking bariatric surgery: prevalence and related features. Surg Obes Relat Dis 2:153–158, 2006

Allison KC, Lundgren JD, O'Reardon JP, et al: Proposed diagnostic criteria for night eating syndrome. Int J Eat Disord 17 April 2009 [Epub ahead of print]

American Academy of Sleep Medicine: Short sleep duration linked to obesity, consistently and worldwide. May 2, 2008. Available at: http://www.sciencedaily.com/releases/2008/05/080501062808.htm. Accessed March 17, 2009.

American Psychiatric Association: Diagnostic and Statistical Manual of Mental Disorders, 4th Edition, Text Revision. Washington, DC, American Psychiatric Association, 2000

Antle MC, Silver R: Orchestrating time: arrangements of the brain circadian clock. Trends Neurosci 28:145–151, 2005

Aronne LJ, Nelinson DS, Lillo JL: Obesity as a disease state: a new paradigm for diagnosis and treatment. Clin Cornerstone 9(4):9–29, 2009

Baird JP, Choe A, Loveland JL, et al: Orexin-A hyperphagia: hindbrain participation in consummatory feeding responses. Endocrinology 150:1202–1216, 2009

Basta M, Lin HM, Pejovic S, et al: Lack of regular exercise, depression, and degree of apnea are predictors of excessive daytime sleepiness in patients with sleep apnea: sex differences. J Clin Sleep Med 4:19–25, 2008

Benca RM, Cirelli C, Tononi G: Basic science of sleep, in Kaplan and Sadock's Comprehensive Textbook of Psychiatry, 9th Edition, Vol I. Edited by Sadock BJ, Sadock VA, Ruiz P. Philadelphia, PA, Lippincott Williams & Wilkins, 2009, pp 361–374

Boivin DB, Tremblay GM, James FO: Working on atypical schedules. Sleep Med 8:578–589, 2007

Boston RC, Moate PJ, Allison KC, et al: Modeling circadian rhythms of food intake by means of parametric deconvolution: results from studies of the night eating syndrome. Am J Clin Nutr 87:1672–1677, 2008

Bray MS, Young ME: Circadian rhythms in the development of obesity: potential role for the circadian clock within the adipocyte. Obes Rev 8:169–181, 2006

Burwell CS, Robin ED, Whaley RD, et al: Extreme obesity associated with alveolar hypoventilation—a Pickwickian syndrome. Am J Med 21:811–818, 1956

Cappuccio FP, Taggart FM, Kandala NB, et al: Meta-analysis of short sleep duration and obesity in children and adults. Sleep 31:619–626, 2008

Castillo MR, Hochstetler KJ, Tavernier RJ Jr, et al: Entrainment of the master circadian clock by scheduled feeding. Am J Physiol Regul Integr Comp Physiol 287:R551–R555, 2004

Chaput JP, Després JP, Bouchard C, et al: The association between sleep duration and weight gain in adults: a 6-year prospective study from the Quebec Family Study. Sleep 31:517–523, 2008

Colles SL, Dixon JB, O'Brien PE: Night eating syndrome and nocturnal snacking: association with obesity, binge eating and psychological distress. Int J Obes (Lond) 31:1722–1730, 2007

de Castro JM: Circadian rhythms of the spontaneous meal pattern, macronutrient intake, and mood of humans. Physiol Behav 40:437–446, 1987

de Castro JM: The time of day of food intake influences overall intake in humans. J Nutr 134:104–111, 2004

Fadel J, Bubser M, Deutch AY: Differential activation of orexin neurons by antipsychotic drugs associated with weight gain. J Neurosci 22:6742–6746, 2002

Froy O: The relationship between nutrition and circadian rhythms in mammals. Front Neuroendocrinol 28:61–71, 2007

Fuller PM, Lu J, Saper CB: Differential rescue of light- and food-entrainable circadian rhythms. Science 320:1074–1077, 2008

Gangwisch JE, Heymsfield SB, Boden-Albala B, et al: Sleep duration as a risk factor for diabetes incidence in a large U.S. sample. Sleep 30:1667–1673, 2007

Gau SF, Soong WT: The transition of sleep-wake patterns in early adolescence. Sleep 26:449–454, 2003

Gavrila A, Peng C-K, Chan JL, et al: Diurnal and ultradian dynamics of serum adiponectin in healthy men: comparison with leptin, circulating soluble leptin receptor, and cortisol patterns. J Clin Endocrinol Metabol 88:2838–2843, 2003

Goel N, Stunkard AJ, Rogers NL, et al: Circadian rhythm profiles in women with night eating syndrome. J Biol Rhythms 24:85–94, 2009

Halberg F: Chronobiology and nutrition. Contemporary Nutrition 8:1–2, 1983

Harris GC, Aston-Jones G: Arousal and reward: a dichotomy in orexin function. Trends Neurosci 29:571–577, 2006

Harvey AG: Sleep and circadian rhythms in bipolar disorder: seeking synchrony, harmony and regulation. Am J Psychiatry 165:820–829, 2008

Hastings MH, O'Neill JS, Maywood ES: Circadian clocks: regulators of endocrine and metabolic rhythms. J Endocrinol 195:187–198, 2007

Hastings MH, Maywood ES, Reddy AB: Two decades of circadian time. J Neuroendocrinol 20:812–819, 2008

Haus R, Smolensky M: Biological clocks and shift work: circadian dysregulation and potential long-term effects. Cancer Causes Control 17:489–500, 2006

Hippocrates: Aphorisms VII, lxxii, in Works, Vol IV. Translated by Jones WHS. Loeb Classical Library. Cambridge, MA, Harvard University Press, 1967, p 213

Howell MJ, Schenck CH, Crow SJ: A review of nighttime eating disorders. Sleep Med Rev 13:23–34, 2009

Hu FB: Metabolic consequences of obesity, in Obesity Epidemiology. Edited by Hu FB. New York, Oxford University Press, 2008, pp 149–173

Jenkins JB, Omori T, Guan Z, et al: Sleep is increased in mice with obesity induced by high-fat food. Physiol Behav 87:255–262, 2006

Jørgensen EA, Knigge U, Warberg J, et al: Histamine and the regulation of body weight. Neuroendocrinology 86:210–214, 2007

Knipling R, Wang J: Crashes and fatalities related to driver drowsiness/fatigue. Research Note from the Office of Crash Avoidance Research. Washington, DC, National Highway Traffic Safety Administration, 1994, pp 1–8

Knutson KL, Van Cauter E: Associations between sleep loss and increased risk of obesity and diabetes. Ann N Y Acad Sci 1129:287–304, 2008

Knutson KL, Ryden AM, Mander BA, et al: Role of sleep duration and quality in the risk and severity of type 2 diabetes mellitus. Arch Intern Med 166:1768–1774, 2006

Knutson KL, Spiegel K, Penev P, et al: The metabolic consequences of sleep deprivation. Sleep Med Rev 11:163–178, 2007

Kohsaka A, Bass J: A sense of time: how molecular clocks organize metabolism. Trends Endocrinol Metab 18:4–11, 2007

Kohsaka A, Laposky AD, Ramsey KM, et al: High-fat diet disrupts behavioral and molecular circadian rhythms in mice. Cell Metab 6:414–421, 2007

Kolstad HA: Nightshift work and risk of breast cancer and other cancers—a critical review of the epidemiologic evidence. Scand J Work Environ Health 34:5–22, 2008

Kretschmer DB, Schelling P, Beier N, et al: Modulatory role of food, feeding regime and physical exercise on body weight and insulin resistance. Life Sci 76:1553–1573, 2005

Laposky AD, Bradley MA, Williams DL, et al: Sleep-wake regulation is altered in leptin-resistant (db/db) genetically obese and diabetic mice. Am J Physiol Regul Integr Comp Physiol 295:R2059–R2066, 2008

Leibowitz SF, Weiss GF, Walsh UA, et al: Medial hypothalamic serotonin: role in circadian patterns of feeding and macronutrient selection. Brain Res 503:132–140, 1989

Leidy HJ, Williams NI: Meal energy content is related to features of meal-related ghrelin profiles across a typical day of eating in non-obese premenopausal women. Horm Metab Res 38:317–322, 2006

Levi F, Schibler U: Circadian rhythms: mechanisms and therapeutic implications. Annu Rev Pharmacol Toxicol 47:593–628, 2007

Lundgren JD, Allison KC, Crow S, et al: Prevalence of the night eating syndrome in a psychiatric population. Am J Psychiatry 163:156–158, 2006

Marshall NS, Glozier N, Grunstein RR: Is sleep duration related to obesity? A critical review of the epidemiological evidence. Sleep Med Rev 12:289–298, 2008

Martin SL: Mammalian hibernation: a naturally reversible model for insulin resistance in man? Diab Vasc Dis Res 5:76–81, 2008

Masaki T, Yoshimatsu H: The hypothalamic H1 receptor: a novel therapeutic target for disrupting diurnal feeding rhythm and obesity. Trends Pharmacol Sci 27:279–284, 2006

Mendoza J: Circadian clocks: setting time by food. J Neuroendocrinol 19:127–137, 2007

Mendoza J, Angeles-Castellanos M, Escobar C: A daily palatable meal without food deprivation entrains the suprachiasmatic nucleus of rats. Eur J Neurosci 22:2855–2862, 2005

Miller BH, Olson SL, Turek FW, et al: Circadian clock mutation disrupts estrous cyclicity and maintenance of pregnancy. Curr Biol 14:1367–1373, 2004

Moore-Ede MC: Physiology of the circadian timing system: predictive versus reactive homeostasis. Am J Physiol 250 (5 pt 2):R737–R752, 1986

Napolitano MA, Head S, Babyak MA, et al: Binge eating disorder and night eating syndrome: psychological and behavioral characteristics. Int J Eat Disord 30:193–203, 2001

National Institute of Neurological Disorders and Stroke: Brain basics: understanding sleep. Bethesda, MD, National Institutes of Health. Updated May 2007. Available at: www.ninds. nih.gov/disorders/brain_basics/understanding_sleep.htm. Accessed September 30, 2009.

Neel JV: Diabetes mellitus: a "thrifty" genotype rendered detrimental by "progress"? Am J Hum Genet 14:353–362, 1962

Ohno K, Sakurai T: Orexin neuronal circuitry: role in the regulation of sleep and wakefulness. Front Neuroendocrinol 29:70–87, 2008

O'Reardon JP, Ringel BL, Dinges DF, et al: Circadian eating and sleeping patterns in the night eating syndrome. Obes Res 12:1789–1796, 2004

Pack AI, Gislason T: Obstructive sleep apnea and cardiovascular disease: a perspective and future directions. Prog Cardiovasc Dis 51:434–451, 2009

Parry BL, Meliska CJ, Sorenson DL, et al: Plasma melatonin circadian rhythm disturbances during pregnancy and postpartum in depressed women and women with personal or family histories of depression. Am J Psychiatry 165:1551–1558, 2008

Patel SR, Hu FB: Short sleep duration and weight gain: a systematic review. Obesity (Silver Spring) 16:643–653, 2008a

Patel SR, Hu FB: Sleep deprivation and obesity, in Obesity Epidemiology. Edited by Hu FB. New York, Oxford University Press, 2008b, pp 320–341

Patel SR, Malhotra A, White DP, et al: Association between reduced sleep and weight gain in women. Am J Epidemiol 164:947–954, 2006

Patel SR, Blackwell T, Redline S, et al; Osteoporotic Fractures in Men Research Group; Study of Osteoporotic Fractures Research Group: The association between sleep duration and obesity in older adults. Int J Obes (Lond) 32:1825–1834, 2008

Perfetto F, Tarquini R, Cornélissen G, et al: Circadian phase difference of leptin in android versus gynoid obesity. Peptides 25:1297–1306, 2004

Plante DT, Winkelman JW: Sleep disturbance in bipolar disorder: therapeutic implications. Am J Psychiatry 165:830–843, 2008

Prasai MJ, George JT, Scott EM: Molecular clocks, type 2 diabetes and cardiovascular disease. Diab Vasc Dis Res 5:89–95, 2008

Precope J: Hippocrates on Diet and Hygiene. London, Zeno, 1952

Ramsey KM, Marcheva B, Kohsaka A, et al: The clockwork of metabolism. Annu Rev Nutr 27:219–240, 2007

Rana JS, Mukamal KJ, Morgan JP, et al: Circadian variation in the onset of myocardial infarction: effect of duration of diabetes. Diabetes 52:1464–1468, 2003

Rand CS, Macgregor AM, Stunkard AJ: The night eating syndrome in the general population and among postoperative obesity surgery patients. Int J Eat Disord 22:65–69, 1997

Reite M, Weissberg M, Ruddy J: Clinical Manual for Evaluation and Treatment of Sleep Disorders. Washington, DC, American Psychiatric Publishing, 2009

Roenneberg T, Wirz-Justice A, Merrow M: Life between clocks: daily temporal patterns of human chronotypes. J Biol Rhythms 18:80–90, 2003

Sack RL: The pathophysiology of jet lag. Travel Med Infect Dis 7:102–110, 2009

Sack RL, Auckley D, Auger RR, et al; American Academy of Sleep Medicine: Circadian rhythm sleep disorders, part I: basic principles, shift work and jet lag disorders. Sleep 30:1460–1483, 2007

Sakurai T: Roles of orexins and orexin receptors in central regulation of feeding behavior and energy homeostasis. CNS Neurol Disord Drug Targets 5:313–325, 2006

ScienceDaily: Sleep deprivation doubles risks of obesity in both children and adults. July 13, 2006. Available at: http://www.sciencedaily.com/releases/2006/07/060713081140.htm. Accessed March 17, 2009.

Scott EM, Grant PJ: Neel revisited: the adipocyte, seasonality and type 2 diabetes. Diabetologia 49:1462–1466, 2006

Sleipness EP, Sorg BA, Jansen HT: Contribution of the suprachiasmatic nucleus to day:night variation in cocaine-seeking behavior. Physiol Behav 91:523–530, 2007

Spiegel K, Knutson K, Leproult R, et al: Sleep loss: a novel risk factor for insulin resistance and type 2 diabetes. J Appl Physiol 99:2008–2019, 2005

Stephan FK, Davidson AJ: Glucose, but not fat, phase shifts the feeding-entrained circadian clock. Physiol Behav 65:277–288, 1998

Strollo PJ Jr, Rogers RM: Obstructive sleep apnea. N Engl J Med 334:99–104, 1996

Strubbe JH, Woods SC: The timing of meals. Psychol Rev 111:128–141, 2004

Stunkard AJ, Grace WJ, Wolff HG: The night-eating syndrome; a pattern of food intake among certain obese patients. Am J Med 19:78–86, 1955

Stunkard AJ, Allison KC, O'Reardon JP: The night eating syndrome: a progress report. Appetite 45:182–186, 2005

Stunkard AJ, Allison KC, Lundgren JD, et al: A paradigm for facilitating pharmacotherapy at a distance: sertraline treatment of the night eating syndrome. J Clin Psychiatry 67:1568–1572, 2006

Stunkard A, Allison K, Lundgren J: Issues for DSM-V: night eating syndrome (editorial). Am J Psychiatry 165:424, 2008

Subramanian S, Strohl KP: Obesity and pulmonary function, in Handbook of Obesity: Etiology and Pathophysiology, 2nd Edition. Edited by Bray GA, Bouchard C. New York, Marcel Dekker, 2004, pp 935–952

Szentirmai E, Hajdu I, Obal F Jr, et al: Ghrelin-induced sleep responses in ad libitum fed and food-restricted rats. Brain Res 1088:131–140, 2006

Tanofsky-Kraff M, Yanovski SZ: Eating disorder or disordered eating? Non-normative eating patterns in obese individuals. Obes Res 12:1361–1366, 2004

Tasali E, Leproult R, Ehrmann DA, et al: Slow-wave sleep and the risk of type 2 diabetes in humans. Proc Natl Acad Sci U S A 105:1044–1049, 2008

Trento M, Broglio F, Riganti F, et al: Sleep abnormalities in type 2 diabetes may be associated with glycemic control. Acta Diabetol 45:225–229, 2008

Van Cauter E, Holmback U, Knutson K, et al: Impact of sleep and sleep loss on neuroendocrine and metabolic function. Horm Res 67 (suppl 1):2–9, 2007

Vgontzas AN: Does obesity play a major role in the pathogenesis of sleep apnoea and its associated manifestations via inflammation, visceral adiposity, and insulin resistance? Arch Physiol Biochem 114:211–223, 2008

Vgontzas AN, Bixler EO, Chrousos GP, et al: Obesity and sleep disturbances: meaningful sub-typing of obesity. Arch Physiol Biochem 114:224–236, 2008

Wadden TA, Phelan S: Behavioral assessment of the obese patient, in Handbook of Obesity Treatment. Edited by Wadden TA, Stunkard AJ. New York, Guilford, 2002, pp 186–226

Warren MW, Gold MS: The relationship between obesity and drug use (letter). Am J Psychiatry 164:1268 [reply: 1268–1269], 2007

Weikel JC, Wichniak A, Ising M, et al: Ghrelin promotes slow-wave sleep in humans. Am J Physiol Endocrinol Metab 284:E407–E415, 2003

Wirz-Justice A: Chronobiology and psychiatry. Sleep Med Rev 11:423–427, 2007

Wittmann M, Dinich J, Merrow M, et al: Social jetlag: misalignment of biological and social time. Chronobiol Int 23:497–509, 2006

World Health Organization: Obesity and overweight. Fact sheet #311. September 2006. Available at: http://www.who.int/mediacentre/factsheets/fs311/en/index.html. Accessed November 3, 2009.

Yang S, Liu A, Weidenhammer A, et al: The role of mPer2 clock gene in glucocorticoid and feeding rhythms. Endocrinology 150:2153–2160, 2009

Yannielli PC, Molyneux PC, Harrington ME, et al: Ghrelin effects on the circadian system of mice. J Neurosci 27:2890–2895, 2007

Yoshimatsu H: Hypothalamic neuronal histamine regulates body weight through the modulation of diurnal feeding rhythm. Nutrition 24:827–831, 2008

Zee PC, Manthena P: The brain's master circadian clock: implications and opportunities for therapy of sleep disorders. Sleep Med Rev 11:59–70, 2007

Zvonic S, Ptitsyn AA, Conrad SA, et al: Characterization of peripheral circadian clocks in adipose tissues. Diabetes 55:962–970, 2006

Zvonic S, Floyd ZE, Mynatt RL, et al: Circadian rhythms and the regulation of metabolic tissue function and energy homeostasis. Obesity (Silver Spring) 15:539–543, 2007

10

DIET AND WEIGHT

*Cues to foods that are high in sugar, fat, and salt create emotional tension—
a psychic itch, if you will—and eating becomes a strategy for
easing the stimulus-induced tension.*

David A. Kessler, *The End of Overeating* (2009, pp. 198–199)

GENERAL PRINCIPLES OF DIET

Dieting Within Our Environment

Back in the late 1970s, Hirsch (1978, p. 2) suggested that the current dietary regimens to which we subject our obese patients are "the modern-day equivalent of beating the insane to keep them quiet." In other words, the dietary regimens then available did not work very well and were perhaps even overtly cruel, and if they did work, the results were short-lived and hardly curative. Unfortunately, more than 30 years later, we have not come much farther.

First of all, as we have emphasized, weight loss and maintenance are about much more than diet. As Newbold et al. (2007) succinctly put it, "The exact etiology of obesity remains uncertain." As a result, it has to be approached from a multidimensional perspective—including genetic, evolutionary, physiological, psychological and behavioral, environmental, and possibly even infectious (most recently referred to as *infectobesity;* Ifland et al. 2009) perspectives—of which diet is only one element.

A recent environmental theory is that prenatal or childhood exposure to toxic synthetic chemicals is potentially *obesogenic* and may be one of the factors involved in the recent increase of the rates of obesity seen in children, as described below (Newbold et al. 2007; Trasande et al. 2009). These toxic environmental compounds—which have been called *endocrine disruptors* because they may adversely interfere with our complex endocrinological systems—include drugs given years ago to pregnant women to prevent miscarriage (e.g., diethylstilbestrol); bisphenol A, used currently in the manufacture of plastic food and beverage containers; and phthalates,

335

used to manufacture items like shampoos, cosmetics, and nail polish). There is some suggestion that such compounds are found in higher percentages in the urine of obese children (Newbold et al. 2007; Trasande et al. 2009). Suggested environmental factors affecting children are of particular concern given the increase in childhood obesity rates. According to statistics from the World Health Organization (WHO; 2006), at least 20 million children under the age of 5 were overweight worldwide in 2005, as determined by new WHO Child Growth Standards. Ogden et al. (2006) reported that between 1980 and 2002, overweight prevalence in children and adolescents ages 6–19 years had tripled. And "the heaviest children have been getting heavier" (Ogden et al. 2008). Almost 32% of children and adolescents had a body mass index (BMI) value "at or above the 85th percentile" for the years 2003–2006 (Ogden et al. 2008).

Despite the fact that researchers continue to offer novel speculations regarding the etiology of obesity, we would be remiss if our comprehensive approach to obesity did not include a study of the role of diet—exactly what and how much we choose to eat—in weight control and maintenance. After all, "a negative energy balance is the most important factor affecting weight loss amount and rate" (Seagle et al. 2009). A negative energy balance can be achieved, of course, through a decrease in calories, an increase in exercise, or, most effectively, a combination of both diet and exercise. In this chapter we focus on diet. Diet can involve a restriction of calories generally and/or a prescription to eat or avoid certain food groups (protein, fat, or carbohydrates in various combinations).

Years ago, Mireille Guiliano came out with a book that became an extremely popular bestseller. With the captivating title *French Women Don't Get Fat* (Guiliano 2004), she sought to give advice on a way of life based on French culture. Apparently French women can eat anything, including typically fattening French meals, wine, and pastries, but in very small quantities, and French women walk everywhere. That is their secret to why they don't become fat. Of course, genetics plays a major role (see "Genetics and Obesity" in Chapter 2, "Obesity in the United States"), and the fact that French women also tend to smoke may, unfortunately, be another part of the equation. Nevertheless, moderation and portion control can have significant impact on whatever diet you choose, as we and many others have emphasized (e.g., Hill 2009; Wansink 2006). For example, Hill (2009) suggests the *small change approach*, with the notion that small changes in lifestyle are "more feasible to achieve and maintain" over time than much larger changes. Hill applauds the food industry's addressing package size by creating snacks in 100-calorie packages, and he recommends taking an extra 2,000 steps a day that would burn off about 100 calories a day—the "energy gap" between intake and expenditure that fosters a potential yearly weight gain. It is that small upward creep in weight day after day that causes most people to become overweight. And it is the opposite of the typical American idea that bigger is better, portrayed so well in *Super Size Me*, Morgan Spurlock's scathing 2004 film about the fast-food industry.

Wansink and Van Ittersum (2007) have coined the term *portion distortion* to refer to our tendency to think that fast food jumbo-sized portions, which may actually be 250% larger than a regular portion, are actual serving sizes. No one is immune to this: "When it comes to biasing how much food a person eats, portion size is no respecter of person, position, or profession," and most studies over the years "have shown that portion size influences people of all weights," not just those who are obese (Wansink and Van Ittersum 2007). And these researchers note that portion distortion has no regard for a person's state of hunger—they report on a study in which even after people had finished their lunch, they ate 51% more *stale* popcorn from large containers than medium ones. Wansink and Van Ittersum (2007) speculate that because the amount we can eat is flexible, all of us can be influenced by consumption norms—what we think is "appropriate, typical, reasonable, and normal to serve." And the large portions in restaurants and large boxes in supermarkets influence these norms; we tend to get confused and pay less attention to how much we are eating with such large portions. The all-you-can-eat buffet is an example of how easily we can lose track of consumption monitoring, especially when our dirty plates are gone each time we return to the table after another trip to the buffet (see "The Psychology of Temptation and Self-Control" in Chapter 4, "The Psychology of the Eater"; see also Wansink 2006, pp. 37–40).

In regard to the effect of increased portions, Bogusky (2008) has written a book, mostly in pictures, that is a visual tour de force in demonstrating exactly how significant these increased servings can become. Bogusky, an advertising executive, explains that he had no intention of writing a diet book but became fascinated with the notion of dieting when he and his wife purchased a 60-year-old house by the lake in which his modern-day dishes did not fit in the house's original kitchen cabinets (2008, pp. 12–13). And so the 9-inch "Diet" was born. In fact, not only had plate sizes changed over the years (from under 9 inches to an average of 12 inches or more now), but so had just about everything else, including the portion size of French fries, sodas, bagels, muffins, et cetera. Bogusky explains, in the language of advertising, this is "value marketing," or the fact that it costs the seller just "pennies" more to increase the size of a portion sold (p. 37). Notice, in fact, that in most restaurants now we are eating off plates that years ago would have been serving-sized plates for an entire table. And Bogusky (p. 94) tells of how Americans, so used to super-sizes, thought they were buying "normal" drinking glasses when they were actually purchasing flower vases from the Swedish company Ikea!

One of the major difficulties with maintaining a diet is the culture and environment in which we live. For most people in the United States, there is just too much inexpensive and relatively tasty food available. And Rodin (1978) makes the point that obese people may be more sensitive and responsive to external environmental food stimuli—sights and smells and tastes of food—than slimmer people, who eat when they are hungry. This is the concept of *cognitive salience*. Barkeling et al. (2003), in investigating the impact of vision on eating, found, for example, that obese people when they were blindfolded during eating ate considerably less food (24% less) and ate more slowly. Two of the subjects were quoted as saying that actually seeing food increased their appetites. But in general, people of all weight categories can be tempted by (and highly responsive to) these cues, says Rodin. Says David Kessler, former commissioner of the U.S. Food and Drug Administration, "Once you begin to debate 'Should I or shouldn't I?' you've lost the battle" (Kessler 2009, p. 221).

Furthermore, a pattern involving both scarcity and unpredictability is more likely to lead to increased dependence on external eating cues and can lead to "hungry eyes" in both humans and animals (Rodin 1978, p. 585). The notion "your eyes are bigger than your stomach" expresses the same idea. As Hill et al. (2003) explain, "Our biology, which evolved in times of frequent famine, is now essentially maladaptive in our environment of food abundance and sedentariness." Kessler also acknowledges the genetic predisposition that has evolved over time in humans and animals, but it is our "conducive environment" today that creates and specifically triggers what he labels our pattern of "hypereating" (Kessler 2009, p. 168).

Another factor is that we do not always have fresh foods available as often as we like, and sometimes not at all. We are no longer an agrarian society. And our foods themselves contain chemicals. Eric Schlosser, in his book *Fast Food Nation* (2005, pp. 124–127), vividly describes how unnatural our so-called natural flavors can be: "The distinction between artificial and natural can be somewhat arbitrary and absurd, based more on how the flavor has been made than on what it actually contains.... Natural and artificial flavors sometimes contain exactly the same chemicals, produced through different methods" (p. 126). In other words, the word *natural* on a label does not ensure that it is healthier and, in fact, so-called natural products are sometimes produced in the same manufacturing plants as artificial products. Adds Schlosser, "Calling any of these flavors 'natural' requires a flexible attitude toward the English language and a fair amount of irony" (p. 127).

Furthermore, many people get their meals eating out, where calories, let alone grams of fat, carbohydrates, and protein, are not posted, unless the restaurant belongs to a chain that is now required to post nutritional ingredients and calorie counts. As noted in Chapter 7 ("Medical Conditions and Weight"), Currie et al. (2009) found, in a large sample of 3 million school children and 1 million pregnant women, the proximity to a fast food restaurant increased the risk of obesity rates—for ninth graders, for example, when a school was within 0.1 mile of a fast food restaurant there was a 5.2% increase in obesity rates, and when a pregnant woman was within 0.5 mile of one, she had a 2.5% greater chance of gaining more than 40 pounds during her pregnancy. And eating at home is not easier. Says *New York Times* columnist Frank Rich (2009): "What are Americans still buying? Big Macs, Campbell's soup, Hershey's chocolate, and Spam—the four food groups of the apocalypse." Said comedian Jon Stewart, in interviewing Robert Kenner, the director of the film *Food, Inc.*, on his *The Daily Show With Jon Stewart*: "Salt, sugar, fat—aren't they the three basic food groups? I haven't seen the [food] pyramid in a long time" (July 2, 2009). And if we have ever tried to add up the number of grams of food from each food group that we consume in a day, we know how daunting the process is, even if we are sufficiently motivated and have all the information available to us. Even converting to grams from other measurements like ounces or number of pieces of food can be overwhelming.

Wansink and Chandon (2006) also suggest that "low-fat" nutrition labels may encourage some people to overeat and can lead to "overconsumption of nutrient-poor and calorie-rich foods." Furthermore, such labels tend to "reduce anticipated consumption guilt." In fact, many packages describe their product as guilt-free (e.g., baked potato chips) despite the fact they still have many calories, though fewer than the full-fat product. Wansink and Chandon (2006) found experimentally that people do tend to have less guilt when eating these products and do tend to read-just upward their sense of what is an appropriate portion size, whether they are eating candy or granola, when the term *low-fat* appears on the label. And as they point out, people tend to think being low in fat is equivalent to having substantially fewer calories, even when the actual calorie count is not so very different and the fat is sometimes replaced with products that "tend to make people hungrier," such as fat-free cookies loaded with sugar. These researchers call this the "health halo effect." Just labeling the candy M&M's as "low-fat" (even though no such version is marketed) led people to eat 28% more—and those who were obese ate 47% more. Mostly, though, those without a weight problem tended to eat more of so-called healthy products with low-fat labeling, whereas obese people tended to eat more of *all* products with a low-fat label.

The Science of Calorie Counting

An important part of dieting, though, is accountability, as we have noted. Techniques like daily weighing and keeping a food journal of everything one eats, or reporting in to a nutritionist or even to a friend or spouse on a regular basis, can all be of assistance in weight maintenance. But all of that is work and requires considerable memory as well as discipline, and unfortunately, we all have a tendency to underestimate just how much we eat. See Chapter 2, "Obesity in the United States," on the "eye-mouth gap" (Tataranni and Ravussin 2002, pp. 48-49).

Furthermore, calorie counting is often more complicated than it first appears. Buchholz and Schoeller (2004) acknowledge that "a calorie is just a calorie" thermodynamically because "the human body cannot create or destroy energy but can only convert energy from one form to another." But they also note that the human body is "not a perfect engine." In other words, there is actually a slight difference between "the gross energy . . . of consumed food (called 'metabolizable energy') and the energy contained in feces and urine." So when we say that there are 4 calories per gram for either protein or carbohydrates and 9 calories per gram for fat, we are actually giving average values, with slight differences depending on the specific food itself. Perhaps we can paraphrase a famous saying as "All carbohydrates are equal, but some are more equal than others." This is particularly true with dietary fiber, a carbohydrate that is broken down by gut flora. Transit time in the gut, as well as the actual number of gut flora in the bowel, can all affect just how many calories can be extracted from fiber at any one time. The point is that daily calorie counting, outside a laboratory, and particularly when the typical diet has different classes of foods, is hardly an exact science. Grossly, though, as we have said previously, we have to eliminate 3,500 calories from our diet per week just to lose only 1 pound (see "Factors Involved in Daily Energy Requirements" in Chapter 3, "Food: The Basic Principles of Calories").

Just how many calories a person needs per day varies widely. That number depends not only on body frame size, which is by custom determined by wrist size and height, but also on activity level—not just exercise, but all activity—from very light (e.g., sitting) to heavy (e.g., digging ditches). (See Chapter 8, "Exercise," for more discussion of activity levels.) The number of calories needed per day is also based on gender. Ancel Keys , in an article from the late 1940s, believed the term *nutritional requirement* had "no clear and constant meaning" despite its popular use (Keys 1949). To the list already noted (e.g., basal metabolism, size of the person, occupation, and general activity level), Keys added the importance of considering climate, gender, and age. He said that typically in colder climates, for example, our basal metabolism elevates "in a significant" though "small" way compared to levels in warmer climates and would affect how many calories we require. He noted too that women typically need fewer calories than men and that we tend to need fewer calories as we age.

In their book *The New Living Heart Diet*, DeBakey et al. (1996) use tables adapted from the 1959 Metropolitan Life Insurance Company charts (and not later versions of the Metropolitan Life charts, which allowed for heavier and less healthy weights) to calculate the number of calories appropriate for a healthy regimen. For example, a medium-framed, moderately active man who is 6 feet tall and whose healthy weight is between 158 and 175 pounds is able to eat 2,850 calories a day and maintain his weight; that same man, though, engaged in only light activity could eat only 2,500 calories a day without putting on weight. A medium-framed, moderately active woman who is 5 feet 5 inches tall and whose healthy weight is between 124 and 139 pounds can eat 2,250 calories a day and maintain her weight. That same woman engaged in light activity should eat only 1,950 calories a day in order to maintain her weight. Those calorie counts may not seem very different, but as we have repeatedly said, and as has been noted especially by Wansink (2006, p. 31), relatively small differences in calorie counts can make a substantial difference over the course of a year. Furthermore, because activity level is often difficult to measure accurately, figuring out exactly how many calories we need can be more challenging than it seems. The tables provided by DeBakey et al. (1996, pp. 357–359), though, are helpful guidelines.

The Regimen of Diet

The word *diet* comes through the ʀomance languages of Spanish, Portuguese, Italian, and French from the ancient Greek word meaning "mode of life" and even possibly from the Greek word for "to live" (Oxford English Dictionary 1989). Hippocrates wrote four books on the subject, translated into English as *Regimen* (Hippocrates 1967), from which we have quoted throughout this book, including some of the specifics of what to eat, the importance of moderation in food intake, and the importance of exercise as a means of maintaining one's health. Chaucer was probably the first to use our word *diet* ("diete") to mean a prescribed and restricted course of food intake (Oxford English Dictionary 1989).

The history of diets is really the history of medicine and is beyond our scope here. For those interested, Bray (2004, pp. 1–31) gives an overview, including early work on metabolism and the physiology of the human body and diets of the early twentieth century. Suffice it to say that almost everything has been tried over the years, and certainly, many readers will have found by personal experiment that many diets, at least initially, can lead to weight loss. Weight maintenance, as we have noted, is another matter (e.g., see Chapter 2, "Obesity in the United States," and Chapter 5, "The Metabolic Complexities of Weight Control"). Brownell et al. (1986) speak of a *safe point* in the course of dieting. This is the time before a person tends to relapse and "beyond which relapse is unlikely." They acknowledge that, at least anecdotally, those who tend to struggle early with adhering to a diet are more likely to succeed in the long run. These dieters have learned to deal with the inevitable slips that occur when dieting whereas those who are "perfect adherers" are less immune and more likely to have that self-destructive all-or-none attitude. Van Itallie (1978) makes the point that successful dietary adherence involves not only motivation and a knowledge of calorie counts, but also "endurance, persistence, and the capacity to endure frustration and discouragement"—all qualities of cognitive self-regulation, as we have noted earlier. (For more on self-regulation, see Chapter 4, "The Psychology of the Eater").

> Reduced-calorie diets result in weight loss, regardless of the nature of the diet.

Over the years, some researchers have told us that calories do matter, then that they don't matter, and now, most recently, that they actually do matter. For example, almost all diets, regardless of their nutrient composition, can help people lose weight as long as they reduce calories. A recent randomized, prospective study of over 800 overweight or obese men and women (Sacks et al. 2009) compared four diets of varying fat, protein, and carbohydrate compositions over the course of 2 years. Two of the diets were low in fat and two were high in fat; two of them were average in protein content, whereas two were high in protein. Subjects were offered group and individual instructional sessions. The researchers also encouraged the participants to engage in moderate exercise, but only 90 minutes per week (lower than what most researchers in weight maintenance would recommend; see Chapter 8, "Exercise"). What they found was that subjects in all the dietary groups had similar responses to the diets in terms of feelings of satiety, hunger, and even "satisfaction with the diet," and similar attendance in group instructional sessions. Most importantly, Sacks et al. (2009) found that "reduced-calorie diets result in clinically meaningful weight loss regardless of which macronutrients they emphasize." What these researchers also found, though, was that in the first 6 months, subjects in each group lost about 6 kilograms (~13 pounds), but by 1 year, they began to gain the weight back. On average, weight loss among the 80% who completed the study was only 4 kilograms (~9 pounds). And at most, only 15% of participants lost 10% or more of their initial weight.

Nevertheless, the researchers found that all the diets were able to reduce the risk factors for both diabetes and cardiovascular disease (e.g., cholesterol levels, triglyceride levels, blood pressure, and fasting insulin levels), and they concluded that any diet, "when taught for the purpose of weight loss with enthusiasm and persistence, can be effective." So despite the facts that diet is only one component of weight control and maintenance and both enthusiasm and persistence often wane over time for many people, we suggest that it is worthwhile to understand some of the principles behind dietary practice. After all, according to statistics from Esposito and Giugliano, in 2005 more than 54 million Americans were dieting.

Because there are so many books supporting one diet or another, diet books often have inventive, clever, attention-getting titles—such as Guiliano's *French Women Don't Get Fat*, or *Did You Ever See a Fat Squirrel?* (Adams 1972), *The New Living Heart Diet* (DeBakey et al. 1996), *Beyond a Shadow of a Diet* (Matz and Frankel 2004), *Thin Tastes Better* (Gullo 1995), *The Thin Commandments* (Gullo 2005), *The 9-Inch "Diet"* (Bogusky 2008), and *The Skinny* (Aronne 2009)—or have a place name in the title, such as *The South Beach Diet* (Agatston 2003), *The Complete Scarsdale Medical Diet* (Tarnower and Baker 1982), or *The New Beverly Hills Diet* (Mazel et al. 1996). After all, who wouldn't want to be associated with South Beach, Scarsdale, or Beverly Hills?

Judith Beck's new book *The Complete Diet for Life* (Beck 2008) is essentially a diet treatment manual and will be discussed in Chapter 11, "Psychological Treatment Strategies and Weight." In addition to cognitive treatment approaches for weight loss and maintenance, her book, though, contains information on calorie-conscious portion control, menus, and even recipes.

The point of this chapter, though, is that one diet, just like one size, could not possibly work for everyone. We hope we have made it clear that our internal physiological milieus and external environments are different for us all. In other words, we all have our own unique genetics, circadian rhythms, metabolic complexities, and psychological makeups with unique reward pathways in our brains, defense structures in our minds, and different abilities to resist temptation—all in the context of a complex, overwhelming, and sometimes even toxic environment. And the diet industry does not help. Says Naomi Wolf (1992, p. 102), "The 'supportive' rhetoric of the diet industry masks the obvious: The last thing it wants is for women to get thin once and for all."

Another point is that the word *diet* is not just a noun but also a verb, by which we mean it is an action word. To diet is to engage in an active, lifetime process. The Greeks, and particularly Hippocrates, had it correct: If people want

> "The last thing [the diet industry] wants is for women to get thin once and for all."
>
> **Source: Wolf 1992, p. 102**

to lose weight and maintain a loss over time, even as they age and their metabolism slows, they have to think of diet as a *mode of life*—a *regimen*—that incorporates moderate to vigorous daily exercise. As Hippocrates stated, "Excess or deficiency in food or exercise, however small the disproportion on either side, will ultimately lead to disease" (Precope 1952, p. 32), and "Eat less, exercise more" (Precope 1952, p. 90).

Michael Pollan (2008), in his book *In Defense of Food: An Eater's Manifesto*, speaks of our confusing Western ideology of "nutritionalism," as we have mentioned (see Chapter 3, "Food: The Basic Principles of Calories"), that is, our preoccupation with nutrition as a science rather than with food itself. Pollan believes that food has become a delivery system for nutrients, rather than something to eat. His advice is to eat "real" food, that is, "mostly plants and not too much" (Pollan 2008, p. 1)— and avoid those center lanes in the supermarket with all our modern, packaged, processed so-called food. He says, "When corn oil and chips and sugary breakfast cereals can all boast being good for your heart, health claims have become hopelessly corrupt" (p. 156). Hippocrates gave the same advice in the middle 400s B.C., namely, "Fresh foods in all cases give more strength than others, just because they are nearer to the living creature" (Hippocrates 1967, p. 343).

EARLY RESEARCH

Clara Davis

The self-selected diet experiment. In the late 1920s, researcher and pediatrician Clara Davis studied initially three infants (Davis 1928) and ultimately a group of 15 infants, all "newly weaned" and younger than 1 year old, for a period of up to 6 years to assess what foods the infants would *choose* to eat over time, as well as how their nutritional status fared (Davis 1939). Davis (1928) initially had been particularly concerned with the digestive troubles and nutritional status of infants "who after weaning are set up at the family table and allowed to eat the pastries, preserves, gravies, white bread, sugar, and canned foods that are commonly found there."

Instead, Davis allowed her group of infants to self-select from a group of foods she provided for them: "Food was not offered to the infant either directly or by suggestion" (Davis 1939). Her food choices contained all natural, fresh foods—no canned goods—and no salt, sugar, cream, butter, or cheese was on her list. What the list did include were foods like fresh fruits, vegetables, fish, and chicken, but also unusual foods including bone marrow, sweetbreads, brains, and liver. She found over time they all chose a balanced diet, even though each of the 15 diets was somewhat different and definite tastes developed. Specific tastes "were developed by sampling, which is essentially a trial and error method." She also found that "there was a tendency in all the infants to eat certain foods in waves," that is, eating larger and larger quantities of a certain food or food group followed by a decline in that particular choice. Members of Davis's kitchen staff called this *egg jags* or *meat jags*, for example. (Today we might call this *sensory-specific satiety*, as mentioned in Chapter 4.) Furthermore, Davis's group of infants was without constipation and had no serious illnesses for the entire 6 years of the study; she found "after the first six months' period...no noticeably fat or thin children, but a greater uniformity than often obtains among those of the same family."

Davis was quite ahead of her time for noting that both sugar and white flour brought with them "a train of nutritional evils" (Davis 1939). She raised a question that is particularly relevant now, 80 years later, in our fast-food world: "Whether the evils are due to innate fallibilities of appetite with respect to these products, or whether appetite in such cases is merely overruled by extraneous considerations of novelty, cheapness, ease of procurement, and preparation, etc., has not been determined." It is still not clear whether we can, all these years later, answer the question she raised. Her contention was that "natural, unprocessed, and unpurified foods" such as those eaten by "primitive peoples" provide "scientifically sound diets and excellent nutrition." Davis would be turning over in her grave now if she knew how much those evils have permeated the diets of most Americans, and particularly our children.

The study would hardly pass ethical research protocols today inasmuch as these were institutionalized infants, and her writings do not discuss what happened to the mothers. Davis (1939) did note that several infants had the bone disease rickets, and others were poorly nourished or undernourished on admission. But this study has often been quoted in the literature to show that if left to our own devices, we would all choose balanced diets. After all, even babies could do so. But these infants and children were given a specific array of foods—"the 'trick' in the experiment...was in the food list" (Davis 1939)—from which to choose. There was not a candy bar or cookie or pretzel among the choices. When these tempting choices are neither known nor available, children have to choose among healthy choices. If, however, the typical sweets are available, healthy foods often do not stand a chance among most adults, let alone among children. Greg Critser says, in his book *Fat Land* (2003, p. 42), "A perpetually snacking child is...literally a walking, talking, fat-making machine."

Ancel Keys

The history of man is in large part the chronicle of his quest for food.

Ancel Keys et al., *The Biology of Human Starvation* (1950, p. 3)

The Minnesota semistarvation experiment. In the mid 1940s, in the middle of World War II, when there were reports of starvation in Europe, physiology researcher Ancel Keys asked for volunteers among wartime conscientious objectors for an experiment on the physical and psychological effects of severe food restriction. Keys advertised for study subjects in a brochure titled "Will You Starve That They Be Better Fed?" (Kalm and Semba 2005). Of the 100 men he interviewed, he chose 36 physically and mentally healthy applicants (ages 20–33 years) for his 6-month, continuous-residence, semistarvation experiment. The results of his research were published in an enormous two-volume treatise, *The Biology of Human Starvation* (Keys et al. 1950), and the project came to be known as the Minnesota semistarvation experiment. Over the course of the experiment, the men were to lose 25% of their body weight (daily calories were adjusted accordingly) and then undergo a 3-month period of refeeding rehabilitation. In general, the average calorie intake daily was about 1,570 calories, with 50 grams of protein and 30 grams of fat. The diet was designed to simulate the diet of the famine areas in Europe, with only "token amounts of meats and dairy [products]" (Keys et al. 1950, p. 74). The men were also expected to engage in about 22 miles of walking each week.

Apparently, humans can tolerate a weight loss of about 5%–10% of their body weight "with relatively little functional disorganization" (Keys et al. 1950, p. 18). But when weight loss approaches 35%–40% of body weight, most people cannot survive. A severe famine might result in weight losses of 15%–35% of body weight (Keys et al. 1950, p. 18). Keys et al. distinguished the process of total starvation (or fasting) from a prolonged phase of calorie deficiency: significantly, when a person is not eating any food, Keys found, hunger feelings dissipate within a few days; with prolonged undernutrition, hunger sensations are "progressively accentuated." But in both conditions, humans have a lowered heart rate and a lowered metabolism (p. 29). People do experience edema in semistarvation; Keys, though, made the point that patients with anorexia nervosa tend not to have edema because they often have a very low intake of water and other liquids, and thus are more likely to be dehydrated than nonanorexic individuals (p. 101).

> Humans can tolerate a weight loss of up to 10% of their weight without the functional disorganization that starvation causes.

Of course, Keys was well aware that the conditions for his men hardly reflected war-torn Europe: the men in his experiment were under no physical threat; they had comfortable living conditions, adequate warm clothing, and nothing to fear. They could still attend university classes and they knew that they would always be served meals. As one participant later said, "We were starving under the best possible medical conditions. And most of all, we knew the exact day on which our torture was going to end" (Kalm and Semba 2005).

During the 6 months of semistarvation, Keys' subjects developed "striking changes" physically and mentally. They had a gradual wasting of muscle and subcutaneous fat, and showed "marked emaciation" in their faces and bodies. They developed muscle pains and soreness and felt cold much of the time. Furthermore, they became irritable, felt weak and tired, and lost all libido (Keys et al. 1950, pp. 827–828). They became totally preoccupied with food (not unlike patients seen clinically with anorexia nervosa) and were interested in recipes and cookbooks (p. 833). Said Keys, "The Minnesota subjects were often caught between conflicting desires to gulp their food down ravenously and to consume it slowly so the taste and odor of each morsel would be fully appreciated. Toward the end of the starvation period, some men would dawdle for almost two hours over a meal" that would previously have been eaten in a few minutes (p. 833).

Emotionally, the men developed instability, with periods of depression, social withdrawal, temper outbursts, and inability to concentrate. And their personal appearance began to deteriorate over time: they stopped shaving, brushing their teeth, or combing their hair, though they did continue to bathe (Keys et al. 1950, pp. 835–836). Said Keys, "Perhaps the outstanding feature in both famine and the Minnesota Experiment is depression and apathy" (p. 907). Keys even called the syndrome a *semistarvation neurosis* (p. 908).

Psychological and physical rehabilitation, including refeeding, lasted 3 months, after which the subjects were still "not back to normal." Apparently, the rehabilitation period was extremely difficult and for some was the most difficult part of the experiment (Kalm and Semba 2005). Kalm and Semba interviewed 18 of the men from the experiment who were alive 60 years later. These men remained passionate about being conscientious objectors. Some of the men looked back on the experience as being "one of the most important and memorable activities in their lives," and most seemed to feel glad they had participated.

Dulloo et al. (1997) revisited Keys' original data to investigate why Keys' subjects in the refeeding, rehabilitation stage had such an enormous pattern of food ingestion—some eating thousands of additional calories a day—a "poststarvation hyperphagia." They found that contrary to common belief that this hyperphagia is related exclusively to the amount of fat depletion from the semistarvation phase, rather, it is related as well to the body's attempts to recover the loss of lean body tissue that had occurred simultaneously when fat mass was depleted. Dulloo et al. (1997) found that fat mass is recovered at a faster rate than lean body tissue such that the poststarvation hyperphagia will continue until there is replacement of both fat and lean body mass. In fact, there is often an "overshooting" of fat mass (i.e., people

---

PSYCHOLOGICAL EFFECTS OF A SEMISTARVATION DIET

- In 6 months of semistarvation, volunteers (men) lost about 2.5 pounds a week by limiting protein and total calorie intake and walking 22 miles a week.

- As they lost up to 25% of their initial weight, they became increasingly irritable, weak, dizzy, tired, and less tolerant to cold, with hair loss, reduced coordination, muscle soreness, and no interest in sex.

- Food became a major preoccupation and even an obsession.

- During the rehabilitation phase, some needed about 4,000 calories a day and still did not get relief from their hunger.

Source: Kalm and Semba 2005

---

gain more weight than they had been originally) before the body can recover its lost lean tissue. This study may have clinical implications in our understanding of why some people tend to regain more weight (above their pre-diet weight) after a loss of weight, and why exercise (to preserve lean body tissue) becomes so important in the weight maintenance phase.

Keys's work established some of the basic ground rules for refeeding people after starvation. Palesty and Dudrick (2006) speak of the importance of the *Goldilocks paradigm*, in which optimal nutritional support has to be "just right"—not too hot, not too cold, not too much of anything.

THERAPEUTIC CALORIE RESTRICTION

When on a starvation diet, a patient should not be fatigued.

Hippocrates, *Aphorisms* II, xvi

Fasting for Weight Control

Fasting, or the temporary abstinence from food for a period of time, can be part of a religious ritual (e.g., Yom Kippur in the Jewish religion or Ramadan in the Muslim religion), a plan to lose weight quickly (medically supervised or otherwise), or a political statement (e.g., a hunger strike). Interestingly, during Ramadan, Muslims fast from sunrise to sunset daily for an entire month but they generally do not lose weight or decrease the number of calories they eat, even though they are eating only one meal a day (Johnstone 2007).

Medical fasting, or *therapeutic starvation* to facilitate rapid weight loss, was a technique made popular in the 1950s and 1960s as a treatment for intractable obesity (Johnstone 2007). Melanson and Dwyer (2002, p. 255) believe total fasting has no place in weight reduction under any circumstances because of the significant health risks it may cause. For example, fasting has been associated with loss of muscle (i.e., lean tissue rather than fat); metabolic abnormalities such as ketosis; electrolyte disturbances such as loss of sodium and potassium; ventricular fibrillation; and even sudden death (Melanson and Dwyer 2002, p. 255). Furthermore, because patients often feel weak, dizzy, and faint, they tend to decrease their energy expenditure so they use fewer calories than they might otherwise.

> Fasting has been associated with loss of muscle, ketosis, electrolyte imbalances, ventricular fibrillation, and even sudden death.

Nevertheless, temporary, intermittent fasting, despite its risks, has been touted as a kind of detoxification for the body. One of the most popular recently, though it dates back to the 1940s apparently, is Master Cleanse, a regimen in which the dieter consumes only water, 2 tablespoons of fresh lemon juice, 2 tablespoons of dark amber maple syrup, and a touch of cayenne pepper—a sort of spicy lemonade (Stein 2007). Joel Stein, of *Time* magazine, reported firsthand on his experience: "I'm feeling really light-headed. That feeling of clarity that fasters talk about? That is the loss of peripheral vision. I am also cold even though my 86-year-old grandmother is not. This cannot be healthy....I feel actual hunger pangs."

Johnstone (2007) found that following a 36-hour fast, research subjects lost about 1%–2% of their body weight (but it was probably more due to loss of water and glycogen stores than to loss of fat), and in this short-term fast they reported feelings of hunger as Joel Stein (2007) did. His conclusion, even when his research subjects underwent a longer total fast of 6 days' duration, consuming nothing except water or non-caloric beverages, and lost 5% of their initial body weight, was that "starvation was only a quick fix, with minimal impact on reducing [fat]." And feelings of hunger did not dissipate, even over 4–5 days of fasting. If anything, Johnstone believes that hunger feelings increase over time and that the faster the weight loss, the greater the accompanying feelings of fatigue.

> - "The official daily ration in the Auschwitz concentration camp was one liter of watery soup, 250 grams of bread and about 25 grams of margarine or imitation honey." (Keys et al. 1950, p. 777)
>
> - "During the great famine that began in May 1940 during the German occupation of the Netherlands, the Dutch authorities maintained rations at between 600 and 1,600 calories a day, or what they characterized as the level of semistarvation....In the Lodz Ghetto in 1941, besieged Jews were allotted starvation rations of 500 to 1,200 calories a day. At Treblinka, 900 calories was scientifically determined to be the minimum necessary to sustain human functioning. At 'the nation's top weight-loss clinics,' where 'patients' are treated for up to a year, the rations are the same." (Wolf 1992, p. 195)

Fessler (2003), an ethicist, reviewed the psychological changes that occur during prolonged fasting as seen in hunger strikes.

According to Fessler, hunger striking can result in mental deterioration and loss of competence. Personality changes may include increased irritability, impulsivity, and overvaluation of the potential benefits of the hunger strike and undervaluation of the potential harm, as well as "alarming levels of aggressivity." These changes, under certain conditions of food shortages that might occur in nature, might seem adaptive. After all, "meek individuals will lose out in the scramble for food." But the same pattern of changes, when they occur in the context of self-imposed fasting, may be quite maladaptive because "starving people are not in control of their actions." Because of the extensive publicity hunger strikers often receive, particularly with the Internet and other media sources, Fessler believes hunger striking will become more common, and though the situations are different, Fessler sees an analogy to patients with anorexia nervosa, who also may have "disordered decision making." The point is that severe food restriction, as seen in total fasting for whatever reason, has both physical and mental consequences without much benefit.

Very-Low-Calorie Diets

As we mentioned in Chapter 3, a calorie is just a measure of energy, or specifically, the amount of heat required to raise 1 gram of water by 1 degree on the Celsius scale. Particularly in the United States (and throughout this book), we refer to food *calories*, though we really mean kilocalories, or 1,000 calories (Buchholz and Schoeller 2004).

Very-low-calorie diets are those in which calories are restricted to less than 800 per day. They are usually recommended for individuals who are obese (body mass index [BMI] value of > 30 kg/m^2), and they are meant to lead to a weight loss of 1.5–2.5 kilograms per week, or, on average, about 20 kilograms after 8–12 weeks of the diet (Strychar 2006). Wadden and Osei (2002, pp. 236–237) noted these very-low-calorie diets are often very high in protein (70–100 g/day) in order to avoid loss of muscle. And it is very important that the protein be of high biological value, namely high in essential amino acids, in order to avoid a loss of lean tissue (Strychar 2006). Often these diets are in the form of a liquid diet. The problem with very-low-calorie diets is that they can lead to gallstones, as well as cardiac arrhythmias, ketosis, and abnormal water balance, so medical supervision is absolutely essential and the diet should not be used for more than 16 weeks (Melanson and Dwyer 2002, pp. 255–256; Strychar 2006). Furthermore, Wadden et al. (2002, pp. 157–158) reviewed studies and found there are conflicting reports about a higher incidence of binge eating after use of these diets. And Wadden and Osei (2002, p. 237) note that patients are more apt to regain substantially more weight by 1-year follow-up than with higher-calorie diets, and also that the very-low-calorie diet products can be particularly expensive. These researchers do not recommend use of these very-

> Very-low-calorie diets can lead to gallstones, cardiac arrhythmias, and water imbalance.

low-calorie formulations (e.g., Optifast 800) on their own; instead, they recommend supplementing them with a low-calorie dinner so that the total calorie intake for the day ranges instead from 900 to 1,000 calories. Booth et al. (2004) also support the view that these very-low-calorie diets are counterproductive in the longer term. For example, these diets may interfere with a dieter's need to acquire his or her own self-management skills for weight control by depending too heavily on external controls. Furthermore, the dieter may feel too deprived, particularly in social gatherings, which are so often centered on eating.

Heymsfield et al. (2003) reviewed low-calorie meal plans that involve prepackaged foods and snacks, particularly when offered as a partial meal replacement plan. The researchers, in reviewing the limited number of these partial plans, acknowledge that no one has actually established definitions of *meal replacement* or *partial meal replacement.* In general, though, patients are provided one or two meals that are portion controlled and fortified with vitamins and minerals, and are asked to eat a "sensible" dinner. These structured plans may work better because patients tend to develop greater behavioral strategies and gain more nutritional information, and they are often associated with behavior modification techniques, but Heymsfield et al. (2003) report that within 1 year of follow-up in the few studies available, there was an almost 50% dropout rate. Those who did complete the year lost up to 16 pounds, but no longer-term follow-up data were cited.

Along those lines, Heymsfield et al. (2007) examined why dieters on low-calorie diets (>800 cal/day and usually ~1,200–1,600 cal/day) fail to lose the weight they are expected to lose over time. Even though low-calorie diets have been the cornerstone of the treatment of obesity, they have been consistently shown over the past 50 years to fall far short of expectations. The pattern is typically a rapid weight loss over the first 1–2 weeks, then a slower weight loss, with maximal weight loss between 6 months and a year, and then a gradual weight regain over time. Heymsfield and his colleagues concluded that the low efficacy characteristic of these diets is most likely due to poor adherence to the diet rather than to major metabolic changes or adaptations. In other words, it seems that lack of compliance is what leads to the disappointing and surprising results such that patients typically lose less than half the weight that might be expected given their presumed calorie intake. This is not surprising inasmuch as there are two major components to control of eating: the homeostatic (short-term and long-term physiological signals of satiety) and the hedonic (cognitive, emotional, and reward signals). Because these two systems do not seem to be integrated, though they clearly interact, they must be taken into account separately (Seagle et al. 2009). Failure to consider the hedonic aspects of food intake will almost inevitably lead to failure to control weight.

> The hedonic components of eating control override the homeostatic ones and diets fail.

Calorie Restriction and Longevity

Fontana (2009) makes the point that to date, we have nothing "that can prevent, stop, or reverse the aging process" either in humans or animal models. The best we can do is *slow down* the process of aging and increase the natural life span, which can be done by as much as 60% in animals with a long-term program of calorie restriction without malnutrition (Fontana 2009). Speakman and Hambly (2007) clarify that this calorie restriction "depends solely on the reduction of calorie intake, rather than intake of specific dietary nutrients," and it is currently the only experimental manipulation of the environment that produces a change in the rate of the aging process. Furthermore, the process preserves nutritional status, unlike other states of calorie restriction such as that in the semistarvation experiment of Keys et al. (1950) described above, or the eating disorder anorexia nervosa.

The idea of calorie restriction has been around since the mid 1930s, when it was shown that this process prolonged the life span in rats. More recently, even when genetically altered obese mice (with twice the normal amount of fat) were put on a calorie-restricted diet, they had a longer life span than genetically normal, lean mice (Speakman and Hambly 2007). Many different species (e.g., yeast, insects, and fish) have yielded similar results. Interestingly, though, Speakman and Hambly (2007) note that it does not work in houseflies and even the specific genotype and strain of a mouse may determine how effective the process is and what response occurs. Though results suggest that calorie restriction with adequate nutrition may prolong the human life span, we have no evidence for it. And in fact, Fontana (2009) emphasizes we do not understand or know exactly why calorie restriction might extend the life span of a species nor do we even have evidence that calorie restriction extends life in nonhuman primates. There is ongoing research but, says Fontana, "as rhesus monkeys have an average and maximum lifespan of 27 and 40 years respectively, it may be another 10 years before maximal lifespan data become available on these primates."

We know that long-term calorie restriction with adequate nutrition can prevent or delay many diseases, such as obesity, cancer, diabetes, kidney disease, and cardiac disease, in rodents and may have similar effects in humans, presumably by producing many beneficial metabolic changes. When mammals are on a calorie-restricted diet, they have a sustained decrease in their body temperature (Mattson 2005a). There is also greater insulin sensitivity, lower levels of hormones such as leptin, norepinephrine, and insulin, and higher levels of hormones such as adiponectin, ghrelin, and cortisol—which decrease inflammation—according to Fontana (2009), who also says that recent studies in humans have shown that calorie restriction exerts a powerful anti-inflammatory effect. Furthermore, calorie restriction may work by being what is called a *hormetic agent;* Fontana defines *hormesis* as a "beneficial biological process by which a low-intensity stressor increases resistance to another, more intense stressor." The theory is that calorie restriction, as a chronic low-grade stressor, creates a survival response that enables an organism to endure adversity. Apparently animals exposed to calorie restriction are better able to withstand (i.e., are more resistant to) stressors like surgery, radiation, heat, and others than those that have not experienced calorie restriction. Speakman and Hambly (2007) enumerate three hypothetical mechanisms to explain why calorie restriction with adequate nutrition may be effective: 1) that the process slows down growth; 2) that it curbs excess fat from accumulating and hence averts the comorbid diseases associated with excess fat; and 3) that it initiates certain other processes (e.g., modulates the metabolism of protein) that reduce damage to an organism, such as damage caused by oxidative stress.

> Long-term calorie restriction with adequate nutrition can prevent many diseases and may even extend life.

Although the process of calorie restriction with adequate nutrition raises many questions, some people have already voluntarily begun to engage in calorie restriction with adequate nutrition, in the hope of delaying their own aging and prolonging their lives substantially. For example, the CALERIE (Comprehensive Assessment of Long-term Effect of Reducing Intake of Energy) studies, randomized and controlled, are currently being conducted in different sites and in various phases across the United States (e.g., Fontana et al. 2007). Two of the major questions are, how much calorie restriction is actually required, and how long does someone have to be exposed to calorie restriction with adequate nutrition to gain substantial benefit? Speakman and Hambly (2007) report that many of the animal studies have involved an almost 65% reduction and that has led only to a 20% extension of the life span. And the physiological changes associated with calorie restriction seem to occur fairly quickly, so they ask, "If it is never too late to start, then why would one ever start early?" Aging damage over time is cumulative, though, so there are in fact fewer benefits when calorie restriction with adequate nutrition begins later in life. For example, these researchers point out that a man who begins restricting his calorie intake in his late 40s by about 70% and continues to do so for the next 30 years might prolong his life by less than 3 years (Speakman and Hambly 2007). In other words, such a late start would probably not provide significant benefit in humans. And of course the obvious joke is, is it really a life span extension or does life just *seem* longer when we so restrict our calorie intake?

Another question is whether those who substantially restrict their calories for a prolonged period of time still experience hunger. Experiments with mice have shown that *after* a 50-day period of restriction (which is equivalent to about 2½ human years), mice become hyperphagic, which researchers interpret to mean that these animals remain hungry even after prolonged periods of restriction (Speakman and Hambly 2007). Maintaining a program of calorie restriction requires considerable motivation and much support and has not been particularly effective as a treatment for obesity. People do much better when all their meals are provided and they are involved in a scientific study. However, calorie restriction in the real world is extremely difficult, according to Speakman and Hambly; they suggest that drug-assisted calorie restriction (to alleviate hunger) may ultimately be a possibility, though they acknowledge that it may not have the same effect, and pose the question, "If there is no hunger pain, can there still be a longevity gain?"

Clearly, studies of the effects of long-term calorie restriction in humans are in their infancy. Researchers are also now comparing calorie restriction with the effects of exercise on metabolic functioning. For example, Weiss and Holloszy are part of the CALERIE study and found, contrary to their hypothesis, that calorie restriction (20% in this study) was as effective as exercise in improving both insulin sensitivity and glucose tolerance (Weiss and Holloszy 2007). Redman et al. (2007) compared calorie restriction and calorie restriction with exercise. They found that calorie restriction with or without exercise did not alter the *distribution* of fat in the body, a fact they attribute to genetics. They also found, contrary to their original hypothesis, that exercise did not improve metabolic functioning beyond the benefits obtained with calorie restriction, though it was helpful for weight loss and cardiovascular fitness.

A study by Martin et al. (2007) evaluated the effects of calorie restriction (25% restriction) on cognitive functioning as part of the CALERIE study. They note that dieters often complain of cognitive impairment, but this is probably a function of dieters' preoccupations with thoughts about their weight as well as about food. In their small study of 48 subjects (randomized to four groups including weight maintenance, 12.5% calorie restriction plus exercise, and a very-low-calorie diet), they found no evidence for any consistent pattern of cognitive decline in those on a calorie-restricted diet with testing at 3 and 6 months.

Calorie restriction, though, is not without its problems. For example, Jahng et al. (2007) exposed rats to 50% calorie reduction for 5 weeks and found, along with a marked weight loss, evidence for both anxiety and depression-like signs, a fact they attributed to disturbances in the serotonin system. Plasma corticosterone levels increased significantly in these rodents, and serotonin levels in certain areas of the brain decreased.

Alternate-Day Fasting

An alternative to daily calorie restriction is a pattern of alternate-day fasting, which involves a pattern of intermittent decrease in calorie intake, often with 24-hour periodicity (Varady and Hellerstein 2007). The theory is that it might be easier to maintain calorie restriction if a person is able to eat more normally every other day. In other words, overall calories are not necessarily fewer, but the pattern of consumption is different. Alternate-day fasting, like calorie restriction with adequate nutrition, is apparently affected by genotype. For example, depending on genetics, some people are able to oxidize fat more easily and, if so, they are more likely to lose weight with alternate-day fasting than people with other genotypes (Varady and Hellerstein 2007).

It is not clear how this alternate pattern affects the many hormones that are secreted in a circadian rhythm pattern. Bogdan et al. (2001) found statistically significant changes in the diurnal patterns and blood levels of melatonin, cortisol, testosterone, and prolactin in those fasting during Ramadan, when Muslims are prohibited from eating, drinking, smoking, or having sex from sunrise to sunset daily for a month.

Varady and Hellerstein (2008) reviewed studies comparing the effects of calorie restriction to alternate-day fasting. They found reports of animal studies in which leptin levels were higher on the days of feeding and lower on days that the animals did not eat but, overall, leptin levels were generally lower with alternate-day fasting than with regular, everyday eating, as they are with calorie restriction. In effect, it may work as well as calorie restriction does by decreasing fat cell size (but not numbers) and hence decreasing secretion of proinflammatory cytokines produced by adipose cells. But human studies and animal studies are apparently not consistent: alternate-day fasting can prevent certain cancers (e.g., lymphoma) and diabetes in animals, but this has not been seen in humans (Varady and Hellerstein 2008). However, human studies are often short term. Furthermore, animals are often not able to consume twice as much food on their feast days as they normally would, whereas humans clearly can. And Chandler-Laney et al. (2007) found that a pattern of cyclic calorie restriction and refeeding in rodents led to changes in the animals' behavior and neurochemistry consistent with depression. They speculate that this pattern led to impaired regulation of feeding, brain reward mechanisms, and mood that continued even after the rats had resumed their body weight and normal feeding pattern. Obviously, more studies are warranted.

MEAL FREQUENCY AND RATE OF EATING

In a discussion of the question of impact of meal frequency patterns on weight control, Seagle et al. (2009), in their recent position paper from the American Dietetic Association on weight management, reported that the evidence is inconsistent due to inadequate research, especially a lack of randomized, controlled studies. They observe that there is not even a standard definition of "an eating occasion." They also note that people who routinely have regular eating patterns and consistent meal frequency may differ from those who do not in other ways, such as in their work or exercise schedules or even hormonal patterns. As a result, it is difficult to separate the effects of meal frequency from the effects of other personal characteristics.

Jenkins et al. (1989), comparing "nibbling" versus "gorging," found that nibbling throughout the day produced lower total cholesterol and low-density lipoprotein (LDL) levels as well as reductions in blood insulin levels. They caution, though, that encouraging obese people to eat more frequently may lead them to greater calorie intake throughout the day. Nevertheless, for some people, frequent, small meals may be beneficial for weight control and their metabolic profile. Rodin also suggests that those who eat less frequently tend to be heavier (Rodin 1978, pp. 581–582).

In a more recent study, Frecka and Mattes (2008) measured the secretion of the gastrointestinal hormone ghrelin to evaluate whether the timing of meals affects this hormone. (See Chapter 5, "The Metabolic Complexities of Weight Control," for more details on ghrelin and other hormones.) Typically, ghrelin levels rise prior to eating and have been thought to be an actual signal of hunger. The researchers found, instead, that ghrelin secretion was entrained (conditioned) to customary patterns of eating and that its rise prior to eating was related to anticipation of a meal. Furthermore, Frecka and Mattes speculate that the characteristic rise in ghrelin prior to eating, when there is a regular meal pattern, may be related to alterations in insulin and glucose levels and occur secondarily to these alterations. Ghrelin, therefore, does not seem to be a hunger signal, as thought, although there was a positive association between hunger and ghrelin levels in both obese and nonobese people. Their speculation is that ghrelin and hunger are under separate controls and that the rise in ghrelin prior to eating may help prepare our gastrointestinal systems for food in order to optimize digestion, absorption, and utilization of nutrients. Chaotic, disordered eating patterns, therefore, may have an impact on these processes and hormone secretion. The researchers conclude that habitual meal patterns may be an important variable in human eating (Frecka and Mattes 2008). (See also Chapter 9, "Circadian Rhythms, Sleep, and Weight.")

As we have previously mentioned, many studies, including those from the National Weight Control Registry emphasize the importance of eating breakfast daily (see Chapter 2, "Obesity in the United States"). Significantly, individuals with the night eating syndrome are more likely to have excessive weight and typically eat the majority of their calories at night, have subsequent morning anorexia, and skip breakfast (see Chapter 9, "Circadian Rhythms, Sleep, and Weight"). The vast major-

THE IMPORTANCE OF EATING BREAKFAST

- Eating breakfast every day of the week has been found consistently in studies of people who lose weight and are able to maintain their weight loss: regular breakfast eaters constituted 78% of those who had maintained their weight loss in one large study with almost 3,000 subjects.

- Only 4% of that same study population were able to maintain a weight loss without ever eating breakfast.

- Those who ate breakfast tended to do somewhat more physical activity in a day. In those with binge eating disorder, eating breakfast led to fewer binges and significantly fewer calories consumed per day than in binge eaters who did not eat breakfast.

Source: Wyatt et al. 2002; see also Masheb and Grilo 2006; Sitzman 2006; Wing 1992

ity of participants in the National Weight Control Registry, though, who have maintained a substantial weight loss of over 30 pounds for at least 1 year, are breakfast eaters (most commonly cereal and fruit). Seagle et al. (2009) note that breakfast is often recommended by dietitians because it is a meal that frequently includes fiber and calcium, both important for health. Furthermore, they note that many of the studies that support the importance of breakfast are based on self-reports of breakfast eating. They acknowledge, though, that there is an association between having a high BMI value and eating breakfasts that contain high-fat foods. As with almost everything in this field, we recommend an individual approach. Say Seagle et al. (2009), "Helping a client to find a meal pattern that prevents the times when high hunger coincides with an environment of high-energy food choices seems pertinent."

The evidence-based guidelines from the American Dietetic Association (2009) recommend four or five meals or snacks per day including breakfast, although this is not ranked among their strongest recommendations. They also recommend greater calorie intake during the day as being preferable to eating in the evening.

Mattson (2005a) suggests that, theoretically, there should be a "window of energy intake that promotes optimum health, and this should be true for meal frequency." But unfortunately, we do not yet have enough data to justify recommending any particular schedule. Furthermore, individual differences based on age, sex, and activity level, for example, may also factor into recommendations. But Mattson (2005b) says that it makes sense that there are patterns suitable for human eating other than our typical patterns: evolutionarily, humans probably ate food much more sporadically and may have had one meal per day or may even have had to go without food for days. Says Mattson, "Thus, from an evolutionary perspective, human beings were adapted to intermittent feeding rather than to grazing." Mattson (2005b) finds it remarkable that such a fundamental aspect of eating, the number of meals eaten a day, "has not yet been subject to rigorous scientific investigation."

Not only the frequency of meals but also the rate at which we eat them may affect our weight. Significantly, rapid intake of food within a discrete time period is part of the symptoms complex of and diagnosis for binge eating disorder (DSM-IV-TR; American Psychiatric Association 2000). And even as an expenditure of energy through activity (i.e., nonexercise activity thermogenesis; see Chapter 8, "Exercise"), slower eating may entail more chewing motion and hence more utilization of calories. Perhaps both longer mealtimes to develop satiety and increased chewing to utilize more calories are important factors. There are many research criteria used to measure eating rate, such as our chewing time, chewing movement, number of swallows, bite size, rate, and number, and the number of pauses between bites (Chapelot and Louis-Sylvestre 2008, p. 148).

Ebbeling et al. (2007) suggest that studies indicate that not only large portions but also a rapid rate of eating may lead to obesity. They speculate that this eating style "may not allow adequate time for development of physiologic satiety signals involved in meal termination" although they acknowledge that study results are inconsistent. In their own small study of adolescents who tended to gorge on fast food (swallowing food in large mouthfuls or quantities), they found that neither slowing down eating nor portioning out the food had any impact on how much these adolescents ate.

Otsuka et al. (2006) studied the rate of eating in a large study of healthy Japanese civil servants (> 5,000 men and > 1,400 women). They found that rapid eating was associated with increased calorie intake and higher BMI values. Furthermore, a rapid eating pattern seems to be a consistent behavior over the course of one's life. They note that no one knows at what point in life a rapid eating pattern is actually acquired, but once it is acquired in childhood, it seems to persist through adulthood. These researchers reported that obese patients could lose weight when they ate more slowly, but this slower pattern was difficult for the subjects to maintain even during a behavioral program for weight control. Their conclusion was that a person's eating rate might be a significant key factor in weight control and therapeutic efforts should be made to maintain behavioral modifications.

> "The bulk of the meal eaten over a relatively short period of time remains in the stomach for more than an hour after eating … [so] gastric distention is involved in the short-term inhibition of eating."
>
> **Source: Koopmans 2004**

POPULAR DIETS

General Principles

The same power does not belong to all sweet things, nor to all fat things, nor to all particulars of any other class.

Hippocrates, *Regimen*, Book II

There is considerable competition among the various diet programs, even though there is hardly a shortage of dieters. One effective means of gaining converts to a particular program or diet philosophy is the use of before-and-after diet photo advertisements. Geier et al. (2003) point out that these advertisements frequently lack credibility. Even more important, though, is that their "potential for harm is vast." For example, they tend to increase negative stereotypes about obese people in general and in particular foster a belief that a person's weight is easily controllable, a belief that is "more resistant to change than other beliefs about obesity."

Gina Kolata, in her book *Rethinking Thin* (2007), says that nothing in the world of dieting (or exercise, for that matter) is particularly new. Says Kolata, "It is like the world of fashion, where, women tell each other, if you save your clothes and wait long enough, they'll come into style again" (Kolata 2007, p. 32). Some diets, of course, have particular staying power. For example, Dwyer (1978) reviewed 12 popular diets of the late 1970s. The Pritikin diet, recommending reduced calories and extremely low fat intake (only 10%) in order to live longer (Pritikin 1985), and the Atkins diet, recommending very low carbohydrate intake (Atkins 2002), remain today. Less popular today are the Stillman water diet, recommending 8 glasses of water a day (Stillman 1968), and the Ayds Plan diet, which recommends its candies be eaten prior to each meal (a scientifically unsubstantiated approach) (Dwyer 1978, p. 625). Over the years, we have had the *grapefruit diet* (Thompson and Ahrens 2004), the *cabbage soup diet*, in both the "new" (Danbrot 2004) and the "ultimate" (Cooper 2003) versions, and the *Eat Right 4 Your Type* diet (utilizing an eating plan based on the dieter's blood type; D'Adamo and Whitney 1996), among thousands of others.

> Blood type is a genetic marker, and it is feasible that one day we will be able to identify certain biological markers that will establish a more individualized diet for each of us.

Many of these diets work by monotony: prescribe one food and by the principle of sensory satiety a person may tire of the particular food, eat less of it, and lose weight, at least temporarily. But these diets are not feasible to maintain for life, and many of them are clearly nutritionally unbalanced. Matz and Frankel (2004, pp. 101–103), along somewhat similar lines, speak of the paradoxical concept of *stocking*, the principle of bringing an abundance of foods, including the "forbidden" ones, into our homes. The idea is that "scarcity makes people anxious, and abundance makes people calm."

Dieting by blood type, though, is worth noting. To date, there is no scientific research to confirm that our blood type should in any way determine the foods we eat. Blood type, though, is a genetic marker, and it is feasible that one day we will be able to identify certain biological markers that will establish "a more perfect individual diet" for each of us.

Kolata (2007, p. 60) raises the question, "Are people struggling because the goals, the ideal body weights, have become unrealistic, or are they struggling because the perfect diet just has not been discovered?" Of course, that poses the question, is there really a perfect diet? The answer lies individually: there is no perfect diet for everyone. It may even be that one of the reasons different studies sometimes yield such opposite results is that we are dealing with subsets of populations with metabolic differences that are perhaps too small to measure at this time.

Examples of Dietary Supplementation

Most diets recommend some combination of protein, fat, and carbohydrates, but other diets recommend a particular kind of supplement or even a specific food. For example, Sabaté (2003) found that people who eat nuts, a food high in fat, tend to have a lower BMI value. Nuts are high in protein, fiber, and unsaturated (healthy) fat and, for some people, increase a sense of satiety. Even though nuts range from about 45% to 75% fat content, with macadamia nuts having 74% and pistachios having 48% fat, they do not tend to lead to an increase in body weight if they are a replacement food that does not increase the total amount of calories a person consumes that day. Furthermore, Sabaté (2003) noted that there are some preliminary data indicating that those who eat a nut-rich diet tend to excrete more fat in their stools (and hence do not process all the calories) because nuts are not completely absorbed. For example, those who ate whole peanuts excreted 17% fat whereas those who ate peanut butter excreted only 4%–7%.

Ahuja et al. (2006) recommends a diet supplemented with chili peppers (cayenne or red pepper, with capsaicin as the active ingredient) to increase fat oxidation as well as to increase metabolic energy expenditure. Chili peppers also contain antioxidants like vitamin C, β-carotene, and lutein, all associated with a decreased risk of atherosclerosis (Ahuja et al. 2006). In their small, randomized, crossover study of 22 women and 14 men with a mean BMI value in the slightly overweight category (26.3 kg/m^2), these researchers found that subjects consuming a chili-supplemented diet regularly for 4 weeks had improved insulin sensitivity and reduced insulin secretion postprandially, and those with higher BMI values had a "more definitive" response. Though more research is indicated and study length should perhaps exceed 4 weeks, this study suggests that "regular consumption of chili may attenuate postprandial hyperinsulinemia." For those who are overweight and enjoy spicy food, this may be a useful and pleasant adjunct in controlling insulin levels after eating.

There has also been some suggestion that use of dietary calcium may have a role in weight control. Zemel (2004) found that "dairy sources of calcium...markedly attenuate weight and fat gain and accelerate fat loss." This is much less so with calcium supplements, possibly due to the presence in dairy products of other compounds such as whey. Zemel, who reviewed studies in humans and animals, calls this the *antiobesity effect* of calcium due to calcium being a regulator of lipid metabolism in fat cells (Zemel 2004). Zemel (2004) found that obese people given a diet including three to four daily portions of milk, cheese, or yogurt for 24 weeks—up to 1,300 mg of calcium per day—lost considerably more weight on a reduced-calorie diet (almost 11% of their weight) than control subjects did on the same diet with only 500 mg of calcium daily (6.4% of their weight).

Trowman et al. (2006), on the other hand, conducted a systematic meta-analysis of randomized, controlled trials to assess the effects of calcium supplementation on weight. Ultimately, they were able to include 13 trials, conducted from 1990 to 2004, of subjects older than age 18. The studies were quite discrepant: some were on postmenopausal women, some on younger; some were on obese subjects and others were not. The majority of trials included only female subjects, and ages ranged from the mid 20s to the early 70s. The calcium doses also varied (and one study did not even report how much calcium supplementation was given), as did the lengths of the studies included. Unlike Zemel (2004), these researchers could not find any statistically significant impact on weight with either calcium supplements or actual dairy products. They did note that they unexpectedly found evidence of flawed randomization that could have affected the results of the studies. Interestingly, this meta-analysis did not include information regarding the fat content of the dairy products used. Perhaps future research will be able to sort out these discrepancies. In the meantime, those so inclined (and particularly people concerned about osteoporosis) might want to try supplemental, nonfat dairy products to see whether this method has any effect on their own weight loss efforts.

The Advantages and Perils of High-Protein Diets and Their Relationship to Low Carbohydrate and High Fat Intake

One of the most recent scientifically conducted studies mentioned above, the Sacks et al. study reported in 2009, suggests that it is calorie counting rather than specific percentages of protein, fat, and/or carbohydrates that is essential for weight loss. Many other studies, however, including those by Paddon-Jones et al. (2008), Batterham et al. (2006), Simpson and Raubenheimer (2005), Weigle et al. (2005), Halton and Hu (2004), and Westerterp-Plantenga et al. (2004), sanction the use and importance of high-protein diets. We speculate that an individual's genetics probably determines (or at least has a major role in determining) exactly what proportion of protein, fat, and carbohydrates works best for that person in the context of reduced calories.

> "It seems plausible that for maintenance of reduced body mass, the right diet needs to be matched with the right patient. Ultimately, a 'nutrigenomic' approach most likely will be helpful. At present, there are no data to help clinicians match a diet to an individual patient's 'diet response genotype.'"
>
> Source: Eckel 2005

Protein, however, usually constitutes the smallest percentage of calories consumed per day. Because we tend to eat less protein than fat or carbohydrates, Simpson and Raubenheimer (2005) make the point that even a small decrease in the amount of protein eaten results in large changes in the percentage of carbohydrate or fat intake. This is called *protein leverage*. And apparently, according to these researchers, the amount of protein humans eat has remained far more constant than our intake of either fat or carbohydrates, both over time and in different populations. Our typical U.S. diet contains about 16% protein, 49% carbohydrates, and 35% fat (Batterham et al. 2006). If we are eating 2,000 calories a day, 16% of that would be 320 calories, or about 80 grams.

Simpson and Raubenheimer (2005) speculate that the more we replace protein with energy-dense carbohydrates or fats, which is easy to do with our refined sugars and processed foods, the more inclined we will be toward obesity. Furthermore, the food industry tends to season these low-protein processed foods with sodium and umami, tastes that are typically associated with protein. Our taste buds can distinguish sweet, salt, bitter, and sour. Many researchers, though, believe we also taste the protein-like flavor umami, a savory "glutamate" taste (Duffy and Bartoshuk 1996, pp. 145–146). Simpson and Raubenheimer (2005) suggest that the addition of sodium and umami to food may actually subvert our protein regulatory systems such that we overconsume fat and carbohydrates at the expense of protein.

Paddon-Jones et al. (2008) note that what we consider a high-protein diet can vary, with protein constituting from 27% to 68% of daily calorie intake; expressed in terms of grams, such diets may vary from over 90 to 284 grams of protein per day. These researchers also note that one of the reasons that diets moderately higher in protein tend to lead to greater weight loss is that they lend themselves to better compliance among dieters.

Protein is recognized by most researchers as (and to many dieters, is) the most satiating of the food groups. Paddon-Jones et al. (2008) make the point that carbohydrates are also quite satiating acutely but protein seems to remain satiating for a longer time. These researchers also note that some proteins may be more satiating than others (e.g., animal protein vs. protein from plants like soy). Of course, many things can influence satiety, such as the amount of fiber eaten concurrently, whether the food is in liquid or solid form, what combination of foods is eaten, the quantity of food presented, and, as we have seen repeatedly, the psychology of the eater (especially how much we think we should be eating; see Chapter 4, "The Psychology of the Eater"). Halton and Hu (2004) note that interpreting some of the research on the satiating effects of protein can become a nearly impossible task because of all the variables, including different study designs, subjects, foods, and other factors involved.

The theory behind the satiating effects of protein is that ingesting protein releases in the gut peptide tyrosine-tyrosine (PYY), a hormone that decreases food intake (see Chapter 5, "The Metabolic Complexities of Weight Control"). PYY is also released after ingestion of fat in those who are of normal weight, but according to Batterham et al. (2006), obese rodents and humans seem to have attenuated PYY release. In general, rodents eat less when on a high-protein diet. However, Batterham et al. (2006) found that mice genetically engineered without PYY did not become satiated when given a high-protein diet and actually became obese. When exogenous PYY was given to these mice, they lost weight. The researchers suggest that this kind of dietary manipulation (higher protein content to stimulate the satiating hormone PYY) may have a role in weight control in humans. But they also speculate that the reduced PYY response in obese subjects may be involved in causing and maintaining obesity.

High-protein diets also seem to have a greater thermogenic effect (i.e., utilizing more calories for the processes of digestion and absorption) than fat or carbohydrates. Halton and Hu (2004) note that protein has a typical thermogenic effect of 20%–35%, depending on the amount of protein, whereas carbohydrates have a thermogenic effect of 5%–15%; the effect for fat "is a subject of debate." These researchers also suggest that the thermogenic effect of protein seems to last longer than the effect for fat or carbohydrates. The point is that high-protein diets may work for some through a complex interaction of many factors, including an individual's genetics, protein's thermogenic and satiating effects, and some dieters' ability to sustain greater compliance.

High compliance, though, is not necessarily an outcome over the long term. For example, Due and colleagues found that by 24 months in a study of 50 subjects who were initially overweight or obese, of those in the high-protein group (25% protein, 30% fat), 56% had dropped out (Due et al. 2004). There was an even higher dropout rate—over 75%—in the lower-protein group (12% protein, 30% fat). Due et al. (2004) found that after 24 months, the number of subjects who had remained and who had lost more than 5 kilograms of weight was similar in the high-protein and low-protein groups. Interestingly, however, the subjects in the high-protein group "had a greater reduction in their waist circumference" than those in the lower-protein group at follow-up. In other words, the high-protein group had lost more abdominal fat, and even when there was some weight regain, this group maintained "a reduction" in abdominal fat. Due et al. (2004) commented that it is not known why a high-protein diet should reduce abdominal (i.e., visceral) fat.

High-protein diets are often consequently lower in carbohydrates. Weigle et al. (2005) investigated whether it is the higher protein percentage or the lower percentage of carbohydrates that is responsible for decreased appetite and for weight loss with these diets. In their small study of 19 people, these researchers placed their subjects sequentially on varying percentages of protein while maintaining a consistent percentage of 50% for carbohydrates. Protein percentages were 15% and 30%; fat percentages were 35% and 20%, respectively. They found that the higher percentage of protein, even with 50% carbohydrates, resulted in a sustained decrease in calorie intake and subsequent weight loss. Weigle et al. (2005) speculated that it is the effect of the protein itself, perhaps through the medium of increased central nervous system leptin sensitivity, that is responsible for weight loss when people are on low-carbohydrate diets. In other words, they found that when protein is substituted for fat, this seems to produce a greater weight loss than when carbohydrates are substituted for fat intake in the diet. As a result, carbohydrate restriction itself seems less important than controlling fat intake.

And, as we have said (see Chapter 3, "Food: The Basic Principles of Calories"), our diets should have enough protein to provide essential amino acids (those that our bodies do not produce naturally), protein's building blocks, and be high enough in carbohydrates to sustain blood glucose levels. That means that in general we should consume a minimum of 65–70 grams of protein and a minimum of 50–100 grams of carbohydrates per day. Once we have achieved those minimums, many researchers do not believe the actual percentages of protein, fat, and carbohydrates are as relevant to either weight loss or a healthy diet (Melanson and Dwyer 2002, pp. 250–251).

Katz, though, notes that extreme carbohydrate restriction (<10%) and high protein intake (as recommended by the Atkins diet, which also has a high level of saturated fat and cholesterol) can have their own adverse metabolic effects (Katz 2008, pp. 71–73).

For example, a low-carb, high-protein diet can lead to constipation, nausea, dehydration, kidney stones, bad breath, and even depression, among other symptoms. And when carbohydrate intake is very low, the initial weight loss is often water loss rather than loss of adipose tissue, as we have said. Furthermore, as we have said, ketone bodies are produced, which can lead to dizziness, headache, and fatigue in the short term and to long-term effects such as osteoporosis and an abnormal lipid profile (Katz 2008, p. 71) (the reader is again referred to Chapter 3, "Food: The Basic Principles of Calories"). The potential adverse effects of extreme restriction of carbohydrate intake are outlined in Table 10–1.

Table 10–1. Known and potential adverse effects of extreme restriction of dietary intake of carbohydrates

Adverse effect	Mechanism
Constipation	An established effect attributable to low intake of dietary fiber
Dehydration	Caused by gluconeogenesis consuming water along with glycogen, and ketone bodies causing increased renal excretion of sodium and water
Depression/dysthymia	A theoretical risk due to impaired delivery of tryptophan to the brain and impaired serotonin production
Halitosis	An established effect of ketosis
Hepatic injury	A potential sequela of high protein intake over time
Increased cancer risk	A potential sequela of increased consumption of animal products and decreased consumption of grains and fruit
Increased cardiovascular disease risk	A potential sequela of increased consumption of animal products and decreased consumption of grains and fruit
Nausea	An established effect of ketosis
Nephropathy	A potential consequence of high protein intake over time
Osteopenia	An established effect of ketosis; hypercalciuria is induced by high intake of dietary protein
Renal calculi	A known sequela of ketosis; risk is increased by dehydration

Source. Adapted from Katz DL (with Friedman RSC): *Nutrition in Clinical Practice: A Comprehensive, Evidence-Based Manual for the Practitioner*, 2nd Edition. Philadelphia, PA, Wolters Kluwer Health/ Lippincott Williams & Wilkins, 2008, p. 73. Used with permission.

The Advantages and Perils of High-Carbohydrate Diets and Their Relationship to Fat Intake

As we can see from the statistics in Schlosser's *Fast Food Nation*, fast food restaurants have become a fixture in the American diet. Dumanovsky et al. (2009) report there is "strong evidence of a positive correlation" between eating at fast food restaurants and increased caloric intake. These researchers studied what people actually ordered at fast food restaurants in New York City in 2007, before posted calorie counts were required. They found that on average, the more than 7,700 people surveyed purchased 827 calories worth of food and beverage for lunch. And one-third purchased more than 1,000 calories for this one meal! The researchers are currently collecting data to see whether the new regulation requiring calorie posting will have any effect on consumers' purchases.

FAST FOOD NATION

- On any given day in the United States, about one-quarter of the population visits a fast food restaurant.

- Chicken McNuggets contain twice as much fat per ounce as a hamburger.

- "Americans now spend more on fast food than on higher education, personal computers, computer software, or new cars. They spend more on fast food than movies, books, magazines, newspapers, videos, and recorded music—combined." (p. 3)

Source: Schlosser 2005

Diets extremely high in carbohydrates also have their own adverse effects, particularly in some people. For one thing, they create an abnormal blood lipid profile and lead to increased triglycerides. Ifland et al. (2009), most recently, as well, suggest that highly refined sugar-flour unnatural combinations are addictive substances over which many people will lose control. These researchers call this syndrome the *refined food addiction* and believe those who are addicted have exactly the same DSM-IV-TR patterns of tolerance (requiring more of the substance to satisfy); unsuccessful attempts to cut back ("I can't believe I ate the whole thing"); excessive time spent in attempting to acquire these unnatural substances; reduction of other activities because of their use (e.g., embarrassed to go out socially); continuation of use despite adverse consequences (e.g., presence of a disease such as diabetes); and even withdrawal (e.g., anxiety). Not everyone would agree there is such a syndrome. Obviously, for those who do believe they have evidence of this pattern, a diet high in carbohydrates may lead to out-of-control intake of refined carbohydrates, usually with high glycemic index values (even with the low-fat varieties), and will hardly lead to calorie control—the mainstay of any diet regimen.

Further, Hellerstein (2001) makes the point that when both carbohydrates and fats are present, as in a typical mixed diet, carbohydrates are oxidized preferentially and fat oxidation is suppressed. What this means is that any excessive fat intake (from calories that are not utilized) is stored in the body as adipose tissue.

Carbohydrates are not actually converted to fat (and fat is not converted to carbohydrates), but it seems as though they are because fat oxidation is interfered with and as a result fat accumulates in our bodies. Horton et al. (1995) suggested that when we overfeed on carbohydrates, about 75%–85% of the excess calories are stored as fat, but when we take in an excess of calories from fat, we store 90%–95% of the excess calories as adipose tissue. These researchers overfed a small group of nine normal-weight and seven obese adult male subjects, giving them 150% of their usual intake, with either 50% more fat or 50% more carbohydrates. Their conclusion was that in the context of excessive calorie intake (a positive energy balance), our diet composition can have important effects on how much fat we actually store: "fat leads to more body fat accumulation than [do] carbohydrate[s]," but only when we eat more calories than we expend. Horton et al. (1995) also found, though, that their obese subjects tended to oxidize proportionally more carbohydrates and less fat than those subjects who were of normal weight, and they speculated that those who tend to utilize carbohydrates at higher rates (in the context of consuming too many calories) are at most risk of becoming obese.

Along those lines, Kessler and his group (Naleib et al, 2008) "deconstructed" a vanilla milkshake to ascertain what elements—sugar, fat, or flavoring—are most reinforcing. Though the researchers used fully satiated rats as their subjects, we can hypothesize that humans are not so different. What they found is that sucrose was the most reinforcing element but the presence of even a small amount of fat made the food even more rewarding. Surprisingly, the flavor vanilla "neither enhanced nor attenuated responding" to the fat and sugar mixture. The researchers emphasize, though, that the substitution of sucrose for fat in low-fat foods for humans, as is commonly done, may unfortunately lead to overconsumption of these products.

Horton et al. (1995) believe "it is important to consider individual differences in the influence of diet composition on body weight regulation. Individual differences in fat compared to carbohydrate oxidation may underlie differences in fat storage," particularly when fat is given in excess.

They also found that the actual pattern of overeating may also affect fat accumulation. Excessive fat storage is more likely to occur when there are acute multiple periods of overeating fatty foods over one day or several days than with a more steady intake of fat in the diet (and with high fat intake rather than with high carbohydrate intake).

Minehira et al. (2004) also found that eating dietary fat led to fat accumulation in the body, but so did overfeeding with carbohydrates for 4 days in both their normal-weight and overweight subjects. They acknowledge, though, that their subjects were given meals of "pure glucose" and their results might not necessarily

> "There is little functional capacity for storage of additional protein or carbohydrate in the body, but capacity for fat storage is essentially unlimited."
>
> **Source: Hill 2006**

apply to the mixed diets that people typically eat, or to meals that might contain complex carbohydrates rather than a simple sugar with a high glycemic index value.

Although too much fat, particularly in the context of excessive calorie intake, seems to lead to preferential accumulation of adipose tissue, Willett (2002) believes the focus on reduction of total fat has been "a serious distraction" in all our efforts to reduce obesity. Willett (2002) noted that in the previous two decades in the United States, there was an actual decrease in the percentage of fat typically eaten while simultaneously there was a "massive increase" in the rates of obesity. Furthermore, presumably because fat adds flavor and texture to food, those on diets too low in fat tend not to maintain them over time. In fact, Willett (2002) believes that short-term, modest weight losses achieved on low-fat diets are "difficult to sustain" long term. And because very-low-fat diets are often much higher in carbohydrates, they run the risk of leading to increased abnormal triglyceride levels in dieters. Willett's solution is a diet with moderate fat intake (with 18%–40% of calories from fat), such as what is referred to as the Mediterranean diet. For some people, though, that level of fat in the diet may be too great. Willett (2002) believes, as we do, that genetic susceptibility varies, so that some individuals gain weight on high-fat diets and others do not.

Bray et al. (2004) reviewed research from animal studies. They found that animals fed a high-fat diet developed a greater number of fat cells (i.e., became fat), and when these animals were switched to a lower-fat diet, they did not necessarily lose the weight: even after rats were switched to a lower-fat diet for 7 months, their weight did not drop to their initial weight. In animal experiments, Bray et al. (2004) note that "an increase in fat intake may be particularly important in inducing obesity, whereas a reduction in dietary fat has less of an effect on weight loss," and that these two may even work through different metabolic mechanisms.

> Regardless of the composition of the diet, all overeating eventually leads to obesity.
>
> Source: Horton et al. 1995

Nevertheless, Bray et al. (2004) support the role of lowering fat consumption for humans—even a 10% reduction of fat in our diets, from 36% to 26% of our calorie intake, can lead to weight loss in those who are obese. They note that higher-fat diets (remember that fat yields about 9 cal/g, as compared to 4 cal/g for protein and most carbohydrates) can make it more difficult for dieters to consume fewer calories.

The type of fat in our diet may also have significance. Artmann et al. (2008) exposed rats to different dietary fats (38% of their diet) equivalent to palm oil (high in saturated fat), olive oil (as in the Mediterranean diet; high in monounsaturated fat), and safflower oil (linoleic acid, one of the essential fatty acids and high in polyunsaturated fat). They found that even short-term feeding of these different oils affected tissue levels in the liver and small intestine (but not in the brain) of certain lipid mediators, including the endocannabinoids, which have a role in the brain reward system and affect food intake. The significance of this work for humans is not yet known, but it is suggestive that exposure in our diets to different oils may affect our food intake by their anorectic actions.

A Review of Some Popular Diets

Basic features of the most common weight loss diets are outlined in Table 10–2.

The Ornish diet (Ornish and Brown 2002) is typically very low in fat, as is the Pritikin diet (Pritikin 1985); they call for about 10%–15% of daily calories as fat, and were originally suggested to reverse cardiac disease and atherosclerosis (Strychar 2006). The problem with these diets is that they are then very high in carbohydrates (60%–80%) that can raise triglyceride levels (Lichtenstein and Van Horn 1998) and sometimes too high in fiber—which can cause its own difficulties for the dieter, such as uncomfortable abdominal fullness and even decreased absorption of zinc, calcium, and iron, according to Strychar (2006). As we have mentioned in Chapter 3 ("Food: The Basic Principles of Calories"), the daily recommended guideline for fiber intake is up to 38 grams a day (Institute of Medicine 2008). Strychar also makes the point that the Ornish diet itself, which is essentially a vegetarian diet and has been associated with beneficial cardiac effects, has been difficult to evaluate because it has been studied in the context of exercise and behavior techniques.

Katz (2005) conducted an extensive and thorough literature review and synthesis to assess the "competing dietary claims" offered by the "seemingly limitless market for weight loss approaches" available to today's dieter. He found no evidence to support the superiority of one diet over another for "sustainable weight loss" other than calorie restriction. Unfortunately, extreme caloric restriction, such as is used for rapid weight loss, is "intrinsically unsustainable." Furthermore, Katz found a "prevailing gullibility" among a public "beguiled by a belief in weight-loss magic" such that "virtually any weight-loss claim is accepted at face value."

Both the 2007 *Consumer Reports* review and Brian Wansink (*Mindless Eating*, 2006, pp. 221–224) have compared the advantages and disadvantages of some of the most common diets. For example, Wansink notes that the Sugar Busters diet works because of calorie restriction, rather than the magic of its ratio of 40% fat, 30% protein, and 30% carbohydrates. Many other researchers support the notion that diets with these ratios are oversimplifying complex metabolic processes.

Wansink (2006, p. 223) is also critical of the high-protein Atkins diet, because it condones high consumption of saturated fats. Likewise, he finds the South Beach diet too restrictive for those who do not want to restrict carbohydrates so dramatically (Wansink 2006, p. 221). Wansink's own approach of cutting 100–200 calories a day "mindlessly" is a sensible (and balanced) dietary approach because it focuses on portion control and does not emphasize or exclude any major food group (Wansink 2006, p. 224).

Luis Balart (2005), a gastroenterologist, is another physician critical of the Atkins diet and its "lo-carb mania." He points out that the Atkins diet does not differentiate

Table 10–2. Basics of the most common diets

	Nature of the diet	Advantages	Disadvantages
Atkins diet Robert Atkins, M.D. (low glycemic profile; Atkins 2002)	Initially no carbohydrates, high protein; later low in carbohydrates. Concept of net carbohydrates: carbohydrates minus fiber content	Quick results	Stress on the liver and kidneys; ketone bodies that can cause nausea, bad breath; high saturated fat intake; hard to maintain over time
"Mindful Eating plan" Brian Wansink, Ph.D.	Reduce calorie intake by 100–200 cal/day	No specific food deprivation; dieter can choose what calories to eliminate	Slow loss of weight
Sonoma diet (Gutterson 2005)	Mediterranean style, low in carbohydrates; small plates	Healthy eating plan; no calorie counting	Too restrictive and difficult to execute in restaurants
South Beach diet Arthur Agatston, M.D. (low glycemic profile)	Restricted fat and carbohydrates (except fruits, vegetables, nuts, and grains)	Simple after phase 1; balanced; no calorie counting	Expensive and depriving; hard to maintain over time
Sugar Busters diet (low glycemic profile; Steward et al. 1965)	30/40/30 protein/fat/carbohydrate proportions	No calorie counting; decreases sugar intake; encourages exercise	No scientific basis for specific proportions
UltraMetabolism Mark Hyman, M.D. (low glycemic profile; Hyman 2006)	No refined grains or processed food; "detox your system"; think of food as medicine	Healthy eating; encourages exercise	Expensive and depriving
Weight Watchers (Rippe 2005)	Portion control	Support system; no food restriction	Cumbersome daily point calculations; expensive
Zone diet Barry Sears, Ph.D. (low glycemic profile; Sears 1995)	Control of portions and reduced sugar; percentage of protein, fat, carbohydrate intake (30/30/40) to manage insulin release	Balanced	Not practical; no scientific basis for specific proportions

Source: Consumer Reports 2007; Moyad 2004; Wansink 2006.

between carbohydrates with a high glycemic profile (which create a surge of insulin) and those with a low glycemic profile (which produce a slower rise of glucose and subsequent insulin levels). He also notes that there has been "virtually no scientific evidence to back such a restrictive approach to dieting" and reports that in some of the studies comparing the Atkins diet to other diets, the dropout rate both with Atkins and with the other diets was 40%, because many of these diets are very hard to maintain even for a year, let alone for a lifetime.

Balart (2005) is more supportive of the Sugar Busters diet because it "offers a more complete dietary approach" and does not severely limit one food group over another. It does, though, also emphasize the importance of both differentiating high-glycemic from low-glycemic carbohydrates and reading labels of processed foods to avoid unintended sugars (e.g., in salad dressings) (Balart 2005). Of note, though, is that Gilman (2008, pp. 262–263), in his "encyclopedia" of dieting, reports that Balart (with Andrews, Bethea, and Steward—all physicians from New Orleans) was actually one of the originators of the Sugar Busters diet. The diet's message, says Gilman (p. 262) is that refined sugar is "toxic" and "less sugar"—especially avoiding refined sugar and processed grains—is best.

Nordmann and colleagues (2006) conducted a meta-analysis of six studies (including 447 people) to compare low-carbohydrate with low-fat diets. Their study found substantial dropout rates: after 1 year of follow-up, up to 48% of individuals randomly assigned to low-carbohydrate diets and up to 50% of those on low-fat diets had dropped out. They also found that the low-carbohydrate diets led to greater weight loss at 6 months but not at 12-month follow-up, and that neither diet showed clear benefit in terms of cardiovascular risk factors.

A very high dropout rate (low dietary adherence) was also noted earlier by Dansinger and colleagues (2005), who sought to compare the Atkins, Ornish, Weight Watchers, and Zone diets for adherence. Their randomized study (of 160 subjects initially) relied, as usual, on self-reports of calorie intake and adherence to the diets. Those on the Atkins and Ornish diets had higher dropout rates. For those who continued in the study, the researchers found all these diets could result in weight loss, without much difference among them, at 1 year. Said Dansinger et al. (2005), "All diets achieved modest, although statistically significant, improvements in several cardiac risk factors at one year...but only a minority of individuals can sustain a high dietary adherence level."

Halton and colleagues (2006) evaluated information comparing different diets. In an article published in the *New England Journal of Medicine*, these researchers reviewed data on more than 80,000 female nurses with 20 years of follow-up to assess dietary effects on coronary artery disease. They found that diets lower in carbohydrates and higher in protein and fat were not associated with an increased risk of coronary artery disease; in fact, when the protein and fat came from vegetable sources, these diets were actually helpful in reducing the risk of coronary artery disease in the women studied. They also noted that carbohydrates with a high glycemic profile were particularly associated with an increased risk of heart disease. Further, they found that of their subjects, all of whom used food frequency questionnaires, few used the "strict version" (i.e., <20% carb intake a day) of the Atkins diet.

Gardner et al. (2007) compared the Atkins diet (severe carbohydrate restriction), the LEARN regimen (a name that stands for *lifestyle, exercise, attitudes, relation-ships, and nutrition*—this is the regimen with the greatest emphasis on behavior modification strategies), the Ornish diet (severe fat restriction), and the Zone diet (balanced proportion, in a specific formula, of carbohydrates, proteins, and fats) in a randomized 12-month study of over 300 premenopausal, nondiabetic, overweight and obese women. For obvious reasons, they called this the A to Z Weight Loss Study. It had a fairly low dropout rate of 20% at 1 year. Women on the Atkins diet, with its severe carbohydrate restriction (initially 20 g/day, then 50 g/day), actually lost more weight and, surprisingly, had better metabolic profiles than women on the other diets: lower triglyceride levels, higher high-density lipoprotein cholesterol lev-els, and even lower blood pressure. These researchers' findings differed from those of the Dansinger et al. (2005) study, and Gardner et al. (2007) suggested this may have been due to different inclusion criteria for each of the studies as well as the different dropout rates.

The Gardner et al. (2007) report, appearing in the *Journal of the American Medi-cal Association* (as had the report of the Dansinger et al. study), received considerable media coverage at the time, even though it did not discuss the actual calorie counts or provide detailed information on exercise used with any of the diets. Diet and exercise information was obtained through unannounced telephone calls to the subjects that required them to recall their food and exercise intake. The researchers did note that the Zone and LEARN groups "incorporated specific goals for energy restriction," whereas neither the Atkins nor the Ornish diet restricted calories. Gardner et al. (2007) reported that the actual weight loss for the Atkins group, after 12 months, was only just over 10 pounds (4.7 kilograms), which, for most people with a substantial weight problem, is fairly modest and somewhat disappointing. They concluded that the Atkins diet with its severe carbohydrate restriction (and hence greater fat con-tent) did not lead to substantiated adverse metabolic effects, at least at 1 year, but they also acknowledged that they did not know whether the benefits of the Atkins diet were due to its high protein content or its carbohydrate restriction.

A more recent randomized study (Miller et al. 2009) examined the weight main-tenance phase after weight stabilization with the Atkins diet (high in fat, low in carbohydrates), the South Beach diet (the Mediterranean diet), or the Ornish diet (high in carbohydrates, low in fat) in a group of normal-weight adults in their 30s. Of 26 subjects initially enrolled, nine men and nine women completed the study. The researchers reported that surprisingly few data are available to assess this long-term and extremely important phase of dieting. Their goal was to assess the impact of biochemical and physiological parameters that may have a role in cardiovascular disease with these diets. Particularly, they were curious to ascertain whether the

Atkins diet—high in saturated fats known to increase harmful LDL cholesterol levels and disturb endothelial functioning—would, over a maintenance phase, have a deleterious effect on blood lipid levels. Their study lasted 24 weeks and was divided into six different phases: each subject was exposed to each diet for 4 weeks and had a washout period (length not specified) prior to beginning the next diet trial. Weight loss was not a goal of the study. Miller et al. (2009) found that the Atkins diet yielded higher total cholesterol levels as well as higher harmful LDL levels than either the South Beach or the Ornish diet. Further, those in the Atkins phase of the study had disturbed endothelial functioning (reduced endothelial vasoreactivity). Their conclusion is that, at least after weight stabilization, the Atkins diet, with its high component of saturated fat, may not be as advantageous in terms of cardiovascular risk markers as other studies have suggested.

Sofi et al. (2008) performed a meta-analysis of 12 studies (including more than 1.5 million healthy people and lasting up to 18 years) to assess the health benefits of a Mediterranean-style diet—a diet that is low in red meat and includes olive oil as the major fat, vegetables, fish, fruits, legumes, grains, and moderate amounts of red wine with meals. These researchers found that greater adherence to this type of diet has been significantly associated with health benefits, including a decreased risk of overall mortality, cancer incidence and cancer-related mortality, and cardiovascular mortality. Further, it has been associated with a decreased incidence of both Parkinson disease and Alzheimer disease. Sofi et al. (2008) suggest that the focus on a "dietary pattern as a whole" (i.e., the way people actually eat), rather than focusing on one type of food group or nutrient, is particularly important. They do acknowledge, though, that the Mediterranean-style diet is "not a homogeneous pattern of eating."

An Israeli study (Shai et al. 2008) compared the effects of the Mediterranean diet or a low-carbohydrate diet versus a low-fat diet for 2 years on 322 overweight or moderately obese subjects (>80% men and 26 with diabetes). There were three categories: 1) low fat intake and restricted calories (1,500 cal/day for women and 1,800 cal/day for men), with 30% fat (10% from saturated fat) and no more than 300 mg of cholesterol daily; 2) a Mediterranean-style, moderate-fat diet, high in vegetables and fish and low in red meat, with olive oil as the major fat and nuts added (total of 35% dietary fat); and 3) a low-carbohydrate, nonrestricted-calorie diet with only 20 grams of carbohydrates daily initially, eventually up to 120 grams (modeled on the Atkins diet). Subjects in all three groups lost weight over the first 6 months, but subjects on the low-carbohydrate and Mediterranean-style diets lost more weight—an average of 4.7 and 4.4 kilograms, respectively—than those on the low-fat diet, who lost an average of 2.9 kilograms of weight. As is typically reported in weight loss studies, maximum weight loss occurred in the first 6 months. In this study, researchers found that both the Mediterranean-style diet and the low-carbohydrate diets "were effective alternatives" to the low-fat diet. They suggest that a low-carbohydrate diet, without calorie restriction, may be an optimal alternative for dieters who will not restrict their calorie intake.

More recently, Scarmeas et al. (2009) reported on the relationship between cognitive impairment and diet. In a study of over 1,300 people (a multiethnic and community-based population), they found that those who followed a Mediterranean-style diet were less likely to have mild cognitive decline (i.e., there was "a trend for reduced risk"), which is considered either a predictor for or a transition phase to the eventual development of Alzheimer disease, over the course of about 4.5 years (range, 0.9 to >16 years). They acknowledge that several mechanisms may be involved in this protective effect. For example, individuals not following this diet may have comorbid vascular abnormalities (e.g., diabetes, hypertension, or an abnormal lipid profile), greater oxidative stress, or even inflammatory conditions, all of which have been associated with mild cognitive impairment. In fact, the researchers report that the Mediterranean diet has been linked to lower levels of C-reactive protein and lower levels of interleukin-6, both inflammatory markers, as well as decreased glucose and insulin levels. They are aware, though, that other factors may be involved in the seemingly protective effect of this diet, including activity levels of the dieters and the so-called *healthy person bias*, namely that these people may also engage in many other healthy habits that may contribute to their cognitive functioning.

Another study, by Féart et al. (2009), found that a "high adherence" to a Mediterranean diet was associated with a slower decline on one test, the Mini-Mental State Examination (MMSE), that assessed cognitive functioning in their study of over 1,400 older adults (mean age of 75.9). Interestingly, though, three other tests of global cognitive functioning were not associated with a slower decline. The researchers defined greater adherence as "characterized by higher intake of vegetables, fruits, legumes, cereals, and fish, and particularly a high consumption of olive oil, as well as a decreased intake in meat and dairy products." The researchers speculate there may be a "window of opportunity" for this diet's beneficial effects: once a person is on the road to cognitive decline, the diet may no longer be protective and cannot reverse any previous damage done. Though there are many reasons why a Mediterranean diet may be protective, such as decreasing oxidative stress, inflammation, or vascular disease, the researchers, like those in the Scarmeas et al (2009) study, caution that those who eat a healthier diet may have, in general, an overall healthier lifestyle.

Furthermore, Mente et al. (2009) systematically reviewed the evidence worldwide (studies from the United States, Europe, and Asia for the period 1950 through June 2007, involving over 29,000 people with a median length of follow-up of 11 years) for the protective benefits of a Mediterranean-style diet on coronary heart disease. Mente et al. (2009) found "strong evidence" for the benefits of this dietary pattern (e.g., fruits, vegetables, nuts, monounsaturated fats) on the heart. These researchers also found "strong evidence" for the dangers of trans fats and foods with a high glycemic index, particularly since high-glycemic foods are associated with increased fasting triglyceride levels. Mente et al. (2009), however, caution that coronary heart disease is "a complex condition involving numerous physiologic systems, which makes it unlikely that modifying the intake of a few nutrients would alter these systems and influence clinical outcomes." They stress the importance of an overall dietary pattern, in the context of a healthy lifestyle, as essential for coronary health. Though Mente et al. (2009) do not specify what they mean by lifestyle changes, we can emphasize, as we have throughout this book, the importance of regular exercise and portion control.

RECOMMENDATIONS FOR A HEALTHY DIET

The studies on which we have reported are an infinitesimal number of those available for review. The data are often conflicting and confusing, and many researchers continue to suggest further studies. As we mentioned in Chapter 2, there are many methodological difficulties in evaluating studies on obesity. For example, some studies are conducted in the laboratory, where all food intake and weight changes are monitored carefully, but these tend to involve very few subjects and are usually conducted over a fairly short period of time. Others may be large, possibly community-based studies, over which researchers have very little control. They are at the mercy of subjects' self-reports, not only of calorie counts, foods, and even heights and weights, but also of whether the subjects are adhering to a particular protocol—and self-reports are notoriously inaccurate. Sometimes the inaccuracies may be inadvertent, but other times subjects may tell the researchers what they think the researchers want to hear. Further, researchers may not know what other behaviors their subjects are engaging in, healthy or unhealthy, or even what psychological stresses they are experiencing that may be interfering with the study.

Nevertheless, with all these inherent difficulties and confounding variables, we can offer certain recommendations at this point (summarized in Table 10–3). We emphasize that despite all the many thousands of studies, the field of weight control is still very much in its infancy, and these suggestions may not hold up over time as more research, particularly with genetic markers, enables us to be more exact in our dietary recommendations.

Any recommendations, though, must take lifestyles into account. Wansink (2006, pp. 225–234) writes of *diet danger zones*. As he says, "These are traps that catch all of us at one time or another, but most people fall into only one or two on a regular basis" (p. 225). The *meal stuffer* is the one who takes more than one helping at meals—the person who "cleans everything on [his or her] plate." The *snack grazer* is usually the nervous snacker, who "reaches for whatever food is available," whether hungry or not. The *party binger* is the one who tends to overeat at buffets or parties, that is, in situations where there is much distraction. The *restaurant indulger* is one who tends to frequent restaurants more than most and overeats in this atmosphere. The *desktop* or *dashboard diner* is a multitasker and tends to eat quickly, eating in his or her office or even while driving, and is less likely to eat a "real" meal.

Table 10–3. Principles of a healthy regimen: nothing in excess

Maintain a certain consistent range of calories per day (depends on activity level, height, frame, and weight)

Avoid fasting and very-low-calorie diets without medical supervision

Eat foods high in fiber

Maintain low fat intake: restrict intake of saturated fat found in red meat to less than 7% of calories; use olive oil as major fat in diet

Eat low-glycemic carbohydrates and avoid any processed carbohydrates

Avoid foods with chemicals, even if they are labeled "natural"

Eat high-quality, lean protein (fish, chicken, legumes, grains, nuts); non-animal protein is preferable

No more than two glasses of wine, or equivalent amount of alcohol, per day

Avoid any foods that trigger you to eat more

Eat breakfast and aim for three meals a day; eat at the same time each day and eat most food earlier in day rather than at night

Eat slowly (more chewing uses more calories and allows for fullness to develop)

Remember portion control

Monitor food intake by keeping a food diary

Weigh yourself regularly—even daily

Do aerobic exercise of at least moderate intensity ≥30 minutes each day for cardiovascular fitness and weight loss (and >1 hour to avoid regaining lost weight)

Sleep ≥6½ hours each night, but not >9 hours

Another "trap" is that food labeling can be very confusing and deceptive. For example, even knowing how much carbohydrate sweetener is in a food is not always easy. Kessler (2009, p. 103) points out that food manufacturers get around federal regulations by listing several different kinds of sweeteners separately in order to avoid having to list sugar first when it is actually the primary ingredient in a particular product. As always, let the buyer beware!

Lowe and Levine (2005), similar to Kessler, focus on our toxic food environment, where many people are chronically "eating less than they want." They suggest that the most effective way to reduce our exposure to the "perception of chronic deprivation" is not to try to convince us that we are not hungry, but rather to limit our exposure to those highly palatable foods that activate our "hedonic motivation" in the first place.

Fundamentally, the best diet, as with the best exercise, is the one a dieter will maintain as a way of life—a regimen, as Hippocrates would say—as weight control and maintenance require chronic adherence. And it is one that will fit into the dieter's lifestyle, as we see from Wansink's diet traps. As we have seen from many of the studies, the adherence factor can lead to the downfall of almost any diet. Further, some kind of regular monitoring of weight and food intake does seem an essential part of any diet, at least for most people. And support from either professionals or family and friends is crucial, particularly in the maintenance phase. (As we have noted, this phase is much less reinforcing psychologically because fewer people give encouragement beyond the initial weight loss period.) Professional groups like Weight Watchers may be particularly helpful for those who enjoy the camaraderie of fellow dieters. For those who prefer a solo approach, some structured meals daily, with portion control and food supplied (requiring less choice), can provide certain external regulation.

> "At approximately six months, weight loss begins to plateau across nearly all interventions, but with continued professional support…weight loss can be maintained."
>
> **Source: Franz et al. 2007**

Other than that, we recommend a diet that is balanced nutritionally, is high enough in calories for adequate nutrition and health, and does not put stress on our complex metabolic functioning. There seems to be nothing magical about and no scientific basis for using certain proportions of nutrients, but an extremely lopsided preference for or exclusion of one food group is not advisable. Furthermore, diets that are idiosyncratically unbalanced are much more difficult to maintain over time, particularly in our food-oriented culture.

We have learned that for most people, some calorie monitoring should be an essential part of a regimen. As Makris and Foster (2005) said, "energy in versus energy out" remains the cornerstone of obesity treatment. They also noted it is still not clear whether specific macronutrients differ in their effects on satiety and adherence. The degree to which one is sensitive to fats or to certain carbohydrates or is more satiated by protein probably varies with the individual, and a trial period of any diet may be warranted.

"Nothing in excess"—neither food nor exercise—is what Hippocrates said in the fifth century B.C. That advice cannot be improved on in the twenty-first century A.D.

REFERENCES

Adams R: Did You Ever See a Fat Squirrel? How to Eat Naturally So You'll Never Be Overweight, Never Feel Hungry. Emmaus, PA, Rodale, 1972

Agatston A: The South Beach Diet: The Delicious, Doctor-Designed, Foolproof Plan for Fast and Healthy Weight Loss. Emmaus, PA, Rodale, 2003

Ahuja KD, Robertson IK, Geraghty DP, et al: Effects of chili consumption on postprandial glucose, insulin, and energy metabolism. Am J Clin Nutr 84:63–69, 2006

American Dietetic Association: Adult weight management evidence-based nutrition practice guideline: executive summary of recommendations. 2009. Available at: http://www.adaevidencelibrary.com/topic.cfm?cat=3014. Accessed April 19, 2009.

American Psychiatric Association: Diagnostic and Statistical Manual of Mental Disorders, 4th Edition, Text Revision. Washington, DC, American Psychiatric Association, 2000

Aronne LJ: The Skinny: On Losing Weight Without Being Hungry. New York, Broadway Books, 2009

Artmann A, Petersen G, Hellgren LI, et al: Influence of dietary fatty acids on endocannabinoid and N-acylethanolamine levels in rat brain, liver and small intestine. Biochim Biophys Acta 1781:200–212, 2008

Atkins RC: Dr. Atkins' New Diet Revolution. New York, HarperCollins, 2002

Balart LA: Diet options of obesity: fad or famous? Gastroenterol Clin North Am 34:83–90, 2005

Barkeling B, Linné Y, Melin E, et al: Vision and eating behavior in obese subjects. Obes Res 11:130–134, 2003

Batterham RL, Heffron H, Kapoor S, et al: Critical role for peptide YY in protein-mediated satiation and body-weight regulation. Cell Metab 4:223–233, 2006

Beck JS: The Complete Beck Diet for Life. Birmingham, AL, Oxmoor House, 2008

Bogdan A, Bouchareb B, Touitou Y: Ramadan fasting alters endocrine and neuroendocrine circadian patterns: meal-time as a synchronizer in humans? Life Sci 68:1607–1615, 2001

Bogusky A: The 9-Inch "Diet": Exposing the BIG Conspiracy in America. New York, PowerHouse Books, 2008

Booth DA, Blair AJ, Lewis VJ, et al: Patterns of eating and movement that best maintain reduction in overweight. Appetite 43:277–283, 2004

Bray GA: Historical framework for the development of ideas about obesity, in Handbook of Obesity: Etiology and Pathophysiology, 2nd Edition. Edited by Bray GA, Bouchard C. New York, Marcel Dekker, 2004, pp 1–31

Bray GA, Paeratakul S, Popkin BM: Dietary fat and obesity: a review of animal, clinical and epidemiological studies. Physiol Behav 83:549–555, 2004

Brownell KD: The LEARN (Lifestyle, Exercise, Attitudes, Relationships, Nutrition) Program for Weight Control. Dallas, TX, American Health Publishing, 1991

Brownell KD, Marlatt GA, Lichtenstein E, et al: Understanding and preventing relapse. Am Psychol 41:765–782, 1986

Buchholz AC, Schoeller DA: Is a calorie a calorie? Am J Clin Nutr 79:899S–906S, 2004

Chandler-Laney PC, Castaneda E, Pritchett CE, et al: A history of caloric restriction induces neurochemical and behavioral changes in rats consistent with models of depression. Pharmacol Biochem Behav 87:104–114, 2007

Chapelot D, Louis-Sylvestre J: The role of orosensory factors in eating behavior as observed in humans, in Appetite and Food Intake: Behavioral and Physiological Considerations. Edited by Harris RBS, Mattes R. Boca Raton, FL, CRC Press, 2008, pp 133–162

Consumer Reports: New diet winners: we rate the diet books and plans. Plus: 8 strategies that work. Consumer Reports, June 2007. Available at: http://www.consumerreports.org/health/healthy-living/diet-nutrition/diets-dieting/diets-6-07/overview/0607_diets_ov.htm. Accessed September 16, 2009.

Cooper M: The Ultimate Cabbage Soup Diet. London, John Blake, 2003

Critser G: Fat Land: How Americans Became the Fattest People in the World. Boston, MA, Houghton Mifflin, 2003

Currie J, DellaVigna S, Moretti E, et al: The effect of fast food restaurants on obesity. NBER working paper #214721, National Bureau of Economic Research, February 2009. Available at: http://www.nber.org/papers/w14721. Accessed October 29, 2009

D'Adamo P, Whitney C: Eat Right 4 Your Type: The Individualized Diet Solution to Staying Healthy, Living Longer & Achieving Your Ideal Weight. New York, GP Putnam, 1996

Danbrot M: The New Cabbage Soup Diet. New York, St Martin's Press, 2004

Dansinger ML, Gleason JA, Griffith JL, et al: Comparison of the Atkins, Ornish, Weight Watchers, and Zone diets for weight loss and heart disease risk reduction. JAMA 293:43–53, 2005

Davis CM: Self-selection of diet by newly weaned infants: an experimental study. Am J Dis Child 36:651–679, 1928

Davis CM: Results of the self-selection of diets by young children. Can Med Assoc J 41:257–261, 1939

DeBakey ME, Gotto AM Jr, Scott LW, et al: The New Living Heart Diet. New York, Simon & Schuster, 1996

Due A, Toubro S, Skov AR, et al: Effect of normal-fat diets, either medium or high in protein, on body weight in overweight subjects: a randomized 1-year trial. Int J Obes Relat Metab Disord 28:1283–1290, 2004

Duffy VB, Bartoshuk LM: Sensory factors in feeding, in Why We Eat What We Eat: The Psychology of Eating. Edited by Capaldi ED. Washington, DC, American Psychological Association, 1996, pp 145–171

Dullo AG, Jacquet J, Girardier L: Poststarvation hyperphagia and body fat overshooting in humans: a role for feedback signals from lean and fat tissues. Am J Clin Nutr 65:717–723, 1997

Dumanovsky T, Nonas CA, Huang CY, et al: What people buy from fast-food restaurants: caloric content and menu item selection, New York City 2007. Obes 17:1369–1374, 2009

Dwyer J: Twelve popular diets: brief nutritional analyses. Psychiatr Clin North Am 1:621–628, 1978

Ebbeling CB, Garcia-Lago E, Leidig MM, et al: Altering portion sizes and eating rate to attenuate gorging during a fast food meal: effects on energy intake. Pediatrics 119:869–875, 2007

Eckel RH: The dietary approach to obesity: is it the diet or the disorder? JAMA 293:96–97, 2005

Esposito K, Giugliano D: Obesity, the metabolic syndrome, and sexual dysfunction. Int J Impot Res 17:391–398, 2005

Féart C, Samieri C, Rondeau V, et al: Adherence to a Mediterranean diet, cognitive decline, and risk of dementia. JAMA 302:638–648, 2009

Fessler DMT: The implications of starvation induced psychological changes for the ethical treatment of hunger strikers. J Med Ethics 29:243–247, 2003

Fontana L: The scientific basis of caloric restriction leading to longer life. Curr Opin Gastroenterol 25:144–150, 2009

Fontana L, Villareal DT, Weiss EP, et al; and the Washington University School of Medicine CALERIE Group: Calorie restriction or exercise: effects on coronary heart disease risk factors: a randomized, controlled trial. Am J Physiol Endocrinol Metab 293:E197–E202, 2007

Franz MJ, VanWormer JJ, Crain AL, et al: Weight-loss outcomes: a systematic review and meta-analysis of weight-loss clinical trials with a minimum 1-year follow-up. J Am Diet Assoc 107:1755–1767, 2007

Frecka JM, Mattes RD: Possible entrainment of ghrelin to habitual meal patterns in humans. Am J Physiol Gastrointest Liver Physiol 294:G699–G707, 2008

Gardner CD, Kiazand A, Alhassan S, et al: Comparison of the Atkins, Zone, Ornish, and LEARN diets for change in weight and related risk factors among overweight premenopausal women: the A to Z Weight Loss Study: a randomized trial. JAMA 297:969–977, 2007

Geier A, Schwartz M, Brownell K: "Before and after" diet advertisements escalate weight stigma. Eat Weight Disord 8:282–288, 2003

Gilman SL: Diets and Dieting: A Cultural Encyclopedia. New York, Routledge (Taylor and Francis Group), 2008

Guiliano M: French Women Don't Get Fat. New York, Knopf, 2004

Gullo SP: Thin Tastes Better. New York, Carol Southern Books, 1995

Gullo SP: The Thin Commandments: The Ten No-Fail Strategies for Permanent Weight Loss. Emmaus, PA, Rodale, 2005

Gutterson C: The Sonoma Diet. Des Moines, IA, Meredith Books, 2005

Halton TL, Hu FB: The effects of high protein diets on thermogenesis, satiety and weight loss: a critical review. J Am Coll Nutr 23:373–385, 2004

Halton TL, Willett WC, Liu S, et al: Low-carbohydrate-diet score and the risk of coronary heart disease in women. N Engl J Med 355:1991–2002, 2006

Hellerstein MK: No common energy currency: de novo lipogenesis as the road less traveled. Am J Clin Nutr 74:707–708, 2001

Heymsfield SB, van Mierlo CA, van der Knaap HC, et al: Weight management using a meal replacement strategy: meta and pooling analysis from six studies. Int J Obes Relat Metab Disord 27:537–549, 2003

Heymsfield SB, Harp JB, Reitman ML, et al: Why do obese patients not lose more weight when treated with low-calorie diets? A mechanistic perspective. Am J Clin Nutr 85:346–354, 2007

Hill JO: Understanding and addressing the epidemic of obesity: an energy balance perspective. Endocr Rev 27:750–761, 2006

Hill JO: Can a small-changes approach help address the obesity epidemic? A report of the Joint Task Force of the American Society for Nutrition, Institute of Food Technologists, and International Food Information Council. Am J Clin Nutr 89:477–484, 2009

Hill JO, Wyatt HR, Reed GW, et al: Obesity and the environment: where do we go from here? Science 299:853–855, 2003

Hippocrates: Aphorisms II, xvi, and Regimen II, xxxix, in Works, Vol IV. Translated by Jones WHS. Loeb Classical Library. Cambridge, MA, Harvard University Press, 1967, pp 113, 307

Hirsch J: Obesity: a perspective, in Recent Advances in Obesity Research. Edited by Bray GA. London, Newman, 1978, pp 1–5

Horton TJ, Drougas H, Brachey A, et al: Fat and carbohydrate overfeeding in humans: different effects on energy storage. Am J Clin Nutr 62:19–29, 1995

Hyman M: UltraMetabolism: The Simple Plan for Automatic Weight Loss. New York, Scribner, 2006

Ifland JR, Preuss HG, Marcus MT, et al: Refined food addiction: a classic substance use disorder. Med Hypotheses 72:518–526, 2009

Institute of Medicine of the National Academies: Dietary Reference Intake for Energy, Carbohydrate, Fiber, Fat, Fatty Acids, Cholesterol, Protein, and Amino Acids. Washington, DC, National Academies Press, 2008

Jahng JW, Kim JG, Kim HJ, et al: Chronic food restriction in young rats results in depression- and anxiety-like behaviors with decreased expression of serotonin reuptake transporter. Brain Res 1150:100–107, 2007

Jenkins DJ, Wolever TM, Vuksan V, et al: Nibbling versus gorging: metabolic advantages of increased meal frequency. N Engl J Med 321:929–934, 1989

Johnstone AM: Fasting—the ultimate diet? Obes Rev 8:211–222, 2007

Kalm LM, Semba RD: They starved so that others be better fed: remembering Ancel Keys and the Minnesota experiment. J Nutr 135:1347–1352, 2005

Katz DL: Competing dietary claims for weight loss: finding the forest through truculent trees. Ann Rev Public Health 26:61–88, 2005

Katz DL (with Friedman RSC): Nutrition in Clinical Practice: A Comprehensive, Evidence-Based Manual for the Practitioner, 2nd Edition. Philadelphia, PA, Wolters Kluwer Health/Lippincott Williams & Wilkins, 2008

Kessler DA: The End of Overeating: Taking Control of the Insatiable American Appetite. Emmaus, PA, Rodale, 2009

Keys A: The caloric requirement of adult man. Nutr Abstr Rev 19:1–10, 1949

Keys A, Brozek J, Henschel A, et al: The Biology of Human Starvation, Vols 1 and 2. Minneapolis, University of Minnesota Press, 1950

Kolata G: Rethinking Thin: The New Science of Weight Loss—and the Myths and Realities of Dieting. New York, Farrar, Straus & Giroux, 2007

Koopmans HS: Experimental studies on the control of food intake, in Handbook of Obesity: Etiology and Pathophysiology, 2nd Edition. Edited by Bray GA, Bouchard C. New York, Marcel Dekker, 2004, pp 373–425

Lichtenstein AH, Van Horn L: Very low fat diets. Circulation 98:935–939, 1998

Lowe MR, Levine AS: Eating motives and the controversy over dieting: eating less than needed versus less than wanted. Obes Res 13:797–806, 2005

Makris AP, Foster GD: Dietary approaches to the treatment of obesity. Psychiatr Clin North Am 28:117–139, 2005

Martin CK, Anton SD, Han H, et al: Examination of cognitive function during six months of calorie restriction: results of a randomized controlled trial. Rejuvenation Res 10:179–190, 2007

Masheb RM, Grilo CM: Eating patterns and breakfast consumption in obese patients with binge eating disorder. Behav Res Ther 44:1545–1553, 2006

Mattson MP: Energy intake, meal frequency, and health: a neurobiological perspective. Annu Rev Nutr 25:237–260, 2005a

Mattson MP: The need for controlled studies of the effects of meal frequency on health. Lancet 365:1978–1980, 2005b

Matz J, Frankel E: Beyond a Shadow of a Diet: The Therapist's Guide to Treating Compulsive Eating. New York, Brunner-Routledge, 2004

Mazel J, Wyatt M, Sokol A: The New Beverly Hills Diet. Deerfield Beach, FL, Health Communications, 1996

Melanson K, Dwyer J: Popular diets for treatment of overweight and obesity, in Handbook of Obesity Treatment. Edited by Wadden TA, Stunkard AJ. New York, Guilford, 2002, pp 249–282

Mente A, de Koning L, Shannon HS, et al: A systematic review of the evidence supporting a causal link between dietary factors and coronary heart disease. Arch Intern Med 169:659–669, 2009

Miller M, Beach V, Sorkin JD, et al: Comparative effects of three popular diets on lipids, endothelial function, and C-reactive protein during weight maintenance. J Am Diet Assoc 109:713–717, 2009

Minehira K, Vega N, Vidal H, et al: Effect of carbohydrate overfeeding on whole body macronutrient metabolism and expression of lipogenic enzymes in adipose tissue of lean and overweight humans. Int J Obes Relat Metab Disord 28:1291–1298, 2004

Moyad MA: Fad diets and obesity—part III: a rapid review of some of the more popular low-carbohydrate diets. Urol Nurs 24:442–445, 2004

Naleid AM, Grimm JW, Kessler DA, et al: Deconstructing the vanilla milkshake: the dominant effect of sucrose on self-administration of nutrient-flavor mixtures. Appetite 50:128–138, 2008

Newbold RR, Padilla-Banks E, Snyder RJ, et al: Developmental exposure to endocrine disruptors and the obesity epidemic. Reprod Toxicol 23:290–296, 2007

Nordmann AJ, Nordmann A, Briel M, et al: Effects of low-carbohydrate vs low-fat diets on weight loss and cardiovascular risk factors: a meta-analysis of randomized controlled trials. Arch Intern Med 166:285–293, 2006

Ogden CL, Carroll MD, Flegal KM: High body mass for age among U.S. children and adolescents, 2003–2006. JAMA 299:2401–2405, 2008

Ogden CL, Carroll MD, Curtin LR, et al: Prevalence of overweight and obesity in the U.S., 1999–2004. JAMA 295:1549–1555, 2006

Ornish D, Brown SH: Eat More, Weight Less: Dr. Dean Ornish's Program for Losing Weight Safely While Eating Abundantly. New York, HarperCollins, 2002

Otsuka R, Tamakoshi K, Yatsuya H, et al: Eating fast leads to obesity: findings based on self-administered questionnaires among middle-aged Japanese men and women. J Epidemiol 16:117–124, 2006

Oxford English Dictionary, 2nd Edition, s.v. "diet." Oxford, UK, Oxford University Press, 1989

Paddon-Jones D, Westman E, Mattes RD, et al: Protein, weight management, and satiety. Am J Clin Nutr 87:1558S–1561S, 2008

Palesty JA, Dudrick SJ: The Goldilocks paradigm of starvation and refeeding. Nutr Clin Pract 21:147–154, 2006

Pollan M: In Defense of Food: An Eater's Manifesto. New York, Penguin Press, 2008

Precope J: Hippocrates on Diet and Hygiene. London, Zeno Publishers, 1952

Pritikin N: Pritikin Program for Diet and Exercise. New York, Bantam Doubleday Dell, 1985

Redman LM, Heilbronn LK, Martin CK, et al: Effect of calorie restriction with or without exercise on body composition and fat distribution. J Clin Endocrinol Metab 92:865–872, 2007

Rich F: Herbert Hoover Lives. The New York Times, Sunday Opinion, February 1, 2009

Rippe JM: Weight Watchers Weight Loss That Lasts: Break Through the 10 Big Diet Myths, Hoboken, NJ, Wiley, 2005

Rodin J: Environmental factors in obesity. Psychiatr Clin North Am 1:581–592, 1978

Sabaté J: Nut consumption and body weight. Am J Clin Nutr 78:647S–650S, 2003

Sacks FM, Bray GA, Carey VJ, et al: Comparison of weight-loss diets with different compositions of fat, protein, and carbohydrates. N Engl J Med 360:859–873, 2009

Scarmeas N, Stern Y, Mayeaux R, et al: Mediterranean diet and mild cognitive impairment. Arch Neurol 66:216–225, 2009

Schlosser E: Fast Food Nation. New York, Harper, 2005

Seagle HM, Strain GW, Makris A, et al: Position of the American Dietetic Association: weight management. J Am Diet Assoc 109:330–346, 2009

Sears B, Kotz D: A Week in the Zone: A Quick Course in the Healthiest Diet for You. New York, HarperCollins, 2004

Shai I, Schwarzfuchs D, Henkin Y, et al: Weight loss with a low-carbohydrate, Mediterranean, or low-fat diet. JAMA 359:229–241, 2008

Simpson SJ, Raubenheimer D: Obesity: the protein leverage hypothesis. Obes Rev 6:133–142, 2005

Sitzman K: Eating breakfast helps sustain weight loss. AAOHN J 54:136, 2006

Sofi F, Cesari F, Abbate R, et al: Adherence to Mediterranean diet and health status: meta-analysis. BMJ 337:a1344, 2008

Speakman JR, Hambly C: Starving for life: what animal studies can and cannot tell us about the use of caloric restriction to prolong human lifespan. J Nutr 137:1078–1086, 2007

Steward HL, Bethea MC, Andrews SS, et al: Sugar Busters! New York, Ballantine, 1965

Stewart J: The Daily Show with Jon Stewart, episode 14091. Executive Producer Jon Stewart. July 2, 2009

Stein J: Notes on a food-free diet: an intrepid reporter's firsthand account of how he survived for 48 hours on nothing but a liquid mixture of lemons, cayenne pepper and maple syrup. Time Magazine, June 11, 2007, p 82

Stillman IM: The Doctor's Quick Weight Loss Diet. New York, Dell Publishing, 1968

Strychar I: Diet in the management of weight loss. Can Med Assoc J 174: 56–63, 2006

Super Size Me (documentary film). Written, produced, and directed by Spurlock M. Kathbur Pictures, 2004

Tarnower H, Baker SS: The Complete Scarsdale Medical Diet: Plus Dr. Tarnower's Lifetime Keep-Slim Program. New York, Bantam Books, 1982

Tataranni PA, Ravussin E: Energy metabolism and obesity, in Handbook of Obesity Treatment. Edited by Wadden TA, Stunkard, AJ. New York, Guilford, 2002, pp 42–72

Thompson DL, Ahrens MJ: The Grapefruit Solution: Lower Your Cholesterol, Lose Weight and Achieve Optimal Health With Nature's Wonder Fruit! Great Falls, VA, Linx Corp, 2004

Trasande L, Cronk C, Durkin M, et al: Environment and obesity in the National Children's Study. Environ Health Perspect 117:159–166, 2009

Trowman R, Dumville JC, Hahn S, et al: A systematic review of the effects of calcium supplementation on body weight. Br J Nutr 95:1033–1038, 2006

Van Itallie TB: Dietary approaches to the treatment of obesity. Psychiatr Clin North Am 1:609–619, 1978

Varady KA, Hellerstein MK: Alternate-day fasting and chronic disease prevention: a review of human and animal trials. Am J Clin Nutr 86:7–13, 2007

Varady KA, Hellerstein MK: Do calorie restriction or alternate-day fasting regimens modulate adipose tissue physiology in a way that reduces chronic disease risk? Nutr Rev 66:333–342, 2008

Wadden TA, Osei S: The treatment of obesity: an overview, in Handbook of Obesity Treatment. Edited by Wadden TA, Stunkard AJ. New York, Guilford, 2002, pp 229–248

Wadden TA, Womble LG, Stunkard AJ, et al: Psychosocial consequences of obesity and weight loss, in Handbook of Obesity Treatment. Edited by Wadden TA, Stunkard AJ. New York, Guilford, 2002, pp 144–169

Wansink B: Mindless Eating: Why We Eat More Than We Think. New York, Bantam Books, 2006

Wansink B, Chandon P: Can "low-fat" nutrition labels lead to obesity? J Mark Res 43:605–617, 2006

Wansink B, Van Ittersum K: Portion size me: downsizing our consumption norms. J Am Diet Assoc 107:1103–1106, 2007

Weigle DS, Breen PA, Matthys CC, et al: A high-protein diet induces sustained reductions in appetite, ad libitum caloric intake, and body weight despite compensatory changes in diurnal plasma leptin and ghrelin concentrations. Am J Clin Nutr 82:41–48, 2005

Weiss EP, Holloszy JO: Improvements in body composition, glucose tolerance, and insulin action induced by increasing energy expenditure or decreasing energy intake. J Nutr 137:1087–1090, 2007

Westerterp-Plantenga MS, Lejeune MP, Nijs I, et al: High protein intake sustains weight maintenance after body weight loss in humans. Int J Obes Relat Metab Disord 28:57–64, 2004

Willett WC: Dietary fat plays a major role in obesity: no. Obes Rev 3:59–68, 2002

Wing RR: Weight cycling in humans: a review of the literature. Ann Behav Med 14:113–119, 1992

Wolf N: The Beauty Myth: How Images of Beauty Are Used Against Women. New York, Anchor/Doubleday, 1992

World Health Organization: Obesity and Overweight. Fact sheet #311, September 2006. Available at: http://www.who.int/mediacentre/factsheets/fs311/en/index.html. Accessed November 3, 2009.

Wyatt HR, Grunwald GK, Mosca CL, et al: Long-term weight loss and breakfast in subjects in the National Weight Control Registry. Obes Res 10:78–82, 2002

Zemel MB: Role of calcium and dairy products in energy partitioning and weight management. Am J Clin Nutr 79:907S–912S, 2004

11

PSYCHOLOGICAL TREATMENT STRATEGIES AND WEIGHT

*The management of obesity is notoriously a frustrating business....But however
we rate the emotional factor in the scale of the causes of obesity, it is clear that
the successful management of obesity demands awareness of the psychological
situation. Plenty of patients insist they want to reduce, know that calorie
imbalance is the problem, understand the rudiments of calorie values, of food and
exercise, and still cannot, or at least do not, reduce. Obviously, psychological as
well as dietetic problems must be solved.*

Ancel Keys (1965)

OUR PSYCHOLOGICAL RELATIONSHIP TO WEIGHT AND FOOD

As we have said, there is no specific physical sign or symptom, other than excess
adipose tissue, that is characteristic of everyone with a weight problem. It is likely
that we should really speak of *obesities* plural, chronic disorders of varying severity that may have multiple physiological and genetic etiologies and must be seen
within a multidimensional framework that includes environmental influences. It is
very probable, for example, that a person with class 3 obesity (morbid obesity; i.e.,
with a body mass index [BMI] value of $\geq 40 \text{ kg/m}^2$) has a very different disorder than
someone who has trouble losing those extra 10 pounds.

As we have also noted, researchers have not found one personality type or psychiatric diagnosis characteristic of everyone who is either overweight or obese. In other
words, there is no unique obese personality (Collins and Ricciardelli 2005, p. 305;
Hirsch 2003; Stunkard 1958). Overweight or obesity itself is essentially categorized as

a medical condition and thus would be classified on DSM-IV-TR Axis III (American Psychiatric Association 2000); it is neither an eating disorder nor any other Axis I or II diagnosis, for that matter. Particularly in the United States, in a culture that values thinness, people with weight problems may have considerable psychological distress. Their distress may be due either to a concomitant psychiatric disorder (there is a high rate of comorbidity with depressive or anxiety disorders; personality disorders; eating disorders; and body image disorders) or to issues of self-esteem related to the stigma and discrimination these patients experience, subtly or overtly, as a result of their excessive weight (see Chapter 6, "Psychiatric Disorders and Weight"). Often a person's daily weight on a scale can determine mood for the entire day, as if that number had certain inordinate, magical significance by itself. For some dieters, the reading on the scale is like receiving a failing report card, even when they gain only a pound or a fraction of a pound.

Though no psychopathologies are specific to those with weight problems, there are subgroups within the obese population. For example, Friedman et al. (2002) make the distinction between those who seek treatment for weight loss and those who do not: treatment seekers are more apt to be depressed and have other psychiatric symptoms, are more likely to binge eat, and are more apt to have dissatisfaction with their body. These researchers define *body image* as "an individual's psychological experience of the appearance and function" of his or her body. As such, it is "one aspect of an individual's mental representation of him/herself" and includes both perceptual aspects (e.g., body size) and aspects of attitudes (e.g., how one feels, behaves, and thinks about one's body). And when treatment seekers with a weight problem also have body image issues, they are more likely to have low self-esteem and depression. Friedman et al. (2002) studied 110 people (80 women and 30 men) to assess the connection between psychological distress (as measured by levels of depression and self-esteem) and obesity in those who seek treatment. In their study, unlike some others with more diverse populations, they did find that the more obese the person, the more likely he or she was to have psychological distress. These researchers argue not only for a thorough evaluation of body image dissatisfaction in those seeking treatment but also that this should be a target of intervention efforts. They suggest that body image, at least in their sample, "played a central role in psychological outcome and treatment adherence," but the researchers noted that body image distress may be "quite population specific." For example, those who present for "costly residential treatment" for their obesity may be "particularly sensitive" to the impact of their weight "on their social and personal outcomes" (Friedman et al. 2002).

Other studies, as well, support the notion that there may be an underlying psychological basis in some patients that exacerbates their tendency, genetic or otherwise, toward obesity. For example, Felitti and Williams (1998), in a study of 190 patients with morbid obesity who were on a very-low-calorie diet (weight loss of >100 pounds), found that most of the patients had experienced depression and traumatic life events. They also noted that success or failure in weight loss maintenance "was predicted by adverse family experiences, including spousal alcoholism" (Felitti and Williams 1998, p. 17). But the translations of these findings to the psychological treatment of obesity have not been as practical and convincing.

Though there are many different etiologies for overweight and obesity, most involve eating more calories than are expended. From the time of early childhood, people develop very complicated emotional responses toward eating, often related to how our families dealt with food. And unlike other substances such as alcohol or other drugs that may involve impulse control or even addiction, we obviously can never completely give up food.

Lowe and Butryn (2007) have noted that there is "substantial variability" in how much people actually think about food "even when eating is not imminent or underway." Their research group has devised the Power of Food Scale (PFS), a 21-item questionnaire that rates (on a 5-point scale) people's preoccupation with and susceptibility to food (e.g. thoughts, motivations, feelings). Their scale, particularly relevant in our current climate that encourages eating and even makes food abundantly "psychologically available" so much of the time, does not focus on actual food intake or even overeating. Rather, it has items such as "I find myself thinking about food even when I am not physically hungry" or "If I see or smell food I like, I get a powerful urge to have some." More recently, Lowe et al. (2009) have found their Power of Food Scale has internal consistency and test-retest reliability. The researchers suggest that their scale may have a place in evaluation preoperatively as well as postoperatively in those patients about to undergo bariatric surgery. (For more on bariatric surgery, see Chapter 12, "Pharmacological and Surgical Treatments for Weight.")

Many of our preferences and aversions for certain foods stem from our childhood experiences. So-called comfort foods are often those we came to associate with the warmth and love of special people or special situations in our lives. Foods can be used not only as comfort, but also as *reward* (e.g., "If you do well on your report card, I will take you for ice cream"), *punishment* ("If you don't eat all your lunch, you won't be able to go play"), or even *guilt* ("People are starving in Europe. How can you not finish all your food?") (Wansink 2006, p. 176).

We also all have genetic predispositions regarding tastes. For example, in the first few hours of life babies show different facial expressions for sugar (relaxation of the facial muscles and sucking) as opposed to bitter substances (grimacing) (Mennella and Beauchamp 1996, p. 90). And some people are supertasters, more sensitive genetically to bitter substances (Duffy and Bartoshuk 1996, pp. 160–161). Even the root of our word *disgust* comes from the word for taste. Also, we use words like *honey* or *sweetie* as terms of endearment, or an expression like *apple of his eye* to express a special relationship.

And think how our English language uses the word *tongue*. Our tongue is both for talking and eating, but Kass (1999, p. 81) points out these usages: we learn "to speak the mother tongue; things hard to say are tongue-twisters; those who are speechless are tongue-tied." And we use the word to express "duplicity and lying (forked tongue), verbal assault (tongue-lashing), disrespect ('Hold your tongue') humor and irony (tongue in cheek); eloquence (golden tongued), mystery (speak in tongues), diffidence or surprise ('Cat's got your tongue')." For Kass, "the human tongue, like the human mouth, bespeaks all aspects" of our humanity (Kass 1999, p. 81).

Rozin (1996, p. 235) makes the point that for humans, our meals are often part of social occasions such that "food is a very social entity…a form of social exchange" or even a social instrument (p. 244) that involves three principles: 1) the importance of the mouth as the gateway to the body; 2) the concept of "you are what you eat"; and 3) the *law of contagion,* that is, "once in contact, always in contact" (Rozin 1996, pp. 244–245). This law of contagion, typical of more primitive beliefs, "operates clearly among Western, educated adults." For Rozin, this concept is important because "it links the human preparers or handlers of food to the eaters" such that we tend to value or enjoy food or clothing that has been prepared or tasted or worn by someone we value. On the contrary, we tend to reject something prepared or worn by someone "unsavory" (Rozin 1996, p. 245). Park et al. (2007), in fact, studied how people, particularly those who are germ phobic and fear infection, have more negative and prejudicial feelings toward obese people, as if the obese literally carry infection. That certain kinds of obesity may in fact be spread by viral infection, as we have noted (see "Infectious Agents and Weight Gain" section in Chapter 7, "Medical Conditions and Weight"), of course does not help matters (Whigham et al. 2006).

PSYCHOLOGICAL TREATMENT MODALITIES FOR WEIGHT

Because weight problems are chronic, any treatment, psychological or medical, must take into account the chronic and even relapsing nature of these disorders. Bean et al. (2008) summarize the three major treatment modalities for patients with weight problems based on recommendations from the National Institutes of Health: behavioral, pharmacological, and surgical. Those with BMI values of 25 kg/m^2 or greater should have a program of behavior modification that includes diet, exercise, and behavioral therapy. When a person's BMI value is 30 kg/m^2 or higher (or ≥ 27 kg/m^2 if the patient has weight-related comorbidity or has not responded to a course of behavioral therapy), pharmacotherapy is added to the behavioral therapy. But if the BMI value exceeds 40 kg/m^2 (≥ 35 kg/m^2 when there are serious comorbid medical conditions), bariatric surgery is the treatment of choice. Whatever the treatment modality, if patients do not modify their eating habits and exercise routine, they regain their lost weight over time. As we noted in Chapter 6 ("Psychiatric Disorders and Weight"), many patients with weight problems may not have an official eating disorder but they may have disordered patterns of eating, among their myriad other physical symptoms. Many of those whose eating habits (and calorie consumption) require substantial modification may experience *dieting depression* (Stunkard 1957; Stunkard and Rush 1974) or even more severe psychological symptoms (Bruch 1952) (see Chapter 6).

As a result, psychological treatment strategies should have at least an adjunct role (and sometimes a major role) at any level of overweight or obesity. These psychological strategies may range from self-help groups and programs for behavioral modification to more formal psychotherapy. These strategies, although they are not necessarily curative, are useful to address patients' feelings and conflicts about eating, food, exercise, and health in general, as well as their feelings about body image and self-esteem, issues relating to weight loss specifically, and issues dealing with weight maintenance over time.

Psychotherapeutic treatments—various forms of psychotherapy or psychoanalysis—for the management of weight and eating disorders have been around for years. Stunkard (1958), for example, emphasized what he called the "non-specific factor" in the treatment of obesity, and to him the psychology of the doctor-patient relationship was important. Stunkard went as far as to say that the treatment of obesity would be more successful if physicians concerned themselves less specifically with the patient's obesity and more with the patient him- or herself. The goal of psychotherapeutic treatments, whether related to weight problems specifically or other symptoms, is to help patients access the roots of their problems and conflicts. These conflicts may be conscious but more commonly they are neither conscious nor immediately obvious. Some psychological treatment strategies offer direct encouragement and support whereas others aim to help patients bring about actual changes in their feelings, thoughts, and behaviors. As far back as 1986 there were more than 400 types of psychotherapy available in the United States (Karasu 1986). The types of therapy discussed in this section are those most commonly practiced in this country. Patients, in consultation with an expert, need to find the type of therapy that best suits their individual needs.

The Psychodynamic Therapies

The psychodynamic (i.e., psychoanalytic) approaches, of which there are four primary types—drive psychology, ego psychology, object relations, and self psychology—are geared to making structural changes in the patient's mind. These approaches share the basic stance that early development influences later psychology, although they vary in emphasis on the developmental cause leading to psychopathology (Karasu 1994). Table 11–1 outlines the major points of each of the four types of psychodynamic therapies discussed in this chapter.

Fonagy and Target (2009, pp. 4–6) cite eight assumptions as central to psychodynamic therapy today. They advise that although these assumptions are not unique to the psychodynamic approach, it is unlikely that all eight would be adopted by other treatment modes. The assumptions are:

Table 11–1. Four types of psychodynamic therapies			
	Drive psychology	**Ego psychology**	**Object relations**	**Self psychology**
Theorists	S. Freud	S. Freud A. Freud H. Hartmann	M. Klein W.R.D. Fairbairn O. Kernberg	H. Kohut
Traditional diagnoses	Neuroses and mild personality disturbances	Severe personality disturbance	Mild borderline personality and narcissistic disorders	Severe borderline personality and narcissistic disorders
Basic problem	Structural conflict	Ego defect	Object relations conflict	Self-deficiency
Major maturational issues	Sexuality; competition; formation of ideals and gender identity	Socialization mastery	Separation; individuation; formation of object constancy	Attachment; dependency; formation of self-identity

Source.   Adapted from Karasu TB: "A Developmental Metatheory of Psychopathology." *American Journal of Psychotherapy* 48:581–599, 1994.

1. Assumption of psychological causation

2. Assumption of limitations of consciousness and the influence of unconscious mental states

3. Assumption of internal representations of interpersonal relationships

4. Assumption of ubiquity of psychological conflict

5. Assumption of psychic defenses

6. Assumption of complex meanings

7. Assumption of emphasis on the therapeutic relationship

8. Assumption of the validity of a developmental perspective

The Freudian School (Drive Theory)

Sigmund Freud (1856–1939) was a neurologist by training, but when confounded and inspired by patients whose symptoms were not cured by treatment of the physical, he turned to the notion of curing symptoms by addressing mental causation. Freud credited his inspiration to Josef Breuer, a medical colleague, who was attempting to trace patients' "hysterical" symptoms back to their origins through *psycho-analysis*—a word chosen to reflect the work of chemists who isolated single compounds (Karasu and Karasu 2009, p. 2746). This oldest and most traditional school of psychodynamic therapy is geared toward the exploration of childhood conflicts, drives, and defenses that cause the formation of symptoms and character pathologies. For Freud, psychoanalysis was a "procedure for the investigation of mental processes which are almost inaccessible in any other way," as well as a treatment method and a psychological theory—"a new scientific discipline"—of mental functioning (Freud 1923/1955, p. 235).

> Drive theory–oriented psychotherapy may be considered if the obesity is a manifestation of the patient's intrapsychic conflicts.

Freud espoused the idea that during infancy and early childhood, we advance through states of psychosexual (i.e., libidinal) development and if deprived or overstimulated during any of these stages, we might find our psychological and physical health likewise impaired. The unresolved psychic (i.e., psychological) conflicts resulted in neuroses.

As a means of helping a patient and freeing him or her from neurotic conflicts, Freud envisioned a type of talking therapy in which the patient freely explores and describes *all* thoughts, feelings, experiences, no matter how painful, frightening, or embarrassing—a technique dubbed *free association*. Through this exploration, the patient gains insight into his or her psyche and is equipped to resolve issues in the present. Lynn and Vaillant (1998) summarized three recommendations Freud felt were imperative, in addition to the free flow of information, regarding the analyst's behavior in relation to the individual who was being analyzed. The first is anonymity. The analyst should never reveal emotions or reactions to the patient's disclosures or discuss the analyst's own experiences. Second, the analyst is to remain neutral. In other words, although retaining an empathic role, the analyst should neither give opinions on the patient's associations nor be drafted into the role of guru or teacher (Nemiah 1984, p. 325). Third, the analyst must retain patient confidentiality. A core feature of Freud's psychoanalytic process is transference, the unconscious projection of a past experience or relationship with one person by the patient onto the therapist, who then acts as a bare stage on which the play of the patient's life is reviewed (Ursano et al. 2008, pp. 1182–1183).

To facilitate a free flow of his or her thoughts, the analysand, in a typical psychoanalytic session, lies on a couch, with the analyst out of sight. Although the analyst encourages the exploration of feelings and thoughts and may clarify a point, he or she often remains silent, listening for patterns or distortions in the analysand's repertoire of memories that will be mined further in the analysis (Nemiah 1984, p. 326). Originally Freud met with his patients 6 times per week for an hour at each visit. Later in his career, to make room for more patients, Freud shortened his sessions to the classic "50-minute hour" and saw his patients 5 days per week.

Over the years, some psychoanalysts began conducting psychoanalysis 4 days per week (Nemiah 1984, p. 325). More recently, the International Psychoanalytical Association has even sanctioned the use of 3 sessions per week for the psychoanalytic technique.

Patient populations have evolved over the years from the kinds of patients Freud saw in his clinical practice in Vienna. For practical and even financial reasons, psychodynamically oriented analysts may see patients in psychotherapy with a frequency of once or twice per week. Patients are less likely to use the psychoanalytic couch and more likely to discuss present concerns in their daily life, including issues related to eating and weight, rather than focusing on their childhood memories with the typical analytic pendulum swinging from past to present. Their relationship with the therapist, though, remains an important part of the therapy. (For a discussion of the differences between psychoanalysis and psychotherapy, see Karasu and Karasu 2009, pp. 2761–2771.)

One of the first therapists to deal psychotherapeutically with issues of weight and eating disorders was Hilde Bruch in the 1950s and 1960s. Bruch (1970) conducted psychotherapy with patients who had eating disorders, and particularly those with anorexia nervosa. She took issue with Freud's view that instincts are inborn: she believed, for example, that hunger awareness is not innately present at birth, but rather "develops, accurately or distortedly, through reciprocal transactional feedback patterns of experience" primarily with caretakers who feed the infant (Bruch 1969). She noted that *hunger* has many meanings, one of which is a "physiological state of severe food deprivation, starvation, or widespread famine." But it also denotes a psychological experience involving "the complex, unpleasant, and compelling sensation" someone feels when deprived of food, as well as denoting "a symbolic expression of a state of need in general" (Bruch 1969). Bruch believed that many of her patients, through "incorrect and confusing early learning," were not able to differentiate "hunger—the urge to eat—from signals of bodily discomfort that had nothing to do with food deprivation," but rather with emotional tension. In fact, she thought that "people show great differences in the accuracy of recognizing and conceptualizing bodily needs," and she believed that food itself had many symbolic meanings, including an unsatisfied wish for love or even a substitute for sexual gratification (Bruch 1969).

Ego Psychology

Within the realm of psychoanalysis, but differing in perspective from classical Freudian drive theory, ego psychology focuses on the response (or lack thereof) to stressors. In this view, explored in depth by Anna Freud and Heinz Hartmann, the ego—the negotiator between the drives of id and the over-principled conscience of the superego—contains unconscious defense mechanisms that enable us to adapt to conflicts. These defenses have evolved to keep repressed impulses out of conscious awareness. But "unlike unconscious id impulses...unconscious ego defenses gain nothing from being exposed. Their unobtrusive, seamless presence in the patient's psychic life is perfectly acceptable (ego syntonic) to the patient; they often function as a central feature of the patient's larger personality organization" (Mitchell and Black 1995, p. 26).

> Ego psychology may be considered if the individual's ego needs strengthening to develop adaptive defenses against self-indulgence.

Early work on the function of ego by Anna Freud in the 1930s delved further into how the ego facilitates defenses that enable the individual to function in the world (see Chapter 4, "The Psychology of the Eater," on defenses). Heinz Hartmann moved forward with Anna Freud's concept, giving the ego a larger, more independent role in behavior. He stipulated that not only did the ego function as negotiator of the id's drives, it also worked independently to adapt to the environment. To Hartmann, when aggressive drives or instincts overwhelm the ego, the individual encounters problem behaviors and psychosis.

The role of the therapist in ego psychology mirrors that of the drive theory therapist as an observer–interpreter who remains objective, neutral, and relatively anonymous in the clinical situation (Buckley et al. 2006).

For the ego psychologist, the infantile deprivations and/or overstimulations discussed by Sigmund Freud lead to an arrest in ego development, hampering the individual's ability to master inner conflicts. Therefore, unlike the goal of psychoanalysis in drive theory, the goal in ego theory is not to resolve the source of conflict, but rather to strengthen the ego's capacity to cope and adapt. The therapist, for example, might assist the patient in developing the ego to negotiate the inner conflicts and external realities that may contribute to dysfunctional eating patterns.

Object Relations

The ego psychology school continued to evolve, moving the cause of psychopa-thologies from the idea of a maladapted negotiator of instincts to the representation of self (the ego) and its relationships with objects (i.e., people; usually caretakers) or a drive. This school posits that an individual carries not only instincts, but also cer-tain internal dramas that develop in early childhood in response to the caregiver and become more complex as the child grows. The individual enacts one or more of all these roles in the drama of life.

> Object relations therapy may be considered if the obesity is a manifestation of the patient's family dramas.

The object relations school does not dis-pense completely with the drive/libido concept, but emphasizes its role in the person's relation-ship. In object relations theory, the aim of the instinctual energy is not to relieve ten-sion as Freud conceptualized, but to satisfy the basic human need to relate. Melanie Klein, one of the progenitors of object relations theory, viewed pathology as focused "self-destructive and persistent behaviors," building on Sigmund Freud's idea of a self-destructive death drive. There are two positions of mental function that the indi-vidual may adopt in response to the caregiver: 1) the paranoid-schizoid, in which the individual holds an emotionally immature worldview, separating all into opposites of black and white, good and bad, and 2) the depressive, in which the individual holds a more mature worldview that is interrelated and balanced (Fonagy and Target 2009, pp. 16–18). W. R. D. Fairbairn in the 1950s, like Melanie Klein, postulated that the primary drive is not to derive pleasure, but to search for an object to satisfy needs (Beattie 2003).

One of the most important theorists who came from the theoretical perspec-tive of the object relations school is Otto Kernberg, who has focused on treating patients with borderline personality disorder (Clarkin et al. 2006; Kernberg 1983). These patients are characterized by symptoms that include a fluctuating sense of self, tremendous fears of abandonment, a pattern of unstable personal relation-ships with a tendency to devalue and idealize, strong feelings of rage, and recurrent self-destructive feelings and actions (e.g., cutting, suicidal threats and gestures). Patients with these symptoms often have concomitant disorders of impulse control, including disordered patterns of eating, overt eating disorders, and substance abuse disorders, as well as symptoms of anxiety and depression (DSM-IV-TR; American Psychiatric Association 2000). More recently, Kernberg has focused on a therapy that has grown out of the object relations school, *transference-based psychotherapy*, that is suitable and effective for patients with borderline personality disorder (Clar-kin et al. 2007).

The goal of object relations therapy is to free the person from the constraints of an internalized pathological relationship. Those who carry such a relationship from childhood into adult life may find the object relationship–oriented approach right for them. In this mode of psychotherapy, the therapist provides the patient with a real and corrective emotional experience as an alternative to an early negative developmental experience. The therapist, the caregiver in the clinical situation, helps the patient experience emotions that were lacking in the child-caregiver relationship. Frequency of sessions varies.

Self Psychology

Self psychologists believe that the most fundamental essence of an individual's need is to organize his or her psyche into a cohesive configuration. In the mid twentieth century, psychoanalyst Heinz Kohut developed the theory of self psychology from his work with patients with narcissistic personality disorder. Kohut coined the term *selfobject* (though, early on in his writings, the word appeared as "self-object"). This concept describes how an individual perceives another person in relation to how this other serves the patient. Experiences, especially early in life with parents, either nourish or starve an individual's emotional and physical needs. From these experiences, the individual either develops a healthy cohesive sense of self, in which he or she is cohesive and able

> Self psychology may be considered if the individual has not yet developed a cohesive configuration of the self and if obesity is a breakdown product of this lack of a crystallized self.

to develop as a fully functioning individual, or else develops a self that is depleted, in which case the individual attempts through other people to gain cohesion and the self-esteem needed to function in life. This sometimes leads a person with a depleted self to use drugs to fill a gap in the psyche (Fonagy and Target 2009, pp. 20–22). Likewise, those with a depleted self might also turn to food to fill this psychological void. Fonagy and Target summarize Kohut's vision of self: a) the cohesive self is a goal to be attained, as opposed to there being a self that changes over time; b) the enfeebled self (to whom the selfobject has typically failed to attune emotionally) turns defensively toward pleasure aims (drives); and c) anxiety is primarily the self's experience of a defect or lack of continuity (Fonagy and Target 2009, pp. 20–22).

Self psychology was one of the first psychodynamic therapies to place an emphasis on the importance of the empathy a therapist has for a patient. Unlike the Freudian style of therapy described previously, in self psychology the therapist provides an empathic atmosphere to foster psychological development. The goal here is to help crystallize a patient's sense of self rather than to provide insight per se. Here, the therapist carries an even greater significance than in many other approaches because part of the reorganization of the patient's mind to provide a cohesive self occurs by the transmission of the self from the therapist. But as in the Freudian position, the therapist is abstinent and "does not, for example, affirm the grandiosity of the patient, but rather acknowledge[s] from within the understandable needs of the patient to feel grandiose" (Bachar et al. 1999).

If a patient's self is not fully formed, therapy of the self psychology–oriented school is worth consideration. Frequency of sessions varies.

Interpersonal Therapy

Initially used for treating depression, interpersonal therapy is also one of the newest therapies—manualized, standardized, and well researched. It was developed in the 1980s by Gerald Klerman and Myrna Weissman, with theoretical bases sprung from Harry Stack Sullivan's concept of social psychiatry and humans as social creatures; Adolf Meyer's theory of patient experiences' effects on psychopathology; and John Bowlby's attachment theory. Interpersonal therapy addresses the individual's problem in the broader context of family. Interpersonal therapy places emphasis on relationships occurring in the context of the patient's pathology; for example, it views depression as having three components: symptom formation, social functioning, and personality factors. However, because interpersonal therapy is brief (12–16 weekly, 1-hour sessions), it focuses on improving social functioning as a means to alleviate symptoms. There is, however, no focus on the transference feelings toward the therapist.

> Interpersonal therapy may be considered if interpersonal factors are a contributor to the patient's obesity (e.g., a spouse who enables or encourages the patient to eat).

Interpersonal therapy places problems with social functioning into one or more of the following categories:

- *Interpersonal disputes*—occurring in marital, family, social, or work settings, in which the patient and others have different views on a situation, leading to conflict and distress
- *Role transitions*—occurring when the patient has to make a life change (such as a job change, the end of a relationship, a divorce, or a change of school) that the patient experiences as a loss
- *Grief*—occurring after the death of a loved one, when bereavement has been long-standing or complicated
- *Interpersonal deficits*—occurring when the patient has few or weak relationships

If the patient is the enabler in the family, or overeats as a manifestation of marital unhappiness, or needs the support of his or her spouse for a weight loss program, this may be the appropriate treatment. It is especially useful in marital relationships in which interpersonal conflicts between spouses are potential contributors to an individual's or a couple's obesity.

Treatment sessions for interpersonal therapy are rather structured. The two initial sessions explore and explain the patient's symptoms and describe the therapy's format and process. Sessions 3–14 focus on relationship problems, although the therapist also asks the patient about symptoms and responses to treatment. Sessions 15 and 16 assist the patient with terminating treatment, coping with loss, and evaluating modifications learned in therapy. Interpersonal therapists have adopted strategies from other treatment modalities and have incorporated supportive listening, role-play, communication analysis, and encouragement of expression of affect in this therapy. The focus, though, is not on the therapist or the therapist's relationship with the patient. In fact, a discussion of transference is "avoided at all costs" (John C. Markowitz, personal communication, May 19, 2009, at meeting of the American Psychiatric Association on interpersonal therapy). Markowitz et al. (2006) have found that when patients have symptomatic improvement, there is also a resolution of their interpersonal difficulties.

Neurolinguistic Programming

Neurolinguistic programming is more a technical, linguistic program tool than a school of therapy; it is geared toward analyzing patterns of communication, especially the use of language as a self-identifying process. In a treatment of obesity, this programming might be used as an adjunct method to help make the patient aware of how he or she linguistically relates to the subject of weight. For example, a statement like "I'll try to lose weight" implies some tentativeness or doubts about the outcome; in contrast, "I'll lose weight" signals a clear determination. Tentativeness and ambivalence undermine willpower. If

> Neurolinguistic programming may be considered if the individual is in need of sharpening an awareness of communication patterns related to eating habits.

the patient is unaware of how the linguistic process works in receiving, editing, and conveying information and how that information is processed and expressed, a few neurolinguistic sessions may be appropriate. If nothing else, it may sharpen the patient's consciousness about the subject.

Gestalt Therapy

Gestalt therapy emphasizes one's personal responsibility, whether in one's conscious or unconscious actions. This approach is not interested in resolving the sources of conflicts or remedying deficits. Gestalt

> Gestalt therapy may be considered if the individual needs encouragement to take ownership of the causes of his or her obesity.

therapy is only interested in having the patient take full responsibility for his or her thoughts, feelings, and behavior—and, of course, in the case of obesity, eating habits. Those who tend to blame others, food, or society for their obesity may want to experience a few sessions with a gestalt therapist.

Gestalt therapy was formulated by Friedrich (Fritz) Perls in the 1940s. Perls was originally trained in psychoanalysis before he developed gestalt therapy. Mintz (1973), who studied with Perls, describes gestalt psychology as a theory of personality, a form of psychotherapy, and a philosophy of living. Mintz describes Perls' technique as one-to-one therapy in a group setting, though without encouraging any group interaction: there would be an empty chair next to Perls and group members would take the "hot seat" voluntarily. Perls was apparently a master therapist, adept at noting "the most fleeting gesture, discern[ing] its significance, and [using] it to explore the depths of conflict." Furthermore, Perls thought of anxiety as stage fright and would focus on the patient's fear by asking, "What are you afraid might happen?" (Mintz 1973).

Yontef (1993, p. 125) noted that gestalt therapy concentrates on insight into one's own unconscious mind and is heavily rooted in existentialism. The relationship between therapist and patient is an extremely important element in this type of therapy because an ongoing dialogue is a primary resource for the facilitation of self-discovery. Patients achieve awareness through a systematic exploration of the causes of one's behavior. Strong emphasis is placed on becoming responsible for one's own actions. There is a belief that to eliminate dysfunctional behaviors, one must come to accept them first. Gestalt therapy's groundings in self-awareness and responsibility make it a good treatment option for obese patients.

Gestalt methods are centered heavily on experiencing things in the present and taking ownership of the causes of one's problems. With the problem being obesity, patients would be encouraged to identify the behaviors that contribute to their lives in a negative way. It is not enough to identify these behaviors; gestalt theory suggests controlling the behaviors by helping the patients to recognize that the causes are internal. With obesity and eating disorders especially, an individual might be prone to single out habits that began in childhood, relating the behaviors of accepting poor nutrition or eating for the wrong reasons to parental figures. It would be a logical assumption to most that food intake during childhood is largely dependent on the child's parents or guardians. Although this statement is not entirely untrue, patients must recognize that they have played a significant role in their own obesity, in order to gain the ability to control their behavior. Such admissions of responsibility are extremely important to the process of an individual becoming self-aware.

The therapeutic relationship is essential to the outcome of gestalt therapy as a treatment option. The frequency of sessions may vary, and the relationship between therapist and patient develops over time. The gestalt therapist is encouraged to engage in a dialogue with the patient. There is expected to be a true and authentic relationship, out of which a helpful progression toward the patient's goal will emerge. It is very important that the patient not be led to the goal but come to it out of a natural progression. In this way, gestalt therapy is a team effort. It is extremely helpful for the therapist to come across as genuine in his or her efforts to develop a dialogue with the patient.

Cognitive-Behavioral Therapy

Developed by Aaron T. Beck in the 1960s as a treatment for depression, cognitive-behavioral therapy (CBT) is one of the newest therapeutic approaches. It is also one of the most researched therapies, with a large number of clinical trials completed, because it is outcome oriented and short term. The previous schools of psychodynamic therapy described are much harder to study because they tend to be long-term treatments, have no homogeneous standards of practice for clinicians, and are geared toward patients' subjective experiences. Today, clinicians use CBT to treat a plethora of conditions, including anger, anxiety, phobias, sleep disorders, irritable bowel syndrome, eating disorders, and substance abuse disorders.

> Cognitive-behavioral therapy may be considered if the individual has a distorted view of the self, others, and the world—that is, of body image, food, calories, and eating habits.

CBT is a short-term treatment, often consisting of 8–16 sessions conducted once weekly, geared toward changing symptoms in an objective way. In CBT, treatment focus is tailored to a current problem, in this case overweight/obesity or disordered eating, and treatment challenges distorted views of the self, others, and the world—specifically, incorrect assumptions about food, eating, and self-image. It provides the patient with an alternative cognitive paradigm applicable to life and, more specifically, to eating. It also provides cognitive modifications that target weight-related issues. The therapy espouses the idea that *how* an individual views situations influences how he or she feels. Judith Beck (2007, p. 19) specifically emphasizes that her plan is not a food plan but rather a psychological program. Beck's program focuses on the patient's thoughts that sabotage his or her attempts at controlling symptoms, particularly overeating. These *key distortions* include *rationalization* ("It's all right to eat this cake because ..."), *underestimation of consequences* ("It doesn't matter too much if I eat this"), *self-deluded thinking* ("I've already cheated so it doesn't matter if I eat more"), *arbitrary rules* ("I should not waste food"), *mind reading* ("My husband won't like it if I don't share his food"), and *exaggeration* ("I never feel really full") (Beck 2007, p. 11).

Along those lines, Helmering and Hales (2005, pp. 139–140) speak of common excuses people employ to sabotage their dieting: they describe the *health excuse* ("I'll feel better if I eat"); the *blaming excuse* ("My husband doesn't like it when I diet"); the *giving up excuse* ("I'll never be thin anyway"); the *celebration excuse* ("It's my birthday"); and the *victim excuse* ("I have a slow metabolism").

For Beck, there are also mental triggers (e.g., thinking about or imagining food); emotional triggers (e.g., unpleasant feelings that lead to eating); and social triggers (e.g., people or situations that lead to eating) (Beck 2007, p. 29). Furthermore, she emphasizes that a person has to set realistic weight loss goals, a point emphasized by Perri and Corsica (2002, pp. 370–373), if he or she wants to be successful at weight loss and maintenance over time.

CBT is beneficial for someone who has considerable maladaptive patterns of behavior at work, at home, or in relationships and wants to change those symptoms that are most bothersome. Because CBT is objective in its approach, the therapist helps the patient assess the current difficulty and set a goal that can be measured in terms of improvement. The CBT clinician is quite active in the treatment sessions and interacts with the patient to teach symptom-management skills. One thing the therapist does is assess a patient's mood by taking an inventory of symptoms, such as depression, anxiety, and hopelessness, and at each session the therapist monitors the patient's feelings by comparing them to feelings in previous sessions. The treatment is very directive, and the therapist may ask the patient to consider improving life through pursuing activities, knowledge, or distractions, such as cultural interests or exercise.

The therapist has the role of a teacher or coach, as he or she helps the individual reach specific goals. In treating weight-related issues, the therapist assesses the patient's disordered thinking about food and presents strategies for learning new eating behaviors. This may consist of explaining to the patient that the road to weight loss is not a straight one, but has peaks, valleys, plateaus, and wrong turns, and that most people getting on that road do so without a clear map. The CBT clinician helps the patient develop a map for getting to the goal. In using CBT for weight loss, the clinician may ask the patient to prepare for dieting by reviewing past diets, identifying difficulties, and developing new skills for diet readiness. The therapist may ask the patient to write a list of reasons for wanting to lose weight and to refer to the list daily (or as many times as necessary when tempted to overeat) (Beck 2007, pp. 1–58).

In her book *The Complete Beck Diet for Life*, Beck (2008, p. 35) recommends a "diet buddy," or someone who keeps us accountable on our diet. She also suggests (p. 119) that those who are tempted to continue to eat might want to put leftover food in opaque containers, place rubber bands around containers, and even have a stapler handy in the kitchen to staple shut packages of excess food. Of utmost importance is the concept that the dieter believes he or she has "no choice" in eating this extra food (Beck 2008, p. 44).

Incidentally, even back in the late 1950s, Siegel (1957) spoke of our human need for the "completion compulsion," that is, that we eat in "units." Siegel found, for example, that most of us seem not to be able to leave a fraction of a cookie, so that Beck's approach of hiding or sealing off leftover food may help most of us who see food and want to finish it. And of course, experiments by Wansink (2006, pp. 78-81) have demonstrated that people will eat more when they see food nearby and exposed, as opposed to food or candy wrapped in aluminum foil or placed at a distance. "The more hassle it is to eat, the less we eat," says Wansink (2006, p. 84), and suggests that "pause points" can be created by dividing a large package into smaller segments (p. 200).

CBT is best for the now-oriented, pragmatic, want-to-focus-on-a-specific-topic individual, because it is independent of deeper psychological explanations. It is often worth trying CBT first because it is time- and cost-efficient. It is particularly help-ful for those with disordered patterns of eating and for those who are interested in maintaining their diet regimen over time as a way of life. Significantly, many weight loss programs (including those recommending medication and even surgery) have incorporated cognitive-behavioral techniques as part of their treatment plan.

Dialectical Behavioral Therapy

Dialectical behavioral therapy (DBT) is an adaptation of CBT developed by psy-chologist and CBT-trained therapist Marsha Linehan as a treatment approach for patients with borderline personality disorder. The treatment is based on a specific theory that assumes emotional dysfunction to be the primary pathology of border-line personality disorder. The treatment is de-signed to improve emotional regulation by using behavioral analysis to pinpoint life events that may have contributed to the development of dys-functional behavior. DBT requires that therapists provide empathic feedback or validation. "The dialectic aspect of treatment is that therapists in-

> Dialectical behavioral therapy may be considered if the individual's obesity is closely associated with some real trauma.

form patients that they acknowledge the reasons why they need to stay the same but still expect them to work hard to change" (Paris 2008, p. 140). DBT has also been shown to help patients with problems involving substance abuse. Unlike traditional CBT, DBT is more long-term and as a result can be more costly.

DBT can be modified for use with patients with weight-related issues. If a thera-pist assumes emotional dysfunction and past trauma to be key components in the development of the patient's specific disorder, DBT may be seen as an alternative to traditionally used treatments. DBT can be used to regulate behaviors of obese patients in a way similar to the way it is used to regulate behaviors of patients with borderline personality disorder. The effectiveness of DBT is highly dependent on the patient's willingness to receive treatment and commitment to the treatment. The process is highly introspective, requiring that the patient be willing and able to participate actively in assessing his or her past behaviors and the possible effect those behaviors have on present behavior.

Linehan (Wright et al. 2008, p. 1235) developed DBT because experience taught her that traditional CBT was not effective enough as a tool for treating a popula-tion with severe disorders. Some key characteristics of DBT set it apart from the traditional method. One of these characteristics is acceptance-based interventions, or *validation strategies*. The therapist emphasizes that the patient's behavior, even when self-harming, is a normal reaction to a situation and is understood by the therapist. Therapists can point out the harmful nature of the behavior while giving patients the validation that they need to gain confidence in making decisions. In pointing out that the behavior is understandable and is a normal reaction to a given situation, a therapist begins to teach patients to trust their own judgment and accept that they are capable of making sound decisions in their lives.

Whereas traditional CBT has a much deeper emphasis on change, DBT, although not eliminating the idea of a need for changes in behavior, uses the validation/acceptance strategy, with a focus on changes in behavior, to help the idea of a change in lifestyle become less daunting for the individual. With this idea at the core of therapy, dialectical strategies then create a balance that helps both the patient and therapist avoid getting stuck in a particular thought pattern or set of ideas, which can be common in cases where emotionality is high. This method eases the client into change and acceptance in a way that feels gradual.

With severely disordered patients, traditional CBT, which places expectations and demands on patients (i.e., doing and reviewing homework daily, such as making note card reminders and lists), has a significantly high dropout rate. The idea of a flow in the therapeutic relationship and of incorporating a dialectical world view to hold the treatment process together works well with patients who might otherwise be consistently torn between extreme positions and arguments. The treatment stresses mindfulness and incorporates Zen Buddhism in its techniques. DBT can be highly intense, consisting of skill-building groups and phone coaching. Therapists are usually expected to meet weekly with a team of professionals to prevent burnout and to encourage therapists in treatment of patients. A therapist may also set up meetings with the patient's family in order to ensure that the home environment encourages and reinforces the positive behaviors that are the goal of treatment.

DBT organizes its treatment in stages and traditionally tries to follow a set path and order in addressing each particular problem. The first stage of treatment focuses on eliminating any life-threatening or otherwise harmful behavior. The goal is to have the patient recognize his or her own harmful behavior and become an active participant in changing that behavior. The progression of stages is a logical one, which helps lead the patient from one goal to the next. The next goal is to keep the patient in therapy so that he or she continues to work toward a healthier and more fulfilling life. This stage emphasizes emotional experiencing, including labeling of emotions and "reducing vulnerability to emotional dysregulation" (Rosenthal and Lynch 2009, p. 2887). The patient is encouraged not only to eliminate harmful thoughts and behaviors but also to replace them with positive, life-affirming ones. The third stage focuses on problems in living that are not debilitating (Rosenthal and Lynch 2009, p. 2887); the patient is encouraged to experience moments of happiness and unhappiness as normal and healthy parts of his or her improving life experience. Linehan has introduced a fourth stage for patients who also seek an additional measure of spiritual fulfillment. This fourth stage "targets a sense of completeness, spiritual growth, insight, enhanced awareness" (Rosenthal and Lynch 2009, p. 2887).

Mindfulness is heavily stressed in the practice of DBT. Linehan emphasizes the importance of being mindful in much of her materials exploring the practice of DBT. It involves being in the present and being without judgment as one experiences. The basics of mindfulness are simple. A patient is encouraged to focus in the moment and take in the entire experience. Patients are encouraged to be aware of the moment by using all the senses to take it in. Attention to smell, touch, and taste as well as sight and sound helps patients gain a fuller understanding of their state of being. Mindfulness is rooted in both Eastern and Western medicine and can be highly effective in helping patients avoid suppressing their experiences and become more aware of their experiences and their reactions to them.

Eastern Approaches

Eastern approaches, such as yoga or meditation, are very much in common practice in the West today. There are many, but all are geared toward either a relaxation of the body and mind or a redirection of awareness toward healthy and happy thoughts. For some practitioners, these approaches may even facilitate arrival at the state of nirvana, that is, transcendence. If chronic anxiety contributes to overeating

> Eastern approaches may be considered if the individual is using food as an anxiolytic.

and the patient is reluctant to take medication, Eastern techniques may be useful. If the wish to eat exceeds the will to abstain and defeats all other known approaches, desires might be extinguished through transcendence, an ultimate goal, though achieving it can be a rather severe undertaking. Yoga, as we have mentioned (see Chapter 8, "Exercise"), is also a helpful adjunct for strength training, balance, and posture, as well as toning the body.

Self-Help

Given that most researchers believe overweight and obesity are lifetime problems (e.g., Cooper et al. 2003, p. 158; Wadden et al. 2004), treatment must extend over the course of the patient's life and be cost-effective. But Latner (2007) reports that after 6 months of weight loss therapy, individuals find the cost-benefit ratio of treatment becomes nearly nil. One way of surmounting the 6-month loss of interest is with self-help. Table 11–2 summarizes the key aspects of organized self-help weight loss programs.

> Self-help is a cost-effective treatment approach that should always be part of any therapeutic regimen, for weight-related problems require lifetime vigilance.

We have seen from the research of the National Weight Control Registry, begun in the 1990s, in which thousands of its registrants have lost substantial weight and maintained the losses over years, that there are many ways to control weight effectively over the long term (see Chapter 2, "Obesity in the United States"). Though most people may need the guidance and supervision of professionals, many other people lose weight without any professional help, as seen in some of the Registry participants.

Table 11–2. Key components of selected commercial and organized self-help weight loss programs

Program	Staff qualifications	Diet	Physical activity	Behavior modification	Support
Weight Watchers	Successful lifetime member (successful program completer)	Low-calorie, "Flex Plan"a; clients prepare own meals	"Get Moving" booklet distributed; systematic approach to exercise	Behavioral weight control methods	Group sessions, weekly meetings
Jenny Craig	Company-trained counselor	Low-calorie diet of prepackaged Jenny Craig meals only	Audiotapes for walking	Manual on weight loss strategies provided	Individual sessions, weekly contact
LA Weight Loss Centers	Company-trained counselor	Low-calorie diet; clients prepare own meals	Optional walking videotape	Included in counseling sessions	Individual sessions three times weekly
Health Management Resources	Licensed physician and other health care providers	Low-calorie or very-low-calorie diet provided through meal replacement products	Walking and calorie charts provided in lifestyle classes	Included in lifestyle classes; accountability and skill acquisition emphasized	Group sessions and weekly classes; some telephone support
Optifast	Licensed physician and other health care providers	Low-calorie diet provided through meal replacement products	Physical activity modules taught in lifestyle classes	Included in lifestyle classes; stress management and social support emphasized	Group sessions and weekly classes; some telephone support

Table 11–2. Key components of selected commercial and organized self-help weight loss programs (*continued*)

Program	Staff qualifications	Diet	Physical activity	Behavior modification	Support
Medifast/Take Shape for Life	Not applicable	Low-calorie or very-low-calorie diet provided through meal replacement products	May be included in Take Shape for Life	May be included in Take Shape for Life	Included in Take Shape for Life
eDiets	Company-trained counselor and company dietitians	Low-calorie diet provided through "virtual dietitian" program; clients prepare own meals	Physical activity seminar as part of eDiets.com	Included in eDiets. com; stress management emphasized	Individual and group Internet support
Take Off Pounds Sensibly (TOPS)	Volunteer group leader elected by local chapter (not for profit)	Low-calorie diet exchange plan recommended	Members make plan with their health care provider	Included in curriculum	Group format; weekly sessions
Overeaters Anonymous (OA)	Volunteer chapter leaders (not for profit)	No specific recommendation	Members make plan with their health care provider	12-step program (obesity results from compulsive eating) with spiritual orientation analogous to Alcoholics Anonymous	Group format; weekly sessions; sponsors

[a]Point system with core list of nutritious foods and can eat any food as long as keep track and control portions. Every food has a point value (Rippe and Weight Watchers 2005, pp. 214–222).

Source.   Adapted from Tsai AG, Wadden TA: "Systematic Review: An Evaluation of Major Commercial Weight Loss Programs in the United States." *Annals of Internal Medicine* 142:56–66, 2005. Used with permission.

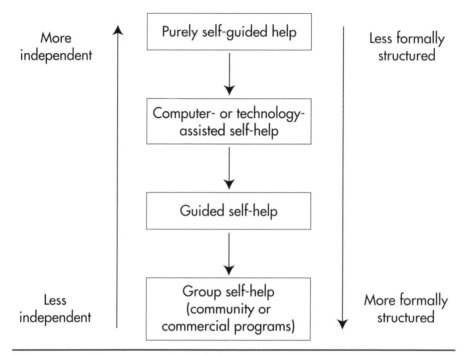

Figure 11–1. Four types of self-help programs.

Source.   Reprinted from Latner JD, "Self-Help for Obesity and Binge Eating. *Nutrition Today* 42:81–85, 2007. Used with permission.

Self-help may be a more financially attainable treatment and one that encompasses a variety of modes, ranging from the structure of a group to the independence of an individual who reads books on diet and nutrition on his or her own; this range is illustrated in Figure 11–1. For example, a search of "diet books" (March 10, 2009) on amazon.com resulted in almost 20,000 books listed. And using the Google search engine to search the words "self-help for obesity" brings 113 million hits within seconds (accessed November 6, 2009). In seeking self-help treatment strategies for weight loss, patients have a plethora of programs from which to choose, ranging from the highly independent self-prompted to the more guided and structured formats of commercial or not-for-profit groups.

A subset of self-help programs consists of computer-guided, technology-based weight loss plans, which may be very effective for some patients. Many reputable Web sites provide newsletters, other publications, and general information regarding health, nutrition, dieting, and even research. (See the Appendix to this volume, "Selected Readings and Web Sites," for more information.)

Figure 11–2 is an example of a food diary, available through the Centers for Disease Control and Prevention Web site (http://www.cdc.gov/healthyweight/pdf/food_Diary_cdc.pdf), that patients can use for assistance in keeping track of their

My Food Diary   Day_____

Meal/Snack (indicate time of day)	What you ate and drank	Where and with whom	Notes (feelings, hunger, etc.)
Breakfast			
Snacks			
Lunch			
Snacks			
Dinner			
Snacks			

Figure 11–2. Example of a food diary.

Source.   Available at: http://www.cdc.gov/healthyweight/pdf/food_diary_cdc.pdf.

eating. Keeping records of food intake (e.g., through food diaries) can be an important part of accountability, much as weighing oneself daily on a scale can be. But it can be easier said than done to remember all that one eats over a period of time. In discussing the self-report food frequency questionnaires required by obesity research studies, Michael Pollan, in his book *In Defense of Food: An Eater's Manifesto* (2008, p. 76), says, "I'm not sure Marcel Proust himself could recall his dietary intake over the last ninety days with the sort of precision demanded." It takes determination, discipline, and motivation to keep a running log of everything one eats (as well as with whom and what one felt) each day, let alone over a period of time.

Several organizations offer online support as part of their paid membership, including Nutrisystem, Weight Watchers, and DietWatch. Consumer Reports, a not-for-profit organization with no commercial affiliations, rates various items and services for safety and reliability. In 2006, it rated the 20 most-accessed diet Web sites on a variety of items, including ease of use and clear disclosure of sponsoring policies. It also evaluated self-help programs to see, for example, whether they supplied relevant details, initial costs, and useful tools for self-management. The following were rated good or very good: WebMD.com, The Biggest Loser Club (biggestloserclub.com), eDiets.com, The Sonoma Diet (sonomadiet.com), South Beach Diet (southbeachdiet.com), and WeightWatchers.com (Consumer Reports 2006).

Latner (2007) describes guided self-help as "bibliotherapy," in which the individual receives a cognitive-behavioral manual designed for weight loss and has minimal contact with an advisor (a therapist, paraprofessional, or assistant) who assesses the individual's progress.

Group-guided self-help runs the gamut from religious communities to well-advertised commercial enterprises that have been in existence for years. These groups provide support; teach about eating habits, exercise, and nutrition; and provide encouragement when a person encounters the difficulties of staying on a reduced-calorie eating plan. Heshka et al. (2003) describe a commercial program to which their patients were assigned as providing "a food plan, a behavior modification plan focused primarily on cognitive restructuring," and weekly weigh-in sessions at which educational materials were distributed and social support was offered.

Take Off Pounds Sensibly (TOPS) is a not-for-profit group that is led by lay-person volunteers, "all of whom have struggled with their weight or with eating problems" (Tsai and Wadden 2005). Its approach is to offer recommendations on a low-calorie diet, increased physical activity, and behavior modification techniques. Overeaters Anonymous is an independent organization that helps individuals advance weight loss through adherence to a 12-step program similar to that used by Alcoholics Anonymous. Although Overeaters Anonymous describes itself as not being religious in nature and having members of various faiths as well as atheists and agnostics, the 12 steps are based "on each member's personal interpretation of a higher power." There are no membership requirements other than a desire to lose weight and admitting the need to stop compulsive eating and food addictions. There are no membership fees, though members are encouraged to make donations through contributions or literature sales. In addition to local, in-person meetings, Overeaters Anonymous offers online meetings at its Web site, as do many other programs now.

With more than 100 groups in the United States, the Trevose Behavior Modification Program originally begun by Albert J. Stunkard (personal communication, October 9, 2009) years ago in Pennsylvania is a volunteer self-help group that potentially provides continuity of care ("lifelong treatment") for those with obesity (Latner et al. 2002). There are no membership fees, but the program has stringent inclusion criteria. For example, people who need to lose more than 100 pounds are not allowed to become members. And only those individuals who are deemed to have the capacity to achieve weight loss are admitted to full membership after a trial period of the first 4 months. There is also a one-time rule—once a person's membership is terminated, he or she can never rejoin the organization. There is strict enforcement of the rules, including mandatory attendance at weekly meetings and weigh-ins, as well as self-monitoring of food intake and physical activity. Membership, though, is offered for life.

Most of the commercial group-guided practices, such as Overeaters Anonymous, Take Off Pounds Sensibly, and the Trevose program, focus on behavior modification, a diet plan, and the support of group members and counselors.

RESEARCH ON PSYCHOLOGICAL TREATMENTS FOR OBESITY

Methodological Issues

During the past two decades, designs and techniques for research in psychotherapy have matured in their application to the treatment of a number of clinical conditions, but studies in weight-related topics have lagged far behind, partly because of the medical/physical variables associated with obese patients that confound the already complex characteristics of average patients receiving psychotherapy.

For example, researchers may have difficulty establishing comparison groups within a study, in that they need to define precisely the patient populations, the psychotherapists, and the nature of the psychotherapy administered. Because it is unethical to withhold a presumed effective treatment, researchers may provide control groups with acceptable alternatives, such as being waiting-list control subjects; sometimes, patients can be used as their own controls.

> Science issues only interim reports.

Next, patients are randomly assigned to one of two or more groups, to ensure that all significant variables are equally distributed and to maximize the statistical probability of attributions. This is followed by implementation of the research, preferably as a pretest/posttest or multivariable design. The latter is a complex and expensive approach and is conducted to investigate the differential effects of the therapy.

The statistical issues can present other problems, with issues such as interrater reliability (all existing coefficients provide ambiguous solutions) and statistical power analysis—that is, the probability of the null hypothesis (a large sample can make even trivial results statistically significant). Furthermore, there are issues related to informed consent, length of therapy, follow-up phase, cost-effectiveness, and cost-benefit ratio. Many of these investigations are large community studies in which researchers have almost no control over other aspects of a patient's life, particularly in long-term studies.

Another issue that is quite significant in obesity research is the high rate of attrition in many studies. Finley et al. (2007) note that most programs do not collect data on the reasons that patients drop out (e.g., issues of scheduling, costs, unrelated illnesses, failure to lose weight, or dissatisfaction with the diet or food) or, for that matter, why other people stay. They found, for example, in a study of the Jenny Craig program for weight loss, that of over 60,000 men and women who enrolled, only 22% remained at 6 months and fewer than 7% stayed with the program for a full year.

There is one significant factor that facilitates research on obesity treatments. That is the outcome measure: its reliability and validity are unquestionable, simple, and inexpensive—one doesn't need a battery of instruments. Outcome is weight loss, determined by changes in BMI values (i.e., measuring weight and height) or change in waist circumference. In other words, a tape measure and an accurate scale can suffice. Of course, there are more sophisticated measurements, such as magnetic resonance imaging, computed tomography, and dual-energy X-ray absorptiometry, as we mentioned in Chapter 2, but most large studies do not use them.

Even though the above issues seem difficult to overcome, it is worthwhile to consider them to create a framework in which to explore the role of psychotherapy in the treatment of obesity.

Research Data on Psychotherapeutic Treatment Strategies

Many of the research studies on specific techniques of psychotherapy were conducted years ago and not repeated. For example, Rand and Stunkard (1983) reviewed the use of psychoanalysis for the treatment of obesity. They followed 84 obese patients (and 63 normal-weight patients) over the course of 4 years (treatment lasted from 3 years to >7 years) in an uncontrolled study. Only 6% of obese patients reported their weight as the primary reason for seeking treatment; however, body image disparagement was reported in 39% of the obese patients at treatment initiation. The treating analysts provided information to the authors on most of the 84 obese patients at 4-year follow-up: 27 were still in analysis; 23 completed analysis; 29 terminated prematurely. Even among the patients who terminated treatment early, 40% had maintained their weight at approximately what it had been at termination; 33% had continued to lose weight; and 27% had regained some weight. The researchers postulate that stress reduction may have been a factor in maintaining weight loss because many of the patients reported eating as a means of coping with stress. The authors concluded that psychoanalysis for patients with obesity is effective for some patients. Long-term treatment, though, "[makes] psychoanalysis an expensive way to lose weight" (Rand and Stunkard 1983).

Sohlberg and Norring (1989), in a study of ego functions in 41 adult patients with disordered eating, found that those who had a preoccupation with weight or shape and had a DSM-III-R (American Psychiatric Association 1987) eating disorder at 1-year follow-up had more severe ego disturbance at initial presentation compared with subjects in the symptom-free cohort.

Some research has shown that severity of object relations deficits and severity of eating disturbances do not necessarily show a correlation. A study by Parrent (1997), on binge eating disorder and dimensions of object relations, evaluated groups of women with eating disorders and compared level of severity of object relations disturbance. Seventy-two women (ages 20–45 years) were divided into groups based on whether they were normal weight, obese, binge-eating obese, or bulimic. Somewhat surprisingly, there was no correlation between a higher level of eating disorder pathology and disturbance in object relations. However, there were significant differences in severity of object relations disturbance when the two control groups (normal-weight and obese subjects) and the two eating-disordered groups (binge eaters and bulimic subjects) were compared. Raynes et al. studied addictions, including "addiction" to food, and concluded that there are "deficits in obese (food dependent) persons similar to those of chemically dependent persons" (Raynes et al. 1989). These researchers support the benefit of multifaceted addiction treatment. Graham and Glickauf-Hughes (1992) discuss treatment of addictions from an object relations perspective. They extrapolate that addictions, in which they include compulsive overeating, are a failure of an individual to separate from the object (i.e., caretaker) from whom he or she had sought comfort as an infant. These individuals are unable to soothe themselves, and they seek comfort from an outside source in their addictions. "Individual therapy concurrent with peer group support can be very beneficial as some patients respond to even the slightest criticism as rejection.... The therapist and the peer group can provide the 'good enough' holding environment to withstand the challenges of early sobriety" (Graham and Glickauf-Hughes 1992).

Bachar et al. (1999) compared self psychology and cognitive orientation therapies for treating eating disorders (anorexia nervosa and bulimia nervosa). The researchers carried out both types of treatment for a year with weekly sessions; the sessions did not focus on patients' attitudes toward eating. Using the self psychology approach, they attributed eating disorders to a pathology of self: these patients could not rely on others to fulfill their selfobject needs (self-esteem regulation, calming, and soothing) so they substituted food to fulfill these needs. The authors concluded that for treating patients with eating disorders, self psychology had a positive outcome. The authors further noted that there were improvements not only in symptoms involving eating, but also in psychological variables such as cohesion of the self.

Research involving interpersonal therapy and eating has been applied to bulimia and anorexia nervosa. Mostly it is based on the presumption that, much like depression, eating disorders may be rooted in problems that individuals have with interpersonal relationships. A study by Tanofsky-Kraff et al. (2007) suggests that interpersonal therapy may be used to curb weight gain among adolescents with a history of binge eating disorder, patients who are at risk for obesity. The authors postulate: "Interpersonal theory posits that interpersonal problems lead to low self-esteem and low mood. Food is used to cope with negative affect and LOC [loss of control] eating ensues. This causes excessive weight gain..., which reinforces interpersonal problems." Interpersonal therapy, according to these researchers, reduces interpersonal problems and results in increases in self-esteem as well as the patient's lessening reliance on food.

In addition, Wilfley et al. (2002) studied 162 overweight patients randomly assigned to participate in either group CBT or group interpersonal therapy sessions for 20 weeks. Interpersonal therapy was found to be a "viable alternative to CBT for the treatment of overweight patients with binge-eating disorder."

Compared to the dearth of information on the other psychotherapeutic treatment modalities, there are many research studies on CBT and disordered eating. However, most of the studies focus on obese patients with concomitant binge eating disorder.

Stahre and Hällström (2005), for example, completed a study of 105 patients with obesity who had been randomly assigned to a (waiting) control group and a CBT group. Of the 57 subjects in the treatment group who completed a 10-week program of CBT, 34 of them continued to participate in the study at 18 months posttreatment. At treatment end, mean weight loss in the treatment group was approximately 8.5 kilograms (18.7 pounds); at 18-month follow-up, mean weight loss was approximately 10.4 kilograms (22.9 pounds), whereas in the untreated control group, weights had increased an average of 2.3 kilograms (5.1 pounds).

Agras et al. (1997), in their study of CBT for obese individuals with binge eating disorder, focused on three treatment goals: minimizing binges, encouraging weight change, and addressing comorbid psychopathology. In this study the researchers followed 93 obese women with binge eating disorder for 1 year after 12-week CBT treatment ended. They found that reductions in binge eating frequency made during CBT were maintained at 1-year follow-up. Cessation or reduction in binge eating did not necessarily equal weight loss during the CBT treatment. In fact, the group gained approximately 1 kilogram (~2.2 pounds). The authors conclude that "cessation of binge eating appears to be an important prelude to maintained weight loss in the obese patient with [binge eating disorder]."

One of the major issues in weight-related research is the need to distinguish between weight loss and weight maintenance once weight has been lost. Cooper et al. (2003, p. 6) point out that assessing long-term weight loss treatment for obesity is problematic for two reasons: "first, the neglect of the contribution of cognitive factors to weight *regain;* and second, the ambiguity over treatment goals…in long-term treatment programs." This idea is supported by a study completed by Ames et al. (2005), who found that patients often regain 30%–50% of lost weight. Some researchers note that weight regain rests on patient failure to use CBT weight control behaviors because over time patients do not believe that they can continue to control their weight. After 4–6 months of weight loss attempts, patients begin to understand that they may not achieve their weight loss goals and that other goals resting on weight loss, such as a desire to improve appearance, will not be attained (Cooper et al. 2003, p. 6). The authors suggest a further adjustment of CBT for obesity so that it becomes a three-step process:

1. Ensure that patients understand the difference between weight loss and weight management.

2. Speak to the patients while they are losing weight about difficulties they may encounter for maintaining their new weight.

3. Teach patients behavioral skills and cognitive responses that will help them control their weight. Practice these skills and responses with them.

These authors also emphasize that since obesity is a chronic disorder, patients should undergo long-term care. This idea is supported by Wadden et al. (2004), who note that it is as impossible to "cure" obesity with short-term treatment as it is to cure other chronic conditions, such as type 2 diabetes. They cite literature reviews that found those patients who received long-term behavioral therapy (an average of 41 sessions) maintained most of their initial weight loss (Wadden et al. 2004). Figure 11–3 compares behavioral treatment (24 weekly sessions) versus behavioral treatment plus long-term maintenance therapy (an additional 48 weeks, biweekly sessions) in helping patients prevent weight regain. The authors, though, warn that extended treatment seems only to delay weight regain and not prevent it.

There is some doubt in the psychiatric community about the newer behavioral therapies. For example, Lars-Göran Öst (2008) believes that there are not enough reliable data to consider DBT or even some other of the recent psychotherapies as empirically supported treatment. Öst notes that there are no stringent rules for evaluating how DBT is practiced, and therefore it is difficult to obtain an accurate measure of its effectiveness. Although randomized, controlled trials have been

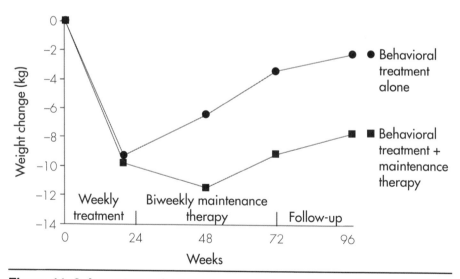

Figure 11–3. Long-term changes in weight for patients who received standard behavioral treatment, with or without biweekly maintenance therapy.

Note. Data from Perri et al. 1986, 1988, 2001.

Source. Reprinted from Wadden TA, Butryn ML, Byrne KJ: "Efficacy of Lifestyle Modification for Long-Term Weight Control." *Obesity Research* 12(suppl):154S, 2004. Used with permission.

conducted, the methodology has not been as strict as with CBT studies. As a result, it is difficult to compare the two therapies with scientific accuracy (Tapper et al. 2009). Nevertheless, DBT does seem to be gaining popularity among behaviorists.

Research Data on Self-Help Treatment Strategies

An early study by Taylor et al. (1991) compared weight loss in 57 overweight women randomly assigned either to a group that only used a pocket computer to list food consumed and to log exercise, or to a group that first followed a guided 1,200-calorie weight loss diet and then used the pocket computer after a loss of weight. Although all subjects met for four 1.5-hour group meetings to review progress, the guided group lost significantly more weight than did the computer-only group (5.3 vs. 3.1 kilograms). The authors summarized that computer-assisted therapy increased weight loss among those individuals who received additional treatment, and suggest its use as an aid to other therapy and for maintenance after weight loss. A study of African American individuals in a church-based setting (Goodman and Blake 2005) showed that a computer-based nutrition education program reduced the number of overweight and obese individuals and increased the number of normal-weight individuals among the 82 adults in the sample. However, the authors suggest that in addition to the computer program, reinforcement of healthy eating guidelines is required.

Although the National Weight Control Registry does not promote any particular type of diet, nor does it make suggestions regarding weight loss strategies, a study of 784 Registry members (Klem et al. 1997) showed that 45% of these individuals lost weight on their own, with no formal program. The research showed that nearly all of the study participants limited food intake and modified physical activity, that is, used exercise to lose and then maintain weight. In addition, approximately three-quarters of the participants weighed themselves more than once weekly and half of them continued to count calories after weight loss. (See Chapter 2, "Obesity in the United States," for more information on the National Weight Control Registry.)

Heshka et al. (2003) randomly assigned individuals to a commercial weight loss program or a guided self-help program. The participants in the guided self-help sample received two 20-minute visits with a dietitian and materials explaining diet and exercise; they were also informed about resources such as the library, Web sites, and organizations offering free information on weight loss. In this particular study of over 420 overweight and obese individuals (predominantly women; 65 men), the commercial weight loss program was Weight Watchers (which included a food plan, an activity plan, and behavioral modification). By 2 years, there was an attrition rate of 27% in each group. Those in the guided self-help group lost up to 1.4 kilograms by the end of the first year but had regained even this modest amount by 2 years. Those in the Weight Watchers group had lost up to 5 kilograms by the end of the first year but were able to maintain a loss of only 3 kilograms by the end of the second year, even among those who had the "highest degree of adherence." Heshka et al. (2003) concluded that weight loss over the 2-year period was "modest" for the commercial weight loss program but greater than for the self-help group.

Tsai and Wadden (2005) conducted a systematic review of the major commercial weight loss programs in the United States and were fairly pessimistic: "With the exception of one trial of Weight Watchers, the evidence to support the use of the major commercial and self-help weight loss programs is suboptimal." They had searched the MEDLINE database for studies from 1966 through 2003 and found 108 studies of commercial weight loss programs, but only 10 of these met their criteria. (Reasons for exclusion included inadequate follow-up, initial study lasting less than 10 weeks, and inadequate data on the number of clients enrolled.) Their review found that many programs were associated with not only high costs but also high attrition rates, and even worse, a "high probability" that people would regain 50% or even more of the weight they had lost within 2 years. Of the three largest commercial programs (Weight Watchers, Jenny Craig, and LA Weight Loss Centers) in the United States, only Weight Watchers had conducted randomized, controlled trials. Those who did best on Weight Watchers (i.e., maintained the largest weight loss), not surprisingly, attended the most group sessions. More recently, as noted earlier, Finley et al. (2007) studied over 60,000 men and women in the Jenny Craig program, which offers prepackaged food (1,200–2,000 cal/day) and recommends that clients exercise at least 30 minutes per day, 5 days per week. Their conclusion was that the program can be effective if a person stays in it for at least 14 weeks, but, as noted, the attrition rate is high.

Tsai and Wadden (2005) also reviewed medically supervised programs, such as Optifast, Medifast, and the Health Management Resources program, that offer meal replacements that are extremely low in calories (only ~400 cal/day!) or low in calories (>800 cal/day), but high in protein (70–100 g/day). Both Optifast and Health Management Resources have mandatory classes on lifestyle modification, as well as a three-phase program that includes an initial phase for rapid weight loss and a maintenance phase, and they insist on medical supervision (Medifast, apparently, does not). Tsai and Wadden (2005) emphasize the dangers, including death, of unsupervised very-low-calorie diets. Earlier, Wadden et al. (1990) reviewed how these very-low-calorie diets are abused by dieters, particularly by those who are only mildly overweight, for quick weight loss results. These diets are recommended only for those who are a minimum of 30% overweight and for a limited period of time. Furthermore, sometimes dieters are supervised by physicians who are not trained to work with these diets. Wadden et al. (1990) noted that some years previously, the unsupervised very-low-calorie Cambridge diet had resulted in 6 deaths. Furthermore, Wadden et al. (1990) reported that when very-low-calorie diets are not combined with "instruction in life-style modification," patients can gain back as much as 67% of the weight they had lost in the year following treatment. Patients on such diets can lose up to 25% of their initial weight within the first 6 months on the program, but by 1 year they can expect to maintain a loss of less than 9% of their initial weight; at 4 years, studies that Tsai and Wadden reviewed indicate that patients maintain a loss of only 5%. These figures represent best-case scenarios because they do not even count subjects lost to attrition, and it is not clear whether these diets provide better long-term results than diets that recommend 1,200–1,500 calories a day.

Latner et al. (2002) evaluated satellite program groups involving 128 members of the Trevose Behavioral Modification Program, the stringently-run self-help group, to assess weight loss and attrition over time. They found that after 2 years of follow-up, almost 44% of their sample remained in treatment and had lost over 35 pounds. At 5 years, almost a quarter of their population still remained in the program and had lost, on average, over 34 pounds from their initial weight. The researchers concluded that this Trevose model that combined "self-help and continuing care" could be "disseminated" successfully to other settings.

Delinsky et al. (2006) also used a Trevose Behavioral Modification Program group population to study the impact of binge eating on obesity in their sample of 136 women and 25 men. The mean age of the group was the mid 40s and the mean BMI value was about 35 kg/m². Significantly, more than one-third (36%) dropped out during the first year. But those who remained lost significant weight (and more than seen with other behavioral programs), and binge eating (a factor in 41% of the sample) did not interfere with weight loss: by 1 year, those who remained in the program had lost more than 18 kilograms (almost 40 pounds).

Dansinger et al. (2007) conducted a meta-analysis of the effects of dietary counseling on weight loss in randomized, controlled trials conducted from 1980 through 2006. They were able to find 46 such studies, involving over 6,300 people. Of the 46 studies, 42 recommended increased exercise as well as dietary counseling. But Dansinger and colleagues found the studies were "generally of moderate to poor methodological quality" with "high rates of missing data": only four studies were considered to be of good quality. Essentially they found that dietary counseling produced a mean weight loss of about 5 kilograms (~11 pounds) by 1 year, but by 3 years, people had regained about half of the weight they had lost. The programs that recommended regular attendance at support meetings and diets with fewer calories had better effects on weight loss.

Though many studies exclude people with type 2 diabetes because they tend to lose less weight (Dansinger et al. 2007), Wadden et al. (2009) reported on the first-year results of the Look AHEAD (Action for Health in Diabetes) study. This ongoing study, examining the long-term effects of weight loss, involves 16 clinical sites and over 5,100 men and women who have type 2 diabetes. This is a randomized, controlled study in which patients are assigned to either a usual care condition (in which they receive information "but not specific behavioral strategies") or an intensive lifestyle intervention (e.g., specific dietary advice of consuming 1,200–1,800 cal/day with < 30% of calories from fat, and meal replacements). Goals of the study are both weight loss (>7% of initial weight) and increased physical activity (>175 minutes/week). The researchers aim to eventually "resolve [in diabetic patients] the conflicting findings from observational studies concerning the cardiovascular consequences of weight loss." By the end of the first year, those in the lifestyle intervention group had lost significantly more weight (8.6% of their initial weight) and the intervention was considered clinically effective in a diverse population, compared with 0.7% of initial weight for the usual care group. Those who did best, not surprisingly, were those who engaged in the most physical activity. Attendance at more group meetings and using more meal replacements (e.g., Glucerna, Slim-Fast, and Optifast products) were also associated with better results. Wadden et al. (2009) caution that their results may not be generalizable to primary practice populations; subjects in the intensive lifestyle intervention group were particularly highly motivated and were given treatment (including meal replacements) free of charge. Even in the intervention group, one-third of subjects were not able to achieve a clinically significant weight reduction (i.e., 5%, which is considered a benchmark) from their initial weight. The researchers also hope to gather information on those who are either nonresponders or suboptimal responders. Interestingly, in the second 6 months, a subgroup of those with poor compliance were given the medication orlistat, which prevents the absorption of dietary fat (see Chapter 12, "Pharmacological and Surgical Treatments for Overweight and Obesity"), with only "marginal" improvement in weight loss.

Despite years of research, outcome studies on psychological treatment strategies for obesity to date leave much to be desired. With the tremendous worldwide increase in obesity, we can only hope that despite the considerable difficulties inherent in obesity research, research will continue to improve, with prospective, randomized, controlled studies of large, diverse populations and with greater standardization.

REFERENCES

Agras SW, Telch CF, Arnow B, et al: One-year follow-up of cognitive-behavioral therapy for obese individuals with binge eating disorder. J Consult Clin Psychol 65:343–347, 1997

American Psychiatric Association: Diagnostic and Statistical Manual of Mental Disorders, 3rd Edition, Revised. Washington, DC, American Psychiatric Association, 1987

American Psychiatric Association: Diagnostic and Statistical Manual of Mental Disorders, 4th Edition, Text Revision. Washington, DC, American Psychiatric Association, 2000

Ames GE, Perri MG, Fox LD, et al: Changing weight-loss expectations: a randomized pilot study. Eat Behav 6:259–269, 2005

Bachar E, Latzer Y, Kreitler S, et al: Empirical comparison of two psychological therapies: self psychology and cognitive orientation in the treatment of anorexia and bulimia. J Psychother Pract Res 8:115–128, 1999

Bean MK, Stewart K, Olbrisch ME: Obesity in America: implications for clinical and health psychologists. J Clin Psychol Med Settings 15:214–224, 2008

Beattie HJ: "The repression and the return of bad objects": W. R. D. Fairbairn and the historical roots of theory. Int J Psychoanal 84:1171–1187, 2003

Beck JS: The Beck Diet Solution. Birmingham, AL, Oxmoor House, 2007

Beck J: The Complete Beck Diet for Life. Birmingham, AL, Oxmoor House, 2008

Bruch H: Psychological aspects of reducing. Psychosom Med 14:337–346, 1952

Bruch H: Obesity and orality. Contemp Psychoanal 5:129–143, 1969

Bruch H: Psychotherapy in primary anorexia nervosa. J Nerv Ment Dis 150:51–67, 1970

Buckley P, Michels R, McKinnon R: Changes in the psychiatric landscape. Am J Psychiatry 163:757–760, 2006

Clarkin JF, Yeomans FE, Kernberg OF: Psychotherapy for Borderline Personality: Focusing on Object Relations. Washington, DC, American Psychiatric Publishing, 2006

Clarkin JF, Levy KN, Lenzenweger MF, et al: Evaluating three treatments for borderline personality disorder: a multiwave study. Am J Psychiatry 164:922–928, 2007

Collins RL, Ricciardelli LA: Assessment of eating disorders and obesity, in Assessment of Addictive Behavior, 2nd Edition. Edited by Donovan DM, Marlatt GA. New York, Guilford, 2005, pp 305–333

Cooper Z, Fairburn CG, Hawker DM: Cognitive Behavior Treatment of Obesity: A Clinician's Guide. New York, Guilford, 2003

Dansinger ML, Tatsioni A, Wong JB, et al: Meta-analysis: the effect of dietary counseling for weight loss. Ann Intern Med 147:41–50, 2007

Delinsky SS, Latner JD, Wilson GT: Binge eating and weight loss in a self-help behavior modification program. Obesity (Silver Spring) 14:1244–1249, 2006

Duffy VB, Bartoshuk LM: Sensory factors in feeding, in Why We Eat What We Eat: The Psychology of Eating. Edited by Capaldi ED. Washington, DC, American Psychological Association, 1996, pp 145–171

Felitti VJ, Williams SA: Long-term follow-up and analysis of more than 100 patients who each lost more than 100 pounds. The Permanente Journal 2:17–21, 1998

Finley CE, Barlow CE, Greenway FL, et al: Retention rates and weight loss in a commercial weight loss program. Int J Obes (Lond) 31:292–298, 2007

Fonagy P, Target M: Theoretical models of psychodynamic psychotherapy, in Textbook of Psychotherapeutic Treatments. Edited by Gabbard GO. Washington, DC, American Psychiatric Publishing, 2009, pp 3–42

Freud S: Two encyclopedia articles, A: Psychoanalysis (1923), in The Standard Edition of the Complete Psychological Works of Sigmund Freud, Vol 18. Translated and edited by Strachey J. London, Hogarth Press, 1955, pp 235–254

Friedman KE, Reichmann SK, Costanzo PR, et al: Body image partially mediates the relationship between obesity and psychological distress. Obes Res 10:33–41, 2002

Goodman J, Blake J: Nutrition education: a computer-based education program. J Health Care Poor Underserved 16:118–127, 2005

Graham A, Glickauf-Hughes C: Object relations and addictions: the role of "transmuting externalizations." Journal of Contemporary Psychotherapy 22:21–33, 1992

Helmering DW, Hales D: Think Thin, Be Thin: 101 Psychological Ways to Lose Weight. New York, Broadway Books, 2005

Heshka S, Anderson JW, Atkinson RL, et al: Weight loss with self-help compared with a structured commercial program: a randomized trial. JAMA 289:1792–1798, 2003

Hirsch J: Obesity: matter over mind? The Dana Foundation. January 1, 2003. Available at: http://www.dana.org/news/cerebrum/detail.aspx?id=2908. Accessed July 6, 2009.

Karasu TB: The psychotherapies: benefits and limitations. Am J Psychother 40:324–342, 1986

Karasu TB: A developmental metatheory of psychopathology. Am J Psychother 48:581–599, 1994

Karasu TB, Karasu SR: Psychoanalysis and psychoanalytic psychotherapy, in Kaplan & Sadock's Comprehensive Textbook of Psychiatry, 9th Edition, Vol 2. Edited by Sadock BJ, Sadock VA, Ruiz P. Philadelphia, PA, Wolters Kluwer/Lippincott Williams & Wilkins, 2009, pp 2746–2775

Kass L: The Hungry Soul: Eating and the Perfecting of Our Nature. Chicago, IL, University of Chicago Press, 1999

Kernberg OF: Borderline Conditions and Pathological Narcissism. Lanham, MD, Rowman & Littlefield, 2000

Keys A: The Management of obesity. Minn Med 48:1329–1331, 1965

Klem ML, Wing RR, McGuire MT, et al: A descriptive study of individuals successful at long-term maintenance of substantial weight loss. Am J Clin Nutr 66:239–246, 1997

Latner JD: Self-help for obesity and binge eating. Nutr Today 42:81–85, 2007

Latner JD, Wilson GT, Stunkard AJ, et al: Self-help and long-term behavior therapy for obesity. Behav Res Ther 40:805–812, 2002

Lowe MR, Butryn ML: Hedonic hunger: a new dimension of appetite? Physiol Behav 91:432–439, 2007

Lowe MR, Butryn ML, Didie ER, et al: The Power of Food Scale: a new measure of the psychological influence of the food environment. Appetite 53:114–118, 2009

Lynn DJ, Vaillant GE: Anonymity, neutrality, and confidentiality in the actual methods of Sigmund Freud: a review of 43 cases, 1907–1939. Am J Psychiatry 155:163–171, 1998

Markowitz JC, Bleiberg KL, Christos P, et al: Solving interpersonal problems correlates with symptom improvement in interpersonal psychotherapy: preliminary findings. J Nerv Ment Dis 194:15–20, 2006

Mennella JA, Beauchamp GK: The early development of human flavor preferences, in Why We Eat What We Eat: The Psychology of Eating. Edited by Capaldi ED. Washington, DC, American Psychological Association, 1996, pp 83–112

Mintz EE: Gestalt therapy and psychoanalysis. Psychoanal Rev 60:407–411, 1973

Mitchell SA, Black MJ: Freud and Beyond: A History of Modern Psychoanalytic Thought. New York, Basic Books, 1995

National Institutes of Health: Computer Retrieval of Information on Scientific Projects (CRISP). Available at: http://crisp.cit.nih.gov. Accessed March 5, 2009.

Nemiah JC: Psychoanalysis and individual psychotherapy, in The Psychosocial Therapies. Edited by Karasu TB. Washington, DC, American Psychiatric Association, 1984, pp 319–336

Öst LG: Efficacy of the third wave of behavioral therapies: a systematic review and meta-analysis. Behav Res Ther 46:296–321, 2008

Paris J: Treatment of Borderline Personality Disorder: A Guide to Evidence-Based Practice. New York, Guilford, 2008

Park JH, Schaller M, Crandall CS: Pathogen-avoidance mechanisms and the stigmatization of obese people. Evol Hum Behav 28:410–414, 2007

Parrent MF: Binge eating disorder and dimensions of object relations. Dissertation Abstracts International: Section B: The Sciences and Engineering, 57:6587, 1997

Perri MG, McAdoo WG, McAllister DA, et al: Enhancing the efficacy of behavior therapy for obesity: effects of aerobic exercise and a multicomponent maintenance program. J Consult Clin Psychol 54:670–675, 1986

Perri MG, McAllister DA, Gange JJ, et al: Effects of four maintenance programs on the long-term management of obesity. J Consult Clin Psychol 56:529–534, 1988

Perri MG, Nezu AM, McKelvey WF, et al: Relapse prevention training and problem-solving therapy in the long-term management of obesity. J Consult Clin Psychol 69:722–726, 2001

Perri MG, Corsica JA: Improving the maintenance of weight lost in behavioral treatment of obesity, in Handbook of Obesity Treatment. Edited by Wadden TA, Stunkard AJ. New York, Guilford, 2002, pp 357–379

Pollan M: In Defense of Food: An Eater's Manifesto. New York, Penguin Press, 2008

Rand CSW, Stunkard AJ: Obesity and psychoanalysis: treatment and four-year follow-up. Am J Psychiatry 140:1140–1144, 1983

Raynes E, Auerbach C, Botyanski NC: Level of object representation and psychic structure deficit in obese persons. Psychol Rep 64:291–294, 1989

Rippe JM and Weight Watchers: Weight Watchers: Weight Loss that Lasts. Break Through the 10 Big Diet Myths. Hoboken, NJ, Wiley, 2005

Rosenthal MZ, Lynch TR: Dialectical behavioral therapy, in Kaplan & Sadock's Comprehensive Textbook of Psychiatry, 9th Edition, Vol. 2. Edited by Sadock BJ, Sadock VA, Ruiz P. Philadelphia, PA, Wolters Kluwer/Lippincott Williams & Wilkins, 2009, pp 2884–2893

Rozin P: Sociocultural influences on human food selection, in Why We Eat What We Eat: The Psychology of Eating. Edited by Capaldi ED. Washington, DC, American Psychological Association, 1996, pp 233–263

Siegel PS: The completion compulsion in human eating. Psychol Reports 3:15–16, 1957

Sohlberg S, Norring C: Ego functioning predicts first-year status in adults with anorexia nervosa and bulimia nervosa. Acta Psychiatr Scand 80:325–333, 1989

Stahre L, Hällström T: A short-term cognitive group treatment program gives substantial weight reduction up to 18 months from the end of treatment: a randomized controlled trial. Eat Weight Disord 10:51–58, 2005

Stunkard AJ: The 'dieting depression': incidence and clinical characteristics of untoward responses to weight reduction regimens. Am J Med 23:77–86, 1957

Stunkard AJ: The management of obesity. N Y State J Med 58:79–87, 1958

Stunkard AJ, Rush J: Dieting and depression reexamined. Ann Intern Med 81:526–533, 1974

Tanofsky-Kraff M, Wilfley DE, Young JF, et al: Preventing excessive weight gain in adolescents: interpersonal psychotherapy for binge eating. Obesity (Silver Spring) 15:1345–1355, 2007

Tapper K, Shaw C, Ilsley J, et al: Exploratory randomised controlled trial of a mindfulness-based weight loss intervention for women. Appetite 52:396–404, 2009

Taylor CB, Agras WS, Losch M, et al: Improving the effectiveness of computer-assisted weight loss. Behav Ther 22:229–236, 1991

Tsai AG, Wadden TA: Systematic review: an evaluation of major commercial weight loss programs in the United States. Ann Intern Med 142:56–66, 2005

Ursano RJ, Sonnenberg SM, Lazar SG: Psychodynamic psychotherapy, in The American Psychiatric Publishing Textbook of Psychiatry, 5th Edition. Edited by Hales RE, Yudofsky SC, Gabbard GO. Washington, DC, American Psychiatric Publishing, 2008, pp 1171–1190

Wadden TA, Van Itallie TB, Blackburn GL: Responsible and irresponsible use of very-low-calorie diets in the treatment of obesity. JAMA 263: 83–85, 1990

Wadden TA, Butryn ML, Byrne KJ: Efficacy of lifestyle modification for long-term weight control. Obes Res 12(suppl):151S–162S, 2004

Wadden TA, West DS, Neiberg RH, et al; Look AHEAD Research Group: One-year weight losses in the Look AHEAD study: factors associated with success. Obesity (Silver Spring) 17:713–722, 2009

Wansink B: Mindless Eating: Why We Eat More Than We Think. New York, Bantam Books, 2006

Whigham LD, Israel BA, Atkinson RL: Adipogenic potential of multiple human adenoviruses in vivo and in vitro in animals. Am J Physiol Regul Integr Comp Physiol 290:R190–R194, 2006

Wilfley DE, Welch RR, Stein RI, et al: A randomized comparison of group cognitive-behavioral therapy and group interpersonal psychotherapy for the treatment of overweight individuals with binge-eating disorder. Arch Gen Psychiatry 59:713–721, 2002

Wright JH, Thase ME, Beck AT: Cognitive therapy, in The American Psychiatric Publishing Textbook of Psychiatry, 5th Edition. Edited by Hales RE, Yudofsky SC, Gabbard GO. Washington, on DC, American Psychiatric Publishing, 2008, pp 1211–1256

Yontef GM: Awareness, Dialogue and Process: Essays on Gestalt Therapy. Gouldsboro, ME, Gestalt Journal Press, 1993

12

PHARMACOLOGICAL AND SURGICAL TREATMENTS FOR OVERWEIGHT AND OBESITY

Although some individuals may never be thin despite heroic efforts to lose weight,
behavioral therapy may help such individuals to develop a set of skills that lead
to attainment of a healthier, though not ideal, body weight...our current potential
to treat obesity with drugs is limited to only a few options in comparison to the
arsenal of drugs available to treat other chronic diseases...

C. P. Cannon and A. Kumar,
Treatment of Overweight and Obesity (2009)

GENERAL CONSIDERATIONS

All treatment of overweight or obese patients begins with a thorough diagnostic assessment. Measures of body fat range from simple (e.g., calipers to pinch the skin, an inaccurate method) to sophisticated (e.g., computed tomography, magnetic resonance imaging, and even bone density scans). But the two most useful—despite their considerable limitations (which we discussed in Chapter 2, "Obesity in the United States")—are the body mass index or BMI (a measure of the relationship of height and weight) and a person's waist circumference. In Chapter 2, the BMI chart is shown in Figure 2–1 and the categories of obesity are listed on page 15.

Once the level of obesity is determined, a health care professional should take a thorough weight and eating history of both the patient and the patient's family, as well as review the patient's medical history. As we have seen (also in Chapter 2), genetics plays a large part in whether a person is overweight or obese, and if a person has obesity in one or both biological parents, that person has a considerably larger chance of being obese and even of having been overweight since childhood or adolescence. There are many reversible (i.e., treatable) conditions that lead to obesity. The most common are endocrine disorders such as thyroid disorder, particularly hypothyroidism, and Cushing syndrome (an excess of cortisol), but polycystic ovary syndrome, growth hormone deficiency, leptin deficiency, hypogonadism, and even an insulinoma (a tumor producing too much insulin) may be etiological as well (Atkinson 2002, pp. 174–175). More commonly, though, medications can lead to weight gain (see Chapter 7, "Medical Conditions and Weight," particularly Table 7–1). A thorough review of all medications a patient is taking is essential. In particular, many antipsychotics (especially the atypical antipsychotics), antidepressants, and lithium and other mood stabilizers can lead to considerable weight gain. Furthermore, corticosteroids, many oral contraceptives, medications for diabetes (e.g., insulin, sulfonylureas), beta-blockers (e.g., propranolol), and even antihistamines can lead to weight gain (Aronne 2002, p. 385). Assessing a patient's history of drug and alcohol use is also crucial. Alcohol use, in particular, may lead to weight gain (due to both its calorie content and its effects inducing failure to monitor accurately how much one is eating), as can regular use of marijuana (known for stimulating the appetite and sometimes leading to hyperphagia).

Table 12–1 lists specific guidelines for a weight-related clinical interview (WRCI)to assist as a guideline in the initial patient assessment. This clinical interview is designed for clinicians, but patients can be given the questionnaire to complete prior to meeting with a professional.

As noted above, an important part of patient evaluation is an assessment of a patient's eating habits. Many of those who are obese do not necessarily have overt eating disorders (e.g., night eating syndrome, bulimia nervosa, binge eating disorder), but most have disordered patterns of eating (e.g., skipping meals; eating very quickly; chaotic, irregular patterns; frequent snacking on food high in sugar and fat).

Aronne (2002, p. 386) makes the point that assessment of a patient's readiness to lose weight should be part of the evaluation. As noted in Chapter 11 ("Psychological Treatment Strategies and Weight") and by Friedman et al. (2002), there are differences between people with weight problems who come for treatment and those who do not. Sometimes, of course, because of medical problems, weight loss is not an option but a necessity. Nevertheless, given that most people want weight loss for cosmetic reasons, a health care professional should assess the patient's reasons and motivation for wanting weight loss now, the patient's support system (family and friends), and the patient's understanding of risks and benefits as well as the time and potential financial commitments involved (Aronne 2002, p. 386). Close family and friends, in particular, may play central roles: we have noted the study by Christakis and Fowler (2007) in which a person's weight was more similar to the weight of his or her spouse and other important people in the person's life (especially those of the same sex) than to the weight of neighbors or others less important in the person's life (see Chapter 4, "The Psychology of the Eater"). This is a person's *social distance* from someone. Assessment should also include the patient's history of previous attempts at weight loss, both successful and unsuccessful, and any history of weight cycling, as well as the patient's daily physical activity.

Because overweight and obesity are overwhelmingly chronic and not curable conditions, weight control (both weight loss and maintenance) requires long-term treatment and monitoring. Though weight control requires constant vigilance, it can be achieved; the thousands of people in the National Weight Control Registry are testament to the fact that such long-term achievement is possible (for more on the Registry see Chapter 2, "Obesity in the United States"). Weight control can be achieved by different means, though there are commonalities. Several general principles are listed below:

1. Treatment and management must be devised on an individual basis: it is obvious that no two people are identical, either by history or by physicality.

2. A patient must have a sense of self-efficacy (Rothman et al. 2004, pp. 140–141); the patient must not only believe that weight loss and maintenance are possible but also have confidence in his or her ability to bring about and continue the changes in behavior required. In other words, mindset is an important part of readiness to control one's weight. Sometimes, that mindset comes about after a person has crossed the so-called diet boundary and reached a *cognitive set point* (Rogers and Smit 2000). This is the point at which one's current weight is no longer acceptable, and it can be triggered by things such as realizing that clothes no longer fit, seeing a specific number on a scale, or seeing oneself in the mirror and being unpleasantly surprised by what one sees. Sometimes, though, it comes about from diagnosis of a concomitant medical disorder.

3. A person has to focus on both the current goal of weight loss and the future goal of weight maintenance. For example, Magen and Gross (2007) have written of how people engage in *delay discounting*—they devalue or discount something that may occur in the future (e.g., developing medical conditions like diabetes and hypertension secondary to overeating and obesity) in favor of immediate gratification (eating delicious but unhealthy food). (See also Chapter 4, "The Psychology of the Eater.")

4. Along those lines, both health care professionals and patients must be aware and be able to appreciate how ambivalent attitudes—both cognitive and affective—can sabotage weight control efforts. For example, Sparks et al. (2001) have spoken of patients having mixed beliefs, torn feelings, or both (e.g., "chocolate is delicious" vs. "chocolate is fattening and even unhealthy").

Table 12–1.   The weight-related clinical interview (WRCI)

Demographics

Age

Ethnicity

Occupation (e.g., sedentary or not)

Level of education

Marital status

Number of children

Current living situation

Any current stressors or changes

Support system

Who lives in the house currently? And for how long?

Medical history

Previous use of medications

Medical hospitalizations

Chronic diseases (especially those related to weight: diabetes, hypertension, cardiac disease, metabolic abnormalities, sleep apnea, osteoarthritis, or cancer)

Age at onset of menses in women and history of any reproductive disorders

Allergies

Asthma

Patient's weight history

Present height and weight

Birth weight, if known; childhood and adolescent weights (e.g., normal, chubby, obese); teased or bullied?

Lowest adult weight (and for how long)

Previous attempts to lose weight (how lost, how much, and how many times)

Do you own a scale?

How often do you weigh yourself?

Do you have a pattern of "yo-yo" dieting where you have regained weight after an intentional weight loss? If so, how frequently and how long does it take?

What led to successful weight loss in the past? What led to subsequent regain?

Were there any physical or psychological consequences (e.g., depression, anxiety, dieting dysphoria, or even psychotic reactions)?

Pregnancy and weight gain (for women); birth weights of children

Table 12–1. The weight-related clinical interview *(continued)*

Weight and medical history in family

Parents' weights and heights and whether parents are still living

Medical history of parents: diabetes, hypertension, cardiac disease, sleep apnea, osteoarthritis, obesity (including distribution—e.g., "pear-shaped," "apple-shaped"), other metabolic abnormalities, cancer history

Spouse and/or significant others in patient's life: weights and heights

Siblings: weights and heights; any history of disordered eating

Eating history

Eating pattern: meal times, snacking habits, habit of skipping meals, night eating, binge eating, gorging; also history of eating patterns in family and during childhood and adolescence

History of overt eating disorder (e.g., anorexia, bulimia, binge eating disorder)

Favorite foods

What would patient eat for his or her last meal?

Who is responsible for meal preparation (including shopping and cooking)?

How often does patient eat out? How many meals does patient eat alone? How often does patient go to fast-food restaurants? How close are fast-food restaurants to home or work?

Is patient more apt to overeat at restaurants? At parties? While alone?

How fast or slowly does patient eat?

Does patient eat while watching TV? At desk at work? While driving?

How much does patient think about food during the day?

Do any specific foods "call out" to you when patient when these foods are in your cabinet or refrigerator?

Are there any foods patient cannot control once he/she starts eating them? ("trigger foods"?)

Other consumption history

Alcohol and drug consumption: what, how much, how often?

Soft drink consumption: what, how much, how often?

Consumption of coffee or tea: how much and how often?

Smoking habits and history of smoking: what, how much, how often? Related to any weight gain or loss?

Gum chewing?

Psychiatric history

Past history of mental illnesses (e.g., anxiety, depression); psychological and/or pharmacological treatments; hospitalizations

Present state of mind (including motivation to lose weight)

Current medications (including over-the-counter medications and off-label uses of prescription drugs)

Table 12–1. The weight-related clinical interview *(continued)*

Psychiatric history *(continued)*

Psychiatric history in family (including substance use)

History of sexual or physical abuse

History of self-injurious behavior (e.g., cutting, nail biting, suicide attempts)

Emotional eating patterns

Is overeating connected with any emotional states such as anxiety, depression, anger, boredom, or happiness?

Do you have any feelings of loss of control when eating?

Describe your feelings after overeating (e.g., guilt, remorse).

Describe your behavior after overeating (e.g., vomiting, use of laxatives or diuretics, excessive exercise).

Exercise and physical activity

What physical activities do you engage in? How often, for how long, and with what intensity per day and per week?

Do you like to exercise?

Describe physical activity required in your work.

Do you take stairs or elevators?

Do you walk to colleagues' offices or send e-mail?

Describe your hobbies.

Body image

Describe five areas of your body that you are not satisfied with.

Describe yourself physically.

How desirable/attractive are you physically?

How active is your current sexual life?

How would you rate your self-esteem and level of self-confidence (on a scale of 1–10, with 10 being the highest level)?

How heavy do you think you are? How much weight do you want to lose?

Reasons for wanting to lose weight and why now

What is the major reason you want to lose weight now (e.g., medical, cosmetic, or both)?

Why will weight loss and maintenance work this time?

What do you need in order to commit to a program?

Physician's assessment of patient's personality and mental status

Ask patient to describe himself or herself in terms of personality (including whether patient is optimistic or pessimistic).

Table 12–1.   The weight-related clinical interview *(continued)*

Physician's assessment of patient's personality and mental status (*continued*)

Determine how you would describe patient (e.g., compulsive, impulsive, free-spirited, rebellious, self-defeating, paranoid, borderline personality), including mood.

What else is important to know about the patient that has not been asked?

Does patient have any questions?

Note.   The weight-related clinical interview is designed to assist clinicians in obtaining the most relevant information they will need to formulate treatment strategies for a patient with excessive weight. Patients can also be given the questionnaire prior to the interview and, for the most part, can fill it out themselves and discuss it later with clinicians.

5.   People must differentiate the phase of weight loss, which is finite and a time when others are likely to notice weight loss and comment favorably, from the chronic phase of weight maintenance, which must continue indefinitely (during which others are unlikely to continue to comment and are apt to take the weight loss for granted, not appreciating the difficulty of maintaining the new weight). It is even possible that future medications for weight loss will be different from medications for weight maintenance.

Health care professionals must be sensitive to their own overt and covert prejudices against the obese as well as to discrimination a patient may have experienced: we have quoted the Wadden and Didie (2003) study that indicated that the word *fatness* is the most undesirable description for obesity (see Chapter 2 of this volume). Those who treat these patients must steer between the Scylla and Charybdis of avoiding any mention of weight and, at the other extreme, focusing exclusively on a patient's obesity. (For further information on prejudice and psychological vulnerability among those with weight problems, see Chapter 2, "Obesity in the United States," and Chapter 6, "Psychiatric Disorders and Weight.")

> Diet, exercise, and psychological strategies must be a part of every weight loss and maintenance program, including those involving pharmacological or surgical therapies.

A TREATMENT DECISION TREE

Brownell and Wadden (1992) and Gatchel and Oordt (2003, pp. 156–159) have proposed a multilevel process for the treatment of obesity. First, determine the level of obesity, with the heaviest patients requiring the most aggressive treatment. Second, begin care with the least intense, least expensive, and least dangerous treatment available, moving those who do not respond to the next level of treatment. Third, help the patient pick the treatment that most closely matches her or his needs. This stepped concept is illustrated by Wadden et al. (2002), who describe four levels of overweight and obesity and how patients enter this stepped-care process (Figure 12–1). Note that these four levels are not to be confused with the categories of obesity outlined in Chapter 2.

Diet, exercise, and psychological strategies must be a part of every weight loss and maintenance program, regardless of the patient's level of overweight or obesity. These modalities and specific recommendations are described in detail in chapters 8 ("Exercise"), 10 ("Diet and Weight"), and 11 ("Psychological Treatment Strategies and Weight").

The following treatment modalities, pharmacological and surgical, are recommended for weight levels 3 and 4 as these are defined in Figure 12–1. Medication does involve a long-term commitment, just as other treatments for obesity do. Wadden et al. (2002) note, "Investigators no longer expect the short-term use of weight loss medications to cure obesity any more than they expect a 3-month trial of medication to cure diabetes."

PHARMACOLOGICAL APPROACHES TO WEIGHT LOSS

My guess is that Americans by and large don't want a drug that makes them eat less. They want a drug that allows them to eat more, but not gain weight.

Michael Fumento, *The Fat of the Land* (1998, p. 249)

What we know about obesity is that it is a chronic condition and that treatment, particularly when it comes to medication, may be required for life. The model is analogous to treating high blood pressure or diabetes. In fact, it is likely that more than one medication will be required for weight loss and even for weight control.

Medication use in obesity has not had an auspicious past. For example, the medications fenfluramine and phentermine were withdrawn from the market several years ago after unexpected reports surfaced of valvular cardiac disease associated with their use (Bray 2005). Ephedra, sometimes called Ma huang (an epinephrine-like compound), as well, was withdrawn from the U.S. market in 2004 when life-threatening cardiac complications (cardiomyopathy, cardiac arrest, myocardial infarction, arrhythmias, and even sudden death) were reported (Nazeri et al. 2009; Seamon and Clauson 2005).

> Modification of lifestyle alone is usually not sufficient to achieve and maintain significant weight loss. Augmentation with drug therapy is becoming an increasingly important option.
>
> **Source: Aronne et al. 2008**

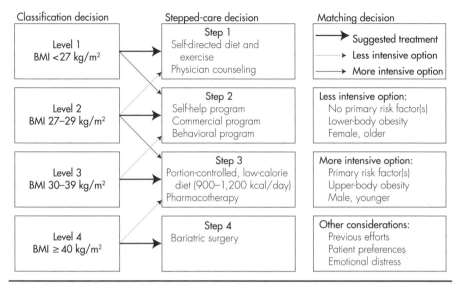

Figure 12–1. A decision tree for selecting treatment.

A conceptual scheme showing a three-stage process for selecting treatment. The first step, the **classification decision,** divides people into four weight categories based on body mass index (BMI) values. The BMI level indicates which of four classes of interventions are likely to be most appropriate in the second stage, the **stepped-care decision.** All individuals are encouraged to control their weight by increasing their physical activity and consuming an appropriate diet. When this approach is not successful, more intensive intervention may be warranted, with the most conservative treatment (i.e., lowest cost and risk of side effects) tried next. The *thick solid arrows* between two boxes show the class of treatments that is usually most appropriate for an individual when less intensive interventions have not been successful. The third stage, the **matching decision,** is used to make a final treatment selection based on the individual's prior weight loss efforts, treatment preferences, and need for weight reduction (as judged by the presence of comorbid conditions or other risk factors). The *dotted lines* point to treatment options for persons with a lesser need for weight reduction because of a lower risk of health complications. The *thin solid arrows* show the more intensive treatment options for patients who, despite having a relatively low BMI level, have a greater risk of health complications. Adjunct nutritional or psychological counseling is recommended for patients who report marked problems with meal planning, depression, body image, or similar difficulties (Wadden et al. 2002).

Source. Reprinted from Wadden TA, Brownell KD, Foster GD: "Obesity: Responding to the Global Epidemic." *Journal of Consulting and Clinical Psychology* 70:510–525, 2002. Used with permission.

FDA-Approved Medications for Weight Loss

Only two medications, sibutramine (Meridia) and orlistat (Xenical, Alli), are currently approved for weight loss by the U.S. Food and Drug Administration (FDA). At this point, medication is recommended only for patients with a BMI value of 30 kg/m² or greater (i.e., in the obese range) or when BMI value is only ≥ 27 kg/m² but the patient has an obesity-related disease or condition (e.g., diabetes, metabolic syndrome) and changes in eating and exercise habits have failed to lead to weight loss after 6 months of these lifestyle changes (Neff and Aronne 2007). Sibutramine inhibits norepinephrine, dopamine, and serotonin reuptake. It acts by reducing appetite and increasing feelings of satiety and hence leads to reduced food intake. Because it is metabolized by the cytochrome P450 enzyme system, it should not be used concurrently with the selective serotonin reuptake inhibitors (Bray 2005; Neff and Aronne 2007), for it may produce the serotonin syndrome, a potentially deadly syndrome manifested by tremor, restlessness, increased reflexes, sweating, shivering, fever, and mental status changes such as confusion (Matorin and Ruiz 2009, p. 1105). Orlistat, by interfering with enzyme activity (e.g., lipase activity), works by inhibiting about 30% of the absorption of fat eaten during a meal (and hence cholesterol intake [Neff and Aronne 2007]). A meta-analysis of double-blind studies of these two medications conducted several years ago (11 studies with orlistat, including >6,000 subjects, and three with sibutramine, including >900 subjects; Neff and Aronne 2007) indicated that attrition rates over the 1-year period for the studies averaged 33% with orlistat and 48% with sibutramine. Weight loss, though better than placebo, was not particularly impressive. About 15% or fewer subjects achieved a weight loss of 10% or more, and this usually occurred within the first 6 months. For most subjects, average weight loss over the year was less than 6 pounds with orlistat and just over 9 pounds with sibutramine. Furthermore, sibutramine apparently does not produce as much weight loss in patients with diabetes as in those without diabetes (Bray 2005). Notably, orlistat was reported to reduce total cholesterol, low-density lipoprotein (LDL) cholesterol, and blood pressure levels as well as improve glucose homeostasis.

In one study, sibutramine led to "small improvements" in high-density lipoprotein (HDL) cholesterol and triglyceride levels but had no clinically or statistically significant effects on glucose control, LDL levels, or total cholesterol levels (Padwal et al. 2003). However, Neff and Aronne (2007) report on other studies that have demonstrated significantly greater improvements in glucose control, HDL cholesterol levels, triglyceride levels, and even waist circumference with sibutramine when compared with placebo. Because it is a sympathomimetic drug, it is not surprising that about 5% of patients taking sibutramine have had evidence of increased systolic and diastolic blood pressure (Bray 2005) and increased pulse. And 7%–20% have had nausea, constipation, dry mouth, or insomnia. The dosage is between 10 and 15 mg once daily with or without food. Wilfley et al. (2008) found in a 24-week study of over 300 patients who met criteria for binge eating disorder that those taking 15-mg doses of sibutramine had significantly fewer binges per week compared with placebo recipients, and mean weight losses of almost 9 pounds. The placebo response in this study, as is sometimes typical in studies of patients with binge eating disorder or other psychiatric disorders, was high: almost one-third in the first (single-blind) phase of the study and over 40% in the second (double-blind) phase were considered placebo responders. The dropout rate was also high, at 38%, though "most dropouts were not due to adverse events" (Wilfley et al. 2008).

Up to 30% of patients taking orlistat had gastrointestinal symptoms, including bloating, oily stools, urgency, and even stool incontinence; decreased levels of β-carotene and fat-soluble vitamins, such as A, D (the most affected), and E were also seen (Padwal et al. 2003). As a result, it is recommended that patients taking orlistat also take a supplemental multivitamin daily. Orlistat has now been approved by the FDA in a reduced dosage form for over-the-counter use. Instead of 120 mg taken three times a day, the dosage of the over-the-counter version, called Alli, is 60 mg taken three times a day. Orlistat has what has been called the "Antabuse effect" Yanovski (2003). Just as patients who drink alcohol while taking Antabuse (disulfiram) become physically ill (with symptoms like throbbing headache, nausea, anxiety, and confusion that can last for several hours [MDConsult 2009]), patients taking orlistat also get an aversive conditioning effect with unpleasant symptoms such as greasy stools and urgency when they do not restrict their fat intake. Yanovski (2003) describes research that suggests that the use of orlistat can lead to a change in a person's fat preferences: people taking it seemed to prefer foods with less fat when given a choice among puddings with different fat content, and this effect was independent of any weight loss.

Off-Label Uses of Medications to Achieve Weight Loss

Many medications in the United States are used for their side effect of weight loss even though they are only approved for other purposes. Two such medications are topiramate (used also to treat migraine headaches) and zonisamide, both approved for treatment of seizure disorders.

Topiramate can produce a weight loss, on average, of about 13 pounds within a year, but it has been associated with cognitive difficulties such as memory problems as well as paresthesias, although these effects are apparently dose related (Powers and Cloak 2007, p. 267). Topiramate may also cause metabolic acidosis, so serum bicarbonate levels must be monitored before and during treatment (Korner and Aronne 2004). Recently, topiramate has been used successfully, in combination with cognitive-behavioral therapy, in the treatment of obesity and binge eating disorder (Claudino et al. 2007).

Zonisamide has been reported to produce a weight loss of about 10 pounds within a year, but it also has been associated with cognitive effects, as well as somnolence and fatigue, rashes (when a patient has a sulfa allergy; L. J. Aronne, personal communication, April 2009), nausea, and taste perversions. Because of its chemical properties, it may increase serum creatinine levels. It has been used in combination with the antidepressant bupropion to increase weight loss, and with fluoxetine to decrease weight gain.

These medications' exact mechanisms of action are not known but are thought to be related to their effects on neurotransmitters, such as serotonin and dopamine in the case of zonisamide, and glutamate blockade with topiramate (Korner and Aronne 2004). Like topiramate, zonisamide has also been used with some effect in obese binge eaters, but attrition rates tend to be as high as 50% (McElroy et al. 2006).

Several medications used in the treatment of type 2 diabetes have unexpectedly been found to produce weight loss. For example, metformin can produce about a 4-pound weight loss and can even be used to forestall the onset of diabetes in individuals at potential risk (Korner and Aronne 2004). Metformin, which seems to decrease food intake, has also been used effectively as an adjunct therapy to control weight gain and even insulin resistance (by increasing insulin sensitivity) in schizophrenic patients given the weight-inducing antipsychotic olanzapine (Wu et al. 2008). Another medication approved to treat diabetes that has some role in controlling food intake and increasing feelings of satiety (and hence can lead to weight loss) is exenatide, a medication given by injection. It is a receptor agonist for glucagon-like peptide 1 (GLP-1), a hormone produced in the small intestine and colon that is released with food intake. Side effects, though, include nausea, diarrhea, and vomiting. When injected twice daily, exenatide can lead to a weight loss of about 6 pounds (Neff and Aronne 2007). The oral medication sitagliptin, a protease enzyme inhibitor, used in type 2 diabetes to enhance insulin secretion, is well tolerated and is "weight neutral" (Neff and Aronne 2007).

Pramlintide is a synthetic preparation of the peptide amylin, which is secreted with insulin by beta cells in the pancreas. Use of pramlintide leads to decreased food intake and subsequent weight loss by suppressing glucagon release and controlling emptying of the stomach (Neff and Aronne 2007). It tends to work locally and more specifically on short-term regulation of food intake, though it binds to receptors in the hindbrain. Over the period of 1 year in which pramlintide was used in conjunction with the LEARN (*lifestyle, exercise, attitudes, relationships, and nutrition*) program—which included the lifestyle interventions of diet (decreasing daily calorie intake by 500) and exercise (walking 10,000 steps per day) plus varying dosages of pramlintide (120, 240, or 360 μg bid or tid)—some patients lost up to 13 pounds and decreased their waist circumference. Pramlintide administration usually involves three injections a day, but when the highest dose of 360 μg was used, two injections were sufficient. Significantly, weight loss was not maintained over the 12-month period when only diet and exercise without medication were used. Though side effects, such as nausea and hypoglycemia, were mild, this study had a high attrition rate (Smith et al. 2008).

In another study, pramlintide was used in combination with a preparation of human leptin, the so-called satiety hormone produced primarily by adipose tissue (Roth et al. 2008; results presented below). When it was first discovered in 1994, researchers believed leptin would be a kind of "magic bullet" breakthrough treatment for weight loss (Roth et al. 2008). Unfortunately, results have been very disappointing. Plasma levels of leptin have to be ten times higher than normal in both human subjects and rodents in order to bring about weight loss. Levels are higher in obese people but, as noted in Chapter 5 ("The Metabolic Complexities of Weight Control"), a state of leptin resistance seems to develop with high leptin levels. Leptin resistance is not well understood, but experiments with mice indicate it may be related to downregulation of receptors, impaired transport across the blood-brain barrier, or even decreased signaling in the hypothalamus (Roth et al. 2008).

What researchers are finding is that although leptin may not work so effectively in the process of weight loss (except in the very few patients who have an actual genetic leptin deficiency), it may work in the weight maintenance phase to prevent weight regain. Experiments by Rosenbaum et al. (2005), for example, demonstrated that giving leptin to patients who had already lost weight reversed changes that the weight loss had brought about in skeletal muscle and the sympathetic nervous system, changes that would normally predispose these patients to regaining weight. Normally, leptin seems to "defend—not reduce" the level of fat in the body, so that after weight loss, lowered leptin levels appear to lead to a person's eating more and decreasing the amount of calories expended in exercise. In other words, when leptin levels fall after weight loss, the body mounts a counterregulation to protect against this perceived threat to survival and seems programmed to regain the lost fat stores. It makes sense, therefore, that medications that induce weight loss initially may ultimately be very different from those that prevent weight regain (Rosenbaum et al. 2005). But when leptin was coadministered with pramlintide, the two medications seemed to work synergistically; together they produced a mean weight loss of more than 25 pounds (more than when either agent is used alone), and the weight loss did not plateau, as tends to occur when each agent is used individually, during the 24-week course of the experiment (Roth et al. 2008).

> Leptin may not be effective for weight loss in most patients, but it may work to prevent weight regain in the maintenance phase. Leptin seems to defend, not reduce, the level of fat in the body.

Medications like the histamine type 2 receptor antagonists that are approved treatments for reducing acidity in the stomach, such as cimetidine, have also been reported to lead to satiety and weight loss in some studies (Zimmermann et al. 2003). And the medication naltrexone, an opiate antagonist, has been shown to reduce food cravings and appetite.

Bupropion is unusual as an antidepressant in that it is associated with statistically significant but "modest" weight loss, rather than weight gain, in some patients. It is not considered a medication for weight loss specifically, but it has a place in the treatment of depression when further weight gain is unwanted. For example, in a study of over 400 depressed patients using 300 mg of the sustained-release formulation, a weight loss of about 3 pounds was maintained throughout the year of the study (Croft et al. 2002). The mechanism for its weight loss effects is not completely known, but is thought to be related to increasing levels of dopamine without affecting levels of serotonin or histamine. Bupropion is also used to aid in smoking cessation and helps reduce weight gain following nicotine withdrawal.

Naltrexone is a medication that has been used in combination with other medications, including bupropion, to produce synergistic effects of weight loss not achieved by either alone. Naltrexone is an opioid antagonist given orally that affects both the β-endorphin system and the pro-opiomelanocortin (POMC) neurons in the hypothalamus that integrate short-term signals related to eating. (POMC is a prohormone that splits into α–melanocyte-stimulating hormone and β-lipoprotein, which becomes β-endorphin; when its levels increase, appetite, food intake, and body weight decrease.) The opioid antagonists seem to work in part by affecting the systems involved in the palatability of foods, especially sugary and fatty foods, thus affecting the "hedonic evaluation"—the liking of food, as opposed to the wanting of food. Indirectly, this process affects appetite and food cravings.

Bupropion, which also stimulates the POMC system, given together with naltrexone led to a greater weight loss in a 24-week study than when either agent is used alone, and the weight loss did not plateau as typically occurs when each agent is used separately. Nausea, usually without vomiting, was the most common side effect, but there were also reports of headache, insomnia, and dizziness (Greenway et al. 2009).

Perhaps one of the most interesting medications for weight loss is rimonabant, a selective cannabinoid type 1 (CB_1) receptor antagonist that has been used for years in Europe but to date is not FDA approved. Interest in the endocannabinoid system developed years ago when it was noted that the active ingredient in marijuana gives people the "munchies"—that is, it increases appetite. Rimonabant is, in effect, an antimarijuana agent (Rumsfeld and Nallamothu 2008).

The endocannabinoid system works both centrally and peripherally with receptors throughout the body, including the brain, gastrointestinal tract, liver, and adipose tissue, and has different functions based on where the receptors are. These receptors apparently "act on demand…depending [on] where and when they are needed" (Cota et al. 2006). For example, in the central nervous system, CB_1 receptors seem to be involved in both homeostatic regulation and the pleasure and reward (hedonic) aspects of energy balance and food intake; in the gastrointestinal tract these receptors increase ghrelin secretion and hence increase appetite and food intake. Studies have indicated that there is a primary dysregulation of the endocannabinoid system in obese individuals (Neff and Aronne 2007).

There have been four phase 3 (human) clinical trials of rimonabant in obesity (RIO) that were randomized, double-blind, and placebo controlled and included once-daily doses of either 20 mg or 5 mg of rimonabant: RIO-Europe (trial for 2 years' duration); RIO-North America (also of 2 years' duration); RIO-Lipids (of 1 year's duration) for those with dyslipidemias; and RIO-Diabetes (of 1 year's duration) for those with type 2 diabetes (U.S. Food and Drug Administration 2007). The medication (i.e. rimonabant) is very effective in producing weight loss over time: it led to a 10% or greater weight loss in up to 39% of people in the RIO-Europe study and was associated with decreased waist circumferences and improved metabolic profiles (e.g., HDL cholesterol, triglyceride, and glucose levels (Van Gaal et al. 2005). In both the RIO-Lipids and RIO-Europe trials, rimonabant increased HDL cholesterol levels by up to 10%, lowered triglyceride levels by up to 30%, and lowered levels of C-reactive protein, a nonspecific marker of inflammation and cardiovascular disease (Vemuri et al. 2008). Rimonabant can increase glucose uptake by the muscles, block de novo lipogenesis in the liver, and increase secretion of adiponectin, a hormone produced by adipose tissue that increases fatty acid oxidation and protects against inflammation (Wright et al. 2008). It also interferes with cravings for palatable foods, particularly sweets (Pacher et al. 2006). Troublesome side effects have been reported, though: depression and suicidal ideation occurred in some studies in almost 3% of subjects receiving a dosage of 20 mg/day.

In the study with the acronym STRADIVARIUS (the Strategy to Reduce Atherosclerosis Development Involving Administration of Rimonabant—the Intravascular Ultrasound Study [Nissen et al. 2008]), symptoms of depression were higher with the 20-mg/day dosage than with placebo (43.% and 28.4%, respectively), and one in seven patients reported psychiatric symptoms such as depression and anxiety. This study apparently did not exclude individuals with a prior history of psychiatric disorders, and it may therefore be more reflective of patients who would be seen in a general clinical setting than studies that exclude such individuals (Rumsfeld and Nallamothu 2008). However, the adverse effects led to the FDA's refusal to approve rimonabant in June 2007 without further research. Nausea, dizziness, anxiety, insomnia, and fatigue have also been reported (Neff and Aronne 2007). In 2007, the FDA published a "Briefing Document" regarding rimonabant 20 mg (U.S. Food and Drug Administration 2007). The FDA (2007) summarized results from the pooled RIO (rimonabant in obesity) studies and found 26% of those on 20 mg of rimonabant (n=1,602) experienced "a psychiatric symptom" versus 14% of the placebo group (n=2,176)—specifically, 9% of those receiving rimonabant reported depression, whereas 5% of those receiving placebo did.

Nevertheless, rimonabant has already been approved for use in more than 40 countries, and in the United Kingdom alone it has been used by more than 40,000 patients (Wright et al. 2008). Aronne et al. (2008) reviewed some of the data regarding suicide risk that had been assessed by the FDA, including studies on the use of rimonabant for smoking cessation. Using the Columbia Classification Algorithm of Suicide Assessment, which evaluates a range of behaviors from self-injurious behavior to completed suicides, they found that the incidence of suicide ideation was actually similar in individuals given placebo and those given rimonabant 20 mg/day—and in fact, the incidence of ideation or attempts was higher in those given placebo.

Gorzalka et al. (2008) take a different approach and focus on the detrimental effects of blocking the endocannabinoid system (as with a drug like rimonabant). Just as marijuana has a calming and stress-reducing effect, so the endocannabinoid system itself seems to function beneficially in habituating a person to chronic stress. We know from animal experiments that when an organism is repeatedly exposed to the same stressor over time, response to that stressor is gradually attenuated. And apparently, as seen in these experiments, rimonabant can interfere with this adaptive process of habituation. Gorzalka et al. (2008) question whether any disruption in this system—even just an inability to upregulate endocannibinoid signals, as might be caused by blocking it with a medication like rimonabant—might be involved in predisposing someone to depression. The tricyclic antidepressant medication desipramine, for example, enhances (upregulates) endocannabinoid signals. There is the suggestion that the endocannabinoid system functions as a kind of gatekeeper for the hypothalamic-pituitary-adrenal stress axis, and future antidepressants may be able to target this system specifically (Gorzalka et al. 2008).

Rimonabant is also now being studied as a potential therapy for people with alcohol addiction (Vemuri et al. 2008). There is speculation that the cannabinoids and the opioids use some of the same mechanisms, including regulation of dopamine release, particularly in regard to behaviors involving motivation such as reward and appetite. Furthermore, it is thought that the endocannabinoids may increase dopamine release by activating the opioid system. Rimonabant has been shown to block the release of dopamine that is caused by both alcohol and nicotine. Rimonabant has also been found to lessen the rewarding effects of morphine and even to lead to withdrawal in rats that are opiate dependent. It seems to have a general role as an anticraving drug in that it stops relapse into drug-seeking behavior regardless of the type of drug abused. And combining rimonabant with the opioid antagonist naloxone seems to have synergistic effects in curbing appetite and hence leading to weight loss (Cota et al. 2006).

Dietary Supplements

Nonprescription drugs have been touted for years as immediate cures for excessive weight. There is no known substance to date that can lead to miraculous weight loss, but patients can be fooled. Again, as noted about diet claims (Chapter 10, "Diet and Weight"), let the buyer beware! One patient recently told us he had heard of a medication that could lead to a pound of weight loss a day, and some people will believe that is possible. Most of these compounds are sold in health food stores as dietary supplements and are not FDA approved or subject to any kind of regulation. Years ago, some supplements contained the herbal stimulant ephedra, but they have been banned because of unsafe cardiovascular side effects including myocardial infarctions, seizures, and even death. Furthermore, it is not always clear whether the products sold even contain the compounds they are purported to contain, let alone in the doses recommended. Many of these products are hardly placebos and may contain impurities, contaminants, illegal drugs, or traces of FDA-approved drugs that are not mentioned on the label's list of ingredients. These products can obviously be dangerous when taken unsupervised or without full knowledge of what they contain. For example, the *New York Times* (Singer 2009) reported that the product sold under the name of StarCaps had contained the drug bumetanide, a diuretic used for patients with heart failure that can lead to dehydration and hypotension as well as untoward reactions with other medications (U.S. Food and Drug Administration 2009). Many other "natural" diet pills, some imported from China, were also found to contain medications that were not listed among the ingredients. Singer noted that Extrim Plus was reported to contain the antiseizure medication phenytoin; Phyto Shape was reported to contain the weight loss medication rimonabant (which as noted above is not approved for use in the United States); and ProSlim Plus and Sliminate were reported to contain the approved weight loss medication sibutramine, which requires a prescription. The marketing research publication *Nutrition Business Journal* found that of the $24 billion spent per year on dietary supplements in the United States, $1.7 billion are spent on weight loss pills alone (Singer 2009).

Summary: Medication Management

To date, medication management for weight loss leaves much to be desired, but there is reason to be optimistic for the future as we understand more about the physiological underpinnings of weight control. For now, medication needs to be seen as an adjunct to other dimensions of weight control, especially environmental influences, namely diet, exercise, and behavioral modifications. For example, Wadden et al. (2005) studied over 200 obese adults (mostly women) in trials comparing the use of sibutramine 15 mg/day and/or lifestyle modification over the course of 1 year. There was an attrition rate of 17%. Lifestyle modification, following the LEARN program, consisted of an exercise regimen, a low-calorie diet of 1,200–1,500 calories per day, and counseling sessions of varying frequency and length. With brief lifestyle modification sessions, the subjects met with a primary care provider; with longer and more frequent sessions, the subjects met with a trained psychologist. Per the LEARN philosophy, subjects were encouraged to keep an exercise and food-intake log for accountability. Not surprisingly, those given sibutramine and more intensive lifestyle counseling lost the most weight: those given sibutramine without any lifestyle modification sessions lost between 11 and 16 pounds, whereas at 1 year, subjects in the combined medication and counseling group lost an average of over 25 pounds. Almost three-fourths of subjects in the combined medication and lifestyle counseling group lost 5% or more of their initial weight, and over half of them lost 10% of their initial weight. Even the counseling-only group lost weight during the first 18 weeks of the study (Wadden et al. 2005). The point is that medication alone, even when effective, becomes more so when there is accountability as provided by keeping careful records of food intake and exercise, and an extended relationship over time to other people, including counselors.

SURGICAL APPROACHES

Plastic Surgery

The Body Contouring of Liposuction

Among the most severely obese, who have considerable medical comorbidities such as hypertension and diabetes, the primary reason people give for wanting to lose weight is to improve their appearance (Sarwer and Thompson 2002, p. 451) (see Chapter 6, "Psychiatric Disorders and Weight"). We seem to be a culture preoccupied with appearance, with the "'good' body versus the 'bad' body" (Napoleon and Lewis 1989). After all, patients seeking cosmetic surgery, including the procedure of liposuction, care enough about their appearance to subject themselves to the pain and discomfort of surgery (Napoleon and Lewis 1989). Cosmetic surgery has even been called *body image surgery* (Bolton et al. 2003).

> Failure to address appropriate psychological screening can result in serious consequences of bariatric surgery, including delayed recovery time, poor compliance, relapses, negative emotional states, and even lawsuits.

In a survey of over 250 plastic surgery practices, Borah et al. (1999) found that psychological complications (most commonly anxiety and depression) occur at least as frequently as physical complications, and those who experience physical complications are much more likely to have psychological complications. They also found a correlation between preoperative anxiety and postoperative anxiety, as well as both mild and severe depression. In other words, those who had psychological distress before surgery were more susceptible to psychological distress postoperatively. Appropriate psychological screening is therefore crucial both prior to and after surgery. Failure to address or manage these psychological complications can have "profound consequences," including delayed recovery time, poor patient compliance with postsurgical instructions, and even hostility to the surgeon and staff.

Sarwer et al. (2002) found that although dissatisfaction with one's body image is the motivation for seeking cosmetic surgery, it is not overall dissatisfaction but rather heightened dissatisfaction with a particular area of his or her body for which a person seeks treatment. Buescher and Buescher (2006) estimate that 10% of individuals seeking cosmetic surgery have body dysmorphic disorder, and Sarwer et al. (2002) found that 7% of those seeking cosmetic surgery in their own study met criteria for this disorder. In general, these patients do not respond well to surgery, with exacerbations or no change in their symptoms (and even violence toward the surgeon or staff), such that it is recommended that cosmetic surgery be contraindicated in this population (Sarwer et al. 2002). Because cosmetic plastic surgery is elective and the notion of patient selection can seem a misnomer, plastic surgeons must be able to screen to distinguish those who simply wish to improve their body contour or their appearance (i.e., they have some specific and realistic reason for being dissatisfied with their body) from those who border on obsession and have overt psychopathology, with serious misperceptions about their body. (See "Body Image and Body Dysmorphic Disorder" section in Chapter 6, "Psychiatric Disorders and Weight," for more on this disorder.)

One of the screening techniques that plastic surgeons can use is to ask a patient to list in order the major five areas she or he thinks need improvement and compare this to the surgeon's own list. If the surgeon's list is substantially different and does not even include areas the patient has singled out, the surgeon may see these discrepancies as a potential red flag warning that this patient warrants special consideration (Napoleon and Lewis 1989). A referral for psychiatric consultation may be necessary before any serious consideration of surgery.

> Plastic surgeons must distinguish patients who have some specific and realistic reason for body dissatisfaction from those who border on obsession and have overt psychopathology and serious misperceptions about their body.

Liposuction is a cosmetic surgical procedure, developed some years ago, that involves the removal of some of the subcutaneous fat (fat beneath the skin as opposed to visceral fat around the organs), or adipose tissue, in the body. About 80% of all the fat in the body is considered subcutaneous (Spalding et al. 2008). Researchers Esposito et al. (2006) acknowledge there is controversy in the literature regarding the metabolic effects of liposuction, but they nevertheless believe that liposuction has a place in obesity treatment in an effort to improve patients' metabolic profiles. As plastic surgeons, they removed the equivalent of almost 3 kilograms (~7 pounds) of fat per patient (considered *large-volume liposuction*) in 45 premenopausal obese women; these women did not yet have full-blown type 2 diabetes, hypertension, or cardiovascular disease, although they did have decreased insulin sensitivity and increased levels of markers for inflammation (e.g., C-reactive protein and tumor necrosis factor alpha [TNF-α]). Esposito et al. followed these patients from 6 months to 1 year and found that, on average, the women had lost 3.5 kilograms (~8 pounds) of body weight and had "significant amelioration" of the markers for inflammation, including increased insulin sensitivity. The study report did not specify whether the subjects were instructed in diet and exercise regimens, as the physicians had done in other studies that they conducted. They did conclude, however, that liposuction should be incorporated into a program that includes lifestyle changes, and they also recommended larger, controlled studies to confirm their findings (Esposito et al. 2006).

Those who have excessive weight have excessive adipose tissue. As noted in an earlier chapter, fat tissue was originally thought to be merely an inert storage container for lipids, for the body's energy supplies (see Chapter 5, "The Metabolic Complexities of Weight Control"). Now, however, we appreciate that adipose tissue is actually an endocrine organ that actively secretes many adipokines (some as yet unidentified) such as leptin and adiponectin; it may therefore seem strange to think of removing this tissue surgically. But that is what thousands of people do when they choose to undergo the procedure of liposuction.

Liposuction is one of the most common aesthetic plastic surgery operations in the United States. With over 245,000 operations done in 2008, it is also one of the most common surgical procedures in general (American Society of Plastic Surgeons 2009). This 2008 figure is down 31% from a high in 2000 of over 354,000 liposuction procedures (presumably because of changes in the economy in more recent years), but it is up from 200,000 procedures per year performed in the mid 1980s (Napoleon and Lewis 1989). Liposuction is used for contouring the body in specific areas that genetically accumulate fat that seems immune to dieting. There is, after all, no "spot reducing—no matter how many sit-ups a person does" (Joseph Rabson, M.D., personal communication, April 2009). The procedure, though, can be expensive and is not covered by insurance, given that it is an aesthetic procedure. One woman, bothered by the "handles" on her hips, paid $10,000 to a plastic surgeon in New York for what amounted to removal of less than 1 pound of fat; clearly, the degree of body dissatisfaction may be completely unrelated to the amount of extra weight a person has (Sarwer and Thompson 2002, p. 447). Liposuction involves making small holes in a specific area, then injecting a fluid, such as saline fluid, and epinephrine to constrict the blood vessels. The fat removal can be done using several different techniques, including a vibrating power-suction machine that liquefies or breaks up the fat. It can be an office procedure, but depending on how much fat is to be removed, it may require general anesthesia and a hospital setting. Ultrasound has been used, though there is a risk of burning, and more recently a laser-assisted approach has been used that some believe is associated with less morbidity and a shorter recovery time (Parlette and Kaminer 2008).

It should be noted that the number of fat cells tends to remain constant after adolescence in both lean and obese people. When fat cells are lost, apparently new fat cells are produced. Obese people, particularly those who have been obese since childhood, have significantly more fat cells than lean people, and the cells have a higher rate of turnover—but it is the enlarging of fat cells by excessive lipid accumulation, not the greater number, that usually accounts for obesity. Spalding et al. (2008) found that fat cell numbers remained the same even

- It is usually not the number of fat cells but their size that accounts for lipid accumulation.

- Fat cells removed by liposuction can be compensated for by the enlargement of remaining cells.

2 years after bariatric surgery or other means of substantial weight loss had reduced BMI values and fat cell volume. There is, however, a constant turnover of fat cells throughout life, even though the adipocyte number is tightly controlled and not influenced by changes in calorie intake. About half of our adipocytes are replaced

every 8 or so years, a rate that is similar in everyone no matter what a person weighs. Learning what mechanism determines adipocyte turnover may eventually lead to new medications against obesity (Spalding et al. 2008).

Some surgeons recommend dieting prior to scheduling a liposuction procedure. Significantly, Sarwer et al. (1998) found that those who present to plastic surgeons with cosmetic surgery requests tend to be health conscious in general: prospective patients scored higher than a comparison group of a national sample of age-comparable women on the Health Evaluation Scale and the Health, Fitness, and Illness Orientation subscale.

Though pounds of subcutaneous fat can potentially be removed safely, plastic surgeons such as Rohrich and colleagues (2004) and Joseph Rabson of Pennsylvania (personal communication, April 2009) emphasize that liposuction is not considered or recognized as a procedure for weight loss per se. They have seen, though, that after surgery people are often sufficiently motivated to continue to diet and do so successfully, with subsequent weight loss and maintenance over time. Rohrich et al. (2004) surveyed patients from 6 months to over 2 years after liposuction, with over half of respondents having had the procedure done more than 2 years ago. Of the more than 200 respondents, 57% reported no weight gain after surgery and, of those, 46% had actually lost weight (some as much as 10 pounds). Rohrich et al. (2004) believe that successful liposuction depends on three postoperative variables: committing to a healthy lifestyle, following a healthy diet, and exercising regularly. Furthermore, patients who are not committed to eating healthy foods are three times more likely to gain weight, and patients who do not commit to exercising regularly are four times more likely to gain weight: "Successful body contouring surgery requires a patient to embrace positive lifestyle habits" (Rohrich et al. 2004). Incidentally, both men and women undergo liposuction, but the procedure is much more commonly done in women (89% in 2008) (American Society of Plastic Surgeons 2009).

But is the quantity of fat in the body regulated? Some, like Mauer et al. (2001), think it may be so: evolutionarily, given that fat is for energy storage, it might be expected that the body would resist a decrease in total body fat whereas it would not necessarily oppose an increase in this energy storage unit. Even for an animal, though, being too fat has potentially negative consequences, such as being an easy target for a predator. So it makes sense that there could be homeostatic mechanisms, a "lipostat," if you will, involved in regulation. In fact, in rodent experiments, as we have mentioned, rats given highly palatable food (the so-called cafeteria diet) developed both metabolic and behavioral changes that restored their weight to its initial level when they resumed a regular diet (Mauer et al. 2001). Environmental factors such as temperature and light have also been known to contribute to regulation of fat in animals in lipectomy experiments. Interestingly, experiments with animals have also found that in some species, after surgical removal of fat, the animals have sometimes had "recovery" of that fat within months. This fat compensation, as it were, occurred even though the animal did not necessarily increase its eating. This seems to fit with the work of Spalding et al. (2008) that showed that when fat cells are destroyed, new ones are created.

Along those lines, there are reports in the literature that breast enlargement occurs in up to 40% of women months after liposuction, particularly in those who gain weight after the procedure (van der Lei et al. 2007). This unexpected incidental finding has been more common when liposuction is done on the hips and abdomen and when a larger volume of fat is aspirated during the procedure. The mechanism is not known, but there is speculation that changes in the estrogen-androgen balance may occur after liposuction of these areas (Yun et al. 2003).

Another significant question regarding liposuction is whether removal of subcutaneous fat has any effect on the metabolic disturbances commonly seen in patients with excessive weight. Visceral fat (i.e., fat that encases internal organs) is more metabolically active than subcutaneous fat. It produces more of the pathological cytokines like TNF-α and interleukin-6 (IL-6), both of which are associated with inflammation, insulin resistance, endothelial dysfunction, and eventually atherosclerosis, and less of the beneficial hormone adiponectin (Hamdy et al. 2006). Visceral fat is the fat that gives someone—male or female, but usually male—an abnormally large waist (the android pattern of fat distribution) and is usually associated with components of the metabolic syndrome such as abnormal glucose metabolism, hypertension, an abnormal lipid profile (including abnormal triglyceride levels), and even overt type 2 diabetes. These metabolic abnormalities are not typically associated with the gynoid pattern of fat distribution, which is excessive subcutaneous fat on the hips, thighs, and buttocks, where liposuction is most commonly done.

Researchers Esposito et al. (2006) acknowledge the controversy in the literature regarding the metabolic effects of liposuction, but they nevertheless believe liposuction has a place in obesity treatment in an effort to improve the metabolic profiles of patients. As plastic surgeons, they removed the equivalent of almost 3 kilograms of fat (considered "large volume liposuction") in 45 premenopausal obese women, but these women did not yet have full-blown type 2 diabetes, hypertension, or cardiovascular disease, although they did have decreased insulin sensitivity and increased markers for inflammation (C-reactive protein and TNF-α). Esposito et al. (2006) followed their sample from 6 months to 1 year and found that on average, the women had lost 3.5 kilograms of body weight and had "significant amelioration" of the markers for inflammation, including increased insulin sensitivity. The study, though, did not specify whether the subjects were instructed in diet and exercise regimens, as had been done in other studies conducted by them. Esposito et al. (2006) did conclude, however, that liposuction should be incorporated into a program that includes lifestyle changes, and they also recommended further larger controlled studies to confirm their findings.

Though there is some controversy, most studies do support the notion that liposuction of subcutaneous fat, even in the abdominal area (where there can be both visceral fat around organs and subcutaneous fat), does not significantly alter a person's metabolic profile. It does not improve insulin sensitivity of muscle, liver, or fat tissue, insulin levels or glucose homeostasis, blood pressure, or lipid profiles. Nor does it significantly change levels of C-reactive protein, IL-6, TNF-α, or adiponectin (Klein et al. 2004). Even when liposuction removes large quantities of subcutaneous fat (it can remove billions of adipocytes [Mohammed et al. 2008]), decreases waist circumference, and reduces leptin levels, it does not improve these metabolic parameters as bariatric surgery, diet-induced weight loss, and weight loss with the use of medications do. It decreases the number of fat cells temporarily, but it does not decrease fat cell size.

> The metabolic culprit is visceral fat, not subcutaneous fat; thus liposuction removal of subcutaneous fat is less likely to help metabolic disturbances.

Like Rabson (J. Rabson, personal communication, April 2009), Klein et al. (2004) emphasize that liposuction definitely should not be considered a clinical treatment for obesity. Their 2004 report, however, generated considerable discussion in the Letters to the Editor section of the *New England Journal of Medicine*, where it was published. Esposito et al. (2004), Arner (2004), and Busetto et al. (2004) all independently support the notion that large-volume liposuction (e.g., ≥ 10 kilograms), particularly when the fat removed is visceral fat, has provided benefits in terms of metabolic functioning, including insulin resistance, glucose tolerance, and levels of inflammatory markers. Discrepancies in data may be related to confounding variables like lifestyle changes, differences in the populations studied, and level of obesity prior to surgery, as well as factors such as the amount and site of the adipose tissue removed.

Bergman (Aronne 2007) explains further that for patients with excessive subcutaneous fat, as BMI values increase there is a linear reduction in insulin sensitivity, but the more a BMI value increases, the more the linear reduction in insulin sensitivity flattens. This means that if a patient with a BMI value of 35 kg/m^2 undergoes liposuction and the procedure results in a decrease in BMI value to about 31 or 32 kg/m^2, the insulin sensitivity will not increase because "you are in the flat part of the curve." In a small prospective study, though, Ybarra et al. (2008) found that abdominal liposuction did independently improve lipid levels (triglyceride levels decreased and HDL cholesterol levels increased) in healthy normal-weight or slightly overweight people, but did not affect insulin sensitivity or other metabolic parameters such as adiponectin or C-reactive protein levels. Despite the results of improved lipid profiles, Ybarra et al. (2008) also conclude that visceral fat rather than subcutaneous fat is the metabolic culprit.

In another study, Mohammed et al. (2008) studied a small population of women for a period ranging from 1½ years to almost 4 years after extensive subcutaneous fat removal by liposuction. They wanted to assess whether any beneficial effects had been masked by the transient inflammation that typically occurs for weeks after the procedure. In fact, no beneficial effects had been masked: even though their patients lost about 7% of their body weight (and maintained the loss through the course of follow-up), their cardiovascular metabolic profiles did not improve. Mohammed et al. (2008), though, caution that we really do not know enough about the effects of liposuction when patients do regain weight after the procedure. Even though such patients do not gain weight in the aspirated areas, they may gain weight in other areas (e.g., the upper back and breasts). These researchers raise the intriguing speculation that liposuction, at least in those who do ultimately regain weight over the long term, could possibly lead to fat being redistributed to more metabolically problematic areas like the liver and skeletal muscle, such that insulin resistance and inflammation could actually develop.

What about the psychological benefits of surgical body contouring? Not surprisingly, those who are most happy with liposuction (and 90% of patients would recommend it to others) are those who do not regain weight over long-term follow-up (Rohrich et al. 2004). Goyen (2002) reported a survey of patients who had had liposuction; of about 125 respondents (predominantly women), 80.5% said they had more confidence, almost 75% reported having more self-esteem, and 87% said they felt more comfortable in their clothing. In other words, the overwhelming majority felt there were positive psychological benefits from the procedure, which in turn motivated them to maintain their weight loss.

Abdominoplasty

Abdominoplasty is a procedure that involves removing and tightening excessive loose skin (unlike liposuction) such as might exist after extensive weight loss or pregnancy. In 2008, there were over 121,600 of these operations performed in the United States (American Society of Plastic Surgeons 2009). An abdominoplasty is a very different and much more extensive procedure than liposuction. It involves tightening of the abdominal wall muscles, as well as a possible incision ("exteriorization") around the umbilicus. A panniculectomy involves excision and removal of excessive overhanging abdominal skin and some fat only (Rabson, personal communication, September 5, 2009). Both abdominoplasty and panniculectomy are sometimes known in the vernacular as a "tummy tuck," and when statistics are given by the American Society of Plastic Surgeons, they are in the same category. But like liposuction, neither an abdominoplasty nor a panniculectomy is a weight loss procedure.

Saldanha et al. (2009) have devised a specialized surgical technique, called "lipo-abdominoplasty," for combining liposuction and simultaneous abdominoplasty that "respects the complete abdominal anatomy." Typically, said Saldanha et al. (2009), blood vessels in the abdominal area where an abdominoplasty is performed account for 80% of the blood supply for the abdominal wall, and standard abdominoplasty can result in blood vessel or nerve damage there. They reported their own technique was less invasive, with less morbidity (e.g., less incidence of hematoma or necrosis of the skin flap and more preservation of arteries, nerves, and lymphatic vessels), than abdominoplasty. Furthermore, their technique resulted in "better body contouring" and less need for surgical revisions than abdominoplasty performed as a second surgery subsequent to liposuction or even after other abdominal procedures done subsequent to bariatric surgery (i.e., required when postoperative skin is flaccid). Said Saldanha et al. (2009), "Following the surgical steps systematically and carefully reduces considerably such complications as abdominal flap ischemia and skin necrosis, which are difficult to treat and which can jeopardize the doctor-patient relationship." It is of note, though, that their study did not mention the BMI values of their 445 patients.

Bolton et al. (2003) prospectively studied 30 women pre- and postoperatively to assess changes in body image after abdominoplasty. Bolton et al. (2003) found that even though their patients' weights did not change, the patients reported increased satisfaction with their weight and significantly less self-consciousness and more comfort with their bodies during sex. Patient satisfaction, particularly as it relates to body image, involves many factors; these include both objective aesthetic criteria such as those used by plastic surgeons during patient evaluation and, more importantly, the patient's subjective perceptions and expectations (Bolton et al. 2003).

> Unlike liposuction and other cosmetic procedures, bariatric surgery improves metabolic functioning.

Bariatric Surgery

Bariatric surgery (with the root word from the Greek *barys*, meaning "heavy," or "weight") has become the mainstay, the definitive surgical treatment, for those with morbid obesity (also called *extreme obesity*, or *class 3 obesity*), that is, with BMI values of 40 kg/m^2 and higher, as well as for those with BMI values of 35 kg/m^2 and higher (*class 2 obesity*), especially if there are serious comorbid health issues like hypertension, diabetes, respiratory insufficiency (e.g., obstructive sleep apnea), or cardiac disease. Also, unlike liposuction, bariatric surgery has provided consistent, significant benefits in improving metabolic functioning. Bariatric surgery is often considered the treatment of choice when lifestyle changes like diet and exercise,

> Bariatric surgery involves procedures that are primarily malabsorptive (i.e., shortening the small intestine to reduce time for digestion and absorption of nutrients) or restrictive (i.e., reducing the storage capacity of the stomach and resulting in earlier feelings of satiety and decreased caloric intake).
>
> **Source: Cannon and Kumar 2009**

alone or in combination with pharmacotherapy, have not proven sufficient or have not given long-lasting results. Unfortunately, statistics indicate that over 95% of those with class 3 obesity regain their lost weight and then some within 2 years of these nonsurgical treatments (Latifi et al. 2002, p. 340).

Techniques

Some form of bariatric surgery has been used for more than 50 years, but it has become increasingly popular over the past several years as techniques have improved and morbidity and mortality rates have dropped. Several techniques are employed today, though it is beyond the scope of this book to discuss the surgical procedures in detail. According to Sjöström (2000), who is an internist and the principal investigator on the Swedish Obesity Study (SOS), one of the largest long-term follow-up studies on surgical treatments of obesity, there are "literally dozens of surgical anti-obesity techniques" that have been described over the years. He notes that in the 1960s, for example, there was a technique involving a shunt between the jejunum and the colon, but this was abandoned because it could result in severe diarrhea and even liver failure.

It was in the 1970s that banding of the stomach, in which a small pouch is created, was first attempted. Over the years, there have been several variations in banding techniques, including variations in where and how to place the band (e.g., vertical, horizontal, flexible, fixed, reversible) and even in how the band is fastened and how a pouch is created (e.g., staples, balloon, silicon tubing) (Sjöström 2000). One form of banding is a vertical banded gastroplasty (VBG), introduced in the 1980s, in which the upper stomach is actually stapled vertically to create a small stomach pouch. Over time, though, the staple line may deteriorate and a second surgery is required in a large proportion of patients (Vaidya et al. 2009, p. 2281). In general, the banding techniques are considered restrictive; that is, they lessen the storage capacity of the stomach and do not involve any malabsorption. Over time, though, a pouch may enlarge, resulting in the need for a second procedure (Vaidya et al. 2009, pp. 2281–2282). Some of these banding procedures can be done laparoscopically (Latifi et al. 2002, pp. 342–345). A more recent restrictive approach is transoral gastroplasty or TOGa, a minimally invasive procedure in which a stapler is guided endoscopically through the oral cavity into the stomach, which is then made smaller by stapling (Fogel et al. 2008). TOGa involves only an overnight stay in the hospital. Patients seem to tolerate this procedure well, and by 6 months of treatment in one study, patients had lost an average of over 25 pounds (Devière et al. 2008).

Gastric bypass surgery, also called the *Roux-en-Y procedure*, involves more extensive surgery and has a restrictive component, a malabsorption component, and a hormonal component. It is the most commonly performed procedure because it has better long-term weight loss results than the stomach banding techniques (see below) (Latifi et al. 2002, p. 343). A small pouch is created in the upper part of the stomach along its lesser curvature so that it can hold only about an ounce of food without a person feeling full, but over time the pouch stretches to hold about a cup of food; it is attached to the jejunum, bypassing the largest part of the stomach, the proximal jejunum, and the duodenum. The surgery also involves dividing the small intestine and creating a route for the food to drain—an operation that essentially "rearranges gastrointestinal anatomy" (Cummings and Flum 2008). Significantly, gastric bypass surgery inhibits the secretion of ghrelin, the hormone that makes a person feel hungry, and this inhibition results in decreased appetite postsurgery. It may also stimulate secretion of GLP-1 from the distal part of the intestine (Cummings and Flum 2008). Unlike some of the other procedures that may require adjustments, the Roux-en-Y, which can be done either abdominally or laparoscopically, does not allow for that possibility and has been considered a "one size fits all" procedure (Vaidya et al. 2009, p. 2282). For more detailed descriptions of these surgical procedures, as well as cosmetic procedures that might be required after bariatric surgery, the reader is referred to Vaidya et al. (2009, pp. 2281 ff).

Gastric bypass surgery is not necessarily a benign procedure. Stephen J. Dubner and Steven D. Levitt, in an article based on their popular book *Freakonomics*, suggest that people choose this procedure because it is what economists call a "commitment device." In other words, "retreat was not an option." They jokingly suggest that instead of such drastic surgery, we carry around our necks a Ziploc bag with a "towelette infused with an aroma of, well, of something deeply disgusting" every time we are tempted to eat too much (Dubner and Levitt 2007, pp. 26, 28).

Potential Complications of Bariatric Surgery

Bariatric surgery does indeed involve a major commitment. Serious complications can arise. For example, with gastric bypass, the part of the stomach that is bypassed may become distended and even perforate. The most serious surgical complications, though, involve infections, such as when there is a leak after surgery from the anastomosis of the stomach to the jejunal part of the intestine: the "abdominal catastrophe" of peritonitis can result. Other postoperative complications can include deep vein thrombosis and pulmonary embolism (Latifi et al. 2002, p. 348). Furthermore, the *dumping syndrome*—a set of "neurohumoral" symptoms including light-headedness, flushing, nausea, sweating, abdominal pain, palpitations, and diarrhea that can occur after eating sugary foods—can be present in as many as 70% of patients after the Roux-en-Y (gastric bypass) procedure (De Maria 2007). Patients should therefore avoid fruit juices and other beverages and foods with excessive amounts of sugar (Shah et al. 2006). Vomiting also occurs fairly commonly in the postoperative period, as it sometimes does after gastric banding surgery, and vomiting and heartburn can persist for more than 10 years after surgery (Bult et al. 2008).

There is even the suggestion (Hagedorn et al. 2007) that gastric bypass surgery significantly changes the way a person metabolizes alcohol, such that peak alcohol levels occur more rapidly, are higher, and last longer. In other words, after the surgery, patients may be more sensitive to alcohol and alcohol may have a greater addiction potential, particularly in those who were binge eaters (Sogg 2007). The speculation is that the smaller stomach pouch facilitates more rapid emptying of liquids, including alcohol, and hence more rapid absorption by the small intestine. Further, the operation circumvents the action of the enzyme alcohol dehydrogenase in the stomach (Hagedorn et al. 2007).

Another concern after bariatric surgery is the possibility of addiction transfer, in which patients replace the addiction to food with other addictions, such as gambling, compulsive shopping, or substance abuse (Sogg 2007).

Morbidity and mortality for patients undergoing these surgical procedures obviously vary with the experience of the surgeons and the medical center as well as with the particular procedure and, of course, patient characteristics such as age, sex, and cardiopulmonary status. For example, the risk of death is reported to be higher in men than in women (Bult et al. 2008). Sjöström et al. (2004) reported the postoperative statistics from the prospective but not randomized Swedish Obese Subjects (SOS) intervention study: 5 of more than 2,000 patients who underwent surgery (gastric bypass or gastric banding) died postoperatively (0.25%); wound complications occurred in 1.8% of patients; deep infections occurred in just over 2%; pulmonary complications occurred in 6%; and in 2.2%, complications were "serious enough" to require another operation. Sjöström (2000), incidentally, noted that one of the reasons their long-term SOS study was not randomized was that when it was started in 1987, the researchers were not given ethical approval for randomization because operative mortality reports (1%–5%) back in the 1970s and 1980s were considered too high. As a result patients had to "decide for themselves" whether they wanted surgery or so-called conventional treatment. Most recently, of course, though there is morbidity as mentioned above, mortality rates have dramatically decreased. In a study by the Longitudinal Assessment of Bariatric Surgery (LABS; 2009), this group looked at 30-day outcomes in 4,776 people (21% men) undergoing first-time bariatric surgical procedures, most commonly the Roux-en-Y (in over 71% of their patients) and laparoscopic adjustable gastric band surgery (in over 25%) during the 2-year period 2005–2007 at 10 different clinical locations. (The remaining 3.5% had other bariatric procedures and were not part of the study.) Significantly, the patients in this study had very high BMI values, with a mean of 46.5 kg/m².

In this study, at 30 days, 0.3% of their total sample of patients had died (though none in the adjustable gastric banding group). In this total sample, 4.3% had at least one major adverse outcome (e.g., deep vein thrombosis, tracheal reintubation). Complications in their patient sample were more apt to occur in patients who had a history of deep vein thrombosis or pulmonary embolus, had obstructive sleep apnea, or had exceptionally high BMI values (e.g., 75 kg/m²).

Complications can arise even years after surgery, such as gallstone formation and hernias at the site of the surgical incision. Once patients have lost substantial weight, they may require an abdominoplasty, the tummy tuck procedure to excise excessive skin. This surgery carries its own risk of complications (Latifi et al. 2002, p. 350; see the "Abdominoplasty" section).

There can also be vitamin deficiencies, including deficiencies in iron and particularly in vitamins D and B_{12}, as well as calcium deficiencies that may require supplementation. In fact, Duran de Campos et al. (2008) report that 8 years after gastric bypass surgery, the 30 women they sampled—whose average age was in the mid 40s—had a considerably higher incidence of osteopenia and vitamin D deficiency and lower levels of urinary calcium (indicating malabsorption) than age-matched control subjects, and most had a lower intake of calcium than recommended for their age (~500 mg/day vs. the 1,000 mg/day recommended). Four of the 30 women had evidence of osteoporosis, although the researchers note that no bone density scans were done preoperatively with which to compare the postoperative scans. For supplementation, researchers recommend calcium citrate rather than calcium carbonate, because calcium carbonate requires acid for absorption, and after surgery stomach acid levels are reduced (Shah et al. 2006).

> Uncomplicated bariatric surgery still requires postoperative follow-up as well as diet and exercise. In particular, vitamin D, vitamin B_{12}, iron, and calcium deficiencies should be anticipated.

Weight Loss After Bariatric Surgery: Determining the Procedure to Choose

There are several things to consider when determining the bariatric procedure of choice for a particular patient. In general, gastric bypass surgery results in greater weight loss than the banding techniques (as discussed below), and the banding techniques have been associated with an increased frequency of the need for a second surgery. Gastric bypass, though, is "technically more demanding," can result in vitamin deficiencies, and importantly, those who have had gastric bypass cannot have an endoscopic evaluation of their stomach, "which makes examinations of malignancy more complicated" (Sjöström 2000). In general, Sjöström (2000) has recommended gastric bypass for those with BMI values of 40 kg/m^2 or greater and the banding procedures for those with BMI values of 34 to 45 kg/m^2. Significantly, in Sjöström and colleagues' long-term SOS studies (2004, 2007), their surgical patients had one of three surgical procedures: gastric bypass, vertical banded gastroplasty, or what he called either "nonadjustable or adjustable banding." The control group did not have any "standardized" treatment; the control conditions ranged from "sophisticated lifestyle interventions and behavior modifications to, in some practices, no treatment whatsoever." The researchers also noted that there were no approved antiobesity medications in Sweden until 1998 (well after the start of this 10-year follow-up.)

Despite the possibility of complications, patients find they can lose substantial amounts of weight after bariatric surgery and usually sustain the loss, particularly with gastric bypass surgery. Even more important than weight loss per se is that the majority of patients, just days after surgery and before they leave the hospital, have resolution of their diabetes. Obviously, this occurs even before any significant weight loss has occurred.

> The majority of patients, even days after bariatric surgery, have resolution of their diabetes and improved metabolic profiles.

As many as 77% of patients who had diabetes prior to surgery no longer require medication for diabetes after surgery (DeMaria 2007). The results from bariatric surgery are often so positive that some even believe it should be a treatment offered to a wider range of patients, not just those with a specific BMI level (Cummings and Flum 2008). In the SOS study, follow-up at 2 years and 10 years after surgery (gastric bypass in ~5% of subjects and some form of gastric banding in the others— i.e., vertical banded gastroplasty and fixed or variable banding) demonstrated that of those who had one of those surgeries ($n = 342$), 72% had "recovery" from their diabetes, but in the control group ($n = 248$), only 21% had "recovery" at 2 years. At 10 years, among the 118 patients assessed at follow-up who had had surgery, 36% still had "recovery" from their initial diabetes, versus 13% of 84 patients in the control group. For hypertension, at 2 years, 34% of 1,204 patients who had had surgery no longer had hypertension, in contrast to 21% of 880 control subjects. At 10-year follow-up, 19% of 424 patients in the surgical group had no hypertension, while 11% of 342 in the control group still did not have hypertension. The researchers concluded that long-term (e.g., 10-year) effects of maintained weight loss on risk factors cannot necessarily be estimated by short-term observation (e.g., 2 years of follow-up). Of note is that the researchers do not define "recovery" in regard to diabetes or hypertension. The important point, though, is that the surgical groups (and only 5 % of the surgeries were gastric bypass) did better than controls at every point of follow-up (Sjöström et al. 2004).

DeMaria (2007) reports that typical weight losses with the various surgical techniques can range from around 40 to over 100 pounds. In general, weight loss is most significant with gastric bypass surgery rather than the banding techniques. In their subsequent data, with up to 15 years of follow-up, Sjöström et al. (2007) found that the average maximum weight loss in gastric bypass patients was 32% at 1–2 years after surgery, whereas the banding techniques resulted in weight reductions of 20%–25%. Over 15 years, control subjects had weight change (gain or loss) of less than or equal to 2%. At 10 years, gastric bypass patients still had weight losses of about 25%, whereas with the various banding techniques patients maintained weight losses of 14%–16%. Weight regain over years, though, can occur with the surgical procedures. Herpertz et al. (2004) report studies in which 20%–30% of patients who underwent bariatric surgery regained weight within 2 years of surgery. Mechanisms for weight regain can include increased intake of calories as the stomach pouch increases in size; decreases in metabolic rate; and possible changes in hormonal levels over time, such as increases in ghrelin levels. Further, leptin levels do decrease after surgery-induced weight loss, and this may also be a factor in weight regain (Shah et al. 2006).

Sjöström et al. (2007) concluded, with up to 15 years of follow-up on their sample of over 2,000 patients who had had bariatric surgery, that the overall mortality rate was lower than in the control group of over 2,000 subjects who had received conventional (nonsurgical) treatment. Adams et al. (2007) found, in almost 10,000 patients who had undergone gastric bypass surgery, that with a mean follow-up of over 7 years, mortality rates associated with coronary artery disease had dropped 56%; those associated with diabetes had dropped 92%; and those associated with cancer had decreased 60% (perhaps related to earlier screening and detection with weight loss, as patients may be more comfortable with their bodies and hence more amenable to seeking medical care). Significantly, though, death rates from nonmedical causes, including accidents and suicides, were 58% higher in those who had had gastric bypass surgery. Psychological screening evaluation prior to surgery and follow-up afterward are therefore essential (Adams et al. 2007). Incidentally, statistics from this study by Adams et al. (2007) prompted Aronne et al. (2008) to note that the rate of suicide for subjects taking rimonabant (i.e., only one completed suicide, and it was not even determined conclusively whether the death was directly related to its use) was lower than the rate reported in those presenting for bariatric surgery.

Psychosocial Benefits of Bariatric Surgery

Fabricatore et al. (2006) surveyed almost 200 mental health professionals who work with bariatric surgeons to assess the means by which psychological evaluation is conducted in candidates for surgery. They found that assessment practices vary widely but almost always include a presurgical personal interview of the patient. Assessment measures have included symptom inventory scales (e.g., for depression, anxiety, and eating disorders), mental status exams, and even personality tests such as the Minnesota Multiphasic Personality Inventory. There was no consensus among the mental health professionals regarding how psychological evaluation should be done. Furthermore, research could not identify consistent contraindications, nor could they identify what psychosocial criteria would predict a poor postsurgical outcome. And because bariatric surgery is so successful in reducing mortality from obesity, Fabricatore et al. (2006) raise the provocative question of whether it is "even ethical to recommend against surgery in the absence of data-based contraindications."

But back in the mid 1970s, Mills and Stunkard (1976) wrote about some of the behavioral changes found in patients after they had undergone bariatric surgery. At the time, jejunoileal bypass (less common today) was the procedure performed on the 69 patients—56 women and 13 men—in the study. Significantly, 68% of patients in the study had become obese by their teenage years and over 90% were obese by the time they were in their 20s. Patients were interviewed about 3 years after surgery. Patients had lost on average approximately 100 pounds, but 88% had severe postoperative diarrhea that made them restrict their food intake to avoid this. This diarrhea actually lasted for years, and these patients were experiencing up to four (and sometimes even up to eight) bowel movements, with accompanying rectal tenderness, a day. Most importantly, Mills and Stunkard (1976) found that at follow-up, patients' eating patterns had tended to normalize compared with presurgical patterns; that is, fewer calories were consumed at each meal, with less eating between meals and less bingeing at night. Furthermore, patients did not experience the characteristic dysphoria seen with other attempts at weight loss—Mills and Stunkard suggested that "surgery may have provided the subjects with 'medical evidence' that their obesity was not their fault." Stunkard et al. (1986) also found that bariatric surgery ("intestinal bypass") improved the psychosocial functioning of severely obese patients: they experienced less self-consciousness, improved mood, more autonomy, improved sexual relations, and greater assertiveness. Further, patients experienced less body image disparagement and were less likely to avoid looking at themselves in the mirror. These improved feelings about their body image often occurred within the first 6 months after surgery, even before patients had achieved their maximal weight loss. Stunkard et al. (1986) hypothesized that people who decrease the amount of food they eat "in the service of physiological regulation may have less emotional difficulty than those who decrease it in opposition to that regulation." They cautioned that even after surgery, a patient still has to regulate food intake. One patient had said to them, "It is important to remember that it is your stomach that is stapled, not your arms."

> It is a patient's stomach that is stapled, not his or her arms.

Though initial reports have seemed overwhelmingly positive vis-à-vis the psychological benefits of bariatric surgery, Stunkard et al. (1986) also cautioned that patients may not always admit to negative effects, in order not to disappoint their physicians. For example, Black et al. (1992) found a greater incidence of mood and anxiety disorders, bulimia nervosa, and personality disorders, particularly borderline personality disorder, in a sample of 88 morbidly obese patients (most weighing > 300 pounds and ~80% women) who presented to a clinic to request bariatric surgery (gastric banding) compared with control subjects. In a later study, Black et al. (2003) looked at psychiatric diagnosis in a group of 44 morbidly obese subjects (77% women) with a baseline BMI value of 50.0 ± 7.4 kg/m^2 who had undergone vertical banded gastroplasty and been followed for 6 months to assess weight loss. In general, the researchers found that neither Axis I nor Axis II diagnoses (based on DSM-III criteria) were predictive of weight loss in their group. They concluded that "the exclusion of otherwise suitable candidates for bariatric surgery on the basis of psychiatric disorder may be inappropriate." Black et al. (2003) added, "In fact, if subjects were excluded because of a history of psychiatric illness, few patients would be eligible for surgery." The researchers acknowledge limitations of their data in that the follow-up period of 6 months was short and there were few subjects in each category.

Predictors of Successful Weight Loss After Bariatric Surgery

Ray et al. (2003) interviewed about 150 patients, mostly women, 1 year after gastric bypass surgery to evaluate psychosocial factors that could predict successful weight loss. Sixty percent of them had lost more than half of their excess weight within the first year, and they tended to maintain the loss during the second postoperative year according to annual questionnaires. But 40% had more difficulty with weight control, particularly in complying with dietary constraints after surgery. Several factors were associated with more successful weight loss after surgery, including having a large social network and having had previous successes in dieting, though neither of these reached significance. Patients who admitted to less social distress regarding their obesity—that is, people less distressed by extrinsic factors—also seemed to do better. In other words, patients tend to lose more weight when they have a greater sense of "personal security" and "an intrinsic drive to lose weight" and seem better able to "deal with the stress of dietary habit adjustments and changes in body image." A history of sexual abuse, reported in 28% of these patients, was also

> A history of sexual abuse, prior substance abuse, prior psychiatric hospitalization, binge eating, and poor physical health are the largest predictors of unsuccessful weight outcome after bariatric surgery.

seen as a risk factor interfering with weight loss, as was a history of "psychiatric problems," which more than 9% of patients in this sample had experienced (for unspecified reasons).

Kalarchian et al. (2002) evaluated a sample of about 100 patients, mostly female, 2–7 years after they had undergone gastric bypass surgery. Binge eating, defined as a subjective loss of control over eating (unrelated to the actual quantity eaten), was found to be common, seen in 46% of patients, and was related to a tendency in these patients to regain some of the weight they had lost. In 2007 Kalarchian et al. evaluated a group of 288 people who were requesting bariatric surgery, to assess the presence of psychiatric disorders in this population. The average BMI value was greater than 50 (52.2 kg/m^2), which is class 4 obesity (supermorbid obesity); 83% of the subjects were female and 88% were white. The researchers found that psychiatric disorders were prevalent in these candidates for bariatric surgery: about 66% of them had a lifetime history of at least one Axis I disorder (most commonly mood disorders, at about 45%) and 38% met diagnostic criteria (most commonly for anxiety disorders, at 24%) at the time they were evaluated. Further, those with a lifetime history of an Axis I diagnosis had a higher BMI value and poorer physical health than those without such a lifetime history. Almost 30% of the candidates had a history of an eating disorder, usually binge eating disorder, and more than 15% had a binge eating disorder at the time of evaluation. Almost 30% had at least one Axis II personality disorder (most commonly obsessive-compulsive or avoidant personality disorder), which was also associated with poorer physical health, and 25% of the sample had both Axis I and Axis II diagnoses. Almost 33% of the sample had a history of substance abuse or dependence.

> "The holy grail of the bariatric surgeon is to identify those obese individuals who will have the insight, desire, and discipline to be successful partners in the process of weight loss."
>
> Source: Ray et al. 2003

Herpertz et al. (2004) conducted a systematic review to determine whether there are psychological and psychosocial criteria that could predict weight loss success, as well as psychological health, after bariatric surgery. They found that personality traits did not have any predictive value and that it was the severity of a patient's symptoms rather than the specific symptoms themselves that predicted successful weight loss. They emphasized that one of the most important criteria in predicting successful weight loss is not a psychiatric diagnosis per se but how that diagnosis affects a patient's eating behavior. They also distinguished patients who are distressed by a psychiatric illness, who may tend to do poorly, from those who are distressed by being morbidly obese, who may be more likely to do well.

Segal et al. (2004) found that some patients develop an eating disorder after bariatric surgery. These researchers suggest the possibility of a new diagnostic category seen postoperatively in those with morbid obesity: *postsurgical eating avoidance disorder*. Their patients tended to lose weight more rapidly after surgery than generally expected; used purging and excessive restriction of food intake that could be related to bingeing episodes or not; had considerable anxiety about regaining weight to their preoperative level; had negative attitudes toward nutritional advice; and experienced body image dissatisfaction or even distortion. Segal et al. (2004) recommend that the medication olanzapine, used effectively to treat anorexia nervosa, may have a place in treating some patients after bariatric surgery.

Most recently, Marcus et al. (2009) have raised questions about the proposed new eating disorder described by Segal et al. (2004). They found there was "no empirical support" for categorizing it as a separate eating disorder, though they do acknowledge the importance of appreciating that clinically significant eating disorders can develop after bariatric surgery. For example, Marcus et al. (2009) note that reported rates of binge eating, with a subjective sense of loss of control over eating, have been as high as 49% after bariatric surgery.

These studies emphasize that patients with morbid or supermorbid obesity may be in a category by themselves. It is not surprising that this level of obesity would be associated with significant psychopathology, particularly given the social stigma against the obese (see Chapter 2, "Obesity in the United States").

According to estimated statistics gathered by members of the American Society for Metabolic and Bariatric Surgery (2010; personal communication, November 9, 2009) and approved by the organization's executive council, there were 220,000 procedures (in total) in 2008. Of this number, 44% had laparoscopic adjustable gastric banding, and 51% in total had one of four versions of the Roux gastric bypass, making Roux gastric bypass still the most commonly done of the procedures. The remaining 5% were other bariatric procedures (e.g., gastric sleeve, duodenal switch) that we have not discussed. With the increasingly common practice of bariatric surgery, it is especially important to consider the possibility of psychiatric disorders in patients both before and after surgery, inasmuch as they may interfere with surgical outcome, preventing achievement of maximal weight loss, and may lead to more serious psychiatric morbidity.

REFERENCES

Adams TD, Gress RE, Smith SC, et al: Long-term mortality after gastric bypass surgery. N Engl J Med 357:753–761, 2007

American Society for Metabolic and Bariatric Surgery. http://www.asmbs.org. Accessed January 11, 2010.

American Society of Plastic Surgeons: 2000/2007/2008 National Plastic Surgery Statistics: Cosmetic and Reconstructive Procedure Trends. 2009. Available at: http://www.plastic surgery.org/Media/stats/2008-cosmetic-reconstructive-plastic-surgery-minimally-invasive-statistics.pdf. Accessed November 7, 2009.

Arner P: Metabolic effects of liposuction—yes or no? (letter) (comment on Klein et al. 2004). N Engl J Med 351:1354–1355, 2004

Aronne LJ: Treatment of obesity in the primary care setting, in Handbook of Obesity Treatment. Edited by Wadden TA, Stunkard AJ. New York, Guilford, 2002, pp 383–394

Aronne LJ: Roundtable discussion: targeting abdominal obesity to reduce cardiovascular risk in patients with type 2 diabetes mellitus. Am J Med 120 (suppl 1):S29–S34, 2007

Aronne LJ, Pagotto U, Foster GD, et al: The endocannabinoid system as a target for obesity treatment. Clin Cornerstone 9:52–64; discussion 65–66, 2008

Atkinson RL: Medical evaluation of the obese patient, in Handbook of Obesity Treatment. Edited by Wadden TA, Stunkard AJ. New York, Guilford, 2002, pp 173–185

Black DW, Goldstein RB, Mason EE: Prevalence of mental disorder in 88 morbidly obese bariatric clinic patients. Am J Psychiatry 149:227–234, 1992

Black DW, Goldstein RB, Mason EE. Psychiatric diagnosis and weight loss following gastric surgery for obesity. Obesity Surg 13:746–751, 2003

Bolton MA, Pruzinsky T, Cash TF, et al: Measuring outcomes in plastic surgery: body image and quality of life in abdominoplasty patients. Plast Reconstr Surg 112:619–625; discussion 626–627, 2003

Borah G, Rankin M, Wey P: Psychological complications in 281 plastic surgery practices. Plast Reconstr Surg 104:1241–1246, 1999

Bray GA: Drug treatment of obesity. Psychiatr Clin North Am 28:193–217, 2005

Brownell KD, Wadden TA: Etiology and treatment of obesity: understanding a serious, prevalent, and refractory disorder. J Consult Clin Psychol 60:505–517, 1992

Buescher LS, Buescher KL: Body dysmorphic disorder. Dermatol Clin 24:251–257, 2006

Bult MJ, van Dalen T, Muller AF: Surgical treatment of obesity. Eur J Endocrinol 158:135–145, 2008

Busetto L, Bassetto F, Nolli ML: Metabolic effects of liposuction—yes or no? (letter) (comment on Klein et al 2004). N Engl J Med 351:1355–1357, 2004

Cannon CP, Kumar A: Treatment of overweight and obesity: lifestyle, pharmacologic, and surgical options. Clin Cornerstone 9(4):55–71, 2009

Christakis NA, Fowler JH: The spread of obesity in a large social network over 32 years. N Engl J Med 357:370–379, 2007

Claudino AM, de Oliveira IR, Appolinario JC, et al: Double-blind, randomized, placebo-controlled trial of topiramate plus cognitive-behavior therapy in binge-eating disorder. J Clin Psychiatry 68:1324–1332, 2007

Cota D, Tschöp MH, Horvath TL, et al: Cannabinoids, opioids and eating behavior: the molecular face of hedonism? Brain Res Rev 51:85–107, 2006

Croft H, Houser TL, Jamerson BD, et al: Effect on body weight of bupropion sustained-release in patients with major depression treated for 52 weeks. Clin Ther 24:662–672, 2002

Cummings DE, Flum DR: Gastrointestinal surgery as a treatment for diabetes. JAMA 299:341–343, 2008

DeMaria EJ: Bariatric surgery for morbid obesity. N Engl J Med 356:2176–2183, 2007

Devière J, Ojeda Valdes G, Cuevas Herrera L, et al: Safety, feasibility and weight loss after transoral gastroplasty: first human multicenter study. Surg Endosc 22:589–598, 2008

Dubner SJ, Levitt SD: The stomach-surgery conundrum. The New York Times Magazine, November 18, 2007, pp 26–28

Duran de Campos C, Dalcanale L, Pajecki D, et al: Calcium intake and metabolic bone disease after eight years of Roux-en-Y gastric bypass. Obes Surg 18:386–390, 2008

Devière J, Ojeda Valdes G, Cuevas Herrera L, et al: Safety, feasibility and weight loss after transoral gastroplasty: first human multi-center study. Surg Endosc 22:589–598, 2008

Esposito K, Giugliano G, Giugliano D: Metabolic effects of liposuction—yes or no? (letter) (comment on Klein et al. 2004). N Engl J Med 351:1354, 2004

Esposito K, Giugliano G, Scuderi N, et al: Role of adipokines in the obesity-inflammation relationship: the effect of fat removal. Plast Reconstr Surg 118:1048–1057, 2006

Fabricatore AN, Crerand CE, Wadden TA, et al: How do mental health professionals evaluate candidates for bariatric surgery? Survey results. Obes Surg 16:567–573, 2006

Fogel R, De Fogel J, Bonilla Y, et al: Clinical experience of transoral suturing for an endoluminal vertical gastroplasty: 1-year follow-up in 64 patients. Gastrointest Endosc 68:51–58, 2008

Friedman KE, Reichmann SK, Costanzo PR, et al: Body image partially mediates the relationship between obesity and psychological distress. Obes Res 10:33–41, 2002

Fumento M: The Fat of the Land: Our Health Crisis and How Overweight Americans Can Help Themselves. Harmondsworth, UK, Penguin Books, 1998

Gatchel RJ, Oordt MS: Clinical Health Psychology and Primary Care: Practical Advice and Clinical Guidance for Successful Collaboration (chapter: Obesity). Washington, DC, American Psychological Association, 2003, pp 149–167

Gorzalka BB, Hill MN, Hillard CJ: Regulation of endocannabinoid signaling by stress: implications for stress-related affective disorders. Neurosci Biobehav Rev 32:1152–1160, 2008

Goyen MR: Lifestyle outcomes of tumescent liposuction surgery. Dermatol Surg 28:459–462, 2002

Greenway FL, Whitehouse MJ, Guttadauria M, et al: Rational design of a combination medication for the treatment of obesity: integrative physiology. Obesity (Silver Spring) 17:30–39, 2009

Gutheil RJ, Oordt MS: Clinical Health Psychology and Primary Care: Practical Advice and Clinical Guidance for Successful Collaboration. Washington, DC, American Psychological Association, 2003

Hagedorn JC, Encarnacion B, Brat GA, et al: Does gastric bypass alter alcohol metabolism? Surg Obes Relat Dis 3:543–548, 2007

Hamdy O, Porramatikul S, Al-Ozairi E: Metabolic obesity: the paradox between visceral and subcutaneous fat. Curr Diabetes Rev 2:367–373, 2006

Herpertz S, Kielmann R, Wolf AM, et al: Do psychosocial variables predict weight loss or mental health after obesity surgery? A systematic review. Obes Res 12:1554–1569, 2004

Kalarchian MA, Marcus MD, Wilson GT, et al: Binge eating among gastric bypass patients at long-term follow-up. Obes Surg 12:270–275, 2002

Kalarchian MA, Marcus MD, Levine MD, et al: Psychiatric disorders among bariatric surgery candidates: relationship to obesity and functional health status. Am J Psychiatry 164:328–334, 2007

Klein S, Fontana L, Young VL, et al: Absence of an effect of liposuction on insulin action and risk factors for coronary heart disease. N Engl J Med 350:2549–2557, 2004

Korner J, Aronne LJ: Pharmacological approaches to weight reduction: therapeutic targets. J Clin Endocrinol Metab 89:2616–2621, 2004

Latifi R, Kellum JM, De Maria EJ, et al: Surgical treatment of obesity, in Handbook of Obesity Treatment. Edited by Wadden TA, Stunkard AJ. New York, Guilford, 2002, pp 339–356

Longitudinal Assessment of Bariatric Surgery (LABS) Consortium, Flum DR, Belle SH, King WC, et al: Perioperative safety in the longitudinal assessment of bariatric surgery. N Engl J Med 361:445–454, 2009

Magen E, Gross JJ: Harnessing the need for immediate gratification: cognitive reconstrual modulates the reward value of temptations. Emotions 7:415–428, 2007

Marcus MD, Kalarchian MA, Courcoulas AP: Psychiatric evaluation and follow-up of bariatric surgery patients. Am J Psychiatry 166:285–291, 2009

Matorin AA, Ruiz P: Clinical manifestations of psychiatric disorders, in Kaplan & Sadock's Comprehensive Textbook of Psychiatry, Vol 2, 9th Edition. Edited by Sadock BJ, Sadock VA, Ruiz P. Philadelphia, PA, Wolters Kluwer Lippincott Williams & Wilkins, 2009, pp 1071–1107

Mauer MM, Harris RB, Bartness TJ: The regulation of total body fat: lessons learned from lipectomy studies. Neurosci Biobehav Rev 25:15–28, 2001

McElroy SL, Kotwal R, Guerdjikova AI, et al: Zonisamide in the treatment of binge eating disorder with obesity: a randomized controlled trial. J Clin Psychiatry 67:1897–1906, 2006

MDConsult: Disulfiram: adverse reactions. Available (by subscription) at: http://druginfo. goldstandard.com/direct/getinfofext.asp?caller. Accessed April 3, 2009.

Mills MJ, Stunkard AJ: Behavioral changes following surgery for obesity. Am J Psychiatry 133:527–531, 1976

Mohammed BS, Cohen S, Reeds D, et al: Long-term effects of large-volume liposuction on metabolic risk factors for coronary heart disease: intervention and prevention. Obesity (Silver Spring) 16:2648–2651, 2008

Napoleon A, Lewis CM: Psychological considerations in lipoplasty: the problematic or "special care" patient. Ann Plast Surg 23:430–432, 1989

Nazeri A, Massumi A, Wilson JM, et al: Arrhythmogenicity of weight-loss supplements marketed on the internet. Heart Rhythm 6:658–662, 2009

Neff LM, Aronne LJ: Pharmacotherapy for obesity. Curr Atheroscler Rep 9:454–462, 2007

Nissen SE, Nicholls SJ, Wolski K, et al: Effect of rimonabant on progression of atherosclerosis in patients with abdominal obesity and coronary artery disease: the STRADIVARIUS randomized controlled trial. JAMA 299:1547–1560, 2008

Pacher P, Bátkai S, Kunos G: The endocannabinoid system as an emerging target of pharmacotherapy. Pharmacol Rev 58:389–462, 2006

Padwal R, Li SK, Lau DC: Long-term pharmacotherapy for overweight and obesity: a systematic review and meta-analysis of randomized controlled trials. Int J Obes Relat Metab Disord 27:1437–1446, 2003

Parlette EC, Kaminer ME: Laser-assisted liposuction: here's the skinny. Semin Cutan Med Surg 27:259–263, 2008

Powers PS, Cloak NL: Medication-related weight changes: impact on treatment of eating disorder patients, in Clinical Manual of Eating Disorders. Edited by Yager J, Powers PS. Washington, DC, American Psychiatric Publishing, 2007, pp 255–285

Ray EC, Nickels MW, Sayeed S, et al: Predicting success after gastric bypass: the role of psychosocial and behavioral factors. Surgery 134:555–564, 2003

Rogers PJ, Smit HJ: Food craving and food "addiction": a critical review of the evidence from a biopsychosocial perspective. Pharmacol Biochem Behav 66:3–14, 2000

Rohrich RJ, Broughton G 2nd, Horton B, et al: The key to long-term success in liposuction: a guide for plastic surgeons and patients. Plast Reconstr Surg 114:1945–1952, 2004

Rosenbaum M, Goldsmith R, Bloomfield D, et al: Low-dose leptin reverses skeletal muscle, autonomic, and neuroendocrine adaptations to maintenance of reduced weight. J Clin Invest 115:3579–3586, 2005

Roth JD, Roland BL, Cole RL, et al: Leptin responsiveness restored by amylin agonism in diet-induced obesity: evidence from nonclinical and clinical studies. Proc Natl Acad Sci U S A 105:7257–7262, 2008

Rothman AJ, Baldwin AS, Hertel AW: Self-regulation and behavior change: disentangling behavioral initiation and behavioral maintenance, in Handbook of Self-Regulation: Research, Theory, and Applications. Edited by Baumeister RF, Vohs KD. New York, Guilford, 2004, pp 130–148

Rumsfeld JS, Nallamothu BK: The hope and fear of rimonabant. JAMA 299:1601–1602, 2008

Saldanha OR, Federico R, Daher PF, et al: Lipoabdominoplasty. Plast Reconstr Surg 124:934–942, 2009

Sarwer DB, Thompson JK: Obesity and body image disturbance, in Handbook of Obesity Treatment. Edited by Wadden TA, Stunkard AJ. New York, Guilford, 2002, pp 447–464

Sarwer DB, Wadden TA, Pertschuk MJ, et al: Body image dissatisfaction and body dysmorphic disorder in 100 cosmetic surgery patients. Plast Reconstr Surg 101:1644–1649, 1998

Sarwer DB, Wadden TA, Whitaker LA: An investigation of changes in body image following cosmetic surgery: cosmetic follow-up. Plast Reconstr Surg 109:363–369, 2002

Seamon MJ, Clauson KA: Ephedra: yesterday, DSHEA, and tomorrow—a ten year perspective on the Dietary Supplement Health and Education Act of 1994. J Herb Pharmacother 5(3):67–86, 2005

Segal A, Kussunoki DK, Larino MA: Post-surgical refusal to eat: anorexia nervosa, bulimia nervosa or a new eating disorder: a case series. Obes Surg 14:353–360, 2004

Shah M, Simha V, Garg A: Review: long-term impact of bariatric surgery on body weight, comorbidities, and nutritional status. J Clin Endocrinol Metab 91:4223–4231, 2006

Singer N: F.D.A. finds "natural" diet pills laced with drugs. The New York Times, Business section, B1, February 9, 2009. Available at: http://www.nytimes.com/2009/02/10/business/10pills.html. Accessed April 4, 2009.

Sjöström L: Surgical intervention as a strategy for treatment of obesity. Endocrine 13:213–230, 2000

Sjöström L, Lindroos AK, Peltonen M, et al: Lifestyle, diabetes, and cardiovascular risk factors 10 years after bariatric surgery. N Engl J Med 351:2683–2693, 2004

Sjöström L, Narbro K, Sjöström CD, et al: Effects of bariatric surgery on mortality in Swedish obese subjects. N Engl J Med 357:741–752, 2007

Smith SR, Aronne LJ, Burns CM, et al: Sustained weight loss following 12-month pramlintide treatment as an adjunct to lifestyle intervention in obesity: emerging treatments and technologies. Diabetes Care 31:1816–1823, 2008

Sogg S: Alcohol misuse after bariatric surgery: epiphenomenon or "Oprah" phenomenon? Surg Obes Relat Dis 3:366–368, 2007

Spalding KL, Arner E, Westermark PO, et al: Dynamics of fat cell turnover in humans (letter). Nature 453:783–787, 2008

Sparks P, Conner M, James R, et al: Ambivalence about health-related behaviors: an exploration in the domain of food choice. Br J Health Psychol 6:53–68, 2001

Stunkard AJ, Stinnett JL, Smoller JW: Psychological and social aspects of the surgical treatment of obesity. Am J Psychiatry 143:417–429, 1986

The NS, Gordon-Larsen P: Entry into romantic partnership is associated with obesity. Obesity 17:1441–1447, 2009

U.S. Food and Drug Administration: FDA briefing document NDA 21-888 Zimulti (rimonabant) tablets 20mg Sanofi Aventi. Advisory Committee, June 13, 2007. Available at: http://www.fda.gov/OHRMS/DOCKETS/AC/07/briefing/2007/4306b1-fda-backgrounder.pdf. Accessed November 7, 2009.

U.S. Food and Drug Administration: Questions and answers about FDA's initiative against contaminated weight loss products. April 30, 2009. Available at: http://fda.gov/Drugs/ResourcesForYou/Consumers/QuestionsAnswers/ucm136187.htm. Accessed November 7, 2009.

Vaidya V, Steele KE, Schweitzer M, et al: Obesity, in Kaplan & Sadock's Comprehensive Textbook of Psychiatry, 9th Edition, Vol 2. Edited by Sadock BJ, Sadock VA, and Ruiz P. Philadelphia, PA Lippincott Williams & Wilkins, 2009, pp 2273–2288 van der Lei B, Halbesma GJ, van Nieuwenhoven CA, et al: Spontaneous breast enlargement following liposuction of the abdominal wall: does a link exist? Plast Reconstr Surg 119:1584–1589, 2007

Van Gaal LF, Rissanen AM, Scheen AJ, et al; RIO-Europe Study Group: Effects of the cannabinoid-1 receptor blocker rimonabant on weight reduction and cardiovascular risk factors in overweight patients: 1-year experience from the RIO-Europe study. Lancet 365:1389–1397, 2005

Vemuri VK, Janero DR, Makriyannis A: Pharmacotherapeutic targeting of the endocannabinoid signaling system: drugs for obesity and the metabolic syndrome. Physiol Behav 93:671–686, 2008

Wadden TA, Didie E: What's in a name? Patients' preferred terms for describing obesity. Obes Res 11:1140–1146, 2003

Wadden TA, Brownell KD, Foster GD: Obesity: responding to the global epidemic. J Consult Clin Psychol 70:510–525, 2002

Wadden TA, Berkowitz RI, Womble LG, et al: Randomized trial of lifestyle modification and pharmacotherapy for obesity. N Engl J Med 353:2111–2120, 2005

Wilfley DE, Crow SJ, Hudson JI, et al: Efficacy of sibutramine for the treatment of binge eating disorder: a randomized multicenter placebo-controlled double-blind study. Am J Psychiatry 165:51–58, 2008

Wright SM, Dikkers C, Aronne LJ: Rimonabant: new data and emerging experience. Curr Atheroscler Rep 10:71–78, 2008

Wu RR, Zhao JP, Guo XF, et al: Metformin addition attenuates olanzapine-induced weight gain in drug-naive first-episode schizophrenia patients: a double-blind, placebo-controlled study. Am J Psychiatry 165:352–358, 2008

Yager J, Gitlin MJ: Clinical manifestations of psychiatric disorders, in Kaplan & Sadock's Comprehensive Textbook of Psychiatry, 8th Edition, Vol 1. Edited by Sadock BJ, Sadock VA. Philadelphia, PA, Lippincott Williams & Wilkins, 2004, pp 964–1002

Yanovski S: Sugar and fat: cravings and aversions. J Nutr 133:835S–837S, 2003

Ybarra J, Blanco-Vaca F, Fernández S, et al: The effects of liposuction removal of subcutaneous abdominal fat on lipid metabolism are independent of insulin sensitivity in normal-overweight individuals. Obes Surg 18:408–414, 2008

Yun PL, Bruck M, Felsenfeld L, et al: Breast enlargement observed after power liposuction: a retrospective review. Dermatol Surg 29:165–167, 2003

Zimmermann U, Kraus T, Himmerich H, et al: Epidemiology, implications and mechanisms underlying drug-induced weight gain in psychiatric patients. J Psychiatr Res 37:193–220, 2003

APPENDIX

SELECTED READINGS
AND WEB SITES

There are many excellent resources on dieting, nutrition, exercise, and other aspects of weight loss and maintenance. These are some of the ones that have been most helpful to us.

DIETING

Aronne LJ (with Bowman A): The Skinny: On Losing Weight Without Being Hungry. New York, Broadway Books, 2009

Beck JS: The Beck Diet Solution: Train Your Brain to Think Like a Thin Person. Birmingham, AL, Oxmoor House, 2007

Brownell KD: The LEARN (Lifestyle, Exercise, Attitudes, Relationships, Nutrition) Program for Weight Control. Dallas, TX, American Health Publishing, 1991

DeBakey ME, Gotto AM Jr, Scott LW, et al: The New Living Heart Diet. New York, Simon & Schuster, 1996

Gullo SP: Thin Tastes Better. New York, Carol Southern Books, 1995

Gullo SP: The Thin Commandments: The Ten No-Fail Strategies for Permanent Weight Loss. Emmaus, PA, Rodale, 2005

Hyman M: UltraMetabolism: The Simple Plan for Automatic Weight Loss. New York, Scribner, 2006

Kolata G: Rethinking Thin: The New Science of Weight Loss—and the Myths and Realities of Dieting. New York, Farrar, Straus & Giroux, 2007

Roizen MF, Oz MC: You on a Diet: The Owner's Manual to Waist Management. New York, Free Press, 2006

Rolls B: The Volumetrics Eating Plan: Techniques and Recipes for Feeling Full on Fewer Calories. New York, HarperCollins, 2005

Wansink B: Mindless Eating: Why We Eat More Than We Think. New York, Bantam Books, 2006

Zinczenko D (with Goulding M): Eat This, Not That: Thousands of Simple Food Swaps That Can Save You 10, 20, 30 Pounds—Or More! New York, Rodale, 2008

GENERAL NUTRITION

Bowden J: The 150 Healthiest Foods on Earth: The Surprising Unbiased Truth About What You Should Eat and Why. Beverly, MA, Fair Winds Press, 2007

Critser G: Fat Land: How Americans Became the Fattest People in the World. Boston, MA, Houghton Mifflin, 2003

Katz DL (with Friedman RSC): Nutrition in Clinical Practice: A Comprehensive, Evidence-Based Manual for the Practitioner, 2nd Edition. Philadelphia, PA, Wolters Kluwer Health/Lippincott Williams & Wilkins, 2008

Kessler DA: The End of Overeating: Taking Control of the Insatiable American Appetite. Emmaus, PA, Rodale, 2009

Nestle M: What to Eat. New York, North Point Press, 2006

Pollan M: In Defense of Food: An Eater's Manifesto. New York, Penguin, 2008

Precope J: Hippocrates on Diet and Hygiene. London, Zeno, 1952

Schlosser E: Fast Food Nation. New York, Harper, 2005

EXERCISE

Craig M: Miss Craig's 21-Day Shape-Up Program for Men and Women: A Plan of Natural Movement Exercises for Anyone in Search of a Trim and Healthy Body. New York, Random House, 1968

Howley ET, Franks BD: Fitness Professional's Handbook, 5th Edition. Champaign, IL, Human Kinetics Publishers, 2007

Root L: No More Aching Back: Dr. Root's New Fifteen-Minute-a-Day Program for a Healthy Back. New York, Signet, 1991

SELF-REGULATION

Baumeister RF, Vohs KD (eds): Handbook of Self-Regulation: Research, Theory, and Applications. New York, Guilford, 2004

SLEEP DISORDERS

Reite M, Weissberg M, Ruddy J: Clinical Manual for Evaluation and Treatment of Sleep Disorders. Washington, DC, American Psychiatric Publishing, 2009

EATING DISORDERS

Yager J, Powers PS (eds): Clinical Manual of Eating Disorders. Washington, DC, American Psychiatric Publishing, 2007

MORE DETAILED INFORMATION ON OBESITY

Pathophysiology

Bray GA, Bouchard C (eds): Handbook of Obesity: Etiology and Pathophysiology, 2nd Edition. New York, Marcel Dekker, 2004

Epidemiology

Hu FB: Obesity Epidemiology. New York, Oxford University Press, 2008

Treatment

Wadden TA, Stunkard AJ (eds): Handbook of Obesity Treatment. New York, Guilford, 2002

WEB SITES PROVIDING WEIGHT-RELATED HEALTH INFORMATION

http://www.eatright.org. American Dietetic Association. The association's EatRight site provides food and nutrition resources for both consumers and professionals.

http://www.nutritionupdates.org. Arbor Clinical Nutrition Updates. This pharmaceutical and food industry–related site reports research findings on nutrition; free and for-fee subscriptions.

http://www.cdc.gov/nccdphp/dnpa/obesity. Centers for Disease Control and Prevention (part of the U.S. Department of Health and Human Services). The CDC's Overweight and Obesity site offers information on nutrition and exercise in the prevention of obesity and assists individuals with beginning a weight loss program (including a food diary).

http://www.nhlbi.nih.gov/health. National Heart, Lung, and Blood Institute (part of the National Institutes of Health). Provides health information for both consumers and professionals.

http://www.ars.usda.gov/ba/bhnrc/ndl. U.S. Department of Agriculture, Agriculture Research Service. Provides nutrient information.

http://win.niddk.nih.gov. Weight-control Information Network (sponsored by the National Institute of Diabetes and Digestive and Kidney Diseases, or NIDDK). Offers consumers and professionals access to publications such as newsletters, research, and data about obesity and weight management programs.

Professional Sites

The following two Web sites for medical professionals are accessible only via subscription, but they are outstanding references on obesity, nutrition, diet, exercise, and related topics.

http://www.mdconsult.com
http://www.uptodate.com

INDEX

Page numbers printed in *boldface* type refer to tables, figures, or sidebars.